Delmar's
CRITICAL CARE

NURSING CARE PLANS

2nd Edition

Delmar's
CRITICAL CARE

NURSING CARE PLANS

2nd Edition

SHEREE COMER, RN, MS

THOMSON
———*———
DELMAR LEARNING

Australia Canada Mexico Singapore Spain United Kingdom United States

THOMSON

DELMAR LEARNING

Delmar's Critical Care Nursing Care Plans, 2nd Edition
by Sheree Comer

Vice President,
Health Care Business Unit:
William Brottmiller

Editorial Director:
Cathy L. Esperti

Acquisitions Editors:
Matthew Filimonov, Melissa Martin

Senior Developmental Editor:
Elisabeth F. Williams

Marketing Director:
Jennifer McAvey

Marketing Coordinator:
Kip Summerlin

Editorial Assistant:
Patricia Osborn

Technology Director:
Laurie K. Davis

Art and Design Coordinators:
Connie Lundberg-Watkins, Alex Vasilakos

Production Coordinator:
Bridget Lulay

Project Editor:
Jennifer Luck

Library of Congress Cataloging-in-Publication Data

Comer, Sheree.
   Delmar's critical care nursing plans / Sheree Comer.—2nd ed.
      p.   ; cm.
   Rev. ed. of: Critical care nursing plans. c1998.
   Includes bibliographical references and index.
   ISBN 0-7668-5995-9 (alk. paper)
I. Intensive care nursing. 2. Nursing care plans.
   [DNLM: 1. Critical Care—Nurses' Instruction.
2. Patient Care Planning.   WY 154 C732d 2005]
I. Title: Critical care nursing care plans. II. Comer, Sheree. Critical care nursing care plans. III. Title.
   RT120.I5C576 2005
   610.73'61—dc21

                                          2003051513

Notice to the Reader

Publisher does not warrant or guarantee any of the products described herein or perform any independent analysis in connection with any of the product information contained herein. Publisher does not assume, and expressly disclaims, any obligation to obtain and include information other than that provided to it by the manufacturer.

The reader is expressly warned to consider and adopt all safety precautions that might be indicated by the activities described herein and to avoid all potential hazards. By following the instructions contained herein, the reader willingly assumes all risks in connection with such instructions.

The publisher makes no representations or warranties of any kind, including but not limited to, the warranties of fitness for particular purpose or merchantability, nor are any such representations implied with respect to the material set forth herein, and the publisher takes no responsibility with respect to such material. The publisher shall not be liable for any special, consequential, or exemplary damages resulting, in whole or part, from the readers' use of, or reliance upon, this material.

CONTENTS

PREFACE

CONCEPTUAL APPROACH

The nursing process serves as a learning tool for readers and as a practice and documentation format for clinicians. Based on a thorough assessment, the nurse formulates a specific plan of care for each individual patient. The care plans in this book are provided to facilitate that process for readers and practitioners. To that end, these care plans have been developed to reflect physical and functional symptomatology that are listed according to body systems and disease processes. Included are some of the most common problems associated with the adult patient in the Critical Care Unit. Each disorder includes, as appropriate, an overview of the disease process, medical care associated with the particular problem that may be prescribed for the condition, drug actions, diagnostic procedures, laboratory tests with expected values, essential nursing diagnosis care plans that are identified with the particular disease process, as well as discharge and outcome criteria. Each disorder has its own pathophysiology chart that shows how the body system is affected by causative factors, pathology, complications, and resultant signs and symptoms. The essential nursing diagnoses and care plans may be cross-referenced with plans for conditions within the system or with plans for conditions within other body systems if they apply. A notation cross-referencing a care plan may be found under the listing for the nursing care plan that directs the reader to a diagnosis, where the main care plan can be found. Signs and outcomes specific to the particular condition will be notated under the specific diagnosis, utilizing the main care plan, with noted expansion of interventions and rationales.

It is not uncommon for the critical care patient to have more than one condition requiring treatment and care, nor uncommon for a condition to contribute to the complication of another diagnosis. It may be necessary to combine care plans or portions of care plans that are applicable to the patient's individual case.

ORGANIZATION

Delmar's Critical Care Nursing Care Plans, 2nd edition, includes care plans by body system for disorders often seen in the critical care unit. Nursing care begins with a comprehensive review and assessment of each individual patient. The data is then analyzed and a specific plan of care developed. The format of each nursing care plan in this book is summarized below.

- Nursing diagnoses as approved by the North American Nursing Diagnosis Association (NANDA) taxonomy (2003–2004); the complete NANDA listing is found in Appendix A (new to this edition).
- Related factors (etiology) for each diagnosis are suggested and the user is prompted to choose the most appropriate for the specific patient.
- Defining characteristics for each actual diagnosis are listed with prompts to the user to include specific patient data from the nursing assessment.
- Goals are related to the nursing diagnosis and include a time frame for evaluation to be specified by the user.
- Appropriate outcome criteria specific for the patient are suggested. In keeping with current practice, this edition includes a Nursing Outcome Classification (NOC) label for each nursing diagnosis. Appendix B offers a complete listing of NOC labels.
- Nursing interventions and rationales are comprehensive. They include pertinent continuous assessments and observations. Common therapeutic actions originating from nursing and those resulting from collaboration with the primary caregiver are suggested with prompts for creativity and individualization. Patient and family teaching and psychosocial support are provided with respect for cultural variation and individual needs. Consultation and referral to other caregivers is suggested when indicated.
- Nursing Intervention Classification (NIC) labels are provided in this new edition for each nursing

diagnosis. These are inserted after the interventions and rationales to assist the user in becoming familiar with this classification process for nursing interventions. Appendix C provides the complete listing of the NIC labels.

- Evaluation of the patient's goal and presentation of data related to the outcome criteria is followed by consideration of the next step for the patient.

A new, descriptive introductory chapter outlines how to customize care plans for an individual patient based on the standardized care plans found in this book.

A CD is included in the back of the book which contains electronic files for all the care plans in this book.

ACKNOWLEDGMENTS

I would like to thank the people, without whom this book would not have been possible. I am thankful for the ability and circumstances that led to the writing of this book, for the opportunity to be able to give back some of the knowledge I've been shown and the chance to make a difference, and for the people in my life who have truly been a blessing to me. I thank my husband and daughter, Allen and Ashley, for giving up their time with me (as well as the computer), for never giving up on me when I wondered if I could really do this project, and for managing to love me throughout all the trials and tribulations we've endured. Thanks to Raymond Goodwin Hubbard, my dad, Lysta Garver Eppele ("Miss Garver"), and Joseph Anton Eppele ("Uncle Joe"), who always thought that I was, and would be, someone special in the world. I thank Annie Lincoln for being the friend that she has been, through really thick and thin times, and her parents, Bill and Ann Lincoln, who wanted to adopt me into their family. I thank my other friends, Beverly (the consummate ICU nurse), Estelle (the encourager), and Diane (the eternal optimist). Thanks to Dr. Paul Little for showing me that there are still some individuals who can demonstrate true caring and compassion for patients, and for his courageousness and dignity in the face of adversity. Thanks to my own personal physicians who have taken me seriously. Thanks to all the patients that I've cared for over the years that have taught me so much about what real nursing was, and to Janie Trojcak, R.N., my first head nurse for helping to mold me into the kind of nurse I turned out to be. I thank Alexandra Swann, my very first editor, as well as all the editors and people I've worked with at Delmar. Thanks to you all.

Sheree Raye Comer, R.N., M.S.

REVIEWERS

Rebecca Dahlen, Ed.D, MSN, RN-CS, CCRN
Assistant Professor
California State University
Long Beach, California

Cindy McCoy, RN, PhD
Assistant Professor
Troy State University
Troy, Alabama

Bonnie R. Sakallaris, RN, MSN
Director, Cardiac Services, Division of Nursing
Washington Hospital Center
Washington, DC

AN INTRODUCTION TO THE USE OF THE NURSING CARE PLANS

INTRODUCTION

The benchmarks towards excellence in nursing practice are encompassed in the nursing diagnostic processes of assessment, diagnosis, planning, outcome identification, intervention, and finally, evaluation. The nursing process provides a strong framework that gives direction to the practice of nursing. Nursing care planning is the product of the application of the nursing diagnostic process. Without the planning process, quality and consistency in patient care would be lost. Nursing care plans provide a means of communication among nurses, their patients, and other health care providers to achieve health care outcomes. Nursing diagnoses provide the basis for selection of interventions to achieve outcomes for which the nurse is accountable (NANDA, 2003). "Now, as never before, today's nurses must make more complex professional decisions, determine what things to do and what things not to do for which clients. Priorities are critical: often the nurse must make hard choices between what is essential and what is merely beneficial" (Barnum, 1999). The primary purpose of the nursing diagnostic processes applied by nurses is to design a plan of care for and in conjunction with the patient that results in the prevention, reduction or resolution of the client's health problem (Harkreader, 2004).

In the current health care environment, specifically the thrust into an interdisciplinary delivery of care model, nurses are positioned for a level of accountability not seen in prior health care practice climates. In addition to requiring more independent decision making by the nurse, the current health care environment engages various disciplines in working together and jointly sharing responsibility for patient outcome achievement. The changes that are occurring offer nursing the opportunity to define its boundaries and to use the nursing process to deliver care. Nurses need the tools to assist them in accurately predicting achievable patient outcomes for a given primary condition, and they also need the skill to tailor interventions to the individual patient and his or her unique circumstances. This text is designed to provide that guidance.

NURSING CARE PLANS AND INDIVIDUAL PATIENT CARE NEEDS

This book is intended to facilitate the care planning process for nurses working with critical care patients. The nursing diagnoses that are used throughout this book are taken from the NANDA's Taxonomy II (NANDA, 2003). The outcome statements may be made in two ways: using the Nursing Outcome Classification (NOC) or writing an outcome statement. This text also contains suggested Nursing Intervention Classifications (NIC) for each nursing diagnosis to assist the reader in applying the two classifications to the clinical setting. For each primary condition all the care plans include introductory information about the primary condition and the current medical management followed by:

1. nursing diagnoses with their related to (etiological) factors and defining characteristics

2. expected behaviorally measurable outcome criteria or patient goals

3. nursing interventions. Rationales are included for the nursing interventions to assist the nurse in building a knowledge base to apply the information, make clinical decisions, and to think how best to respond to the patient's needs.

4. evaluation, as the final piece of the nursing process. The ability of the patient to meet the evaluative criteria indicates the patient is moving toward resolution of the identified nursing diagnosis.

The nursing care plans provided in this text are intended to serve as a catalyst for reflection and a guideline to the standards of care. In order to apply them to your patient's situation you must critically think about what you know about your patient and his or her history. You must actively pursue all parts of the patient information base, examining the evidence the client has brought forth to define specific problems and then arrive at specific goals to manage those problems. You will make decisions about how to actualize those goals by choosing or selecting interventions which will assist in meeting the goals and resolving the problem. Standardized care plans provide the practitioner with minimum expectations and predictable patterns of responses. The nurse can then compare these with the patient's presentation and then move forward to design a plan of care that is responsive to that individual and also reflects current management modalities.

The process for planning individualized care involves the same steps as the nursing process.

1. Collect and review the patient assessment data. Typically, the information will be found on the standardized facility assessment sheet, the patient medication administration record, laboratory reports, and in the progress notes. Interview the patient and complete your own assessment record either from school or the focused assessment provided by the facility. After studying the health record, you need to organize the information into a summary of patient issues.

2. Identify viable nursing diagnoses and potential "risk for" situations. Review the nursing diagnoses provided by the standardized care plan. Choose those which fit the patient data base you've collected. The diagnostic process is individualized by identifying "related to" factors and "defining characteristics" which the patient has identified in the assessment process. For example: "Acute pain related to bowel cramping supported by the patient verbalizing pain at a 9 on the scale of 0–10." The patient's own words and pain rating allow the nurse to match the defining characteristics and interventions in the standardized plan to the patient's own perceptions.

3. Plan to meet specific outcomes/client goals. The goals should pertain to the specific patient interventions and move the patient toward resolution of the problem. The outcomes provided in the text will support this and allow for specific qualifiers such as time frames, target times, and patient variables to

be added to allow for individualization of the plan. "Client verbalizes pain at a level 3 or less" would be a standardized outcome. "*Within the next 24 hours*" sets an achievable target time and individualizes the plan.

4. Design interventions to meet the goal and resolve the nursing diagnosis. Choose interventions which are pertinent to the patient and are consistent with the medical orders. Ongoing evaluation of the pain level and the administration of pain medications would be examples of both independent and collaborative nursing interventions which would achieve the outcome and resolve the "Acute Pain" diagnosis.

5. Evaluate the effectiveness of the plan. By setting patient-specific, observable outcomes, the plan communicates the need for ongoing evaluation and updating. This allows for resolution of the problem or revision using the standardized care plan for potential interventions to address the problem.

CRITICAL THINKING, THE NURSING PROCESS, AND CARE PLAN DEVELOPMENT

Critical thinking and decision making skills are used in identifying nursing diagnoses. Critical thinking entails purposeful, goal-directed thinking. It aims to make clinical judgments based on evidence (Alvaro, 2004). The nurse uses critical thinking to synthesize the information from the assessment data collection and then makes judgments about how to put the information together into a meaningful whole. In this way, the nurse applies the patient assessment information to a new clinical situation. The standardized nursing care plans in this book will allow you to review the patient assessment and history, and then assist you in formulating a new individualized nursing care plan.

The following case study illustrates how to apply individual patient data to a care plan in this book.

MYOCARDIAL INFARCTION CASE STUDY

Mrs. Dora Mendez, age 52, was admitted to the CCU from her husband's physician's office with a diagnosis of atypical chest pain. She was attending her husband while he visited his physician for management of his diabetes. She is a Hispanic overweight female.

She is diaphoretic, complains of vague chest pain, anxiety, shortness of breath, indigestion, and dizziness. She rates her pain 5 on the scale of 0 to 10. She states "she doesn't know why she is here, this has happened before and there is nothing the matter. It is just her "change of life." She says she doesn't need this and her husband will be very angry with her. She should be home taking care of him. She doesn't understand why they gave her aspirin at the doctor's office. They even asked her to chew it! Upon arrival to the emergency room her twelve lead EKG showed sinus tachycardia with ST segment elevation in leads II, III, AVF and depression in V2 and V3. She was alert and oriented. Her heart rate was 120 beats per minute, BP 152/88 and her respirations were 25 bpm with a temperature 99F. Oxygen was administered at 5 L per minute, and her oxygen saturation was 95%. Lung sounds were clear and heart sounds S1 and S2 are audible with no murmurs or clicks. No peripheral edema was noted, her extremities were cool and clammy, pulses were present bilaterally. She is 60 inches and weighs 160 lbs. with central obesity. Bowel sounds are present in all quadrants.

She denies any significant medical history but her father and her uncles all died young of heart attacks. She had a total abdominal hysterectomy after the birth of her last child. She denies smoking or alcohol use and doesn't know her cholesterol levels. Occasionally she gets headaches. She denies any allergies. Laboratory and diagnostic screening showed Na 145 meq/L, Cl 102 meq/L, K 3.3 meq/dl, Mg 2.0 meq/dl, Ca (ionized) 4.3 mg/dl, CO2 19, BUN 9 mg/dl, creatinine .8 mg/dl, WBC 145.5 thou/dl, Hct 44.3%, and HgB 14.5 g/dl, cholesterol 210 mg/dl.

Cardiac enzymes: Troponin 12.0 ng/dl, CPK-MB
    10 ng/dl
Coagulation studies: PT 11.9 / INR = 1.02   PTT
    26.9 seconds

Mrs. Mendez was unresponsive to NTG spray .4 mg in the ER. She stated her chest still felt heavy and was asking for a heating pad which is what she put on her arm and side of her chest at home. She was placed on a NTG drip titrated at 5 mcg/min every five minutes, Heparin 5000 units was given IVP and a drip started at 2500 u/hr. Reteplase (Retavase) is given as a 10 million unit IVP and repeated 30 minutes later. She was transferred to the CCU where they noted a 6 beat run of ventricular tachycardia attributed to the reperfusion. Ten hours after admission, her chest pain returned and she became hypotensive

and went into cardiogenic shock. An intraaortic balloon pump is inserted with the resulting diminishment of her chest pain and the Mrs. Mendez is prepared for an emergency cardiac catheterization and potential cardiac surgery.

NURSING DIAGNOSIS #1
Acute Pain

Related to: Decreased blood flow to myocardium, myocardial ischemia or infarct, post-procedure discomfort, chest wall pain post surgery, or pericarditis.

Defining Characteristics: Chest pain with or without radiation, facial grimacing, clutching of hands to chest, restlessness, diaphoresis, changes in pulse and blood pressure, dyspnea, dizziness, arm pain, shoulder pain, shortness of breath, fatigue, tachycardia, changes in CVP, PAP, PCWP, TPR, SVR, decreased cardiac output, and cardiac index.

Outcome Criteria:

✔ Chest pain will be relieved or controlled.
✔ Hemodynamic status will be stable.

NOC: *Pain Control*

INTERVENTIONS

Evaluate chest pain as to type, location, severity relief and gauge with activity or rest and other symptoms concurrently noted, such as pallor, diaphoresis, radiation of pain, nausea, vomiting, shortness of breath and vital sign changes, arm pain, shoulder pain, shortness of breath, fatigue tachycardia, changes CVP, PAP, PCWP, TPR, SVR, decreases cardiac output, and cardiac index.

Evaluate chest pain encouraging client to report any return of chest sensations, indigestion, dizziness, and shortness of breath.

Obtain a description of the intensity using a 0–10 scale, with 0 being no pain and 10 being the worst pain experienced.

Obtain quantification of pain using pain scale to gauge improvement or relief of pain every 5 minutes to 1 hour as indicated.

Obtain a history (when possible) of previous cardiac pain and family history of cardiac problems.

Prepare for the administration of thrombolytic therapy or for primary post-transluminal coronary angioplasty.

Monitor the client's response to Retavase assessing for bleeding, reperfusion arrhythmias, and a return of chest pain. Maintain Heparin infusion per protocol.

(continues)

INTERVENTIONS

Insert IV lines and obtain samples as ordered.

Monitor hemodynamic status by use of pulmonary artery catheter, if available, and notify MD of significant changes.

Monitor for increasing hemodynamic instability by evaluating BP, HR, cardiac rhythm, lung sounds, heart sounds every 4 hrs, or as indicated. Report significant changes immediately. Report return of chest pain while on IABP or a decrease in cardiac index below 2.2 L/min/m2, PcWP greater than 18.

Administer oxygen by nasal cannula or mask as indicated.

Administer oxygen at 4 L/minute maintaining O2 saturation at or greater than 95%.

Administer analgesic as ordered.

Administer Morphine Sulfate 5 mg IVP and nitroglycerine titration per protocol prn for pain relief and hemodynamic stability.

Administer beta-blockers as ordered.

Administer antiemetics as ordered.

Administer anxiolytics as ordered.

Maintain bedrest during pain, with position for comfort; nurse to stay with patient during pain.

Provide bedside commode as tolerated, return to bed with onset of pain.

Maintain relaxing environment to promote calmness.

Maintain relaxing environment, provide patient with reassurance about her husband and his care at home.

Instruction:

Instruct patient to notify nurse immediately of any chest pain.

Instruct patient that pain is significant and not just menopausal, encourage her to report chest sensations immediately. Assess cardiac rhythm for ischemic changes.

Instruct patient in relaxation techniques, deep breathing, guided imagery, visualization, etc.

Assist patient to identify strategies that comfort her, turn lights down in room, maintain a quiet environment, and administer anxiolytics as needed.

Instruct patient in nitroglycerine SL administration after hospitalization; 1 p5 minutes up to 3 times and if pain unrelieved, patient should seek emergency care.

Instruct patient to report pain immediately, reinforcing the meaning of the pain and the importance of using medications to alleviate it.

Instruct patient/family in medication effects, side effects, contraindications, and symptoms to report.

Instruct and reassure patient and family about effectiveness of medication and the expected responses to medication administered.

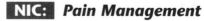 **NIC:** *Pain Management*

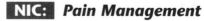 NURSING DIAGNOSIS #2
Decreased cardiac output

Related to: *Damaged myocardium, decreased contractility,* dysrhythmias, conduction defects, alteration in preload, *alteration in afterload, vasoconstriction,* myocardial ischemia, and ventricular hypertrophy.

Defining Characteristics: Elevated or *decreased blood pressure,* elevated mean arterial pressure greater than 120 mmHg, *elevated systemic vascular resistance greater than 1400 dyne-seconds/cm2, cardiac output less then 4 L/minute, or cardiac index less than 2.5 L/min/m2,* tachycardia, cold pale extremities, absent or decreased peripheral pulses, ECG changes, hypertension, S3 or S4 gallops, decreased urinary output, diaphoresis, orthopnea, dyspnea, crackles (rales), jugular vein distention, edema, *chest pain.*

Outcome Criteria:

✔ Vital signs and hemodynamic parameters will be within normal limits for the patient with no dysrhythmias noted.

NOC: *Vital Sign Status*

INTERVENTIONS

Auscultate apical pulses and monitor heart rate and rhythm.

Monitor BP in both arms.

Monitor vital signs and hemodynamic parameters every 15 to 30 minutes.

Monitor ECG for dysrhythmias and treat as indicated.

Monitor lead with the greatest R wave to trigger balloon pump inflation.

Determine level of cardiac functioning and existing cardiac and other conditions.

Measure CO and perform other hemodynamic calculations.

Monitor difference in patient's end diastolic and balloon assisted end-diastolic pressure indicating afterload reduction.

Monitor for the development of new S3 or S4 gallops.

Auscultate for the presence of murmurs or rubs.

Observe lower extremities for edema, distended neck veins, cold hands and feet, mottling, oliguria. Notify MD if urine output is less than 30 mL's for two consecutive hours.

Observe lower extremities, especially the extremity with the intraaortic balloon catheter for edema, mottling, diminished pulses, temperature, motion, sensation, and color every 15 minutes to 1 hour. Report urine output less than 30 mL's per hour promptly.

INTERVENTIONS

Position in semi-fowlers position.

Position patient between 15 and 30 degrees in bed, especially with IABP catheter in place, and restrict movement of catheterized limb.

Administer cardiac glycosides, nitrates, vasodilators, diuretics, and antihypertensives as ordered.

Correlate pharmacologic interventions with the patient hemodynamic status, pain relief and changes in ECG.

Titrate vasoactive drugs as ordered per MD parameters.

Correlate pharmacologic interventions with the patient hemodynamic status, pain relief and ischemic changes in ECG.

Weigh every day.

Arrange activities so as to not overwhelm patient. Maintain reduced activity for at least 12 hours with use of bedside commode only, and then increase activity as tolerated within the first 48 hours.

Explain reason for frequent monitoring and reassure about physical condition.

Avoid Valsalva-type maneuvers with straining, coughing, or moving. Administer stool softeners as needed/ordered.

Provide small, easy to digest meals.

Monitor patient's nutritional status and provide oral hygiene every 2 hours and as requested.

Have emergency equipment and medications available at all times.

Instruction:
Instruct patient/family to avoid/stop smoking after myocardial infarction.

Instruct in the use of nicotine replacements and methods of stopping smoking.

Instruct patient/family on medications, dose, effects, contraindications and avoidance of over the counter drugs without MD approval.

Instruct patient/family about medications such as morphine sulfate, NTG, heparin, and ASA and their relationship to cardiac perfusion and the reduction of chest pain and the maintenance of oxygen to the cardiac tissue.

Instruct in activity limitations.

Instruct regarding limited movement of affected limb, and turning side to side while on bed rest.

Demonstrate exercises to be done.

Instruct to report chest pain immediately.

Instruct patient regarding the meaning of new onset chest pain and reassure that measures will be taken to alleviate it once it is reported.

Instruct patient/family regarding placement of pulmonary artery catheter, and post procedure care.

Instruct patient/family regarding placement of pulmonary artery catheter, and intraaortic balloon catheter and pump along with the sounds and post procedure care associated with these devices.

INTERVENTIONS

Assist with insertion and maintenance of pacemaker, when needed.

Prepare patient/family for potential Percutaneous Coronary Intervention or CABG procedures.

Reinforce physician's explanation about procedures and their indications. Allow patient and family to express concerns and fears.

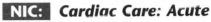 **NIC:** *Cardiac Care: Acute*

 ## CLINICAL PATHWAYS: A METHOD OF ACHIEVING OUTCOMES ACROSS THE CONTINUUM OF CARE

Health care participants are demanding satisfaction with the expensive services they are consuming. Health care organizations publish their outcomes and report them to state, federal, and independent agencies as a method of maintaining practice standards and attracting consumers and health care providers. The demand for the most effective and cost-efficient manner of restoring patients to health has led to the clinical pathway collaborative client care model. Clinical pathways, also known as "care maps," are care management tools that outline the expected clinical course and outcomes for a specific client type (Kelly-Heidenthal, 2003). The manner in which a pathway is constructed is usually agency specific but typically follows the patient's length of stay on a day-by-day basis for the specific disease process or surgical intervention. They are a clinical tool that organizes, directs, and times the major care activities and interventions of the entire multidisciplinary team for a particular diagnosis or procedure. Their design is intended to minimize delays, maximize appropriate resource utilization and promote quality care. "The clinical pathway describes a blended plan of care constructed by all providers, considering the subject together" (Barnum, 1999).

Clinical pathways act as the "gold standard" against which interdisciplinary outcomes and the efficiency of the care may be measured. Institutions may choose to replace the nursing care plan with a clinical pathway. The pathway then guides the nurse along a sequence of interdisciplinary interventions that incorporate standardized aspects such as patient and family teaching, nutrition, medications, activities, and diagnostic studies and treatments. The tool is developed collaboratively by all health team members and includes predictable and established time frames, usually by delineating each hospital day as an event requiring new intervention along a continuum. The issue here is to deliver consistent competent care, and a care map provides this consistency not just on a shift-by-shift basis but also throughout the entire agency. Clinical pathways also, because of their standardization of practice, allow for measuring performance improvement within an agency and between similar agencies over time.

The task here is to appreciate that clinical pathways guide rather than dictate the course of care for an individual. They do not take into account patient problems which are coexisting and are also impacting the patient's recovery process. Therefore, the process of incorporating clinical pathways and the use of this text is the same as in individualizing standard care plans. The nurse must incorporate the individualized needs that exist in conjunction with the clinical pathway. When the patient's needs vary from the outcome achievement time frame, the nurse must assess, report, and manage the variance to meet the patient's needs. The manner of reporting these variances is also frequently agency-specific. At times, the variances are documented on the clinical pathway, at other times the nursing care plan format is incorporated into the document or an individualized care plan is initiated and documentation about the variance is continued until it is resolved. Not all patients' care is incorporated into a clinical pathway model. For more complex patient care situations an individualized care plan format applying the various standardized nursing diagnoses in this text is more appropriate.

Well-designed nursing care plans and/or care maps move the patient from one level of care on the health care continuum to another. They monitor and guide the progress of the patient from the acutely ill phase of illness to the community or outpatient phase of illness. Care planning organizes and coordinates the patient care in a manner which promotes consistency, a current standard of care, and communication, and incorporates the problem solving process which integrates responsiveness to patient needs and cost efficiency.

UNIT 1

CARDIOVASCULAR SYSTEM

1.1

MYOCARDIAL INFARCTION

Myocardial infarction (MI) is a critical emergency that requires timely management to save heart muscle and limit damage that may evolve over several hours. Blood flow is abruptly decreased or stopped through the coronary arteries and results in ischemia and necrosis to the myocardium if not treated. Many people die prior to receiving medical care because of the denial that anything may be wrong and postponement of seeking medical care. Cardiac dysrhythmias, mainly ventricular fibrillation, is usually the cause of death in these individuals. An MI is diagnosed based on type of chest pain, electrocardiographic changes, and increase of cardiac enzymes, such as CK, SGOT, troponin levels, and LDH. Precordial pain is similar to but usually more intense and prolonged than anginal pain, and in the instance of MI, the chest pain is usually constant and not relieved with nitroglycerin or rest.

Atherosclerosis of the arteries is usually the most common finding in patients with an MI. Atherosclerosis and arteriosclerosis are used interchangeably when discussing the fatty plaques that adhere to the inner layer of the arteries. The continuous buildup of these plaques, as well as the potential for hemorrhage at the intimal layer may result in alterations of the blood flow through the coronary arteries and abnormalities in platelet aggregation may contribute to changes in coronary perfusion. Infarction may occur without coronary artery disease or occlusion, and if the patient has developed an adequate collateral circulation, coronary occlusion may occur without infarction.

MI is usually a disease involving the left ventricle but the damage may extend to other areas, such as the atria or right ventricle. A right ventricular myocardial infarction typically has high right ventricular filling pressures and severe tricuspid regurgitation. Transmural infarcts involve the entire thickness of the myocardium and are characterized by Q waves on the electrocardiogram. Nontransmural infarcts are characterized by ST segment and T wave changes. Subendocardial infarcts normally involve the inner portion of the myocardium where wall tension is highest and the blood flow is most vulnerable to circulatory problems. Occlusion of the right coronary artery will result in an inferior infarction that may also include posterior portions of the heart. Occlusion of the left main artery, known as "the widow maker," frequently results in death because of the extensive damage. Occlusion of the left anterior descending artery results in an anterior infarction and may include some inferior parts of the heart, and occlusion of the circumflex artery results in a lateral infarction.

Precipitating factors for MIs include heredity, age, gender, presence of hypertension, presence of diabetes mellitus, cigarette smoking, hyperlipidemia, obesity, sedentary lifestyles, and stress.

The main goals in treating myocardial infarction are to increase blood flow to the coronary arteries and thus decrease infarction size, increase oxygen supply and decrease oxygen demand to prevent myocardial death or injury, and control or correct dysrhythmias.

MEDICAL CARE

Oxygen: used to increase available oxygen supply

Analgesics: morphine is the drug of choice because of its dual role as an analgesic as well as a vasodilator; given in incremental doses IV every 5 minutes as needed; IM injections are avoided because they can raise the enzyme levels and do not act as quickly

Thrombolytic agents: drugs such as streptokinase (Streptase, Kabikinase), urokinase (Abbokinase), anistreplase (Eminase, APSAC), or alteplase (Activase, Tissue Plasminogen Activator, TPA, rtPa) are given either intravenously or intracoronary to activate the body's own fibrinolytic system to dissolve the clot and resume coronary blood perfusion

Cardiac glycosides: digitalis used to increase force and strength of ventricular contractions and to decrease the conduction and rate of contractions in order to increase cardiac output; usually not used in the acute phase

Diuretics: drugs like furosemide (Lasix) used to promote excess fluid removal, to decrease edema and pulmonary venous pressure by preventing sodium and water reabsorption

Vasodilators: hydralazine (Apresoline), nifedipine (Procardia, Adalat), nitroglycerin (Nitropaste, Nitrodur, Nitrostat, Tridil, Nitroglycerine), prazosin (Minipres), captopril (Capoten) used to relax venous and/or arterial smooth muscle to decrease preload, decrease afterload, and decrease oxygen demand

Beta-adrenergic blockers: drugs such as acebutolol (Sectral), atenolol (Tenormin), betaxolol hydrochloride (Kerlone), bisoprolol fumarate (Zebeta), carteolol hydrochloride (Cartrol), carvedilol (Coreg), esmolol (Brevibloc), metoprolol (Toprol XL, Betaloc, Lopressor), labetalol hydrochloride (Normodyne, Trandate), nadolol (Corgard), pindolol (Visken), propranolol (Inderal), and timolol (Blocadren) used to decrease blood pressure, decrease elevated plasma renins, and with nonselective blockers, may do so without related reflex tachycardias; used to treat ventricular dysrhythmias and for the prophylaxis of angina

Heparin: used with thrombolytic protocols, and in the treatment of MI; prevents conversion of fibrinogen to fibrin and prothrombin to thrombin by its action on antithrombin III

Platelet aggregation inhibitors: aspirin helps to decrease aggregation of platelets and helps with vasodilation of the peripheral vessels; clopidrogrel bisulfate (Plavix) helps to reduce atherosclerotic-induced events by binding to ADP receptors on platelets which prevents fibrinogen from attaching to the receptors and, thus, preventing formation of clots

Glycoprotein IIb/IIIa Inhibitors: drugs, such as abciximab (ReoPro), eptifibatide (Integrilin), and tirofiban hydrochloride (Aggrastat), affect the members of the integrin family of receptors found in the membranes of platelets by changing the conformation to be receptive to one end of a fibrinogen dimer which is the final common pathway of platelet aggregation; by this action, the normal binding of fibrinogen and other factor inhibits platelet aggregation and clot formation

Laboratory: leukocyte count, sed rate and blood glucose may be elevated as an effect of stress and tissue necrosis; if leukocytes remain elevated (up to 15,000 cells/mm^3), it may indicate complications such as embolization, infection, or pericarditis; CK–MB values greater than 5% of the total CK indicates myocardial necrosis, but can lack sensitivity and specificity; CK–MB isoforms are another new cardiac marker—an absolute level of CK–MB2 >1 U/L or ratio of CK–MB2 to CK–MB1 of 1.5 have an increased sensitivity and specificity for the diagnosis of an MI within the first 6 hours after the onset of symptoms; the troponin complex has 3 subunits, known as troponin T, troponin I, and troponin C; troponin T and I rise less than 6 hours after the onset of ischemic changes and are the most sensitive and earliest enzyme markers; cardiac-specific troponin T (cTnT) and cardiac-specific troponin I (cTnI) may be present up to 7–14 days after the onset of MI; myoglobin is not a cardiac specific test, but may be detected as early as 2 hours after an MI and used in conjunction with clinical presentation and other tests; creatine phosphokinase (CK, CPK) will normally increase within 4–6 hours, peak between 12–24 hours, and last 2–3 days but should not be used as sole indicator because of possibility of elevation with other problems such as surgery or trauma; lactate dehydrogenase (LDH) will normally increase within 8–12 hours, peak between 2–4 days, and last 7–10 days but should not be used as sole indicator because of possibility of elevation with other problems such as liver failure; serum glutamic oxaloacetic transaminase (SGOT) is occasionally used as an infarct indicator; isoenzymes of CK are very specific with CK–MB most specific for MI, and levels do not rise with transient chest pain or in surgical procedures; a definitive level for CK–MB is greater than or equal to 5% of the total CK; LDH isoenzymes, specifically LDH1 is more specific for MI; if the total LDH is elevated and LDH1 is most predominant, MI is confirmed; both CK–MB and LDH1 will return to normal 72–96 hours after elevation. LDH1/LDH2 ratios that are greater than 1 may indicate tissue necrosis, but can also be noted in hemolyzed serum samples

Chest X-ray: shows any enlargement of the heart and pulmonary vein, presence of pulmonary edema or pleural effusion

Electrocardiography: shows indicative changes associated with sites of acute infarcts using Q waves, ST segment elevation, and T wave inversion; reveals changes with atrial and ventricular enlargement, rhythm and conduction abnormalities, ischemia, electrolyte abnormalities, drug toxicity, and presence of dysrhythmias

Echocardiography: used to study structural abnormalities and blood flow through the heart; M-mode echocardiography measures structures with a single ultrasonic beam that provides a narrow view of the heart; two-dimensional (2D) echocardiography shows a two-dimensional and wider look at the heart that is more useful in diagnosing right ventricular infarcts; documents increased right ventricular size, performance and segmental wall motion abnormalities, and blood flow through the heart; used to assess left ventricular function, atrial or ventricular septal defects, aneurysms, and thrombus formations

Nuclear cardiologic testing: MUGA (multiple gated acquisition study) provides information that approximates ejection fractions and the analysis of the ventricular wall motion; 99mTc (Technetium-99 pyrophosphate scan) shows infarcted areas as increased levels of radioactivity, or "hot spots" that appear 12–36 hours after infarct and remain for 4–7 days; PET (positron emission tomography) allows measurement of myocardial blood flow, fatty acid and glucose metabolism, and blood volume; thallium scans can determine size and location of damage as a "cold spot"

Magnetic resonance imaging (MRI): provides a three-dimensional view that can detect changes in tissues before structural damage is done and is safe for pregnant women and children

Cardiac catheterization: used to assess pathophysiology of the patient's cardiovascular disorder, to provide left ventricular function information, to allow for measurement of heart pressures and cardiac output, to evaluate stenotic lesions, and to measure blood gas content

Intra-aortic balloon pump (IABP): decreases the workload on the heart, decreases myocardial oxygen demand, increases coronary perfusion, decreases afterload, decreases preload, and helps to limit infarct size if quickly initiated; improves cardiac output and tissue perfusion; used in cardiogenic shock, for support following cardiac surgery, for intractable chest pain, and in cardiac catheterizations or other cardiovascular procedures of high-risk patients

Angioplasty: primary PTCA may be used as an alternative to thrombolytic therapy in patients with MI, ST elevation, or new or presumed new left bundle branch blocks who present with symptoms within 12 hours, in patients who present within 36 hours of acute ST elevation or Q wave MIs, or new left bundle

branch block MI patients who develop cardiogenic shock; revascularization can be done within 18 hours of the shock onset in patients who have contraindications to thrombolytic therapy

Ventricular assist device (VAD): used on either or both ventricles to provide total support to the heart and circulation in order to allow recovery to the heart; usually indicated in patients who are awaiting cardiac transplantation or in those patients with cardiogenic shock and ventricular failure; may be used in conjunction with IABP

Pacemakers: either temporary or permanent, used in anticipation of lethal dysrhythmias and/or conduction problems

Surgery: coronary artery bypass grafting to reroute the coronary blood flow around the diseased vessel to enable coronary perfusion

NURSING DIAGNOSES

ACUTE PAIN

Related to: decreased blood flow to myocardium, myocardial ischemia or infarct, postprocedure discomfort, chest wall pain postsurgery, pericarditis

Defining Characteristics: chest pain with or without radiation, facial grimacing, clutching of hands to chest, restlessness, diaphoresis, changes in pulse and blood pressure, dyspnea, dizziness, arm pain, shoulder pain, shortness of breath, fatigue, tachycardia, changes in CVP, PA pressures, PCWP, TPR, SVR, decreased cardiac output and cardiac index

Outcome Criteria

✔ Chest pain will be relieved or controlled to patient's satisfaction.

✔ Hemodynamic status will be stable.

NOC: *Pain Control*

INTERVENTIONS	RATIONALES
Evaluate chest pain as to type, location, severity, relief, change with activity or rest, other symptoms concurrently noted, such as pallor, diaphoresis, radiation of pain, nausea, vomiting,	Variations may occur with patients regarding specific complaints and behavior. Most MI patients look acutely ill and can only focus on their pain. Respirations may be increased as

INTERVENTIONS	RATIONALES
shortness of breath, and vital sign changes.	a result of anxiety and pain. Heart rate may increase because of increased catecholamines, stress, and pain, which can also increase blood pressure.
Obtain description of intensity using 0–10 scale, with 0 being no pain and 10 being the worst pain experienced.	Pain is a subjective experience and personal to that patient. Intensity scales are useful to gauge improvement or deterioration as perceived by the patient.
Obtain history (when possible) of previous cardiac pain and familial history of cardiac problems.	This provides information that may help to differentiate current pain from previous problems, as well as identify new problems and complications.
Prepare for the administration of thrombolytic therapy or for primary posttransluminal coronary angioplasty.	Rapid revascularization minimizes coronary tissue damage and loss.
Insert IV lines and obtain blood samples as ordered.	At least 2 IV sites should be obtained prior to the beginning of thrombolysis because once the drug has been administered, punctures will need to be minimized and the need for concurrent medications require at least two separate lines in case drugs are incompatible with each other or interact with other medications. Blood levels should be drawn for baseline values for comparison posttreatment.
Monitor hemodynamic status by use of pulmonary artery catheter, if available, and notify physician of significant changes.	PA pressures represent the right and left sided heart pressures. The PA systolic pressure corresponds to the right ventricular pressure, and is normally 15–25 mm Hg. PA diastolic pressure corresponds to the left ventricular end-diastolic pressure and is used to identify left ventricular function. Normal values range from 10–18 mm Hg. The PCWP reflects left atrial pressures and correlates with left ventricular end-diastolic filling pressures, and normal values are 5–15 mm Hg. PCWP is elevated with fluid overload, left ventricular failure, and ischemia. Cardiac output (CO) is measured by thermodilution with normal values between

INTERVENTIONS	RATIONALES
	4–8 L/minute and reflect the amount of blood that is circulated in one minute. Cardiac index (CI) is normally 2.5–4 L/min/m².
Administer oxygen by nasal cannula or mask as indicated.	Supplemental oxygen can increase the available oxygen and can relieve pain associated with myocardial ischemia. Hypoxemia may be a result of left ventricular failure and ventilation/perfusion mismatching.
Administer analgesic as ordered, such as morphine sulfate, meperidine (Demerol), or Dilaudid IV.	Morphine is the drug of choice to control MI pain, but other analgesics may be used to reduce pain and reduce the workload on the heart. IM injections should be avoided because they can alter cardiac enzymes and are not absorbed well in tissue that is non- or underperfused. Pain relief decreases an elevated sympathetic response and helps to deter the dysrhythmias that may occur as a result of circulating catecholemines.
Administer beta-blockers as ordered (such as atenolol, pindolol, and propranolol).	These drugs block sympathetic stimulation, reduce heart rate and systolic blood pressure, and thus lowers the myocardial oxygen demand. Beta-blockers should not be given in severely impaired contractility states because of the negative inotropic properties.
Administer calcium-channel blockers as ordered (such as verapamil, diltiazem, or nifedipine).	These drugs can increase coronary blood flow and collateral circulation, reduce preload and myocardial oxygen demands, which can decrease pain due to ischemia.
Administer anti-emetics as ordered prn.	Analgesics may cause nausea and anti-emetics will help control this symptom, as well as assisting with the increased amount of vagal tone seen with myocardial infarction. Anti-emetics may also potentiate the action of the analgesic.
Administer anxiolytics as ordered prn.	These drugs may be helpful if the patient is anxious, agitated,

(continues)

(continued)

INTERVENTIONS	RATIONALES
	or delirious because of pain, sleep deprivation, or ICU psychosis.
Maintain bedrest during pain, with position of comfort; nurse to stay with patient during pain.	Reduces oxygen consumption, and demand; alleviates fear and provides caring atmosphere.
Maintain relaxing environment to promote calmness.	Reduces competing stimuli and reduces anxiety.
Instruct patient to notify nurse immediately of any chest pain.	Delay in notification can delay pain relief and may require increased amounts of medication in order to finally achieve relief. Pain can cause further damage to an already-injured myocardium, and may signal extension of MI, spasm, or other complication.
Instruct patient in relaxation techniques, deep breathing, guided imagery, visualization, and so forth.	Helps to decrease pain and anxiety and provides distraction from pain.
Instruct patient in nitroglycerin SL administration after hospitalization; 1 q5 minutes up to 3 times, and if pain is unrelieved, patient should seek emergency medical care.	Knowledge facilitates cooperation and compliance with medical regimen. Pain unrelieved with NTG may be indicative of MI.
Instruct patient in activity alterations and limitations.	Decreases myocardial oxygen demand and workload on the heart.
Instruct patient/family in medication effects, side effects, contraindications, and symptoms to report.	Promotes knowledge and compliance with therapeutic regimen. Alleviates fear of unknown.

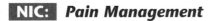 **NIC:** *Pain Management*

Discharge or Maintenance Evaluation

- Blood flow to the myocardium will be restored.
- Patient will report pain being absent or controlled with medication administration.
- Medication will be administered prior to pain becoming severe.
- Patient/family will be able to recall effects, side effects, and contraindications of medications accurately.
- Activity will be modified in such a way as to prevent onset of chest pain.

INEFFECTIVE TISSUE PERFUSION: CARDIOPULMONARY

Related to: tissue ischemia, reduction or interruption of blood flow, vasoconstriction, hypovolemia, shunting, depressed ventricular function, dysrhythmias, conduction defects

Defining Characteristics: chest pain, abnormal hemodynamic readings, dysrhythmias, decreased peripheral pulses, cyanosis, decreased blood pressure, shortness of breath, dyspnea, cold and clammy skin, decreased mental alertness, changes in mental status, oliguria, anuria, sluggish capillary refill, abnormal electrolyte and digoxin levels, hypoxia, ABG changes, ventilation/perfusion imbalances, changes in peripheral resistance, impaired oxygenation of myocardium, ECG changes (ST segment, T wave, U wave), LV enlargement, palpitations

Outcome Criteria

- ✔ Patient will have vital signs within normal parameters with no dysrhythmias on ECG.
- ✔ Blood flow and perfusion to vital organs will be preserved and circulatory function will be maximized.
- ✔ Patient will be free of dysrhythmias.
- ✔ Hemodynamic parameters will be within normal limits.
- ✔ Patient will have increased coronary perfusion with coronary artery blood flow restored and symptoms relieved.
- ✔ ST segment elevation will return to baseline.
- ✔ Cardiac enzymes will normalize more rapidly as a result of reperfusion.

NOC: *Tissue Perfusion: Cardiac*

INTERVENTIONS	RATIONALES
Monitor vital signs. Obtain hemodynamic values, noting deviations from baseline values.	Provides information about the hemodynamics of the patient and facilitates early intervention for problems.
Administer thrombolytic drugs as ordered and as per protocol specific to medication.	Thrombolytic drugs lyse the clot that may be occluding the coronary artery and promote restoration of oxygen and blood flow to the heart in order to increase tissue perfusion.

INTERVENTIONS	RATIONALES
Monitor ECG for disturbances in conduction and for dysrhythmias and treat as indicated.	Decreased cardiac perfusion may instigate conduction abnormalities. Ventricular fibrillation is the most common dysrhythmia following MI. Reperfusion dysrhythmias frequently occur during the initial period after blood flow to the coronary arteries is restored after the administration of thrombolytics.
Prepare for emergent cardioversion, defibrillation, or administration of resuscitative drugs as may be required.	Reocclusion may occur with signs such as ST segment changes, chest pain, decreased blood pressure, or dysrhythmias, and must be treated per protocol.
Administer oxygen by nasal cannula as ordered, with rate dependent on disease process and condition.	Provides oxygen necessary for tissues and organ perfusion.
Observe patient for the development of bleeding to oral mucosa and gums, insertion sites, GI tract, and elsewhere. Monitor coagulation studies.	Thrombolytic drugs may create bleeding complications as a result of their action.
Assess patient for fever, shortness of breath, urticaria, bronchospasm, and flushing.	Streptokinase and anisoylated plasminogen streptokinase activator complex (APSAC) can cause allergic reactions that require urgent treatment.
Auscultate lungs for crackles (rales), rhonchi, or wheezes.	May indicate fluid overload that will further decrease tissue perfusion.
Auscultate heart sounds for S_3 or S_4 gallop, new murmurs, presence of jugular vein distention, or hepatojugular reflex.	May indicate impending or present heart failure.
Monitor oxygen status with ABGs, S_vO_2 monitoring, or with pulse oximetry.	Provides information about the oxygenation status of the patient. Continuous monitoring of saturation levels provide an instant analysis of how activity affects oxygenation and perfusion for the patient.
Monitor for changes in respiratory status, increased work of breathing, dyspnea, and so forth.	Decreased cardiac perfusion may result in pump failure and precipitate respiratory distress and failure.
Determine the presence and character of peripheral pulses, capillary refill time, skin color and temperature.	May indicate decreased perfusion resulting from impaired coronary blood flow.

INTERVENTIONS	RATIONALES
Administer clarithromycin as ordered.	This macrolide antibiotic has been shown in trials to decrease the risk of death in patients who have myocardial infarctions or angina. Infections can cause inflammation and this plays a role in the development of coronary artery disease. Several infective organisms, such as *Chlamydia* and *pneumoniae*, are associated with CAD. Trials have shown that a 3-month course of antibiotic treatment reduces the risk of future heart attacks.
Administer glucose-insulin-potassium infusion if ordered.	In trials, a combination of 25% glucose, 50 IU/L insulin, and 80 mmol/L KCl (GIK) helped with metabolic modulation in acute MI patients and decreased the risk of morbidity when given as an infusion at 1.5 cc/kg/hr for 24 hours.
Administer LMWH (Dalteparin) as ordered.	Low-molecular-weight heparin has an increased degree of inhibition of factor Xa relative to thrombin, prevents thrombin generation, inhibits thrombin formation, and decreases the rate of heparin-associated thrombocytopenia. Hirudin, a recombinant protein found in leech saliva, has been shown to decrease death rates with patients with MIs.
Monitor patient for signs/symptoms of cardiac rupture and treat per protocol.	Cardiac rupture usually occurs within the first 24 hours or from 4–7 days following MI because of expansion of the infarcted ventricular wall. It is usually seen with initial MIs, anterior MIs, in women and the elderly, and in patients who have used corticosteroids or NSAIDs. Early successful reperfusion is the best method of prevention of rupture.
Discourage any nonessential activity.	Ambulation, exercise, transfers, and Valsalva-type maneuvers can increase blood pressure and decrease tissue perfusion.

(continues)

(continued)

INTERVENTIONS	RATIONALES
Assist patient with planned, graduated levels of activity.	Allows for balance between rest and activity to decrease myocardial workload and oxygen demand. Gradual increases help to increase patient tolerance to activity without pain.
Titrate vasoactive drugs as ordered.	Maintain blood pressure and heart rate at parameters set by physician for optimal perfusion with minimal workload on heart.
Auscultate for bowel sounds and monitor for complaints of nausea, vomiting, anorexia, abdominal distention, abdominal pain, or constipation.	Decreased perfusion to mesentery may result in loss or change in peristalsis, resulting in GI use of analgesics, and change in surroundings may contribute to changes in GI status.
Monitor urine output for adequate amounts, character of urine, presence of sediment, and specific gravity.	Decreased perfusion to renal arteries may result in oliguria. Dehydration secondary to nausea and vomiting may affect renal perfusion.
Monitor lab work such as renal or liver profiles. Monitor coagulation studies and notify physician for unexpected abnormalities.	May indicate organ dysfunction and decreased perfusion. Thrombolytic agents will impair coagulation and care must be taken to ensure patient safety because of the increased risk for bleeding and hemorrhage.
Instruct patient/family on medications, dosage, effects, side effects, and contraindications.	Promotes compliance with regimen and knowledge base.
Instruct patient to refrain from smoking.	Smoking causes vasoconstriction which can decrease perfusion.
Instruct patient/family in dietary requirements, menu planning, sodium restrictions, foods to avoid.	Reduction of high-cholesterol and sodium foods will help to control atherosclerosis, hyperlipidemia, fluid retention, and the effects on coronary blood flow.

NIC: *Cardiac Care: Acute*

Discharge or Maintenance Evaluation

- Lung fields will be clear and free of adventitious breath sounds.
- Extremities will be warm and pink, with easily palpable pulses.
- Vital signs and hemodynamic parameters will be within normal limits for patient.

- Oxygenation will be optimal as evident by pulse oximetry greater than 90%, S_vO_2 greater than 75%, or normal ABGs.
- Patient will be free of chest pain and shortness of breath.
- Patient will be able to verbalize information accurately regarding medications, diet and activity limitations.
- Patient will exhibit no signs of bleeding complications and coagulation studies will be within set parameters.
- Patient will be free of dysrhythmias.

DECREASED CARDIAC OUTPUT

Related to: damaged myocardium, decreased contractility, dysrhythmias, conduction defects, alteration in preload, alteration in afterload, vasoconstriction, myocardial ischemia, ventricular hypertrophy

Defining Characteristics: elevated or decreased blood pressure, elevated mean arterial pressure greater than 120 mm Hg, elevated systemic vascular resistance greater than 1400 dyne–seconds/cm^5, cardiac output less than 4 L/min or cardiac index less than 2.5 L/min/m^2, tachycardia, cold, pale extremities, absent or decreased peripheral pulses, ECG changes, hypotension, S_3 or S_4 gallops, decreased urinary output, diaphoresis, orthopnea, dyspnea, crackles (rales), jugular vein distention, edema, chest pain

Outcome Criteria

✔ Vital signs and hemodynamic parameters will be within normal limits for patient, with no dysrhythmias noted.

NOC: *Cardiac Pump Effectiveness*

NOC: *Circulation Status*

INTERVENTIONS	RATIONALES
Auscultate apical pulses and monitor heart rate and rhythm. Monitor BP in both arms.	Decreased contractility will be compensated by tachycardia, especially concurrently with heart failure. Blood volume will be lowered if blood pressure is increased resulting in increased afterload. Pulse decreases may be noted in association with

INTERVENTIONS	RATIONALES
	toxic levels of digoxin. Hypotension may occur as a result of ventricular dysfunction and poor perfusion of the myocardium.
Monitor ECG for dysrhythmias. and treat as indicated.	Conduction abnormalities may occur because of ischemic myocardium affecting the pumping efficiency of the heart. Rapid recognition and treatment of complications is essential to increase perfusion and cardiac output.
Determine level of cardiac function and existing cardiac and other conditions.	Additional disease states and complications may place an additional workload on an already compromised heart.
Measure CO and perform other hemodynamic calculations.	Provides direct measurement of cardiac output function, and calculated measurement of preload and afterload.
Monitor for development of new S_3 or S_4 gallops.	S_3 gallops are usually associated with congestive heart failure but can be found with mitral regurgitation and left ventricular overload after MI. S_4 gallops can be associated with myocardial ischemia, ventricular rigidity, pulmonary hypertension, or systemic hypertension, which can decrease cardiac output.
Auscultate for presence of murmurs and/or rubs.	Indicates disturbances of normal blood flow within the heart related to incompetent valves, septal defects, or papillary muscle/chordae tendonae rupture post-MI. Presence of a rub with an MI may be associated with pericarditis and/or pericardial effusions.
Observe lower extremities for edema, distended neck veins, cold hands and feet, mottling, oliguria. Notify physician if urine output is <30 cc/hr for 2 consecutive hours.	Reduced venous return to the heart can result in low cardiac output. Oliguria results from decreased venous return caused by fluid retention.
Position in semi-Fowler's position.	Promotes easier breathing by allowing for chest expansion and prevents pooling of blood in the pulmonary vasculature.
Administer cardiac glycosides, nitrates, vasodilators, diuretics,	Used in the treatment of vasoconstriction and to reduce heart

INTERVENTIONS	RATIONALES
and antihypertensives as ordered.	rate and contractility, reduces blood pressure by relaxation of venous and arterial smooth muscle which then in turn increases cardiac output and decreases the workload on the heart.
Titrate vasoactive drugs as ordered per physician parameters.	Maintains blood pressure and heart rate at levels to optimize cardiac output function. Reduction of preload and afterload using vasoactive drugs increases cardiac output. Nitroglycerin should not be given until there is sufficient volume with IV fluids achieved because of the risk of hypotension. Inotropic support is helpful when cardiac output fails to improve with volume replacement, and contractility is enhanced. Heart rate can be controlled with beta-blockers, atropine, pacemakers, and/or cardioversion.
Administer IV fluids as ordered.	Up to 1 liter of fluid may be required for right ventricular MIs to provide sufficient circulating volume to maintain cardiac output.
Administer dobutamine immediately in RV MIs after fluid has been given if cardiac output does not improve, per hospital protocol.	May require inotropic support to maintain or achieve adequate cardiac output if fluid resuscitation fails to improve status.
Observe for high-grade heart block or atrial fibrillation, and treat per protocol with AV sequential pacing and/or medications as ordered.	Second and third-degree heart block are common and may require pacing to sustain cardiac output. Atrial fibrillation is common and occurs in approximately one-third of all patients who have hemodynamic compromise. These dysrhythmias worsen the patient's hemodynamic status and require urgent treatment to preserve cardiac function.
Observe for drug-refractory sustained polymorphic ventricular tachycardia ("electrical storm") and treat per protocol.	Episodes of this type of dysrhythmia are rare, but do occur and may be a result of uncontrolled ischemia or increased sympathetic tone.

(continues)

(continued)

INTERVENTIONS	RATIONALES
	Treatment is usually IV β-blockers, IV amiodarone, placement on IABP, or emergent revascularization.
Weigh every day.	Weight gain may indicate fluid retention and possible impending congestive failure.
Arrange activities so as to not overwhelm patient. Maintain reduced activity for at least 12 hours with use of bedside commode only, and then increase activity as tolerated within first 48 hours.	Avoids fatiguing patient and decreasing cardiac output further. Balancing rest with activity minimizes energy expenditure and myocardial oxygen demands by maintaining adequate cardiac output. Early mobilization lowers the risk of development of pulmonary emboli.
Avoid Valsalva-type maneuvers with straining, coughing or moving. Administer stool softeners as needed/ordered.	Increasing intra-abdominal pressure results in an abrupt decrease in cardiac output by preventing blood from being pumped into the thoracic cavity and, thus, less blood being pumped into the heart which then decreases the heart rate. When the pressure is released, there is a sudden overload of blood which then increases preload and the workload on the heart.
Provide small, easy to digest, meals.	Large meals increase the workload on the heart by diverting blood flow from that area. Caffeine directly stimulates the heart and increases heart rate, and used to be restricted, but patients who are regular caffeine drinkers have developed a tolerance and could experience withdrawal symptoms, such as increased heart rate or headache, if caffeine is withheld.
Have emergency equipment and medications available at all times.	Coronary occlusion, lethal dysrhythmias, infarction extensions or intractable pain may precipitate cardiac arrest that requires life support and resuscitation.
Instruct patient/family to avoid/stop smoking after myocardial infarction. Instruct in the use of nicotine replacements and	Nicotine causes vasoconstriction, which can result in decreased perfusion and coronary spasms. Smoking is the leading pre-

INTERVENTIONS	RATIONALES
methods of stopping smoking.	ventable cause of death in the United States. Smoking increases the risk of cancer, damage to the respiratory system, death because of cardiovascular causes, reduces bone mass, and increases the risk for osteoporosis. Cessation of smoking can substantially reduce or reverse the risks that are associated with smoking. Nicotine replacement may be required to prevent withdrawal in the patient who is a heavy smoker, and who is physically and psychologically dependent on cigarettes.
Instruct patient/family on medications, dose, effects, side effects, contraindications, and avoidance of over-the-counter drugs without physician approval.	Promotes knowledge and compliance with regimen. Prevents any adverse drug interactions.
Instruct in activity limitations. Demonstrate exercises to be done.	Promotes compliance. Reduces potential for decrease in cardiac output by lessening the workload placed on the heart.
Instruct to report chest pain immediately.	May indicate complications of decreased cardiac output. Recurrent chest pain after myocardial infarction may indicate that patient has continuing ischemia, which requires prompt attention to limit cardiac damage.
Instruct patient/family regarding placement of pulmonary artery catheter, and post-procedure care.	Alleviates fear and promotes knowledge. Pulmonary artery catheter necessary for direct measurement of cardiac output and for obtaining values for other hemodynamic measurements.
Assist with insertion and maintenance of pacemaker when needed.	Cardiac pacing may be necessary during the acute phase of MI or may be necessary as a permanent measure if the MI severely damages the conduction system.
Prepare patient/family for potential percutaneous coronary intervention (PCI) or CABG procedures.	If thrombolytic therapy is unsuccessful, other reperfusion interventions may be required to limit cardiac damage, especially if patient has multivessel disease.
Prepare patient/family for use of IABP therapy.	IABP may be necessary in patients with decreased cardiac output and ongoing ischemia,

INTERVENTIONS	RATIONALES
	especially with the presence of severe hypotension or cardiogenic shock. IABP therapy frequently acts as a bridge to revascularization procedures.

NIC: *Hemodynamic Regulation*

Discharge or Maintenance Evaluation

- Patient will have no chest pain or shortness of breath.
- Vital signs and hemodynamic parameters will be within normal limits for age and disease condition.
- Minimal activity will be tolerated without fatigue or dyspnea.
- Urinary output will be adequate.
- Cardiac output will be adequate to ensure adequate perfusion of all body systems.

RISK FOR IMBALANCED FLUID VOLUME

Related to: increased sodium and water retention, decreased organ perfusion

Defining Characteristics: edema, weight gain, intake greater than output, increased blood pressure, increased heart rate, shortness of breath, dyspnea, orthopnea, crackles (rales), oliguria, jugular vein distention, pleural effusion, specific gravity changes, altered electrolyte levels

Outcome Criteria

✔ Blood pressure will be maintained within normal limits and edema will be absent or minimal in all body parts.

NOC: *Fluid Balance*

INTERVENTIONS	RATIONALES
Auscultate lungs for presence of crackles (rales).	May indicate pulmonary edema from cardiac decompensation.
Observe for jugular vein distention and dependent edema.	May indicate impending congestive failure and fluid excess.

INTERVENTIONS	RATIONALES
Determine fluid balance by measuring Intake and output, and observing for decreases in output and concentrated urine.	Renal perfusion is impaired with decreased cardiac output, which leads to sodium and water retention and oliguria.
Weigh daily and notify physician of greater than 2 lb/day increase.	Abrupt changes in weight usually indicate excess fluid.
Provide patient with fluid intake of 2 L/day, unless fluid restriction is warranted.	Fluids provide hydration of tissues. Fluids may need to be restricted because of cardiac decompensation.
Administer diuretics as ordered.	Drugs may be necessary to correct fluid overload depending on emergent nature of problem.
Monitor electrolyte for imbalances.	Hypokalemia can occur with the administration of diuretics.
Instruct patient and family regarding dietary restrictions of sodium.	Fluid retention is increased with intake of sodium.
Instruct patient and family to observe for weight changes and report these to physician.	Weight gain may be first overt sign of fluid excess and should be monitored to prevent complications.
Instruct patient and family in medications prescribed after discharge, with dose, effect, side effects, contraindications.	Promotes knowledge and compliance with treatment regimen.

NIC: *Fluid Monitoring*

Discharge or Maintenance Evaluation

- Patient will have no edema or fluid excess.
- Fluid balance will be maintained and blood pressure will be within normal limits of baseline.
- Lung fields will be clear, without adventitious breath sounds, and weight will be stable.
- Patient will be able to verbalize understanding of dietary restrictions and medications.

ANXIETY

Related to: hypoxia, change in health status, fear of death, threat to body image, threat to role functioning, pain, sympathetic stimulation, pain

Defining Characteristics: restlessness, insomnia, anorexia, increased respirations, increased heart rate, increased blood pressure, difficulty concentrating, dry mouth, poor eye contact, decreased energy, irritability, crying, feelings of helplessness, confusion, fear of consequences

Outcome Criteria

✔ Patient will be able to use coping mechanisms effectively, will appear less anxious, and be able to verbalize feelings.

NOC: *Anxiety Control*

INTERVENTIONS	RATIONALES
Identify patient's perception of illness or situation. Encourage expressions of anger, grief, sadness, fear, and loss.	Patient may be afraid of dying and be anxious about his immediate problem as related to his lifestyle and the problems that have been left unattended.
Assess patient for physiologic causes of anxiety.	Hypoxia and hypoxemia can produce the same symptoms, and physiologic dysfunction should be ruled out first.
Explain all procedures to patient in concise and reassuring manner. Repeat information as needed based on patient's ability to comprehend.	Knowledge reduces fear of the unknown. Establishes feelings of trust and concern. Information may need to be repeated or reinforced because of competing stimuli.
Encourage the patient to discuss his fears and feelings. Provide an atmosphere of acceptance without judgment. Accept his use of denial, but do not reinforce false beliefs. Avoid confrontations and upsets.	Assists the patient in verbalizing concerns and provides the opportunity to deal with matters of import to the patient. Accepting the patient's feelings may decrease his anxiety which can facilitate a therapeutic environment for instruction. Denial can be useful to decrease anxiety but can postpone dealing with the reality of the problem. Confrontations can lead to anger and exacerbate the use of denial and decrease cooperation.
Provide opportunities for the family to visit and assist with care if possible. Orient to routines.	Familiar people can decrease anxiety of the patient, as well as provide a more conducive atmosphere for learning and recovery. Predictability can decrease anxiety. Supportive family members can comfort the patient and relieve worries.
Provide private time for patient and family member(s)	Allows time for expression of concerns and feelings, and

INTERVENTIONS	RATIONALES
to verbalize feelings.	relieves tension by establishing a more normal routine.
Provide opportunities for patient to control his environment and activities as much as feasible, based on condition.	Allows the patient to have some control over his situation and facilitates compliance with care of which patient is not in control.
Provide opportunity for patient to rest without interruption as much as possible.	Facilitates coping mechanism by conserving energy, and by providing required rest.
Administer antianxiety drugs as ordered.	Promotes rest and reduces anxiety.
Instruct patient and family as to all procedures, tests, medications, and care in a factual consistent manner. Reinforce as needed.	Accurate information reduces anxiety, facilitates the relationship between patient and nurse, and allows the patient and family to deal with the problem in a realistic manner. Repetition, when needed, helps in the retention of information when the attention span is diminished.
Instruct patient in relaxation techniques, such as guided imagery, relaxation therapy, music therapy, and so forth. Provide for diversionary activities.	Reduces anxiety and stress.
Instruct about post-discharge care, activities, limitations, symptoms to report, problems that might be encountered, and goals.	Reduces anxiety and promotes increased independence and self-confidence; decreases fear of abandonment that can occur with discharge from hospital; assists patient and family to identify realistic goals and decreases the chances of discouragement with limitations during recuperation.

NIC: *Anxiety Reduction*

Discharge or Maintenance Evaluation

■ Patient is able to recognize feelings and identify mechanisms to cope and identify causes.

■ Patient has significant reduction in fear and anxiety and appears less tense, with normal vital signs.

■ Patient/family can appropriately utilize problem-solving skills.

- Patient can verbalize concerns easily and has increased energy.
- Patient can make appropriate decisions based on factual information regarding his condition and is able to discuss future plans.

DEFICIENT KNOWLEDGE

Related to: new diagnosis, lack of understanding, lack of understanding of medical condition, lack of recall

Defining Characteristics: verbalized questions regarding problems, inadequate follow-up on instructions given, misconceptions, lack of improvement of previous regimen, development of preventable complications

Outcome Criteria

✔ Patient will be able to verbalize and demonstrate understanding of information given regarding condition, medications, and treatment regimen.

NOC: *Knowledge: Treatment Regimen*

IINTERVENTIONS	RATIONALES
Determine patient's baseline of knowledge regarding disease process, normal physiology, and function of the heart.	Provides information regarding patient's understanding of condition as well as a baseline from which to base teaching.
Monitor patient's readiness to learn and determine best methods to use for teaching. Attempt to incorporate family members in learning process. Reinstruct/reinforce information as needed.	Promotes optimal learning environment when patient shows willingness to learn. Family members may assist with helping the patient to make informed choices regarding his treatment. Anxiety or large volumes of instruction may impede comprehension and limit learning.
Provide time for individual interaction with patient.	Promotes relationship between patient and nurse, and establishes trust.
Instruct patient on procedures that may be performed.	Provides knowledge and promotes the ability to make informed choices.
Instruct patient on medications, dose, effects, side effects, contraindications, and signs/symptoms to report to physician.	Provides information to the patient to manage medication regimen and ensure compliance.

IINTERVENTIONS	RATIONALES
Instruct in dietary needs and restrictions, such as limiting sodium or increasing potassium.	Patient may need to increase dietary potassium if placed on diuretics; sodium should be limited because of the potential for fluid retention.
Provide printed materials when possible for patient/family to review.	Provides references for patient and family to refer to once patient is discharged, and can enhance the understanding of verbally-given instructions.
Demonstrate and instruct on technique for checking pulse rate and regularity. Instruct in situations where immediate action must be taken.	Self-monitoring promotes self-independence and can provide timely intervention for abnormalities or complications. Heart rates that exceed set parameters may require further medical alteration in medications or regimen.
Have patient demonstrate all skills that will be necessary for postdischarge.	Provides information that patient has gained a full understanding of instruction and is able to demonstrate correct information.
Instruct/demonstrate exercises to be performed, avoiding overtaxing activities, signs/symptoms that may require the cessation of any activity, and to report symptoms that may require medical attention	Exercise programs are helpful in improving cardiac function. Prompt attention to potential complication can assist in limiting damage to organs, and allows for timely intervention.
Refer patient to cardiac rehabilitation as ordered.	Provides for further improvement and rehabilitation postdischarge, using graduated exercise programs while maintaining surveillance of patient's cardiac status.

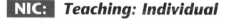

NIC: *Teaching: Individual*

Discharge or Maintenance Evaluation

- Patient will be able to verbalize understanding of condition, treatment regimen, and signs/symptoms to report.
- Patient will be able to correctly perform all tasks prior to discharge.
- Patient will be able to verbalize understanding of cardiac disease, risk factors, dietary restrictions, and lifestyle adaptations.

ACTIVITY INTOLERANCE

Related to: cardiac dysfunction, changes in oxygen supply and consumption, fatigue, weakness, increased work of breathing, hypoxia, hypoxemia, inadequate rest

Defining Characteristics: chest pain, neck and jaw pain, arm pain, dysrhythmias, ischemic ECG changes, increased heart rate, increased blood pressure, dyspnea with exertion, pallor, feelings of weakness and tiredness, decreased oxygen saturation

Outcome Criteria

✔ Patient will be able to increase and achieve desired activity level, progressively, with no intolerance symptoms noted, such as respiratory compromise.

✔ Patient will be able to conserve energy while carrying out self-care activities.

✔ Patient will be able to maintain range of motion within parameters specific to patient.

NOC: *Activity Tolerance*

IINTERVENTIONS	RATIONALES
Assist patient with ambulation, as ordered, with progressive increases as patient's tolerance permits.	Increased activity increases workload on the heart and may compromise perfusion and cellular metabolism. Gradual increases allow the body to compensate for the increase in workload
Monitor heart rate, rhythm, respirations, and blood pressure for abnormalities. Treat lethal dysrhythmias per protocol. Notify physician of significant changes in VS.	Changes in vital signs assist with monitoring physiologic responses to increases in activity. Changes that do not return to normal within a few minutes must be identified and treated. Circulatory compromise may occur if activity level is increased too rapidly.
Identify causative factors leading to intolerance of activity.	Illness can create diminished capacity for compensation of increased workload on the heart. Alleviation of factors that are known to create intolerance can assist with development of an activity level program.
Encourage patient to assist with planning activities, with rest	Participation in planning care enhances compliance and helps

IINTERVENTIONS	RATIONALES
periods as necessary. Instruct in energy conservation techniques.	give the patient a feeling of self-worth and well-being. Rest periods between activities allow for reduction in oxygen demand and help to reduce fatigue and encourage independence.
Perform/assist with active or passive ROM exercises at least QID.	Exercises maintain joint mobility, prevent contractures, and assist with maintenance of muscle strength and tone.
Turn patient at least every 2 hours, and prn.	Improves respiratory function, prevents skin breakdown, and prevents development of complications.
Instruct patient in isometric and breathing exercises.	Exercises will improve breathing and allow patient to gradually increase activity level. Effective breathing patterns while performing activities will assist in reducing exertion.
Instruct patient on energy conservation techniques.	Use of shower chairs, foot rests, gathering required items prior to activity, and so forth will help to decrease energy expenditure and fatigue which may result in increased dyspnea and lack of activity tolerance.
Provide patient/family with exercise regimen, with written instructions.	Promotes self-worth and involves patient and his family with self-care. Use of written materials allows for referral to instructions once patient has been discharged from hospital facility.

NIC: *Exercise Promotion*

Discharge or Maintenance Evaluation

■ Patient will be able to tolerate activity without excessive dyspnea or hemodynamic instability.

■ Patient will be able to perform ADLs within limits of disease process.

■ Patient will be able to recall information accurately, identify causative factors for activity intolerance, and will be able to utilize breathing techniques and energy conservation techniques effectively.

■ Patient will be compliant with prescribed activity regimen.

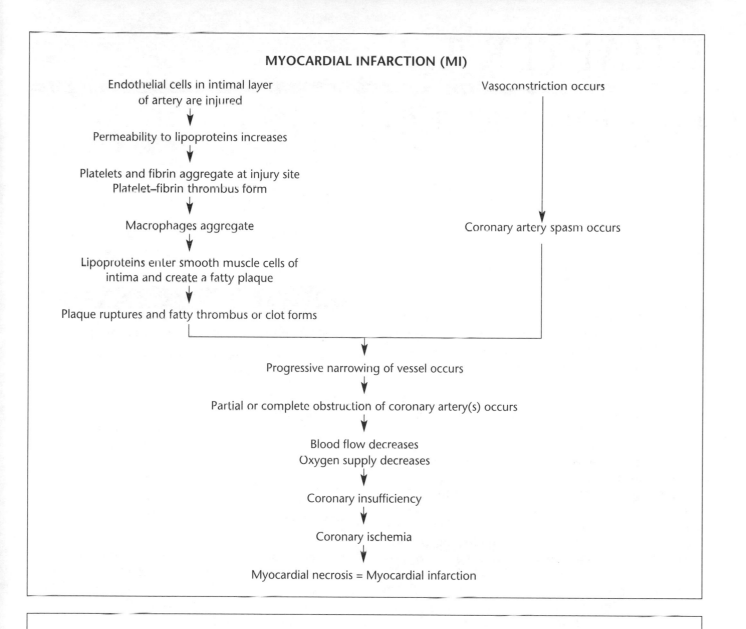

MYOCARDIAL INFARCTION (MI)

Endothelial cells in intimal layer
of artery are injured
↓
Permeability to lipoproteins increases
↓
Platelets and fibrin aggregate at injury site
Platelet–fibrin thrombus form
↓
Macrophages aggregate
↓
Lipoproteins enter smooth muscle cells of
intima and create a fatty plaque
↓
Plaque ruptures and fatty thrombus or clot forms

Vasoconstriction occurs
↓
Coronary artery spasm occurs

Progressive narrowing of vessel occurs
↓
Partial or complete obstruction of coronary artery(s) occurs
↓
Blood flow decreases
Oxygen supply decreases
↓
Coronary insufficiency
↓
Coronary ischemia
↓
Myocardial necrosis = Myocardial infarction

COMPLICATIONS RESULTING FROM MI THAT MAY LEAD TO DEATH IF NOT TREATED

Congestive heart failure

Dysrhythmias

Conduction problems

Cardiogenic shock

Systemic embolus

Pulmonary embolus

Papillary muscle rupture

Dressler's syndrome

Ventricular rupture

Ventricular septal defects

CHAPTER 1.2

CARDIOGENIC SHOCK

Cardiogenic shock is a severe form of pump failure that occurs when damage to the heart muscle is sufficient enough to impair contractility and reduce stroke volume and cardiac output. Usually the patient must necrotize 40% or more of the left ventricular myocardium to result in shock. In this type of shock, blood volume is adequate and fluid challenges will not improve cardiac output because the problem is that the heart fails to pump effectively. This decreases the stroke volume, and eventually tissue ischemia and hypoxia occurs. Cardiac output is decreased and hypotension ensues. Because of inadequate tissue perfusion, anaerobic metabolism produces lactic acid, leading to an acidotic state in the body. Despite treatment, 80% of patients who suffer this shock state will die.

Cardiogenic shock may result from mechanical interference with ventricular filling, from interference with ventricular emptying, from disturbances in heart rate or rhythm, or from inadequate myocardial contraction. Other causes that may predispose the patient to cardiogenic shock include myocardial infarction, myocardial ischemia, acute dysrhythmias, heart failure, cardiac tamponade, papillary muscle rupture, rupture of the interventricular septum or wall of the ventricle, ventricular aneurysm, mural thrombi, cardiomyopathy, pulmonary embolism, tension pneumothorax, or damage to the myocardial valves.

In the early stages of shock, the initial decrease in cardiac output and blood pressure may be masked by the nervous system and compensatory mechanisms from the baroreceptors, which attempt to compensate for the increases in the body's cardiac workload and myocardial oxygen demand. The body eventually becomes unable to maintain these compensatory efforts of vasoconstriction, increased heart rate, and increased metabolic rate, causing increased cellular permeability and obstruction of the microvasculature. Obstruction of blood flow eventually results in organ dysfunction, damage, and death. Unless the cycle is interrupted, the outcome is always death.

MEDICAL CARE

Oxygen: to increase available oxygen supply

Arterial blood gases: used to evaluate hypoxia and hypoxemia, metabolic acidosis, and other imbalances

Laboratory: used to evaluate electrolyte status, especially sodium, potassium, chloride, and magnesium; hematocrit may decrease with hemorrhage; CK isoenzymes may be elevated if MI present, troponin T and I increased

Radiology: X-rays of chest used to assess for cardiomegaly, pleural effusions, and pulmonary congestion, and placement of central venous lines and pulmonary artery catheters

Electrocardiography: used to identify the presence of prior or present MI; right ventricular MI can be noted if ECG done with RV leads (V_4R); identify and document the presence of dysrhythmias, axis deviation, and conduction defects

Echocardiography: 2D, 3D, and TEE may be used to evaluate the cause of shock state, ventricular dysfunction, presence of pericardial effusions or tamponade, septal defects, and to evaluate valve integrity

Alpha-adrenergic agonists: phenylephrine (Neo-Synephrine) used to improve blood pressure through vasoconstriction without inotropic effect

Beta-adrenergic agonists: isoproterenol (Isuprel) and dobutamine (Dobutrex) used to act directly on the myocardium to improve contractility, and to lower preload and afterload

Alpha-beta adrenergic agonists: norepinephrine (Levophed), epinephrine (Adrenalin), and dopamine

(Intropin) used to improve contractility through vasoconstriction and direct action on myocardium

Vasodilators: nitroglycerin (Tridil) and nitroprusside (Nipride) used to reduce venous return to the heart by promoting peripheral pooling of blood, reduces preload, afterload, and myocardial oxygen consumption

Diuretics: furosemide (Lasix) used to reduce cardiac congestion and pulmonary edema

Enzyme inhibitors: amrinone (Inocor) used to inhibit the enzyme phosphodiesterase, increase available calcium, and increases cyclic adenosine monophosphate, or cAMP, levels to strengthen contractions

Cardiac catheterization: used to assess pathophysiology of the patient's cardiovascular disorder, to provide left ventricular function information, to allow for measurement of heart pressures and cardiac output, to measure mixed venous blood gas content, to evaluate coronary artery stenosis, ventricular and valvular function, and presence of shunts

Intra-aortic balloon pump: used to decrease workload on the heart by decreasing preload and afterload, and to improve coronary artery perfusion

Ventricular assist devices: used when other measures have failed; VADs allow blood to bypass the ventricle(s) which allows the heart to rest and lowers myocardial oxygen demands

COMMON NURSING DIAGNOSES

ANXIETY (see MI)

Related to: change in health status, fear of death, threat to body image, threat to role functioning, pain, fear, uncertainty

Defining Characteristics: restlessness, insomnia, anorexia, increased respirations, increased heart rate, increased blood pressure, difficulty concentrating, dry mouth, poor eye contact, decreased energy, irritability, crying, feelings of helplessness

DEFICIENT KNOWLEDGE (see MI)

Related to: new diagnosis, lack of understanding, lack of understanding of medical condition, lack of recall

Defining Characteristics: questions regarding problems, inadequate follow-up on instructions given, misconceptions, lack of improvement of previous regimen, development of preventable complications

ADDITIONAL NURSING DIAGNOSES

DECREASED CARDIAC OUTPUT

Related to: impaired cardiac contractility, can be noted if ECG done with RV leads (V_4R); can observe for presence of dysrhythmias, axis circulatory failure, bradycardia, tachycardia, congestive failure

Defining Characteristics: increased CVP with jugular vein distention, cardiac index less than 2.0 L/min/m^2, systolic blood pressure less than 80 mm Hg, mean arterial pressure less than 60 mm Hg, PCWP greater than 18 mm Hg, increased systemic vascular resistance, oliguria, peripheral edema, and pulmonary congestion, cold, clammy skin, weak, thready pulses, dyspnea, tachypnea, cyanosis, confusion, restlessness, mental lethargy, dysrhythmias, chest pain, S_2 split, S_3 gallop, systolic or diastolic murmur, distant or muffled heart sounds

Outcome Criteria

✔ Patient will have adequate cardiac output to maintain perfusion to all body systems.

NOC: *Circulation Status*

NOC: *Cardiac Pump Effectiveness*

INTERVENTIONS	RATIONALES
Monitor ECG for dysrhythmias and changes in heart rhythm.	Decreased cardiac output will decrease perfusion to the heart and dysrhythmias may occur.
Monitor vital signs every 15 minutes, or every 5 minutes during active titration of vasoactive drugs. Maintain MAP at >60 mm Hg.	Bradycardia may result in decreased cardiac output, which leads to hypotension, increased respiratory rate, and can increase heart rate. Compensatory mechanisms in the body can easily fail within a short time. MAP <60 mm Hg is inadequate to perfuse coronary or cerebral vessels.
Monitor hemodynamic pressures and calculate CI, SVR, TPR, left and right stroke work and stroke work index. Measure CO.	Evaluates effectiveness of treatment and allows for efficient titration of vasoactive drugs. Determines actual cardiac output by measurement. In cardiogenic shock, CVP will be elevated >10 mm Hg, CO will be <2.2 L/min, SVR will be increased, PVR and

(continues)

(continued)

INTERVENTIONS	RATIONALES
	TPR will be increased, and stroke volume will be decreased. A good predictor of mortality is the LVSWI, with significant morbidity if <25 gm m/m².
Administer oxygen as ordered. Monitor oxygenation by use of pulse oximetry or ABGs.	Provides supplemental oxygen to increase available oxygen to tissues and reduces hypoxia. Oxygen saturation should be maintained >90% by oximetry to provide adequate oxygenation to tissues. ABGs should be monitored to ensure adequate ventilation and to allow for prompt correction of hypoxia and acid–base imbalances.
Monitor for mental changes and changes in level of consciousness.	Decreased cardiac output may decrease perfusion to cerebral tissues.
Monitor urine output every hour and notify physician if <30 cc/hr.	Decreased cardiac output results in decreased renal perfusion and may lead to oliguria or renal failure.
Monitor for weak/thready pulses, capillary refill >5 seconds, cool, clammy skin, pallor or cyanosis.	Decreased cardiac output results in decreased peripheral perfusion and tissue compromise.
Auscultate lungs for crackles (rales) or wheezes.	May indicate increasing fluid to lungs and impending congestive heart failure.
Observe for cough and pink frothy sputum.	May indicate pulmonary edema.
Auscultate heart tones for systolic murmur, or presence of S₃ gallop.	May indicate ventricular–septal rupture or mitral insufficiency which may cause cardiogenic shock, or may indicate impending congestive failure.
Observe for abnormal precordial movement at the third through the fifth intercostal space.	May indicate cardiogenic shock.
Place head of bed no higher than 30 degrees if blood pressure is within acceptable parameters. Avoid Trendelenburg position.	Elevation of the head of the bed may promote lung expansion and facilitate easier breathing. Blood pressure may be too low to have HOB elevated and patient should be supine to maintain blood pressure and perfusion to vital organs. Placement in Trendelenburg position may increase preload, increase the workload on the heart, inhibit lung expan-

INTERVENTIONS	RATIONALES
	sion, and prevent baroreceptors from sensing decreases in cardiac output.
Administer vasoactive drugs and titrate to maintain vital signs and hemodynamic pressures within physician-ordered parameters.	Through a variety of actions, these drugs allow alteration of hemodynamic status to achieve and maintain optimal perfusion.
Administer morphine IV as ordered.	Relieves pain and helps to improve blood pressure and cardiac output by decreasing preload.
Administer atropine as ordered.	May be used to reverse bradycardia and help prevent some of the vagal effects from morphine.
Avoid using isoproterenol with MI patients except for temporary use prior to transvenous pacing, and only if shock is associated with severe bradycardia.	Isuprel increases myocardial oxygen consumption and workload of the heart while it increases heart rate.
Prepare patient for placement on IABP or for VAD usage.	Provides knowledge and decreases fear. Patient may require cardiac catheterization, PTCA, CABG, or other interventions to obtain and maintain perfusion to the heart and other vital organs. IABP or VAD may be required to decrease the workload on the heart to maintain perfusion, and sustain life.
Instruct on equipment, procedures, medications, and potential interventions.	Provides knowledge and decreases fear.
Prepare patient/family for use of thrombolytics.	Thrombolytic drugs may be necessary to sustain life by reperfusion in acute MI.

NIC: *Shock Management: Cardiac*

Discharge or Maintenance Evaluation

- Patient will have cardiac output/cardiac index and hemodynamic pressures within normal limits.
- Urine output will be adequate.
- Vital signs will be normal and without overt signs of impaired perfusion to any body system.
- Lung fields will be clear with adequate oxygenation.
- Patient will be alert and oriented, with no mental changes.

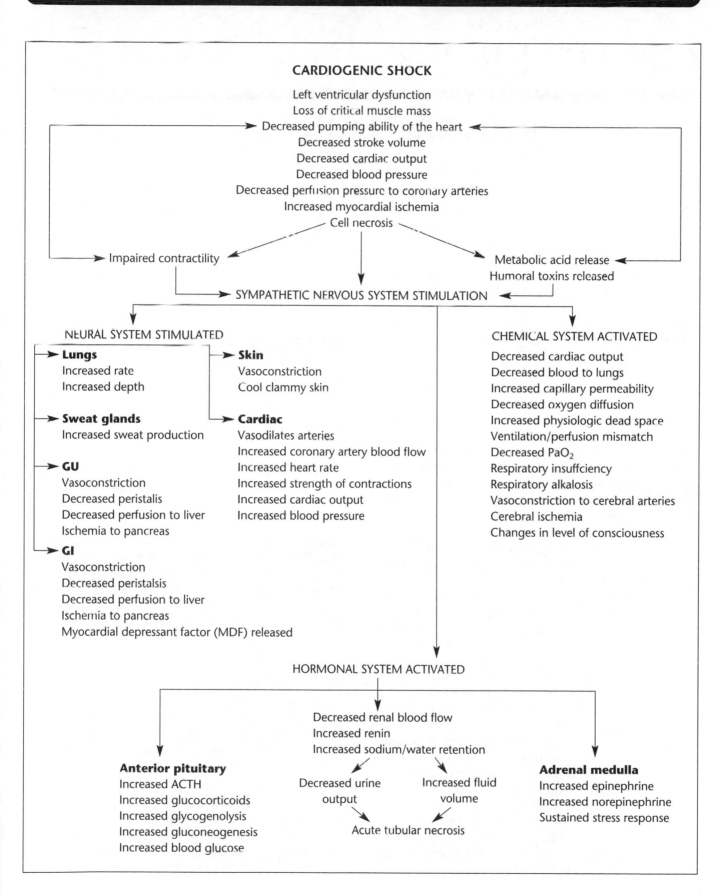

CARDIOGENIC SHOCK

Left ventricular dysfunction
Loss of critical muscle mass
Decreased pumping ability of the heart
Decreased stroke volume
Decreased cardiac output
Decreased blood pressure
Decreased perfusion pressure to coronary arteries
Increased myocardial ischemia
Cell necrosis

Impaired contractility

Metabolic acid release
Humoral toxins released

SYMPATHETIC NERVOUS SYSTEM STIMULATION

NEURAL SYSTEM STIMULATED

Lungs
Increased rate
Increased depth

Sweat glands
Increased sweat production

GU
Vasoconstriction
Decreased peristalis
Decreased perfusion to liver
Ischemia to pancreas

GI
Vasoconstriction
Decreased peristalsis
Decreased perfusion to liver
Ischemia to pancreas
Myocardial depressant factor (MDF) released

Skin
Vasoconstriction
Cool clammy skin

Cardiac
Vasodilates arteries
Increased coronary artery blood flow
Increased heart rate
Increased strength of contractions
Increased cardiac output
Increased blood pressure

CHEMICAL SYSTEM ACTIVATED

Decreased cardiac output
Decreased blood to lungs
Increased capillary permeability
Decreased oxygen diffusion
Increased physiologic dead space
Ventilation/perfusion mismatch
Decreased PaO_2
Respiratory insuffciency
Respiratory alkalosis
Vasoconstriction to cerebral arteries
Cerebral ischemia
Changes in level of consciousness

HORMONAL SYSTEM ACTIVATED

Decreased renal blood flow
Increased renin
Increased sodium/water retention

Anterior pituitary
Increased ACTH
Increased glucocorticoids
Increased glycogenolysis
Increased gluconeogenesis
Increased blood glucose

Decreased urine
output

Increased fluid
volume

Acute tubular necrosis

Adrenal medulla
Increased epinephrine
Increased norepinephrine
Sustained stress response

CHAPTER 1.3

INTRA-AORTIC BALLOON PUMP (IABP)

Placement and use of the intra-aortic balloon pump (IABP) is an advanced procedure that is required in the management of cardiovascular problems that are refractory to routine medical therapeutics. An intra-aortic balloon catheter (IAB) is inserted into the descending aorta, most commonly by way of the femoral artery. The IAB is then attached to the IABP which inflates and deflates the balloon in synchronization with the cardiac cycle. The balloon inflates during diastole when the aortic valve closes and increases the aortic pressure when the blood, distally to the balloon, is displaced forward into the systemic circulation and retrograde to the coronary arteries. The coronary arteries are supplied with additional blood to improve coronary blood flow and perfusion and to decrease preload. Deflation occurs prior to the onset of systole and decreases the aortic pressure and ventricular resistance, and makes it easier for the ventricle to contract and expel its normal volume of blood, thus decreasing afterload. This counterpulsation and displacement of blood decreases myocardial oxygen demand by decreasing myocardial workload and increases coronary perfusion and cardiac output.

Indications for use of IAB counterpulsation include cardiogenic shock, valvular disease, intractable chest pain resistant to medical treatment, prophylactic support during coronary angiography or anesthesia induction, papillary muscle rupture, ventricular septal defects, complications of acute myocardial infarctions, weaning from the cardiopulmonary bypass, septic shock, and as a bridge to cardiac revascularization or transplantation.

Counterpulsation is contraindicated in patients with severe aortic insufficiency, dissecting aneurysms, peripheral vascular disease, organic brain syndrome, irreversible brain damage, absent femoral pulses, trauma that has resulted in internal bleeding, active bleeding ulcers, blood dyscrasias, or previous aorto-femoral or aortoiliac bypass grafts.

Because the potential for complications is high, this procedure should be utilized only by personnel well-versed and competent in all aspects of the IABP function and troubleshooting complications.

One of the major complications associated with the use of the IABP is the compromise of the left circulation. Occasionally, weaning the patient from the IABP is difficult, and other treatment modalities may be utilized.

MEDICAL CARE

Oxygen: used to increase available oxygen supply

Nitrates: drugs such as nitroglycerin (Minitran, Nitrobid, Nitrodur, Nitrogard, Nitrol, Nitrostat, Tridil), isosorbide dinitrate (Iso-bid, Isorbid, Isordil, Novasorbid, Imdur, ISMO, Monoket), and erythrityl (Cardilate) used to relax vascular smooth muscle to produce vasodilation, decrease preload, decrease afterload, decrease venous return, decrease peripheral vascular resistance, decrease oxygen demand

Beta-blockers: drugs such as acebutolol (Sectral), atenolol (Tenormin), betaxolol hydrochloride (Kerlone), bisoprolol fumarate (Zebeta), carteolol hydrochloride (Cartrol), carvedilol (Coreg), esmolol (Brevibloc), metoprolol (Toprol XL, Betaloc, Lopressor), labetalol hydrochloride (Normodyne, Trandate), nadolol (Corgard), pindolol (Visken), propranolol (Inderal), sotalol hydrochloride (Betapace), and timolol (Blocadren) used to reduce myocardial oxygen demand by blocking catecholamine and sympathetic-induced increases in heart rate, contractility and blood pressure; slows AV node conduction; decreases sodium and water retention by reduction of renin secretion; decreases platelet aggregation and may reduce vasospasm

Calcium-channel blockers: drugs such as amlodipine (Norvasc), bepridil (Vascor), diltiazem (Cardizem), nicardipine (Cardene), nifedipine (Procardia, Adalat), verapamil (Calan, Isoptin, Verelan, Covera) used for decreasing myocardial oxygen demand and to enhance relaxation in hypertrophic cardiomyopathies;

reduces blood pressure and afterload, and helps prevent coronary spasm from a decreased oxygen supply

Sympathomimetic drugs: dobutamine (Dobutrex), dopamine hydrochloride (Intropin, Dopamine), metaraminol (Aramine), and norepinephrine (Levophed) used for treatment of hypotension in normovolemic states and in the treatment of severe heart failure and cardiogenic shock

Placement of IAB: necessary for counterpulsation to begin

Cardiac catheterization: used to define lesions and evaluate their severity, to provide information on ventricular function, and to allow for measurement of heart pressures and cardiac output

Laboratory: PT, PTT, and platelets are obtained to monitor anticoagulation status; general chemistry profiles and renal profiles are monitored every day for chemical imbalances and impending hepatic or renal problems; cardiac isoenzymes are used to monitor for heart damage; CBC and WBC differentials are done every day to monitor for infection and changes in hematologic status; cultures of blood, urine and sputum are done for temperature elevations greater than 102 degrees to assess for infection/suspected organisms

Arterial blood gases: used to assess oxygenation status

Chest X-ray: used daily to monitor placement of IAB and watch for migration; to assess enlargement of the heart and/or pulmonary vessels, and to assess pulmonary fluid status and atelectasis

Electrocardiography: reveals changes with atrial and ventricular enlargement, rhythm and conduction abnormalities, ischemia, electrolyte abnormalities, drug toxicity, and presence of dysrhythmias

Pacemakers: either temporary or permanent, used in anticipation of lethal dysrhythmias and/or conduction problems

NURSING DIAGNOSES

INEFFECTIVE TISSUE PERFUSION: CARDIOPULMONARY, CEREBRAL, GASTROINTESTINAL, PERIPHERAL, RENAL

Related to: placement of IAB, cardiac failure, tissue ischemia, vasoconstriction, hypovolemia, shunting, depressed ventricular function, dysrhythmias, conduction defects, hypoxia, reduction or interruption of blood flow

Defining Characteristics: visual disturbances, paresthesias, mental changes, change in level of consciousness, confusion, restlessness, pulse and blood pressure changes, changes in cardiac output, changes in peripheral resistance, impaired oxygenation of myocardium, chest pain, cardiac dysrhythmias, changes in ECG (ST segment, T wave, U wave), left ventricular enlargement, dyspnea, shortness of breath, tachypnea, palpitations, nausea, vomiting, slow digestion, oliguria, anuria, electrolyte imbalance, cold, clammy skin, decreased peripheral pulses, mottling, cyanosis, diaphoresis

Outcome Criteria

✔ Blood flow and perfusion to vital organs will be preserved and circulatory function will be maximized.

✔ Patient will be free of dysrhythmias and hemodynamic parameters will be within normal limits.

✔ Insertion site will be free of infection and limb distal to the insertion site will maintain adequate perfusion.

NOC: *Tissue Perfusion*

INTERVENTIONS	RATIONALES
Monitor vital signs every 15 to 30 minutes until stable, then every hour. Notify physician of deviations from parameters.	IABP timing is based on heart rate, and when rate changes >10 beats/minute, adjustments in timing are necessary to ensure optimal counterpulsation. Dysrhythmias hamper optimal oxygenation and function of the IABP.
Monitor mean arterial blood pressure every hour, or per hospital protocol.	Assesses volume status to help monitor for efficacy of counterpulsation. MABP can be calculated by adding 1/3 (systolic BP-diastolic BP) + diastolic BP. MABP is a function of cardiac output and systemic vascular resistance. Levels <60 have little, if any, perfusion to brain.
Obtain pulmonary artery pressures every hour.	Provides information as to fluid status and heart pressures. PA systolic pressures represent RV pressures with normals ranging

(continues)

(continued)

INTERVENTIONS	RATIONALES
	from 20–30 mm Hg. PA diastolic pressures reflects the LVEDP and is an indirect measurement of LV function with normals ranging from 10–20 mm Hg. PCWP reflects the LA pressure and is used to assess LV filling pressures with normals ranging from 4–12 mm Hg.
Measure cardiac output/cardiac index and perform hemodynamic calculations every 1–4 hours.	Directly measures the volume of cardiac output in L/min, and gives calculated information regarding preload and afterload. Normal CO should range from 4–8 L/min and CI from 2.5–4 L/min/m². SVR which represents afterload should range between 900–1400 dynes/sec/cm⁵.
Monitor for malfunction of IAB and IABP and correct problems rapidly. Manually flutter IAB prn pump failure. Notify physician of problems.	Improper timing of balloon can promote complications and worsen condition. Early inflation leads to regurgitation into the left ventricle or premature closing of the valve, and increases afterload. Late inflation decreases augmentation and reduces coronary perfusion. Early deflation allows the pressure to rise to normal end-diastolic levels preceding systole which does not reduce afterload. Late deflation encroaches on the next systole and increases afterload. IAB cannot be left in patient longer than 30 minutes without movement of balloon because of thrombus formation on the IAB.
Monitor for normal physiologic function of heart and be able to identify correlation between the function and the arterial pressure waveforms during counterpulsation.	In the beginning of the cardiac cycle, prior to a ventricular contraction, the arterial pressure is at the diastolic level that is determined by the vascular resistance and elastic status of the artery. When the ventricle contracts, the pressure quickly exceeds arterial pressure and pushes the aortic valve open to allow blood to flow into the aorta. The speed and volume of the blood flowing into the aorta raises the pressure of the artery to its systolic level. As soon as the left ventricular pressure decreases below the arterial

INTERVENTIONS	RATIONALES
	diastolic pressure, the aortic valve closes, which causes a brief displacement in the blood column of the aorta and a brief drop in aortic pressure. This drop is seen on an arterial pressure tracing as the dicrotic notch, which indicates that ventricular diastole has begun. Most of the coronary blood flow takes place during diastole when the ventricular muscle is in a relaxation state. If diastolic pressure is not maintained to ensure perfusion of the coronary arteries, myocardial oxygen supply will decrease. Heart rate also impacts the blood flow, with increases shortening diastolic time with each beat and filling time for the coronary arteries is reduced, also decreasing myocardial oxygen supply. The IABP assists the heart by increasing aortic pressure during diastole in order to augment the coronary perfusion, and decreases aortic pressure during systole to decrease the workload on the left ventricle. The balloon is inflated during diastole and deflated during systole. Through the combination of augmentation of the aortic diastolic pressure and decrease in aortic end-diastolic pressure, afterload decreases, cardiac output increases, and blood circulation to the coronary arteries increases. Inflation of the balloon should be timed to occur at the dicrotic notch on the pressure tracing and deflation must occur prior to the opening of the aortic valve, or just prior to the next systole. Timing is done to ensure the greatest amount of decrease in aortic end-diastolic pressure, with optimum 5–15 mm drop.
Provide adequate amounts of gas (CO₂ or helium) in IAB; refill IAB every 2 hours, as needed, or more often if fever present.	Underinflation of IAB can result in subtherapeutic effects from minimizing blood displacement. Increased body temperature increases the normal loss of gas from the balloon.

INTERVENTIONS	RATIONALES
Notify physician if augmentation cannot be maintained, afterload is not reduced, or if reddish-brown fluid noted in tubing of IAB.	Signals problems with catheter, pump, or patient requiring immediate attention. Discoloration in IAB tubing signifies that a fracture in the catheter has occurred and the fluid is actually blood. At this point, prepare for removal of the catheter.
Determine level of consciousness, mental changes, neurologic deficits.	Mental changes will result as tissue perfusion to brain decreases.
Monitor urine output every hour. Notify physician if <30 cc/hr, or >200 cc/hr in the absence of diuretics or fluid challenge.	Low cardiac output will cause decreased tissue perfusion to kidneys and oliguria. Migration of the IAB can partially or totally occlude the renal arteries leading to oliguria or anuria. Increased urine may indicate problems with other body systems, such as SIADH.
Monitor presence and equality of peripheral pulses, extremity color, temperature, and sensations. Notify physician of problems.	Decreased or absent pulses may indicate migration of IAB and possible occlusion of arteries.
Elevate head of bed no more than 15 degrees. Do not flex involved leg.	Flexion greater than this may cause catheter to kink and fracture.
Assist with ROM to uninvolved leg as needed, and with flexion/extension of involved foot.	Reduces complications from immobility.
Observe insertion site for bleeding or hematoma.	Concurrent use of anticoagulants may result in hemorrhage.
Check all body secretions for occult blood.	Heparin anticoagulation is required and can result in abnormal coagulopathy and complications.
Monitor general chemistry, renal profile, and CBC.	Provides information about potential blood loss and infection; chemistry profiles provide information about impending hepatic or renal insufficiency, or identify electrolyte disturbances.
Instruct patient/family on procedure, benefits, risks, post-procedure care.	Provides knowledge and allows patient to make an informed choice.
Instruct/demonstrate ROM to uninvolved leg, and flexion/extension to foot of involved leg.	Provides activity as tolerated while on IABP.

INTERVENTIONS	RATIONALES
Prepare patient/family for placement on IABP, post-procedure care.	IABP may be necessary to increase cardiac output, and decrease afterload and preload in order to decrease the workload on the damaged heart.

NIC: *Cardiac Care*

Discharge or Maintenance Evaluation

- Cardiac output will be within normal limits without use of IABP.
- Patient/family will be able to verbalize correct information regarding care, risks, and benefits.
- Patient will have optimum perfusion to all body systems.
- Patient will be able to accurately demonstrate exercises.
- Patient will report no episodes of chest pain or shortness of breath.
- Hemodynamic parameters and vital signs will be within normal limits.
- Lung sounds will be clear and free of adventitious breath sounds with optimal oxygenation.
- Urinary output will be within normal limits.
- Minimal activity will be tolerated without shortness of breath or extreme fatigue.
- Medications will be administered with no undesirable effects.

RISK FOR INFECTION

Related to: IAB placement, invasive lines, catheters, puncture wounds, invasive procedures, environmental exposure from devices left in place for extended periods of time

Defining Characteristics: disruption of skin surfaces, redness, drainage, elevated temperature

Outcome Criteria

✔ Patient will be free of infection with no fever or chills.
✔ All invasive lines will be free of erythema, edema, and drainage.

NOC: *Risk Detection*

INTERVENTIONS	RATIONALES
Inspect all invasive lines for signs of infection and/or bleeding.	Invasive lines provide entry route for pathogens.
Change site dressing using sterile technique every day. Notify physician for signs of infection.	Insertion site provides a direct route for infection, and must be monitored to prevent complications.
Monitor temperature every 2–4 hours. Obtain cultures of urine, sputum, and blood for evaluation as warranted.	Sudden temperature increases may indicate infective process. Cultures can isolate the specific pathogen so as to enable specific antibiotic therapy to be ordered.
Change IV tubing/arterial line tubing per protocol, using aseptic technique. Change peripheral lines every 3 days and prn.	Decreases the incidence of infection. Bacteria begins to grow within 24 hours in IV solution. Replacement of IV lines prevents phlebitis and risks of infective complications.
Inform patient of need for changing peripheral lines, solutions, and care to sites.	Facilitates knowledge, patient comprehension, and compliance with treatment.
Instruct patient to notify nurse of pain to invasive sites, or other symptoms of infection.	May indicate infection.

NIC: *Infection Protection*

Discharge or Maintenance Evaluation

■ Patient will have no signs of infection to invasive line sites.

■ Peripheral lines will be changed within 3 days to avoid risk of infection.

■ Patient will have no signs of systemic infection.

EXCESS FLUID VOLUME

Related to: ineffective pumping of the heart, decreased cardiac output, increased preload, increased afterload, sodium retention, volume shifts from one compartment to another, compromised regulatory mechanisms

Defining Characteristics: altered mental status, changes in respiratory pattern, orthopnea, changes in blood pressure and pulmonary artery pressures, crackles (rales), dyspnea, edema, increased CVP, intake greater than output, jugular vein distention, oliguria, pulmonary congestion, weight gain, S_3 gallop, rest-lessness, anxiety, anasarca, azotemia, changes in urine specific gravity, electrolyte imbalances

Outcome Criteria

✔ Lung fields will be clear and free from auscultation of adventitious breath sounds.

✔ Patient will have no edema and weight will be stable with intake and output equivalent.

NOC: *Fluid Balance*

INTERVENTIONS	RATIONALES
Administer oxygen as ordered.	Provides supplemental oxygen to an already-compromised and poorly-perfused heart.
Monitor cardiac rhythm for changes. Treat per protocol, and notify physician.	Changes in cardiac rhythm or presence of dysrhythmias may result from alterations in fluid or electrolyte status. Peaked or increased T waves, prolonged PR intervals, widened QRS complexes, or depressed ST segments may indicate hyperkalemia.
Monitor I & O q 1–2 hours. Notify physician if urine <30 cc/hr.	Intake greater than output may indicate fluid retention or fluid overload.
Administer IV fluids as ordered.	Provides venous access, hydration, and route for emergency medications. IV fluids should be given at ordered rate via IV pump to maintain flow rate and to avoid inadvertent administration of excessive fluid.
Weigh patient daily, preferably at same time and on same scale.	Provides for consistency of data. Weight gain of >2 lbs/day usually is caused by fluid excess.
Auscultate lungs for presence of crackles (rales), wheezing, or other adventitious breath sounds. Observe for distended neck veins. Notify physician for significant changes.	May indicate excessive systemic fluid volume or worsening heart failure.
Administer morphine sulfate IV as ordered.	Morphine is the drug of choice to decrease preload by decreasing blood return to the heart, decreases pain, decreases myocardial oxygen demand and consumption, and increases venodilation.

INTERVENTIONS	RATIONALES
Monitor lab work, especially electrolytes, renal profile, and specific gravity of urine.	Patients may become hypokalemic with the use of diuretics and the potential for cardiac glycoside toxicity increases with hypokalemia. Increased specific gravity indicates fluid retention. BUN and creatinine provide indications of renal function.
Administer diuretics as ordered.	Diuretics promote fluid excretion by decreasing both intravascular and extravascular fluid volume, and consequently, decreases preload, decreases central venous pressures, and decreases pulmonary capillary wedge pressures.
Observe for complaints of fatigue, headache, dry mouth, muscle cramping, dizziness, nausea, and vomiting.	May be signs and symptoms of complications from electrolyte imbalances, hypovolemia, or renal dysfunction.
Observe for peripheral and sacral edema, and ascites.	Decreases in osmotic pressure or fluid overload can result in edema.
Instruct patient in signs to report, such as shortness of breath, decreases in urinary output, edema, and so forth.	Prompt identification of potential complications allows for rapid treatment and prevention of further problems.
Instruct patient/family in medications, effects, side effects, and so forth.	Promotes knowledge, promotes compliance, and involves patient and family in care.

NIC: *Hypervolemia Management*

Discharge or Maintenance Evaluation

■ Patient will have balanced intake and output.

■ Vital signs will be stable for patient's parameters and baseline.

■ Lab work will be within normal limits for patient.

■ Patient will be able to accurately recall signs and symptoms to report to nurse and/or physician.

RISK FOR DEFICIENT FLUID VOLUME

Related to: potential blood loss from oozing/draining sites of invasive lines

Defining Characteristics: bleeding from puncture sites and wounds, actual blood loss as measured by hemoglobin/hematocrit, hypotension, tachycardia

Outcome Criteria

✔ Patient will have no significant blood loss from invasive lines.

NOC: *Fluid Balance*

INTERVENTIONS	RATIONALES
Measure all sources of intake and output.	Provides information to evaluate fluid status.
Weigh daily.	Weight gain over 24 hours usually indicates fluid gain. Fluid imbalance can be approximated as 1 lb = 500 cc fluid.
Monitor vital signs and hemodynamic pressures.	Tachycardia, hypotension, and changes in hemodynamics may indicate volume depletion.
Test all body fluids for presence of occult blood.	Anticoagulation may place patient at risk for bleeding.
Monitor insertion site for bleeding, hemorrhage, or hematoma. Apply pressure dressing if warranted, and notify physician for sustained bleeding from site.	Bleeding tendencies are increased because of concomitent use of systemic anticoagulants and patient is at risk for bleeding.
Monitor PT, PTT, platelets, and CBC.	PT, PTT, and platelets provide information about coagulation; CBC provides information about potential blood loss.
Administer IV solutions and volume expanders as indicated.	IV solutions and volume expanders may be required to treat rapidly decreasing circulating volume caused by exsanguination.
Administer packed RBCs, blood, or platelets as warranted.	Hemorrhagic volume losses may be life-threatening. Replacement of platelets may be necessary to provide normal coagulation.
Administer vitamin K or protamine sulfate if warranted.	May be required to return coagulation times to normal or reverse effects of anticoagulants.
Instruct patient to report any noted bleeding or oozing on body.	Prompt observation of complications can result in prompt treatment.
Instruct patient to avoid any activity that may promote bleeding.	Prevents accidental injury and decreases chance of hemorrhage.

NIC: *Fluid Management*

Discharge or Maintenance Evaluation

■ Patient will be able to verbalize signs/symptoms of bleeding to report.

■ Patient will be compliant in avoidance of safety concerns.

■ Patient will have stable hemodynamic status with no over hemorrhage from any site.

IABP

Inflation of balloon during ventricular diastole

↓

Increases diastolic pressures

Increases coronary blood flow

Increases myocardial oxygen supply

Increases myocardial contractility

Deflation of balloon just prior to ventricular systole

↓

Decreases afterload

Decreased myocardial oxygen demand

Migration of IAB

Subclavian occlusion

↓

Loss of pulse to upper extremities, especially left arm

Cold, mottled, cyanotic extremity

Renal artery occlusion

↓

Decreased urinary output

Oliguria

Anuria

Femoral occlusion

↓

Loss of pedal pulses

Cold, mottled, cyanotic extremity

Claudication

NORMAL ARTERIAL PRESSURE WAVEFORM

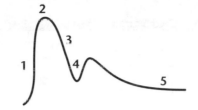

1 = Arterial pulse curve (anacrotic limb)
2 = Peak systolic pressure
3 = Dicrotic limb
4 = Dicrotic notch
5 = Aortic end-diastolic pressure

NORMAL TIMING OF ELECTRICAL/MECHANICAL EVENTS ON THE HEART

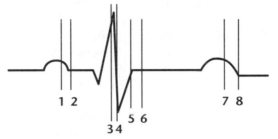

1 = Beginning of right atrial contraction
2 = Beginning of left atrial contraction
3 = Beginning of left ventricular contraction
4 = Beginning of right ventricular contraction
5 = Beginning of right ventricular ejection of blood
6 = Beginning of left ventricular ejection of blood
7 = Ending of left ventricular ejection
8 = Ending of right ventricular ejection

ARTERIAL PRESSURE WAVEFORM USING 1:2 COUNTERPULSATION

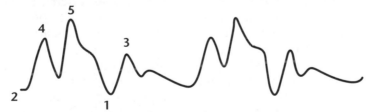

1 = Balloon assisted aortic end-diastolic pressure (AoEDP)
2 = Patient aortic end-diastolic pressure (AoEDP)
3 = Balloon assisted systole
4 = Patient systole, or Unassisted systole
5 = Peak diastolic augmented pressure

Balloon AoEDP should be lower than the patient's AoEDP, and the balloon assisted systole should be lower than the patient's systole.

CHAPTER 1.4

CARDIAC SURGERY

Critical coronary artery disease treatment requires the maximization of cardiac output, which can be accomplished by improvement in heart muscle function and increase of blood flow through coronary artery bypass grafting and/or valvular replacements. Cardiac surgery is commonly performed for three-vessel disease, with ongoing ischemia despite fibrolytic therapy and/or PTCA, left main coronary artery disease, two-vessel disease if the left anterior descending artery is involved, or if the left ventricular function is impaired, post-PTCA occlusions, and in myocardial infarctions in which a complication such as ventricular septal defect or papillary muscle rupture occurs. It is also utilized for valvular dysfunction and congenital heart defects, and for conditions requiring blood to be diverted from the heart and lungs to facilitate a bloodless operative field.

In coronary artery bypass graft (CABG) surgery, a vein or artery graft harvested from the arms or legs is anastomosed to the aorta with the distal portion to the involved coronary artery to bypass the diseased obstruction and supply adequate blood flow to the heart. The internal mammary artery is utilized for CABG surgery because the patency rate is 90–95% over a 10–20 year time period, and there are fewer problems with differences in lumen size as an artery is then anastomosed to an artery without the need for routing from the aorta. In valvular surgery, incompetent or leaking valves are replaced or repaired with prosthetic ones.

Not all patients with coronary artery disease are candidates for CABG surgery. It is usually recommended for those patients with intractable angina, signs of ischemia, or an increased risk of coronary ischemia/infarction as a result of angiographic studies. Complications may occur in almost every body system and may be a result of the disease process or defect, the surgery, or the use of cardiopulmonary bypass, and so the decision for surgery is a multifaceted one.

One of the most important factors in the decision of candidacy for CABG surgery is the ejection fraction. This is the ratio of stroke volume compared to the end-diastolic volume and an ejection fraction greater than 55 reflects a good operative risk. Ejection fraction less than 25% were usually considered inoperable because of the high mortality associated with it, but ejection fractions less than 35% have greater expectation of benefit from CABG than do those with a normal EF. Systolic dysfunction that may be a result of chronic hypoperfusion and not a result of infarction may have large areas of myocardial viability that can benefit from revascularization procedures, even when LV function is especially poor.

The surgery is performed via a median sternotomy incision which provides exposure of the heart and avoids the pleural spaces. A cannula is placed in a vein and an artery and then attached to the cardiopulmonary bypass machine whereby the diverted blood is mechanically oxygenated and circulated to the other parts of the body. The machine, which is operated by a trained perfusionist, substitutes for left ventricular pumping and creates a blood–gas exchange. After the patient's body temperature has been cooled to around 86 degrees, the aorta is cross-clamped and a cold cardioplegic solution, usually containing dextrose, potassium, magnesium and inderal, is placed around the heart and injected into the coronary arteries. This causes an electromechanical arrest and provides an inert operative site. Cross-clamp durations longer than 3 hours usually result in severe complications for the patient. After the grafts have been completed or valves replaced, mechanical perfusion is slowly discontinued and cannulas are removed when arterial blood pressure and cardiac functioning are adequate. Depending on hospital and physician protocol, the patient may have some or all of the following: atrial and ventricular pacing wires are placed, as well as arterial lines, pulmonary artery catheter, left atrial line, and mediastinal or pleural chest tubes.

Common complications associated with CABG surgery include renal failure, respiratory failure, perioperative MI or stroke, vein graft closure, hemorrhage, blood trauma, complement activation, coagulation abnormalities, fluid shifts, increased catecholamine levels, microemboli, dysrhythmias, pericarditis, postpericardiotomy syndrome, embolism, pneumonia, atelectasis, hemothorax, stroke, and postcardiotomy delirium. Other complications that are seen less often include stress ulcer, cardiac tamponade, cardiogenic shock, endocarditis, gastrointestinal bleeding, mediastinitis, and paralytic ileus.

MIDCAB, or minimally invasive direct coronary artery bypass, is also known as "beating heart surgery" or limited access coronary artery surgery. This surgical treatment creates a detour for blood flow around the stenosed coronary artery, usually the LAD, but with a minimal invasion into the chest and does not require the use of cardiopulmonary bypass machine, thereby reducing complications. This type of surgery is not used if multiple arteries are involved, but is less traumatic and less expensive, utilizing a smaller incision than regular CABG procedures. In MIDCAB, the patient's heart is not stopped completely, but is simply slowed down with medications. The operation is performed using a stabilization device that allows for only 1 mm range of motion of the heart. Although the risk of serious complications is reduced because of the avoidance of "cracking the sternum" and the use of smaller doses of heparin, the MIDCAB has some limitations. It has been found that the MIDCAB may not be as successful long term as the standard CABG, and patients who had the MIDCAB were more likely to develop blockages in their new grafts than patients who had undergone the standard CABG. If the mammary artery cannot be utilized, or if the surgeon has difficulty in accessing the left anterior descending artery, the MIDCAB procedure is not a potential treatment.

There are variants of the MIDCAB surgery, such as a port access surgery, keyhole surgery, the off-pump coronary artery bypass (OPCAB), and the use of robotic visualization techniques. The port access surgery involves creating several small incisions in the chest to allow the surgeon to use fiberoptic endoscopes and small surgical instruments to perform the procedure. This type of surgery does require the use of the heart–lung machine so that the heart can be safely stopped and is accomplished by using the femoral vein and/or artery to divert the blood flow to the heart–lung machine.

The keyhole surgery, also known as buttonhole surgery and laparoscopic bypass, is done through a small window cut into the rib cage and is performed on the beating heart. Rerouting the blood from the heart is accomplished through small incisions between the ribs with the beating heart being placed in direct view, and using blood vessels found nearby. This surgery is only being performed on patients who have single blockages.

The OPCAB uses several techniques, and the patient's chest is opened as if to do the conventional CABG, but no cardiopulmonary bypass machine is used and the heart is not stopped. Different types of stabilizing devices may be used to restrain the heart movement one section at a time. This particular type of procedure is used very selectively because the technique is more difficult and the surgeon requires more skill than with conventional CABG surgery.

The use of robotic visualization involves a voice-activated robot in the operating room with the cardiac surgeon in a separate room, who is able to manipulate the hand controls that direct the robotic hands when to cut and sew inside the chest. An endoscope is used so the surgeon can visualize the procedure with the attached camera positioned in the chest cavity. The advantage of this procedure is that the robotic hands can be smaller and requires a smaller incision. It is used currently only in a few test cases and has not been approved by the Food and Drug Administration as of this date.

MEDICAL CARE

Pulmonary function studies: used to ascertain baseline pulmonary function

Laboratory: hemoglobin/hematocrit used to monitor oxygen-carrying capability, need for blood replacement, and to monitor for dehydration status; electrolytes used to monitor for imbalances which can affect cardiac function; BUN and creatinine used to monitor renal function; liver profile used to monitor liver function and perfusion; glucose used to monitor for presence of diabetes, nutritional alterations, or organ dysfunction; cardiac enzymes and isoenzymes used to monitor for presence of acute or perioperative myocardial infarction; coagulation profiles used to determine baseline and monitor for coagulation problems; antibody or complement levels used to monitor for postpericardiotomy syndrome or Dressler's syndrome; type and cross-match for blood to have available blood products on hand in case of hemorrhage; ACT used to monitor heparinization

Arterial blood gases: used to monitor oxygenation and assess acid–base balance and ability to wean off mechanical ventilation

Electrocardiography: used to observe for changes in cardiac function, presence of conduction problems, dysrhythmias, or ischemic changes

Echocardiography: used to evaluate wall motion of the heart, evaluate cardiac structure

Chest X-ray: used to identify heart size and position, pulmonary vasculature, pulmonary changes, verifies position of endotracheal tube, pacing wires, and hemodynamic catheters; monitor for barotrauma

Cardiac catheterization: used to evaluate abnormal pressures preop, to assess for pressure gradients across the valves, and to locate and measure coronary lesions

Serine protease inhibitors: aprotinin (Trasylol) has antifibrinolytic action and is used to decrease post-operative blood loss and transfusions that may be required in high-risk CABG patients, patients who are currently on aspirin, and those patients who require reoperative CABG procedures

Antiplatelet drugs: aspirin and dipyridamole (Persantine) used for their antiplatelet aggregation action to help prevent late graft closure

Antifibrinolytics: E-aminocaproic acid and its analogue, transexamic acid have antifibrinolytic action and help to decrease the amount of mediastinal drainage

Antibiotics, Antimicrobials: used preoperatively, antibiotic agents help to decrease the risk of post-op infection 5-fold; cephalosporins, especially cefuroxime, are usual drugs of choice

Vasoactive drugs: inotropic support with dobutamine (Dobutrex) may be required if cardiac output fails to improve after IVFs are given; nitrates, such as nitroglycerin (Tridil) may be used to increase the left ventricular ejection fraction and reduce preload; dopamine hydrochloride (Intropin, Dopamine) used to increase blood pressure when fluid volume replacement is not adequate to improve cardiac output; depending on dosage, dopamine may increase renal blood flow and improve urinary output and GFR, or may stimulate beta-adrenergic receptors to increase cardiac output yet maintain vasodilation, and at doses over 10 μg/kg/min, causes alpha-adrenergic stimulation that increases renal vasoconstriction and peripheral vascular resistance

Antidysrhythmics: lidocaine hydrochloride (Xylocaine) used as initial treatment for ventricular tachycardia and/or ventricular fibrillation; procainamide hydrochloride (Pronestyl, Procan) is another antidysrhythmic used in the treatment for life-threatening dysrhythmias; class III antidysrhythmics, such as bretylium tosylate (Bretylol) and amiodarone hydrochloride (Cordarone) used to treat life-threatening, refractory ventricular tachydysrhythmias that do not respond to other drugs; digitalis (Digoxin, Lanoxin) may be used to treat atrial fibrillation that frequently occurs

IV fluids: used to maintain hydration and to restore circulating fluid volume to maintain adequate cardiac output, support blood pressure, and preload

Blood products/volume expanders: packed red blood cells and/or whole blood may be used to restore adequate circulating fluid volume, to treat hemorrhage, to increase preload and CVP, and to provide adequate route for oxygen carrying capability; albumin and hetastarch may be given to improve fluid volume status to maintain cardiac output

Intra-aortic balloon pump: may be required to treat cardiogenic shock and for patients who require assistance postoperatively to maintain cardiac function

Ventricular Assist Devices: used to bypass the affected ventricle, which allows the heart to rest and recover; left VAD is used to divert blood from the left atrium and bypass the left ventricle, and have the blood returned to the patient via the ascending aorta; right VAD is used to divert the blood from the right atrium, bypassing the right ventricle, and is returned to the patient via the pulmonary artery; VADs are used for cardiogenic shock, postcardiotomy ventricular failure, inability of weaning from the cardiopulmonary bypass machine during cardiac surgery, and as a bridge to transplantation

COMMON NURSING DIAGNOSES

RISK FOR INJURY (see PACEMAKERS)

Related to: cardiac surgery, pacemaker failure, hemothorax or pneumothorax after insertion, bleeding, lead migration, heart perforation, cardiac failure

Defining Characteristics: decreased cardiac output, hemorrhage, diaphoresis, hypotension, restlessness, dyspnea, cyanosis, chest pain, muscle twitching, hiccoughs, muffled heart sounds, jugular vein distention, pulsus paradoxus, dysrhythmias

ANXIETY (see MI)

Related to: surgery, change in health status, fear of death, threat to body image, threat to role functioning, pain

Defining Characteristics: restlessness, insomnia, anorexia, increased respirations, increased heart rate, increased blood pressure, difficulty concentrating, dry mouth, poor eye contact, decreased energy, irritability, crying, feelings of helplessness

DEFICIENT KNOWLEDGE (see MI)

Related to: surgery, lack of understanding, lack of understanding of medical condition, lack of recall

Defining Characteristics: questions regarding problems, inadequate follow-up on instructions given, misconceptions, lack of improvement of previous regimen, development of preventable complications

IMPAIRED PHYSICAL MOBILITY (see PACEMAKERS)

Related to: pain, immobilization, surgery

Defining Characteristics: inability to move as desired, imposed restrictions on activity, decreased muscle strength and coordination, limited range of motion

DISTURBED BODY IMAGE (see PACEMAKERS)

Related to: cardiac and graft incisions, presence of pulse generator, loss of control of heart function, disease process, presence of scars/wounds

Defining characteristics: fear of rejection, fear of reaction from others, negative feelings about body, refusal to participate in care, refusal to look at wounds

INEFFECTIVE TISSUE PERFUSION: RENAL (see RENAL FAILURE)

Related to: postoperative renal dysfunction

Defining Characteristics: serum creatinine changes from preoperative status >0.7 mg/dl at postoperative status, serum creatinine levels >2.0 mg/dl, increasing BUN, decreased urinary output, decreased GFR, pre-existing renal disease, reduced functioning nephrons,

increased renal vascular resistance, decreased total renal blood flow during surgery

ADDITIONAL NURSING DIAGNOSES

DECREASED CARDIAC OUTPUT

Related to: conduction defects, myocardial depression, dysrhythmias, electrolyte imbalances, hypovolemia, hypervolemia, myocardial infarction, coronary artery spasm, vasoconstriction, impaired contractility, alteration in preload, alteration in afterload, hypoperfusion, microemboli, hypoxia, damaged myocardium, use of PEEP while on ventilatory support

Defining Characteristics: decreased blood pressure, mean arterial pressure less than 60 mm Hg, elevated systemic vascular resistance greater than 1400 dyne–seconds/cm^5, cardiac output less than 4 L/min or cardiac index less than 2.5 L/min/m^2, tachycardia greater than 110, cold, pale extremities, absent or decreased peripheral pulses, ECG changes, hypotension, S_3 or S_4 gallops, decreased urinary output

Outcome Criteria

✔ Vital signs and hemodynamic parameters will be within normal limits for patient, with no dysrhythmias noted.

NOC: *Circulation Status*

NOC: *Cardiac Pump Effectiveness*

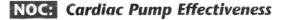

INTERVENTIONS	RATIONALES
Monitor vital signs, especially heart rate and blood pressure. Notify physician of abnormalities. Blood pressure should be taken/ monitored every 15 minutes until stable, or every 5 minutes during active titration of vasoactive drugs.	Tachycardia may occur as a response to pain, anxiety, blood and fluid deficit, and stress, but rates over 130 increase myocardial oxygen consumption and workload on the heart, decreasing cardiac output. Increased blood pressure may promote alterations in heart pressures and increase the risk of complications, as well as placing pressure on suture lines of new grafts. Hypotension may result from fluid deficit, dysrhythmias, and cardiac failure, as well as predispose peripheral vein grafts to close.

(continues)

(continued)

INTERVENTIONS	RATIONALES
Evaluate hypotension that is not responsive to fluid bolus, tachycardia, and distant heart sounds.	May indicate cardiac tamponade in a heart that is unable to fill adequately to maintain cardiac output. Tamponade usually occurs immediately post-op but may occur later during recovery period.
Monitor hemodynamic pressures every 1 hour and prn. Maintain pressures with titration of vasoactive drugs per physician-ordered parameters.	Assists with recognition of complications and allows for manipulation of cardiac pressures by use of fluids and medications. Vasoconstriction is the cause of elevated SVR, and with increases in SVR, may increase left ventricular dysfunction. Cardiac output then becomes dependent on outflow resistance.
Measure cardiac output/cardiac index every 1–2 hours immediately post-op if PA catheter present.	Cardiac output is a measurement that is equal to the product of the stroke volume and the heart rate. Cardiac indexes above 3.0 $L/min/m^2$ are usually adequate except in cases of septic shock. Adequate cardiac output relates to the adequacy of function of other body organs. After CABG surgery, some patients require an increase in CO to meet the stress imposed by the operation and the accompanying increase in oxygen consumption.
Measure left atrial pressure and pulmonary artery wedge pressures if PA catheter present and per hospital protocol.	Determines the left ventricular end-diastolic volume; increases in pressure may indicate congestive heart failure or pulmonary edema, and decreases may indicate low blood volume. Trends and changes in values are of more importance than single readings. Left ventricular dysfunction can elevate left heart filling pressures without a rise in right heart pressures.
Monitor urine output hourly and notify physician if less than 30 cc/hr.	Urine output is an indication of adequate cardiac output and renal perfusion.
Observe for decreased peripheral pulses, cool or cold moist skin, or cyanosis.	May indicate low cardiac output. A low measured CO may be inaccurate because of patient hypothermia.
Monitor for changes in level of consciousness, mental status changes, restlessness, or confusion.	Cerebral perfusion is dependent on adequate cardiac output. Hypoperfusion or microemboli

INTERVENTIONS	RATIONALES
	may result in CNS deficits. Neurologic impairment after CABG has been credited to hypoxia, hypoxemia, emboli, hemorrhage, and metabolic deviations. Postoperative deficits are divided into two main types—those associated with major neurologic deficits, stupor, and coma, and those that are distinguished by intellectual dysfunction or memory impairment. Age of the patient, especially when >70, and history of hypertension were two of the main determining predictors of risk factors for cerebral complications. Microembolization contributes to postoperative cerebral dysfunction after CABG procedures because of surgical manipulation of the ascending aorta and frequently are caused by gaseous emboli. Cerebral edema after extracorporeal circulation by the cardiopulmonary bypass machine potentiates CNS damage and anti-inflammatory drugs may be useful in decreasing interstitial edema.
Monitor for JVD, peripheral edema, and pulmonary congestion. Auscultate for crackles (rales).	May indicate present or impending congestive heart failure.
Observe for shortness of breath, decreases in oximetry, or dyspnea.	May indicate hypoxia and decreased cardiac output.
Monitor ECG for cardiac conduction disturbances, dysrhythmias, or changes in rate/rhythm. Treat per protocol.	Lethal dysrhythmias may occur as a result of electrolyte imbalances, myocardial ischemia or infarction, or problems with electrical conduction, with an associated drop in cardiac output. New onset atrial fibrillation occurs in approximately 30% of patients after CABG surgery, usually on the 2nd or 3rd post-op day, and increases the risk for CVA greatly. This complication usually occurs in those patients with COPD, proximal right coronary artery disease, prolonged cross-clamp time, atrial ischemia, advanced age, and/or withdrawal of beta-blockers.

INTERVENTIONS	RATIONALES
	Aggressive treatment with anti-coagulants and cardioversion may decrease complications that lead to neurologic problems. Treatment of other dysrhythmias should be done per hospital protocol to regulate the heart and its ability to function and heal properly.
Monitor for complaints of severe chest pain.	May indicate a perioperative or postoperative myocardial infarction.
Provide for uninterrupted rest periods and assist with care as needed.	Prevents fatigue and increased workload on the heart leading to decrease in cardiac output and perfusion.
Administer IV fluids as ordered.	Maintains fluid status and hydration, as well as provides access for emergency medications.
Administer blood products as ordered.	Blood or packed red cells may be required to maintain adequate oxygen-carrying capability, and adequate circulating volume for cellular activity. Platelet function and count are decreased with use of cardiopulmonary bypass and proportional to the duration of bypass and depth of hypothermia during surgery.
Administer anticoagulation therapy, such as heparin or low-molecular-weight heparin (LMWH) as ordered.	Dalteparin, a LMWH, has a greater degree of inhibition of factor Xa relative to thrombin, and prevents thrombin generation, inhibits thrombin formation, decreases rate of heparin-associated thrombocytopenia, and also does not require monitoring of coagulation levels as does heparin. Hirudin, which is a recombinant protein found in leech saliva, has been shown to decrease morbidity associated with MIs, and Hirulog is a synthetic direct thrombin inhibitor.
Attempt to reverse any contributing factor such as untreated DKA or endocrine dysfunction.	These may precipitate a low cardiac output state.
Prepare patient for placement on IABP or VAD.	Promotes knowledge and decreases fear. IABP use may be required for cardiogenic shock and heart failure in order to

INTERVENTIONS	RATIONALES
	decrease the workload on the heart. Ventricular assist devices (VADs) bypass the affected ventricle and allow the heart to rest and recover if the patient experiences cardiogenic shock, postcardiotomy ventricular failure, or if the patient is unable to be weaned off cardiopulmonary bypass. If the patient requires a right VAD, hemodynamics and cardiac output values will not be accurate because the blood is being rerouted and bypassing the right ventricle.

NIC: *Cardiac Care: Acute*

Discharge or Maintenance Evaluation

- Patient will have maximal cardiac output and stable hemodynamic pressures.
- Patient will have adequate perfusion of all body systems.
- Patient will be able to recall instructions correctly.

ACUTE PAIN

Related to: mediastinal, leg, or arm incisions, myocardial infarction, angina, inflammation, tissue damage

Defining Characteristics: communication of discomfort or pain, restlessness, irritability, increased heart rate, increased blood pressure

Outcome Criteria

✔ Patient will be free of pain or pain will be controlled to patient's satisfaction.

NOC: *Pain Level*

INTERVENTIONS	RATIONALES
Evaluate complaints of pain—type, location, intensity based on 0–10 scale. Compare preoperative pain perceptions with post-operative pain.	Pain may be perceived in different ways by each individual and is important to differentiate incisional pain from other types of chest pain. CABG patients

(continues)

(continued)

INTERVENTIONS	RATIONALES
	usually do not have severe discomfort to the chest incision but may have increased discomfort with donor site pain. Severe pain should be investigated for possibility of complications.
Monitor vital signs every 1–2 hours and prn.	Heart rates usually increase with pain but bradycardia may occur especially with severely damaged myocardium. Blood pressure may be increased with incisional pain, but can also be labile or decreased when chest pain is severe or if myocardial ischemia/necrosis occurs.
Evaluate complaints of pain in legs or abdomen, or vague nonspecific complaints, especially if associated with changes in mental status or vital signs.	May be indicative of development of thrombophlebitis, infection or GI dysfunction.
Monitor for complaints of pain and/or paresthesia to ulnar area of the hand, or pain to shoulders and arms.	May result from stretching of the brachial plexus during positioning of the arms during surgery and generally resolves over time without specific treatment.
Observe for anxiety, irritability, crying, restlessness, or insomnia.	Nonverbal cues may indicate the presence of pain.
Administer analgesics as soon as discomfort is noticed, or prophylactically prior to painful procedures.	Pain results in muscle tension, which can decrease circulation and intensify pain perception. Medication given prior to procedures known to cause pain may facilitate cooperation with procedures and allow for easier chest movement with respiratory therapy.
Provide back rubs, position changes, and diversionary activities.	Promotes relaxation and helps to redirect attention away from discomfort, thereby reducing the amount of analgesic required.
Encourage deep breathing, visualization, or guided imagery.	Promotes decrease in stress and may reduce analgesic need.
Instruct on methods to reduce strain on muscles when positioning.	Supporting extremities and the maintenance of good body alignment reduce muscle tension and provide comfort.

NIC: *Pain Management*

Discharge or Maintenance Evaluation

■ Patient will be comfortable, pain-free, and be able to recall methods for stress reduction and pain control accurately.

■ Patient will be able to identify differences between postoperative and preoperative chest pain.

■ Patient will be able to maintain optimal body alignment and minimize muscle tension.

IMPAIRED GAS EXCHANGE

Related to: respiratory depression caused by anesthesia, altered oxygen-carrying capability of blood, altered oxygen supply, inadequate ventilation, ventilation/perfusion mismatching, abnormal ABGs, pain, blood loss, atelectasis, pneumothorax, hemothorax, increased pulmonary vascular resistance, increased capillary permeability, chemical mediators, decrease in surfactant

Defining Characteristics: dyspnea, tachypnea, apnea, ventilation/perfusion mismatching, abnormal ABGs, pain, increased hemodynamic pressures, oxygen saturation less than 90%, adventitious breath sounds, hypoxia, hypoxemia, nasal flaring, pale, dusky skin, restlessness, confusion, diaphoresis, tachycardia

Outcome Criteria

✔ Patient will be eupneic with clear breath sounds, and have no evidence of hypoxia/hypoxemia.

✔ Patient will maintain adequate oxygenation and ventilation.

NOC: *Respiratory Status: Gas Exchange*

INTERVENTIONS	RATIONALES
Monitor respiratory rate and depth, presence of dyspnea, use of accessory muscles, nasal flaring, and increasing respiratory work effort. Monitor oxygen saturation by oximetry.	Respiratory rates may be increased by pain, fever, blood loss, fluid loss, anxiety, hypoxia, or gastric distention. Decreases in rate may occur with use of narcotic analgesics. Changes in pulmonary status may result in hypoxemia. Prompt recognition of potential complications can promote prompt treatment.
Monitor VS and cardiac rhythm at least q 1 hour and prn.	Tachycardia and increased respiratory rates may indicate hypoxemia.

INTERVENTIONS	RATIONALES
Auscultate lung fields for diminished or absent breath sounds or for adventitious sounds.	Breath sounds are frequently diminished immediately post-op as a result of atelectasis. Loss of breath sounds in a previously ventilated lung may indicate a partial or total lung collapse, especially when chest tubes have recently been discontinued. Adventitious breath sounds may indicate fluid or secretions have accumulated in the interstitial spaces or airways resulting in a partial occlusion of the airway.
Evaluate chest expansion for symmetry.	Unilateral incomplete chest expansion may indicate that air or fluid is preventing complete expansion of the pleural space, possibly a pneumothorax.
Administer oxygen by cannula or mask as warranted, when extubated.	Provides supplemental oxygen to decrease the workload on the heart and to maximize oxygen delivery to under-perfused tissues.
Observe for pallor or cyanosis, especially to mucous membranes.	Cyanosis of lips, nail beds, or ear lobes, or generalized duskiness may indicate hypoxia as a result of heart failure or pulmonary dysfunction. Pallor is frequently noted immediately postoperatively because of blood loss or insufficient blood replacement.
Observe for presence of cough and sputum character.	Endotracheal tube intubation may promote throat irritation which can result in coughing, but cough may also indicate impending pulmonary congestion or infection. Purulent sputum may reflect pneumonia. Pulmonary edema may result from fluid overload late in recovery, which decreases oxygenation to tissues.
Encourage deep breathing exercises, inspiratory spirometer, or coughing exercises.	Promotes expansion/re-expansion of airways. Adventitious breath sounds may indicate presence of secretions or fluid in lungs.
Observe for signs of respiratory distress, tachycardia, extreme restlessness and feeling of impending doom.	May indicate impending pneumothorax or hemothorax, especially after chest tube removal. May require reinsertion of chest tubes.

INTERVENTIONS	RATIONALES
Monitor respiratory status and ventilatory settings every 1–2 hours while on ventilator.	CABG patients are placed on mechanical ventilation support until awake from anesthesia. FIO_2 is initially 100% and then gradually decreased, while maintaining an adequate PaO_2 above 90. FIO_2 should be decreased to 0.50 as rapidly as possible to prevent actual pulmonary changes that occur with high levels of oxygen. Tidal volumes are usually maintained between 10–15 cc/kg of ideal body weight to allow for less interference with venous return. If patient meets weaning criteria, extubation is usually accomplished within six hours.
Assist with weaning from ventilatory support. Monitor for hemodynamic instability and decreasing oxygen saturation. Monitor ABGs as ordered.	Weaning is usually performed by reducing the rate and then a trial on a T-bar or CPAP mode. Patients who have a history of smoking or COPD often have prolonged need for ventilatory support post-CABG because of their mechanism of breathing. Ventilators provide controlled amounts of oxygen and tidal volumes, and COPD patients have their inert drive to breathe removed by the use of ventilation. Occasionally with use of the cold cardioplegic solution, the phrenic nerve is injured in rare cases, resulting in a loss of function of the diaphragm which is necessary for 60% of the spontaneous tidal volume for the patient.
Suction patient every 2–4 hours and prn. Hyperoxygenate prior to and after suctioning.	Removes mucus that may occlude airways. Oxygen concentration drops drastically with suctioning procedures and leaves the patient compromised with an increased oxygen consumption. Hyperoxygenation helps to reduce the drastic decrease in oxygen concentration and to keep the patient adequately oxygenated and tissues perfused.
Auscultate breath sounds pre- and post-suctioning.	Provides for comparison of breath sounds to evaluate for

(continues)

(continued)

INTERVENTIONS	RATIONALES
	improvement. Occasionally, suctioning will move secretions up the bronchial tree and may cause a partial or total occlusion of an airway. Decreases in previously ventilated lung fields may indicate this phenomenon has occurred.
Monitor use of amiodarone and protamine sulfate. Observe for respiratory impingement.	Some drugs can exacerbate pulmonary problems by their method of action.
Prepare patient for placement on mechanical ventilation if warranted.	Lengthy instruction may not be prudent or possible depending on the severity of the situation. If oxygenation cannot be maintained with the use of supplemental oxygen, the only alternative is intubation/ventilation to increase gas exchange.
Prepare patient for insertion of tracheostomy after 10 days of ETT intubation/ventilation.	Prolonged endotracheal intubation may result in tracheal or nasal necrosis or rupture of ETT cuff. Tracheostomy is considered to prevent ulceration into arteries or other vital tissues, but may need to be avoided because of potential for contamination of sternotomy wound from secretions.
Instruct patient on need for ambulation, movement, and change in position.	Promotes lung expansion and prevents pulmonary congestion and atelectasis.
Instruct on need for respiratory treatments, coughing, deep breathing.	Reassures patient that complying with aggressive pulmonary regimen will not cause injury to surgical sites.
Prepare patient for reinsertion of chest tubes as warranted.	Promotes re-expansion of lung by removing accumulated fluid, blood, or air, and restores normal negative pressure in the pleural cavity.

NIC: *Respiratory Monitoring*

Discharge or Maintenance Evaluation

- Patient will be free of dyspnea with adequate ABGs and oxygenation, and without evidence of cyanosis or pallor.

- Patient will have clear breath sounds to all lung fields with no lung collapse.
- Patient will have vital signs within normal limits and will be able to maintain adequate air exchange.
- Patient will be compliant with respiratory regimen, and will be able to recall all instructions accurately.

IMPAIRED SKIN INTEGRITY

Related to: cardiac surgical incisions, insertion of temporary or permanent pacemaker, alteration in activity, puncture wounds, drains

Defining Characteristics: disruption of skin tissue, insertion sites, pathogenic invasion

Outcome Criteria

✔ Patient will have healed wound sites without signs/symptoms of infection.

NOC: *Tissue Integrity: Skin and Mucous Membranes*

NOC: *Wound Healing: Primary Intention*

INTERVENTIONS	RATIONALES
Inspect pacemaker insertion site, surgical sternotomy site, and graft site for erythema, edema, warmth, drainage, or tenderness.	Prompt detection of problems promotes prompt treatment.
Observe all incisions for healing and progress. Notify physician for incisional areas that are not healing, areas that have reopened or dehisced, edematous and erythematous tissues, bloody or purulent drainage, or hot painful areas.	Chest incisions usually heal first because of the minimal amounts of muscle tissue involved. Donor sites have more muscle tissue, usually are more lengthy incisions and have poorer circulation thereby requiring a longer healing process. Signs may indicate a failure to heal, or the development of complications that require further intervention.
Culture drainage from wound as warranted.	Identifies causative organism that may result in local or systemic infection, and allows for identification of suitable antimicrobial therapy.
Change dressings daily, or per hospital protocol, using sterile technique. Frequently, incisions may be left open to the air after	Allows for observation of site and detection of inflammation or infection. Sterile technique is recommended due to the close

INTERVENTIONS	RATIONALES
24 hours, providing no complications have occurred.	proximity of the portal to the heart increasing the potential for systemic infection. Deep sternal wound infections occur in up to 4% of patients after CABG, with a morbidity rate up to 25%. Obesity and reoperation are the most frequent risk factors that are consistently associated with this complication, but the use of the IMA, the duration and complexity of the surgery, and a history of diabetes have also been noted. Obesity is the strongest predictor for mediastinitis because antibiotics may be inadequately circulated within adipose tissues, the large areas of tissue provides a model environment for bacterial growth, and large skin folds preclude the ability to maintain sterility for wound care.
Utilize Steri-Strips to support incisions when sutures are removed per hospital protocol.	Maintains approximation of healing wound edges to facilitate healing of skin tissues.
Provide adequate nutritional and fluid intake.	Maintains adequate circulating volume, and assists to meet energy requirements to facilitate tissue healing and perfusion.
Monitor lab work, especially CBC and glucose levels.	CBC results can identify infective process and/or hemorrhage. Glucose levels that are elevated may impair healing of the wound. Diabetes, especially insulin-dependent types, has been associated with postoperative mediastinitis, and aggressive medical therapy to maintain blood sugar levels below 200 mg/dl with the use of IV insulin has significantly reduced deep sternal wound infections in diabetics.
Administer antimicrobials as ordered.	May be given preoperatively, perioperatively, and/or postoperatively based on patient's condition. These specific drugs should be given based on culture results when possible to assure maximum efficacy.

INTERVENTIONS	RATIONALES
Instruct on care to wound sites.	Promotes compliance with care to decrease potential for infection. Moisture can promote bacterial growth.
Instruct to observe for and report to physician the following symptoms: redness, drainage, temperature greater than 100 degrees, pain or tenderness to site, or swelling at site.	Provides for prompt recognition of complications and facilitates prompt treatment.
Instruct to avoid constrictive clothing until site has healed.	May cause discomfort at incision site from pressure and rubbing against skin.
Instruct to avoid tub baths until allowed by physician.	Effort needed to get in and out of tub requires use of pectoral and arm muscles which may contribute to placing undue stress on suture lines of sternotomy.

NIC: *Wound Care*

Discharge or Maintenance Evaluation

- Patient will have well-healed incision with no signs/symptoms of infection.
- Patient will be able to recall accurately all instructions given.
- Patient will be able to demonstrate appropriate wound care prior to discharge.

INEFFECTIVE TISSUE PERFUSION: CARDIOPULMONARY, PERIPHERAL

Related to: necessity of having PTCA or stenting procedure done

Defining Characteristics: pain, chest pain, shortness of breath, decreased cardiac output, dysrhythmias, coronary ischemia requiring emergent CABG, restenosis of coronary artery, allergic reaction to contrast dye, hemorrhage, post-CABG graft stenosis, vasovagal reaction to sheath removal, pseudoaneurysm of the femoral artery

Outcome Criteria

✔ Patient will achieve and maintain adequate tissue perfusion to all areas, with no signs or symptoms of complications.

✔ Patient will not require return to surgical suite for 2nd operative procedure.

NOC: *Tissue Perfusuion: Cardiac, Peripheral*

INTERVENTIONS	RATIONALES
Provide explanation to patient and family regarding reasons for need for coronary interventions.	PTCA is used to increase the interior diameter of a stenosed coronary artery in order to improve the coronary blood flow to the heart and prevent ischemia and necrosis. Stenting or atherectomy may be required to maintain patency of the coronary artery, and although the potential for emergent CABG following these procedures may occur in only a small (approximately 2%) number of patients, the possibility should be discussed to prevent anxiety and fear of the unknown and to facilitate knowledge.
Prepare patient for procedure per hospital protocol.	Normally, shaving the groin area is performed, but some facilities will prepare for the eventuality of emergent CABG by shaving the patient from chest to legs. An IV site is obtained to provide IV fluids and emergency medications, and most facilities will begin at least two sites in case direct intracoronary thrombolytics may be given.
After PTCA or other intervention, monitor ECG for rhythm, changes in conduction, or dysrhythmias, and treat per hospital protocol.	Patient may develop coronary vasospasm causing anginal pain, ischemia may result, or coronary occlusion may occur as a result of a dissection and require emergent treatment in order to save patient. Dysrhythmias may occur if patient has a temporary pacemaker because of irritability of the ventricle by the pacing wire. Restenosis may occur after a PTCA as a result of intimal hyperplasia.

INTERVENTIONS	RATIONALES
Maintain IV fluids at ordered rate.	Fluids help to rehydrate patient as well as assist with the excretion of the dye used during the PTCA or other procedure.
Administer heparin drip as ordered after PTCA.	Heparin is normally given as a bolus loading dose, followed by a continuous IV infusion at an ordered rate based upon the patient's coagulation status. Heparin should not be given in the same IV line as nitroglycerin as the nitroglycerin will impair the action of the heparin, nor should heparin be given in the same IV line as any other drug that contains sodium bicarbonate or a phosphate buffer, as many of these drugs are incompatible with heparin. Heparin functions by binding with antithrombin III to help inactivate thrombin and factors Xa and XIa to prevent fibrin formation and clot extension.
Monitor lab work for PTT, ACT, or APTT, and notify physician for ordered parameters.	These lab levels help to identify the preferred anticoagulation levels. ACT should be <150 seconds if the PTCA sheath is to be removed, otherwise the potential for hemorrhage is great.
Monitor patient for bleeding from the sheath insertion site, urine, mouth, nose, or other sources, and notify physician.	May indicate that patient's ability for blood to coagulate has been lost, requiring a decrease or cessation of the drip based on the physician's order. Heparin should be stopped at least four hours prior to the sheath removal post-PTCA to prevent hemorrhage.
Monitor vital signs per hospital protocol, but usually Q 15 minutes initially, then Q 30 minutes, then Q 1 hr, and check peripheral pulses and sheath site for bleeding with each VS check. Notify physician of abnormalities.	Bleeding may occur if seal around the catheter site has broken loose, and may result in hemorrhage. Changes in vital signs may indicate hemorrhage, coronary ischemia, reaction to the dye, or other complication. Loss of a pulse peripherally, or changes in skin temperature or color, may indicate that the sheath has moved and is placing pressure on an artery partially impairing flow, or that a clot has formed to prevent adequate blood flow to the limb. This

INTERVENTIONS	RATIONALES
	symptom requires emergent action to prevent further complications and even, death.
Maintain patient's affected leg in a straight position and immobile, using a sandbag, sheet covering, or leg restraint if needed. The patient should be on bed rest for at least 6 hours up to 12 hours, depending on hospital protocol, and should be repositioned by logrolling.	Proper positioning reduces the chance that bleeding may occur because of a loss of seal at the sheath site.
If bleeding is noted at site, immediately place direct pressure over area, and have another person notify the physician. Pressure should be held until the bleeding has stopped and usually requires at least 10 minutes of direct pressure. If hematoma has formed, it should be marked and observed for changes.	Because the catheter sheath goes directly into the femoral artery, the patient may hemorrhage a significant volume of blood in a short while. Marking the hematoma allows for observation of increasing size. The patient may require blood transfusions depending on the amount of blood loss.
Auscultate site of sheath insertion for systolic bruit every 8 hours, or per hospital protocol, and notify physician if present.	The presence of a bruit, especially in conjunction with pain to site and a pulsatile mass may indicate that a femoral pseudoaneurysm is present, and may require surgical intervention immediately. Patients who are at a high risk for this complication include the obese patient, with whom it is difficult to apply sufficient pressure to halt bleeding, the patient who is receiving anticoagulation therapy, because of hemostasis instability, the elderly patient, in whom the degenerative changes caused by age damage the arterial wall, and those patients who require a larger than No. 8 French sheath size, because of a larger lumen and potential for injury to the artery.
If restenosis of the coronary artery occurs, administer analgesics, heparin, and/or glycoprotein IIb/IIIa receptors as ordered.	Pain may increase anxiety and worsen vasoconstriction and ischemia to the heart. Heparin may be resumed for its thrombolytic action. Glycoprotein IIb/IIIa inhibitors, such as abciximab, may be ordered to inhibit platelet aggregation in high risk PTCA patients, such as diabetics, recent MI or unstable angina

INTERVENTIONS	RATIONALES
	patients, or patients with complicated lesions.
Instruct patient/family in all aspects of coronary interventions planned, including the potential for emergent CABG.	Provides knowledge to decrease anxiety and fear. Assists in maintaining patient compliance.
Instruct patient/family regarding need to maintain bed rest with affected leg kept straight.	Reduces potential for bleeding and allows for patient and family to participate in care by following directions given.
Instruct patient to report any feeling of wetness at sheath site, swelling, increased pain, tingling, paresthesias, weakness in the limbs, chest pain, or shortness of breath.	Ensures prompt notification of potential complications such as hemorrhage or restenosis that will enable prompt intervention to be taken.
Instruct patient/family regarding discharge instructions if PTCA is performed: symptoms to report, such as bleeding, bruising of site, increased pain, masses, shortness of breath, or chest pain, and to call physician or EMS as needed.	Provides for postdischarge knowledge of potential complications and method of dealing with this problem.
Instruct patient/family regarding any medications, diet, activity limitations, and so forth.	Provides for knowledge and compliance. Usually activity is limited for two days with no driving for one day. Dietary modifications may include decreasing cholesterol and sodium to reduce incidence of further atherosclerosis or fluid retention.

NIC: *Cardiac Care*

Discharge or Maintenance Evaluation

- Patient will have PTCA as needed, but will not require emergent surgical intervention for complications.
- Patient will have normal vital signs, with peripheral pulses present and equal bilaterally.
- Patient will have no further chest pain or cardiac dysrhythmias.
- Patient will be able to verbalize understanding of complications to be alert for, and how to deal with them, should they occur.
- Patient will have no complications and will be able to modify diet and lifestyle to avoid further atherosclerosis and coronary stenosis.

CHAPTER 1.5

HEART FAILURE

Heart failure (HF) is the inability of the heart to supply blood flow to meet physiologic demands without utilizing compensatory changes. There may be failure involving one or both sides of the heart as a result of atrial or ventricular dysfunction or increased afterload, and over time, pulmonary and systemic congestion develops and leads to further complications and impaired function. Congestive heart failure, or CHF, is a common complication after myocardial infarction and can be attributed to one-third of the deaths of patients with MIs. Usually following MI, the heart failure is left-sided as most infarctions involve damage to the left ventricle.

There are four stages of heart failure that have been identified. Stage A represents the patients who are at a higher risk for developing heart failure, but do not have any structural disorder of their heart. These could include persons with hypertension, CAD, diabetes, alcohol abuse, or family history of cardiomyopathy.

Stage B represents those patients who have a structural problem with their heart but who have not developed any symptoms of heart failure. Patients in this category may have left ventricular hypertrophy, previous MI, or valvular heart disease.

Stage C represents the patients that have or have had symptoms of heart failure and who also have a basic underlying structural heart disorder. These patients exhibit fatigue and dyspnea as a result of left ventricular dysfunction, or have had these symptoms but are currently receiving treatment for heart failure.

Stage D represents the patients who have end-stage heart failure and whose care may entail the use of mechanical circulatory support, inotropic support, heart transplantation, or end-of-life care. These are the most advanced cases that have significant symptoms even at rest and are receiving maximum medical therapeutics, such as continuous IV support at home, or mechanical circulatory assistance devices, or those who are awaiting a donor for transplantation.

Coronary artery disease is usually the underlying origin of HF in 65% of patients who have left-ventricular dysfunction. The other 35% of patients with HF have either an identifiable cause, such as hypertension or valvular disease, or do not have a specific ischemic cause of systolic dysfunction, such as idiopathic dilated cardiomyopathy.

Heart failure can also be classified as acute or chronic. In chronic heart failure, the body experiences a gradual development of symptoms as compensatory mechanisms fail to continue to offset the reduced ventricular contractility and impaired filling. Chronic heart failure can become acute without any overt cause.

Often, the patient will have no early symptoms of left-sided heart failure. Symptoms of decreased cardiac output will develop once the heart fails to pump enough blood into the systemic circulation. The pressure in the left ventricle increases, which in turn causes retrograde increases of pressure in the left atrium because of the increased difficulty for blood to enter the atrium from the pulmonary veins. Blood backs up in the lung vasculature, and when the pulmonary capillary pressure is exceeded by the oncotic pressure of the proteins in the plasma fluid (usually >30 mm Hg), the fluid leaks into the interstitial spaces. When this fluid moves into the alveoli, shortness of breath, coughing, and crackles (rales) occur. The patient progresses into overt pulmonary edema, with the classic sign of coughing up copious amounts of pink frothy sputum.

Right-sided heart failure is usually caused by left-sided heart failure, but can also be caused by pulmonary emboli, pulmonary hypertension, COPD, right ventricular infarctions, myocardial contusions, atherosclerotic cardiovascular disease, cardiomyopathy, valvular heart disease, atrial or ventricular septal defects, pulmonary stenosis, or sleep apnea.

The lungs can accommodate a small amount of fluid buildup, but eventually, if no intervention is taken, the pressure in the lungs increases to the point whereby the right ventricle has difficulty ejecting blood into the pulmonary artery. The right ventricle fails, the blood in the right atrium cannot drain completely, and, thus, cannot accept the total amount of blood from the vena cavae. Venous pooling occurs with the impairment of venous blood flow, and eventually the organs become congested with venous blood.

Treatment of heart failure involves attempts to improve contractility of the ventricle by use of positive inotropic drugs, decrease of afterload by the use of nitrates and vasodilators, and in some instances, by use of the IABP, and decrease of preload by the use of diuretics, IV nitroglycerin, and fluid/sodium restrictions.

MEDICAL CARE

Oxygen: to increase available oxygen supply

Morphine: used to induce vasodilation, decrease venous return to the heart, reduce pain and anxiety, and decrease myocardial oxygen consumption

Cardiac glycosides: digoxin (Lanoxin) used to increase the force and strength of ventricular contractions and to decrease rate of contractions in order to increase cardiac output

Diuretics: furosemide (Lasix, Furosemide, Luramide), bumetanine (Bumex), chlorothiazide (Diuril), hydrochlorothiazide (Esidrex, Hydrochlorthiazide, HydroDiuril, Thiuretic), chlorthalidone (Chlorthalidone, Hygroton, Hylidone, Thalitone), indapamide (Lozol), metolazone (Diulo, Zaroxolyn), ethacrynic acid (Edecrin), torsemide (Demadex), acetazolamide (Acetazolamide, Diamox), methazolamide (Neptazane), amiloride (Amiloride, Midamor), spironolactone (Aldactone), triamterene (Dyrenium), mannitol (Mannitol, Osmitrol), and urea (Ureaphil) used to promote excess fluid removal and to decrease edema and pulmonary venous pressure by preventing sodium and water reabsorption

ACE inhibitors: enalapril (Vasotec), captopril (Capoten), fosinopril (Monopril), lisinopril (Prinivil, Zestril), quinapril (Accupril), or ramipril (Altace) may be used for afterload reduction; these drugs inhibit angiotensin-converting enzyme and prevent the conversion of angiotensin I to angiotensin II, and are able to decrease the workload on the left ventricle to improve cardiac output; contraindicated in hyperkalemic and shock states

Beta-adrenergic blockers: propranolol hydrochloride (Inderal), nadolol (Corgard), pindolol (Visken), and timolol maleate (Blocadren) are nonselective ß-blockers that are used to reduce blood pressure without a reflex increase or decrease in heart rate; these drugs decrease cardiac excitability and reduce myocardial oxygen demands; bisoprolol (Zebeta), carvedilol (Coreg), and metoprolol tartrate (Lopressor) are the most common, but acebutolol hydrochloride (Sectral), atenolol (Tenormin), along with esmolol hydrochloride (Brevibloc), are selective ß$_1$-receptor blockers that produce chronotropic and inotropic effects by blocking stimulation of ß$_1$-receptors in the cardiac smooth muscle

Vasodilators: diazoxide (Hyperstat), amyl nitrite (Amyl nitrite), cyclandelate (Cyclan, Cyclospasmol), dipyridamole (Persantine), hydralazine (Apresoline), isosorbide dinitrate (Isorbid, Isordil, Sorbitrate), minoxidil (Loniten), nitroprusside (Nitropress, Sodium nitroprusside, Nipride), nitroglycerine, (Minitran, Deponit, Nitro-Bid, Nitrocine, Nitrol, Tridil), and/or tolazoline (Priscoline) used to relax vascular smooth muscle, decrease preload and afterload, decrease oxygen demand, decrease systemic vascular resistance, and increase venuous capacitance

Inotropic agents: dopamine (Dopastat, Intropin), dobutamine (Dobutrex, Dobutamine), and inamrinone lactate (Inocor), and milrinone lactate (Primacor) to increase myocardial contractility, increase cellular levels of camp, produce peripheral vasodilation, decrease preload and afterload, and avoid increasing heart rate

Electrolytes: mainly potassium used to replace that which is lost during diuretic therapy

Laboratory: electrolyte levels to monitor for imbalances; renal profile to monitor for kidney function problems; digoxin levels to monitor for toxicity; platelet count to monitor for thrombocytopenia; liver function studies to monitor for complications from right-sided failure; hemoglobin and hematocrit to monitor for anemia; cardiac enzymes to monitor for myocardial infarction, if suspected

Chest X-ray: shows dilation of cardiac vasculature, and hypertrophy of atria or ventricles, and cardiac valvular calcifications, shows pulmonary vasculature, presence of pulmonary edema, or pleural effusion

Electrocardiography: used to monitor for dysrhythmias which may occur as a result of the heart failure or as a result of nonspecific ECG changes, conduction abnormalities, ischemic changes, drug toxicity or electrolyte effects; this is the single most valuable diagnostic test when coupled with Doppler flow studies

Echocardiography: used to study structural abnormalities and blood flow through the heart, left ventricular function, ejection fraction, wall motion, papillary muscle function, stenotic valves, masses, cardiomyopathy, pericardial effusion, tamponade, calcifications, congenital defects and presence of shunts, or clot formation

Radionuclide imaging, ultrafast CT, and MRI: used to assess left-ventricular systolic function and show ischemia, infarction, structural abnormalities, vascular abnormalities, and tumors

Cardiac catheterization: used to visualize cardiac anatomy, assess cardiac pressures, ventricular contractility, valvular function, and cardiac defects

Surgical intervention: may be required if heart transplantation is necessary or for placement of mechanical assist devices or coronary revascularization in patients with concurrent angina; implantable cardioverter–defibrillators may be placed in patients who also have a history of sudden death, ventricular fibrillation or ventricular tachycardia that is hemodynamically unstable

Intra-aortic balloon pump: decreases the workload on the heart, decreases myocardial oxygen demand, increases coronary perfusion, decreases afterload, decreases preload, improves cardiac output and tissue perfusion

COMMON NURSING DIAGNOSES

ANXIETY (see MI)

Related to: hypoxia, change in health status, fear of death, threat to body image, threat to role functioning, pain

Defining Characteristics: restlessness, insomnia, anorexia, increased respirations, increased heart rate, increased blood pressure, difficulty concentrating, dry mouth, poor eye contact, decreased energy, irritability, crying, feelings of helplessness

DEFICIENT KNOWLEDGE (see MI)

Related to: lack of understanding, lack of understanding of medical condition, lack of recall, hypoxia, hypoxemia

Defining Characteristics: questions regarding problems, inadequate follow-up on instructions given, misconceptions, lack of improvement of previous regimen, development of preventable complications

ADDITIONAL NURSING DIAGNOSES

EXCESS FLUID VOLUME

Related to: ineffective pumping of the heart, increased preload, increased sodium and water retention, decreased organ perfusion, compromised regulatory mechanisms, decreased cardiac output, increased ADH production

Defining Characteristics: edema, weight gain, intake greater than output, oliguria, increased pulmonary artery pressures, increased blood pressure, increased heart rate, shortness of breath, dyspnea, orthopnea, crackles (rales), S_3 or S_4 gallops, rhonchi, wheezing, cough with production of frothy white to pink sputum, diaphoresis, peripheral edema, cool, moist skin, cyanosis, hypoxia, confusion, pulsus alternans, fatigue, anxiety, jugular vein distention, pleural effusion, specific gravity changes, altered electrolyte levels

Outcome Criteria

✔ Lung fields will be clear to auscultation.

✔ Blood pressure will be maintained within normal limits and edema will be absent or minimal in all body parts.

✔ Fluid volume will be stabilized with balanced intake and output.

NOC: *Fluid Balance*

INTERVENTIONS	RATIONALES
Administer oxygen therapy as prescribed.	Supplemental oxygen may be required to prevent hypoxia caused by increased cardiac pressures, fluid increases, and hypoventilation. Depending on the severity of the condition, the patient may require varying amounts of oxygen supplementation to maintain adequate blood saturations, and mechanical ventilation may be required to ensure proper oxygenation.
Monitor vital signs and hemodynamic readings if available.	Fluid volume excess will cause increases in blood pressure, and CVP and pulmonary artery

INTERVENTIONS	RATIONALES
	pressures. These changes will be reflected from the development of pulmonary congestion and heart failure.
Auscultate lungs for presence of crackles (rales), or other adventitious breath sounds. Observe for presence of cough, increased dyspnea, tachypnea, orthopnea or paroxysmal nocturnal dyspnea.	May indicate pulmonary edema from cardiac decompensation and pulmonary congestion. Pulmonary edema symptoms reflect left-sided heart failure. Right-sided heart failure may have slower onset, but symptoms of dyspnea, orthopnea, and cough are more difficult to reverse.
Observe for jugular vein distention and dependent edema. Note presence of generalized body edema (anasarca).	May indicate impending congestive failure and fluid excess. Peripheral edema begins in feet and ankles, or other dependent areas and ascends as failure progresses. Pitting will usually occur only after 10 or more pounds of excess fluid is retained. Anasarca will be seen only with right-heart failure or biventricular failure.
Investigate abrupt complaints of dyspnea, air hunger, feeling of impending doom or suffocation.	Excessive fluid buildup can promote other complications such as pulmonary edema or pulmonary embolus and intervention must be immediate.
Determine fluid balance by measuring intake and output, and observing for decreases in output and concentrated urine.	Renal perfusion is impaired with excessive fluid volume, which causes decreased cardiac output leading to sodium and water retention and oliguria.
Weigh daily and notify physician of greater than 2 lb/day increase.	Abrupt changes in weight usually indicate excess fluid.
Provide patient with fluid intake of 2 L/day, unless fluid restriction is warranted.	Fluids may need to be restricted because of cardiac decompensation. Fluids maintain hydration of tissues.
Administer diuretics as ordered.	Drugs may be necessary to correct fluid overload depending on emergent nature of problem. Diuretics increase urine flow rate and may inhibit reabsorption of sodium and chloride in the renal tubules.
Assess patient response and monitor for complications, such as electrolyte imbalances, renal dysfunction, headaches, dry mouth, dizziness, and so forth.	Diuretics decrease intravascular and extravascular fluid volume, thereby decreasing preload. Electrolytes, especially sodium, potassium, and magnesium, may be decreased and cause complications and organ dysfunction.

INTERVENTIONS	RATIONALES
Administer nutritional supplements and/or hormonal therapy as ordered.	Studies have shown that the use of supplements, such as coenzyme Q_{10}, taurine, and antioxidants, are helpful in the treatment of heart failure. Growth hormone and/or thyroid hormone has also been shown to be helpful in some patients.
Monitor electrolyte imbalances. Note increasing lethargy, hypotension, muscle cramping or mental confusion.	Hypokalemia can occur with the administration of diuretics, and this may increase potential toxicity from concurrent use of cardiac glycosides. Signs of potassium and sodium deficits may occur due to fluid shifts with diuretic therapy.
Administer morphine sulfate 2–5 mg IV as ordered. Observe for complications.	Morphine reduces preload, decreases venous return, decreases myocardial oxygen consumption, reduces pain, and helps to alleviate anxiety. Respiratory depression can occur in some instances resulting in hypoventilation, hypotension, and/or bradydysrhythmias.
Place and maintain patient in semi-Fowler's position.	This position helps to decrease venous return and improves ease of breathing. Diuresis may be enhanced by recumbent position because of increased glomerular filtration and decreased production of ADH.
Auscultate bowel sounds and observe for abdominal distention, anorexia, nausea, or constipation. Provide small, easily-digestible meals.	CHF progression can impair gastric motility and intestinal function. Small, frequent meals may enhance digestion and prevent abdominal discomfort.
Measure abdominal girth if warranted. Assess for ascites.	Progressive right-sided heart failure can cause fluid to shift into the peritoneal space and cause ascites.
Palpate abdomen for liver enlargement; note any right upper quadrant tenderness or pain.	Progressive heart failure can lead to venous congestion, abdominal distention, liver engorgement, and pain. Liver function may be impaired and can impede drug metabolism.
Assist with dialysis or hemofiltration as warranted.	Mechanically removing excess fluid may be performed to rapidly reduce circulating volume in cases refractory to other medical therapeutics.

(continues)

(continued)

INTERVENTIONS	RATIONALES
Instruct patient regarding dietary restrictions of sodium.	Fluid retention is increased with intake of sodium.
Consult with dietitian.	May be required to ensure adequacy of caloric intake with fluid and sodium restriction requirements.
Instruct patient to observe for weight changes daily and report these to physician.	Weight gain may be first overt sign of fluid excess and should be monitored to prevent complications.
Instruct patient/family about heart failure, including necessary changes to lifestyle, compliance with medications, complications with medications, and symptoms that may indicate worsening of condition.	Increases knowledge and helps to ensure compliance with medical regimen. Changes in lifestyle may be required to prevent recurrence of heart failure. Identification of adverse effects from medications or symptoms of worsening condition allows for prompt medical treatment and lessening of complications.
Instruct patient/family in procedure for taking pulse, and parameters for which to notify their physician.	Involves the patient and/or family in the care and allows for potential early identification of dysrhythmias and changes in status.
Instruct patient in medications prescribed after discharge, with dose, effect, side effects, contraindications.	Promotes knowledge and compliance with treatment regimen.
Monitor chest X-rays.	Reveal changes in pulmonary status regarding improvement or deterioration.

NIC: *Hypervolemia Management*

Discharge or Maintenance Evaluation

- Patient will have no edema or fluid excess.
- Fluid balance will be maintained and blood pressure will be within normal limits of baseline.
- Lung fields will be clear, without adventitious breath sounds, and weight will be stable.
- Patient will be able to accurately measure weight and identify changes that may signal impending fluid increase.
- Patient and/or family will be able to accurately demonstrate how to take pulse, verbalize understanding of condition, symptoms of worsening condition, side effects of medications, and dietary restrictions.

DECREASED CARDIAC OUTPUT

Related to: damaged myocardium, decreased contractility, dysrhythmias, conduction defects, alteration in preload, alteration in afterload, vasoconstriction, myocardial ischemia, ventricular hypertrophy, accumulation of blood in lungs or in systemic venous system, conduction defects, impaired filling

Defining Characteristics: dependent edema, elevated blood pressure, elevated mean arterial pressure greater than 120 mm Hg, elevated systemic vascular resistance greater than 1400 dyne–seconds/cm^5, cardiac output less than 4 L/min or cardiac index less than 2.5 L/min/m^2, cold, pale extremities, absent or decreased peripheral pulses, ECG changes, dysrhythmias, hypotension, S_3 or S_4 gallops, decreased urinary output, diaphoresis, orthopnea, dyspnea, crackles (rales), frothy blood-tinged sputum, jugular vein distention, edema, chest pain, confusion, restlessness

Outcome Criteria

- ✔ Vital signs and hemodynamic parameters will be within normal limits for patient, with no dysrhythmias noted.
- ✔ The workload of the heart will be reduced and myocardial oxygen consumption will be decreased.
- ✔ Damage to the heart will be minimal.
- ✔ Patient will be free of pain.
- ✔ Patient will have normal fluid balance.
- ✔ Patient will be eupneic with no adventitious breath sounds or abnormal heart tones.

NOC: *Circulation Status*

INTERVENTIONS	RATIONALES
Determine level of cardiac function and existing cardiac and other conditions by history.	Additional disease states and complications may place an additional workload on an already compromised heart.
Auscultate apical pulses and monitor heart rate and rhythm. Monitor BP in both arms.	Decreased contractility will be compensated by tachycardia, especially concurrently with heart failure. Blood volume will be lowered if blood pressure is increased resulting in increased afterload. Pulse decreases may be noted in association with toxic levels of digoxin, and peripheral pulses may be hard to accurately determine if perfusion

INTERVENTIONS	RATIONALES
	is decreased. Hypotension may occur as a result of ventricular dysfunction and poor perfusion of the myocardium.
Measure cardiac output and cardiac index, and calculate hemodynamic pressures every 4 hours and prn.	Provides measurement of cardiac function and calculated measurements of preload and afterload to facilitate titration of vasoactive drugs and manipulation of hemodynamic pressures.
Monitor ECG for dysrhythmias and treat as indicated.	Conduction abnormalities may occur because of ischemic myocardium affecting the pumping efficiency of the heart. Some vasoactive medications, such as dopamine, dobutamine, milrinone, and amrinone, can cause tachycardias and other dysrhythmias.
Auscultate for development of new S_3 or S_4 gallops.	S_3 gallops are usually associated with congestive heart failure but can be found with mitral regurgitation and left-ventricular overload after MI. S_4 gallops can be associated with myocardial ischemia, ventricular rigidity, pulmonary hypertension, or systemic hypertension, which can decrease cardiac output.
Auscultate for presence of murmurs and/or rubs.	Indicates disturbances of normal blood flow within the heart related to incompetent valves, septal defects, or papillary muscle/chordae tendonae complications post-MI. Presence of a rub with an MI is associated with pericarditis and/or pericardial effusion.
Observe lower extremities for edema, cold hands and feet, mottling, and sluggish capillary refilling.	Reduced venous return to the heart can result in low cardiac output with shunting of blood away from periphery to vital organs, resulting in perfusion deficits such as decreased capillary refill time and cold, mottled, cyanotic extremities. A decrease in venous return leads to fluid retention and edema formation. Use of alpha-adrenergic stimulators cause peripheral vasoconstriction.
Observe for distended neck veins.	May indicate increased fluid retention and overload.

INTERVENTIONS	RATIONALES
Assess patient for changes in mentation and neurologic status.	Decreases in cardiac output can result in decreased cerebral perfusion. Hypoxia, hypoxemia, and fluid and electrolyte imbalances can cause diminished mentation and may often be the first sign of a change in status.
Administer oxygen as ordered. Monitor oxygenation status using oximetry and ABGs as needed.	Supplemental oxygen may be required because of hypoxia and hypoxemia that results from a decrease in cardiac output.
Administer IV fluids as ordered.	Increases and decreases in fluids may be required to maintain left-ventricular end-diastolic pressure (LVEDP) and to maintain adequate cardiac output.
Monitor intake and output, and notify physician if urine output is less than 30 cc/hr for 2 consecutive hours.	Oliguria may result from decreased venous return because of fluid retention. Alpha-adrenergic effects of dopamine at rates greater than 10 mcg/kg/min result in peripheral vasoconstriction, increased afterload, increased blood pressure, and potential decreased cardiac output with diminished renal function.
Position in semi-Fowler's position.	Promotes easier breathing and prevents pooling of blood in the pulmonary vasculature.
Administer cardiac glycosides, nitrates, vasodilators, diuretics, antihypertensives, ACE inhibitors, and beta-blockers as ordered.	Used in the treatment of vasoconstriction and to reduce heart rate and contractility, reduces blood pressure by relaxation of venous and arterial smooth muscle which then in turn increases cardiac output and decreases the workload on the heart.
Titrate vasoactive drugs as ordered per physician parameters.	Maintains blood pressure and heart rate at levels to optimize cardiac output function.
Weigh every day.	Weight gain may indicate fluid retention and possible impending heart failure. Weight loss may reflect improvement in patient's condition by a decrease in excessive fluid retention.
Arrange activities so as to not overtax patient.	Avoids overfatiguing patient and decreasing cardiac output further. Balancing rest with activity minimizes energy expenditure and myocardial oxygen

(continues)

(continued)

INTERVENTIONS	RATIONALES
	demands by maintaining cardiac output.
Avoid Valsalva-type maneuvers with straining, coughing or moving.	Increasing intra-abdominal pressure results in an abrupt decrease in cardiac output by preventing blood from being pumped into the thoracic cavity and, thus, less blood being pumped into the heart which then decreases the heart rate. When the pressure is released, there is a sudden overload of blood which then increases preload, and decreases cardiac output.
Provide small, easy to digest, meals.	Large meals increase the workload on the heart.
Have emergency equipment and medications available at all times.	Coronary occlusion, lethal dysrhythmias, infarct extensions or intractable pain may precipitate cardiac arrest that requires life support and resuscitation.
Assist with placement of IABP, as needed. Prepare patient for placement of LVAD, if needed.	Placement on intra-aortic balloon pump (IABP) therapy decreases the workload on the heart by reducing myocardial oxygen demands, decreasing preload and afterload, and increasing coronary and tissue perfusion. This improves cardiac output and contractility, and can limit the size of infarctions, support circulatory status, and can be used as a bridge to other medical interventions, should they be required. IABP therapy is contraindicated for patients who have severe aortic disease, aortic insufficiency, or peripheral vascular disease that involves the limb affected by placement of the IAB sheath/line. A ventricular assist device (VAD) is a type of pump that can be used on either or both sides of the heart, and allows for partial offloading of a compromised ventricle and permits the heart to rest. VADs are usually indicated for severe cardiogenic shock, as a bridge to transplantation, or for patients who are not able to support ventricular function post-surgery.

INTERVENTIONS	RATIONALES
Assist with insertion and maintenance of pacemaker when needed.	Cardiac pacing may be necessary during the acute phase of MI or may be necessary as a permanent measure if the MI severely damages the conduction system.
Instruct on medications, dose, effects, side effects, contraindications, and avoidance of over-the-counter drugs without physician approval.	Promotes knowledge and compliance with regimen. Prevents any adverse drug interactions.
Instruct in activity limitations. Demonstrate exercises to be done.	Promotes compliance. Reduces decrease in cardiac output by lessening the workload placed on the heart.
Instruct to report chest pain.	May indicate complications of decreased cardiac output.
Instruct patient/family regarding placement of pulmonary artery catheter, and post-procedure care.	Alleviates fear and promotes knowledge. Pulmonary artery catheter necessary for direct measurement of cardiac output and for obtaining values for other hemodynamic measurements.
Instruct patient/family in procedures, such as IABP therapy or need for VAD.	Promotes knowledge of procedures, reduces fear, and involves patient and/or family in treatment plan.

NIC: *Hemodynamic Regulation*

Discharge or Maintenance Evaluation

- Patient will have no chest pain or shortness of breath.
- Vital signs and hemodynamic parameters will be within normal limits for age and disease condition.
- Activity will be tolerated without fatigue or dyspnea.
- Urinary output will be adequate.
- Cardiac output will be adequate to ensure adequate perfusion of all body systems.

IMPAIRED GAS EXCHANGE

Related to: ventilation/perfusion imbalance caused from excess fluid in alveoli and reduction of air exchange area in lung fields, fluid collection shifts into the interstitial space

Defining Characteristics: confusion, restlessness, irritability, hypoxia, hypercapnea, dyspnea, orthopnea, abnormal ABGs, abnormal oxygen saturation

Outcome Criteria

✔ Patient will have adequate oxygenation with respiratory status within limits of normal based on age and other conditions, and ABGs will be within normal limits.

NOC: *Respiratory Status: Gas Exchange*

INTERVENTIONS	RATIONALES
Monitor respiratory status for rate, regularity, depth, ease of effort at rest or with exertion, inspiratory/expiratory ratio.	Changes in respiratory pattern or patency of airway may result in gas exchange imbalances.
Observe for presence of cyanosis and mottling; monitor oximetry for oxygen saturation; monitor ABGs for ventilation/perfusion problems.	Cyanosis results from decreases in oxygenated hemoglobin in the blood and this reduction leads to hypoxia. Reading of 90% on pulse oximeter correlates with pO_2 of 60, depending on the patient's pH, temperature, and other factors.
Monitor for mental status changes, deterioration in level of consciousness, restlessness, irritability, or increased fatigue.	Hypoxia affects all body systems and mental status changes can result from decreased oxygen to brain tissues.
Position in semi- or high-Fowler's position.	Promotes breathing and lung expansion to enhance gas distribution.
Assess for nausea and vomiting.	May indicate effects of hypoxia on gastrointestinal system.
Administer oxygen via nasal cannula at 2–3 L/min, or other delivery systems.	Maintains adequate oxygenation without depression of respiratory drive. CO_2 may be retained with higher flow rates when used in patients with COPD.
Assist with placement of ETT and placement on mechanical ventilation.	Mechanical ventilation may be required if respiratory failure is progressive and adequate oxygen levels cannot be maintained by other delivery systems.
Instruct in breathing exercises as warranted.	Assists to restore function to diaphragm, decreases work of breathing, and improves gas exchange.
Instruct patient to avoid activities that promote dyspnea or fatigue.	Activity increases oxygen consumption and demand, and can

INTERVENTIONS	RATIONALES
Allow for periods of rest between activities.	impair breathing pattern.
Instruct in safety concerns with oxygen use.	Promotes safety with oxygen and provides knowledge.
Instruct patient/family in need for placement on mechanical ventilation, what to expect, what benefits are to be received, what potential problems may be encountered.	Promotes knowledge and decreases anxiety and fear of the unknown.

NIC: *Acid–Base Management*

Discharge or Maintenance Evaluation

■ Patient will exhibit no ventilation/perfusion imbalances.

■ Patient will be eupneic with no adventitious breath sounds.

■ ABGs will be within acceptable ranges for patient with adequate oxygenation of all tissues.

■ Patient will be able to verbalize/demonstrate the correct use of oxygen.

RISK FOR IMPAIRED SKIN INTEGRITY

Related to: bed rest, decreased tissue perfusion, edema, immobility, decreased peripheral perfusion, shearing forces or pressure, secretions, excretions, altered sensation, skeletal prominence, poor skin turgor, altered metabolic rate

Defining Characteristics: disruption of skin surface, pressure areas, reddened areas, blanched areas, mottling, warmth, firmness to area of skin, irritated tissues, excoriation of skin, maceration of skin, lacerations of skin, pruritis, dermatitis

Outcome Criteria

✔ Patient will have and maintain skin integrity.

NOC: *Tissue Integrity: Skin and Mucous Membranes*

INTERVENTIONS	RATIONALES
Monitor mobility status and patient's ability to move self.	Immobility is the primary cause of skin breakdown.

(continues)

(continued)

INTERVENTIONS	RATIONALES
Inspect all skin surfaces, especially bony prominences, for skin breakdown, altered circulation to areas, or presence of edema.	Skin is at risk because of decreased tissue perfusion, immobility, decreased peripheral perfusion, and possible nutritional alterations.
Provide skin care to blanched or reddened areas.	Stimulates blood flow and decreases tissue hypoxia. Excess dryness or moistness of skin can promote breakdown.
Provide eggcrate mattress, alternating pressure mattress, sheepskin, elbow protectors, heel protectors, and so forth.	These items can reduce pressure on skin and may improve circulation.
Reposition frequently, at least every 2 hours. Assist with ROM exercises. Maintain body alignment. Raise head of bed no higher than 30 degrees.	Improves circulation by reduction of time pressure is on any one area. Proper body alignment prevents contractures. Elevations higher than this may promote pressure and friction from sliding down, and shearing force may result in breakdown of skin.
Avoid subcutaneous or IM injections when possible.	Edema and tissue hypoxia impede circulation which can cause

INTERVENTIONS	RATIONALES
	decreased absorption of medication and can predispose patient to tissue breakdown and development of abscess/infection.
Instruct on safety precautions in bed—avoiding bumping against rails, falls, and so forth.	May cause breaks in skin integrity.
Instruct on hazards of immobility; avoid lying or sitting in one position for prolonged time.	Bedrest promotes pressure to skin and tissues.
Instruct on the use of lotions and oil to apply to skin.	Prevents skin dryness and chance of tissue breakdown.

NIC: *Skin Surveillance*

Discharge or Maintenance Evaluation

- Patient will have intact skin, free of redness, irritation, rashes, or bruising.
- Patient will be able to verbally relate measures to reduce chance of tissue injury.

LEFT-SIDED HEART FAILURE

(Burden placed on cardiovascular system by any of the following: ischemic heart disease, coronary artery disease, aortic stenosis or insufficiency, post-pump syndrome, rheumatic fever, diabetes mellitus, thyroid disease, drug abuse, alcohol abuse, left ventricular hypertrophy, mitral stenosis or insufficiency, intracardiac shunting, myocardial contusions, anemia, hypertension, myocardial infarction, valvular heart disease, dysrhythmias, tachy/bradycardia, cardiomyopathy, cardiac tamponade, constrictive pericarditis)

Decreased cardiac output ———————————→ Sympathetic nervous system stimulated
Fatigue, weakness

                                        Heart rate increases
                                          Arteriolar vasoconstriction
                                          Myocardial contractility increases
                                              Venous tone increases
                                              Venous and ventricular filling
                                              pressures increase

Decreased effective arterial blood volume

Renal compensatory changes occur
- Renal blood flow decreases
- Cortical blood flow decreases
- Aldosterone increases
- Glomerular filtration rate decreases
- Renin and angiotensin increase
- Anti-diuretic hormone increases

Sodium reabsorption and free water clearance decreases
Effective blood volume increases

Accumulation of blood in lungs

Left ventricle cannot pump blood from lungs into systemic circulation

Left ventricular pressures and volume increase

Left atrial pressures and volume increase

Fluid backs up into pulmonary vasculature = pulmonary congestion
- Paroxysmal nocturnal dyspnea • Orthopnea

Pulmonary hypertension, PA diastolic and PCWP increases

Fluid leaks into interstitial space and alveoli

Pulmonary edema
- Cough • Frothy, blood-tinged sputum • Crackles (rales)

Decreased oxygen in blood
Impaired gas exchange and hypoxia
- Tachypnea
- Cyanosis
- Confusion
- Restlessness
- Pulmonary effusion
- Pulsus alternans

RIGHT-SIDED HEART FAILURE

(Burden placed on the cardiovascular system by any of the following: left-sided heart failure, pulmonary hypertension, COPD, cor pulmonale, pulmonary embolus, thyrotoxicosis, pulmonary stenosis, mitral stenosis, arteriosclerotic heart disease, right-ventricular myocardial infarction, myocardial contusion, cardiomyopathy, valvular heart disease, atrial or ventricular septal defects, fluid overload, or sleep apnea)

↓

Accumulation of blood in systemic venous system

Lung pressure increases

Pressure in pulmonary vasculature increases

↓

Increased right atrial and ventricular pressures

Increased peripheral venous pressure

↓

Right heart cannot pump blood effectively into pulmonary system

Right-sided heart failure

- Bounding pulses
- Dysrhythmias
- S_3 or S_4 gallop

↓

Venous return decreases

Organs become congested with blood

Peripheral dependent edema occurs

↓

Congestion of portal circulation

Hepatomegaly, hepatojugular reflux

- JVD, weight gain
- Anorexia
- Ascites, abdominal pain, anorexia, nausea
- Fatigue, cyanosis

↓

Advanced heart failure

↓

- Air hunger, gasping
- Tachycardia
- Crackles, frothy blood-tinged sputum
- Skin cool and moist
- Cyanotic lips, nailbeds
- Confusion, stupor
- Enlarged right atrium and right ventricle
- Tricuspid murmur

CHAPTER 1.6

PERICARDITIS

Pericarditis is an inflammation of the pericardium that can occur by a variety of circumstances, such as accumulations of pericardial fluid or decreased compliance caused by neoplasms, fibrosis, or calcifications limiting the ability for ventricular filling during diastole. Gradual pericardial scarring usually results in constrictive pericarditis. The inflammation is usually a manifestation of another disease process, but may be drug induced, from agents such as procainamide, hydralazine, phenytoin, penicillin, phenylbutazone, minoxidil, or daunorubicin. Other causes for pericarditis include idiopathic causes, viral, bacterial, fungal, rickettsial, or protozoal infections, tuberculosis, chest trauma (pacemaker insertion, stabbing, rib fractures), uremia, sarcoidosis, myxedema, neoplasms, acute myocardial infarctions, postsurgical syndrome, autoimmune disorders (lupus, rheumatoid arthritis, scleroderma), inflammatory disorders (amyloidosis), dissecting aortic aneurysms, or radiation treatments to the thorax.

The visceral pericardium is a serous membrane that is separated from a fibrous sac, or parietal pericardium, by a small (less than 50 cc) amount of fluid. If the fluid increases to the point where the heart function is compromised, pericardial effusion occurs and cardiac tamponade becomes a critical concern. The pericardium is important because it holds the heart in a fixed position to minimize friction between it and other structures. Other functions include prevention of exercise- or hypervolemic-induced dilatation of the cardiac chambers and assistance with atrial filling during systole.

Pericarditis may be classified as acute or chronic, as well as constrictive or restrictive. Constrictive pericarditis occurs when fibrin material is deposited on the pericardium and adhesions form between the epicardium and pericardium. Restrictive pericarditis results when effusion into the pericardial sac occurs. Both types cause interference with the heart's ability to fill properly, which causes increases in systemic and pulmonary venous pressures. Eventu-

ally systemic blood pressure and cardiac output decrease.

The main symptoms of pericarditis include increased temperature, increased white blood cell count, sharp, retrosternal and/or left precordial pain that worsens while in a supine position, and a pericardial friction rub best auscultated at the lower left sternal border. The pain may be exacerbated by coughing, swallowing, breathing, or twisting. Other symptoms may be seen depending on the severity of the pericarditis and the rapidity in which the fluid accumulates. Volumes of 100 cc that accumulates quickly may produce a more life-threatening complication, cardiac tamponade, than a larger accumulation of fluid that is generated over a long period of time.

MEDICAL CARE

Oxygen: to increase available oxygen supply

Analgesics: used to alleviate pain

Steroids: given to reduce inflammation and control the symptoms of pericarditis

NSAIDs: Aspirin is the treatment of choice (650 mg q 4–6 hrs); indomethacin may cause increased coronary vascular resistance; ibuprofen helps with the pain but tends to thin the scar and could promote myocardial rupture; used to reduce fever and inflammation

IV fluids: given to help restore left ventricular filling volume and to offset any compressive effects of intrapericardial pressure increases

Inotropic drugs: given for their positive inotropic effects as well as peripheral vasodilating properties

Laboratory: white blood cell count may be elevated, sed rate may be elevated from nonspecific inflammatory response; CK–MB may be mildly elevated;

blood cultures done to identify organism responsible for infective process and to ascertain appropriate drug for eradication; renal profile done to evaluate for uremic pericarditis and worsening renal status; antinuclear antibody test (ANA) will be positive with connective tissue diseases; PPD may be done to evaluate for tuberculosis

Electrocardiography: used to monitor for dysrhythmias, such as tachycardias and atrial fibrillation, and for ST changes with acute pericarditis; there will be diffuse ST elevation in all leads except aVR and V_1, and T wave inversion when the ST segment becomes isoelectric again; PR intervals will be depressed; bradydysrhythmias may be noted in renal insufficiency patients

Echocardiography: used to establish presence of pericardial fluid and an estimate of volume, any vegetation on valves, to observe for right atrium and right ventricular dilatation, constriction with ventricular filling, wall motion abnormalities, right atrial and ventricular diastolic collapse may be signal for pre-tamponade, and to note present cardiac tamponade

Chest X-ray: used to show cardiomegaly and to assess lung fields, to assess for pleural effusion with Dressler's syndrome, and to observe for masses

Cardiac catheterization: although done rarely, can be used to evaluate need for pericardiocentesis, for differentiating diagnoses of constrictive versus restrictive cardiomyopathy, evaluating severity of constriction and for measurement of pulmonary artery pressures, especially filling pressures

Pericardiocentesis: used to relieve fluid buildup and pressure in emergency situations where the patient is deteriorating or is in shock

Surgery: open surgical drainage is usually the treatment of choice for cardiac tamponade

COMMON NURSING DIAGNOSES

ANXIETY (see MI)

Related to: change in health status, fear of death, threat to body image, threat to role functioning, pain

Defining Characteristics: restlessness, insomnia, anorexia, increased respirations, increased heart rate, increased blood pressure, difficulty concentrating, dry mouth, poor eye contact, decreased energy, irritability, crying, feelings of helplessness

DEFICIENT KNOWLEDGE (see MI)

Related to: pain, disease, lack of understanding, lack of understanding of medical condition, lack of recall

Defining Characteristics: questions regarding problems, inadequate follow-up on instructions given, misconceptions, lack of improvement of previous regimen, development of preventable complications

ACUTE PAIN (see MI)

Related to: pericardial inflammation

Defining Characteristics: sharp, stabbing precordial chest pain that increases with inspiration, lying down, swallowing, or turning, and can be relieved by leaning forward, low-grade fever, weakness, weight loss, trapezius pain, facial grimacing, clutching of hands or chest, restlessness, diaphoresis, changes in pulse and blood pressure, dyspnea

ADDITIONAL NURSING DIAGNOSES

INEFFECTIVE TISSUE PERFUSION: CARDIOPULMONARY, RENAL, PERIPHERAL, CEREBRAL

Related to: tissue ischemia, reduction or interruption of blood flow, vasoconstriction, hypovolemia, shunting, depressed ventricular function, dysrhythmias, conduction defects

Defining Characteristics: abnormal hemodynamic readings, dysrhythmias, decreased peripheral pulses, cyanosis, decreased blood pressure, shortness of breath, dyspnea, cold and clammy skin, decreased mental alertness and changes in mental status, oliguria, anuria, sluggish capillary refill, abnormal electrolyte and digoxin levels, hypoxia, ABG changes, chest pain, ventilation perfusion imbalances, changes in peripheral resistance, impaired oxygenation of myocardium, ECG changes (ST segment, T wave, U wave), LV enlargement, palpitations, abnormal renal function studies

Outcome Criteria

✔ Blood flow and perfusion to vital organs will be preserved and circulatory function will be maximized.

✔ Patient will be free of dysrhythmias.

✔ Hemodynamic parameters will be within normal limits.

NOC: *Tissue Perfusion*

INTERVENTIONS	RATIONALES
Obtain vital signs. Obtain hemodynamic values, noting deviations from baseline values.	Provides information about the hemodynamics of the patient.
Determine the presence and character of peripheral pulses, capillary refill time, skin color and temperature.	May indicate decreased perfusion resulting from impaired coronary blood flow.
Discourage any non-essential activity.	Ambulation, exercise, transfers, and Valsalva-type maneuvers can increase blood pressure and decrease tissue perfusion.
Monitor ECG for disturbances in conduction and for dysrhythmias and treat as indicated.	Decreased cardiac perfusion may instigate conduction abnormalities. Dysrhythmias may occur because of compromised function of ventricles due to pressure exerted on them by excess fluid.
Titrate vasoactive drugs as ordered.	Maintain blood pressure and heart rate at parameters set by physician for optimal perfusion with minimal workload on heart.
Administer oxygen by nasal cannula as ordered, with rate dependent on disease process and condition.	Provides oxygen necessary for tissues and organ perfusion.
Administer nonsteroidal anti-inflammatory drugs as ordered.	Helps to decrease inflammation of tissues and relieve pain.
Administer antimicrobials as ordered.	If pericarditis is a result of a bacterial or mycotic infection, the specific antimicrobial drug will be required to eradicate the causative organism.
Auscultate lungs for crackles (rales), rhonchi, or wheezes.	Suggestive of fluid overload that will further decrease tissue perfusion.
Auscultate heart sounds for S_3 or S_4 gallop, new murmurs, presence of jugular vein distention, or hepatojugular reflex.	Suggestive of impending or present heart failure or cardiac tamponade.
Monitor oxygen status with ABGs, S_vO_2 monitoring, or with pulse oximetry.	Provides information about the oxygenation status of the patient. Continuous monitoring of satu-

INTERVENTIONS	RATIONALES
	ration levels provide an instant analysis of how activity can affect oxygenation and perfusion.
Assist patient with planned, graduated levels of activity.	Allows for balance between rest and activity to decrease myocardial workload and oxygen demand. Gradual increases help to increase patient tolerance to activity without pain occurring.
Instruct patient/family on medications, dosage, effects, side effects, and contraindications.	Promotes compliance with regimen and knowledge base.
Instruct patient/family to refrain from smoking.	Smoking causes vasoconstriction which can decrease perfusion.
Instruct patient/family in dietary requirements, menu planning, sodium restrictions, foods to avoid.	Reduction of high-cholesterol and sodium foods will help to control atherosclerosis, hyperlipidemia, fluid retention, and the effects on coronary blood flow.

NIC: *Cardiac Care*

Discharge or Maintenance Evaluation

- Lung fields will be clear and free of adventitious breath sounds.
- Extremities will be warm, pink, with easily palpable pulses of equal character.
- Vital signs and hemodynamic parameters will be within normal limits for patient.
- Oxygenation will be optimal as evidenced by pulse oximetry greater than 90%, S_vO_2 greater than 75%, or normal ABGs.
- Patient will be free of chest pain and shortness of breath.
- Patient will be able to verbalize information correctly regarding medications, diet and activity limitations.

DECREASED CARDIAC OUTPUT (see MI)

Related to: fluid in pericardial sac from pericardial effusion, potential for cardiac tamponade because of effusion, damaged myocardium, decreased contractility, dysrhythmias, conduction defects, alteration in preload, alteration in afterload, vasoconstriction, myocardial ischemia, ventricular hypertrophy, heart failure, hypotension

Defining Characteristics: decreased blood pressure, tachycardia, pulsus paradoxus greater than 10 mm Hg, distended neck veins, increased central venous pressure, dysrhythmias, decreased QRS voltage or electrical alternans, diminished heart sounds, dyspnea, friction rub, cardiac output less than 4 L/min, cardiac index less than 2.5 L/min/m^2, elevated systemic vascular resistance greater than 1400 dyne–seconds/cm^5, ECG changes, S_3 or S_4 gallops, tachycardia, decreased urinary output, diaphoresis, pallor, confusion, restlessness, Kussmaul's sign, peripheral edema, decreased or absent peripheral pulses, cold, pale extremities, chest pain, narrow pulse pressure, pericardial knock, dyspnea, crackles (rales)

Outcome Criteria

✔ Vital signs and hemodynamic parameters will be within normal limits for patient, with no dysrhythmias noted, and no signs of tamponade.

NOC: *Cardiac Pump Effectiveness*

INTERVENTIONS	RATIONALES
Auscultate apical pulses and monitor heart rate and rhythm. Monitor BP in both arms. Assess for pulsus paradoxus.	Decreased contractility will be compensated by tachycardia, especially concurrently with heart failure. Blood volume will be lowered if blood pressure is increased resulting in increased afterload. Pulse decreases may be noted in association with toxic levels of digoxin. Hypotension may occur as a result of ventricular dysfunction and poor perfusion of the myocardium. Pulsus paradoxus can develop as a result of the effect of respiration on the filling of the left ventricle by the flow of blood from the pulmonary veins. During an inspiration there is less pulmonary venous return to the left heart, which is increased by an already-impaired filling caused by elevated intrapericardiac pressure with cardiac tamponade. Pericardial effusion causes heart sounds to be muffled and distant with auscultation of a friction rub. If the fluid

INTERVENTIONS	RATIONALES
	causes a constrictive problem, a "knock" will be able to be heard.
Monitor ECG for dysrhythmias and treat as indicated.	Conduction abnormalities may occur because of ischemic myocardium affecting the pumping efficiency of the heart. Diffuse ST changes will occur in all leads except aVR and V_1 during pericarditis, with T wave inversion occurring when the ST segment becomes isoelectric. Uremic patients may have bradycardias, and sinus tachycardias and atrial fibrillation are common.
Determine level of cardiac function and existing cardiac and other conditions.	Additional disease states and complications may place an additional workload on an already compromised heart.
Measure CO and perform other hemodynamic calculations.	Provides direct measurement of cardiac output function, and calculated measurement of preload and afterload.
Monitor for development of new S_3 or S_4 gallops.	S_3 gallops are usually associated with congestive heart failure but can be found with mitral regurgitation and left ventricular overload after MI. S_4 gallops can be associated with myocardial ischemia, ventricular rigidity, pulmonary hypertension, or systemic hypertension, which can decrease cardiac output.
Auscultate for presence of murmurs and/or rubs.	Indicates disturbances of normal blood flow within the heart related to incompetent valves, septal defects, or papillary muscle/chordae tendonae rupture post-MI. Presence of a rub may be associated with pericarditis and/or pericardial effusions.
Observe lower extremities for edema, distended neck veins, cold hands and feet, mottling, oliguria. Notify physician if urine output is <30 cc/hr for 2 consecutive hours.	Reduced venous return to the heart can result in low cardiac output. Oliguria results from decreased venous return because of fluid retention. Changes may be indicative of impending tamponade or pre-tamponade.
Position in semi-Fowler's position.	Promotes easier breathing by allowing for chest expansion and prevents pooling of blood in the pulmonary vasculature.

INTERVENTIONS	RATIONALES
Administer cardiac glycosides, nitrates, vasodilators, diuretics, and antihypertensives as ordered.	Used in the treatment of vasoconstriction and to reduce heart rate and contractility, reduces blood pressure by relaxation of venous and arterial smooth muscle which then in turn increases cardiac output and decreases the workload on the heart.
Titrate vasoactive drugs as ordered per physician parameters.	Maintains blood pressure and heart rate at levels to optimize cardiac output function.
Weigh every day.	Weight gain may indicate fluid retention and possible impending congestive failure.
Arrange activities so as to not overwhelm patient.	Avoids fatiguing patient and decreasing cardiac output further. Balancing rest with activity minimizes energy expenditure and myocardial oxygen demands by maintaining adequate cardiac output.
Avoid Valsalva-type maneuvers with straining, coughing or moving.	Increasing intra-abdominal pressure results in an abrupt decrease in cardiac output by preventing blood from being pumped into the thoracic cavity and, thus, less blood being pumped into the heart which then decreases the heart rate. When the pressure is released, there is a sudden overload of blood which then increases preload and the workload on the heart.
Provide small, easy to digest, meals.	Large meals increase the work load on the heart by diverting blood flow to that area.
Have emergency equipment and medications available at all times.	Coronary occlusion, lethal dysrhythmias, infarction extensions or intractable pain may precipitate cardiac arrest that requires life support and resuscitation.
If tamponade occurs, do not place patient in Trendelenburg position. Administer oxygen and IV fluids as prescribed. Administer other emergency medications as per protocol.	Trendelenburg position helps to channel the required blood flow to vital organs to maintain perfusion and will increase preload and worsen the constriction of the heart. Fluids increase preload and cardiac

INTERVENTIONS	RATIONALES
	output. Emergency drugs may be required if lethal dysrhythmias occur because of low cardiac output or constriction of heart.
Prepare patient/family for emergency pericardiocentesis and assist with emergent procedure.	Emergent periocardiocentesis will be required to save patient's life by reducing the constriction on the heart and thereby increasing cardiac output to maintain adequate hemodynamic parameters to sustain life.
Instruct patient/family on medications, dose, effects, side effects, contraindications, and avoidance of over-the-counter drugs without physician approval.	Promotes knowledge and compliance with regimen. Prevents any adverse drug interactions.
Instruct patient/family in activity limitations. Demonstrate exercises to be done.	Promotes compliance. Reduces potential for decrease in cardiac output by lessening the workload placed on the heart.
Instruct to report chest pain immediately.	May indicate complications of decreased cardiac output.
Instruct patient/family regarding placement of pulmonary artery catheter, and postprocedure care.	Alleviates fear and promotes knowledge. Pulmonary artery catheter necessary for direct measurement of cardiac output and for obtaining values for other hemodynamic measurements.

NIC: *Hemodynamic Regulation*

Discharge or Maintenance Evaluation

- Patient will have no signs or symptoms of cardiac tamponade or pericarditis
- Patient will be able to accurately recall information.
- Patient will have no chest pain or shortness of breath.
- Vital signs and hemodynamic parameters will be within normal limits for age and disease condition without pulsus paradoxus.
- Minimal activity will be tolerated without fatigue or dyspnea.
- Urinary output will be adequate.
- Cardiac output will be adequate to ensure adequate perfusion of all body systems.

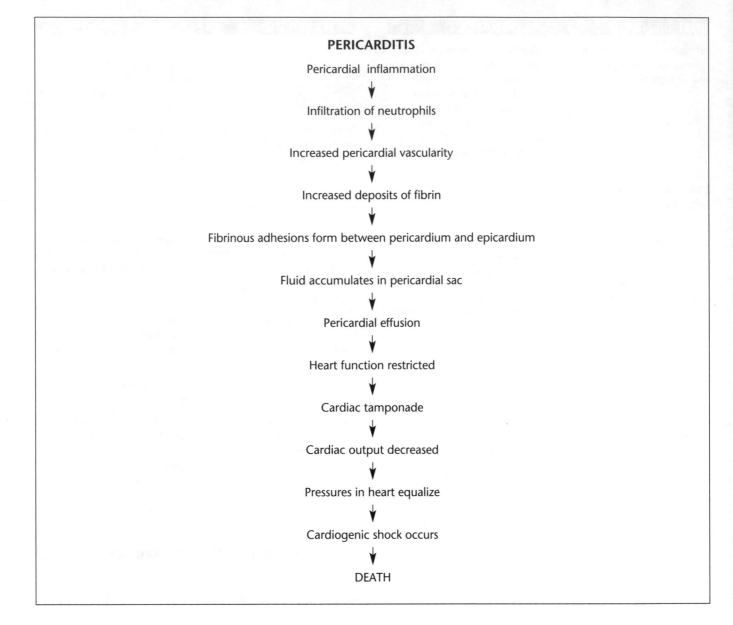

PERICARDITIS

Pericardial inflammation

↓

Infiltration of neutrophils

↓

Increased pericardial vascularity

↓

Increased deposits of fibrin

↓

Fibrinous adhesions form between pericardium and epicardium

↓

Fluid accumulates in pericardial sac

↓

Pericardial effusion

↓

Heart function restricted

↓

Cardiac tamponade

↓

Cardiac output decreased

↓

Pressures in heart equalize

↓

Cardiogenic shock occurs

↓

DEATH

CHAPTER 1.7

PACEMAKERS

Cardiac pacemakers are used to provide an electrical stimulus to depolarize the heart and cause a contraction to occur at a controlled rate. The function of the pacemaker, or pacer, is to maintain the heart rate when the patient's own intrinsic system is unable to do so. The stimulus is produced by a pulse generator and delivered via electrodes/leads that are implanted in the epicardium or endocardium. The electrodes may be unipolar or bipolar and the proximal end attaches to the pulse generator.

In the unipolar electrode, one wire, positioned in the heart, senses and stimulates the electrical heart activity and is connected with the negative terminal on the pulse generator. The other electrode, or ground, is attached to the positive terminal on the pulse generator. This type of lead usually requires a lower threshold of stimulation.

The bipolar electrode has both the sensing and ground electrode in the catheter, and provides better contact with the heart muscle. In the event that one of the bipolar wires malfunctions, it can still be used as a unipolar lead.

The pacemaker will produce a pacer spike on the ECG prior to the depolarized waveform and this indicates pacemaker capture. Continuous observation for problems with the pacemaker should ensure that failure to pace, failure to capture, and failure to sense are treated promptly.

The pacemaker rate is set depending on the patient's requirements. The optimal setting is one in which the lowest rate is used that controls the particular dysrhythmia and provides for adequate cardiac output. The stimulation threshold is the minimal amount of electrical energy required to stimulate the heart to produce a 1:1 capture, and is measured in milliamperes (mA). The sensitivity control reflects the size of the wave that is sensed by the pacemaker and is measured in millivolts (mV), with the smaller number relating to the most sensitivity. Pacemakers are used for varying degrees of heart block, sick sinus syndrome, sinus node dysfunction, overriding of some cardiac dysrhythmias, prophylactically during diagnostic testing, myocardial infarctions, congestive heart failure caused by rhythm disturbances, after open heart surgery or in congenital anomalies of the heart.

Temporary pacers are used when the duration of need is short and permanent pacers are placed for life-long use. Temporary pacemakers can be placed via a transthoracic approach during open heart surgery, transvenous approach into the right atrium or right ventricle, or transcutaneously (external pacer) with skin electrodes while awaiting placement of an internal pacemaker.

Placement of the temporary pacemaker can be performed at the bedside in cases of emergency, but use of fluoroscopy is recommended, when feasible, to ensure proper placement. External pacemaker electrodes can either be placed on the chest, or one to the anterior and one posterior to the chest.

Synchronous pacing, known as demand pacing, is commonly used because the pacer is able to sense the patient's heart impulse. If the patient's rate falls below the rate set on the pacer, the pacer is able to sense this and send an impulse to the desired chamber of the heart and cause the rate to remain at the preset level. Dual chamber synchronous pacing, or AV sequential, is the closest to normal physiologic function and facilitates the atrial kick.

Asynchronous, or fixed-rate, pacing provides impulses to the atrium, ventricle, or both regardless of the patient's intrinsic rate. This should be used solely for those occasions when no electrical activity is present to avoid potential lethal competitive dysrhythmias.

Pacemakers are classified by a 5-letter code developed by the Inter-Society Commission for Heart Disease in which letters are used to denote the chamber paced, the chamber sensed, response to sensing, programmable functions and antitachydysrhythmia functions.

Several complications may occur as a result of pacemakers—pneumothorax, hemothorax, myocardial perforation, hematoma, bleeding, dysrhythmias, pulmonary embolism, electrical microshock, cardiac tamponade, coronary artery laceration, failure to pace, failure to sense, failure to capture, and infection.

MEDICAL CARE

Chest X-ray: used to evaluate placement of lead wires

Electrocardiography: used to monitor for heart rhythm problems, dysrhythmias, and for function/malfunction of pacemakers

Surgery: for placement of permanent pacemakers

COMMON NURSING DIAGNOSES

ACUTE PAIN (see MI)

Related to: pacemaker insertion or transcutaneous pacing

Defining Characteristics: communication of pain, facial grimacing, restlessness, changes in pulse and blood pressure

ANXIETY (see MI)

Related to: need for pacemaker, change in health status, fear of death, threat to body image, threat to role functioning, pain

Defining Characteristics: restlessness, insomnia, anorexia, increased respirations, increased heart rate, increased blood pressure, difficulty concentrating, dry mouth, poor eye contact, decreased energy, irritability, crying, feelings of helplessness

DEFICIENT KNOWLEDGE (see MI)

Related to: need for pacemaker, lack of understanding, lack of understanding of medical condition, lack of recall, new health crisis

Defining Characteristics: questions regarding problems, inadequate follow-up on instructions given, misconceptions, lack of improvement of previous regimen, development of preventable complications

ADDITIONAL NURSING DIAGNOSES

 ### INEFFECTIVE TISSUE PERFUSION: CARDIOPULMONARY, CEREBRAL

Related to: cardiac dysrhythmias, heart blocks, tachydysrhythmias, decreased blood pressure, decreased cardiac output, decreased blood flow

Defining Characteristics: decreased blood pressure, decreased heart rate, decreased cardiac output, changes in level of consciousness, mental changes, cold, clammy skin, cardiopulmonary arrest

Outcome Criteria

✔ Patient will be free of dysrhythmias with adequate cardiac output to perfuse all body organs.

NOC: *Tissue Perfusion: Cardiac, Pulmonary, Cerebral*

INTERVENTIONS	RATIONALES
Monitor ECG for changes in rhythm and rate, and presence of dysrhythmias. Treat as indicated.	Observation for pacemaker malfunction promotes prompt treatment. Pacer electrodes may irritate ventricle and promote ventricular ectopy.
Keep monitor alarms on at all times, with rate limits set 2–5 beats above and below set pacemaker rate.	Provides for immediate detection of pacemaker failure or malfunction.
Obtain and observe rhythm strip every 4 hours and prn. Notify physician for abnormalities.	Identifies proper functioning of pacemaker, with appropriate capture and sensing.
Monitor vital signs every 15 minutes until stable, then every 2 hours.	Assures adequate perfusion and cardiac output. Myocardial perforation can lead to hypotension.
Monitor for signs of failure to capture and correct problem.	Potential causes are low voltage, battery failure, faulty connections, catheter or wire fracture, improper placement of catheter, fibrosis at tip of catheter or ventricular perforation.
Monitor for signs of failure to sense patient's own rhythm and correct problem.	Potential causes are battery failure, improper placement of catheter lead, lead insulation breakage, pulse generator failure, lead fracture, or sensitivity set too high. These things may cause the pacemaker to compete

INTERVENTIONS	RATIONALES
	with the patient's own intrinsic cardiac rhythm.
Monitor for signs of failure to pace and correct problem.	Potential causes are battery failure, lead dislodgment, disconnection, catheter lead fracture, generator failure, or oversensing because some other activity is sensed and misinterpreted as a QRS complex.
Ensure that all electrical equipment is grounded. Avoid touching equipment and patient at same time. Patients should not use radios, shavers, and so forth.	Prevents potential for microshock and accidental electrocution. Electric current seeks the path of least resistance, and the potential for stray current to travel through the electrode into the patient's heart may precipitate ventricular fibrillation.
Place a dry rubber glove over exposed terminals or leads. Wear rubber gloves when handling the electrodes, terminals, etc.	Provides insulation to prevent stray current contact. Static electricity may pass from person to person through the leads.
Pacemaker batteries should not be changed while the pacer is in use. In cases of hardship, batteries should be changed as quickly as possible, wearing rubber gloves, and using utmost caution to avoid touching the battery terminals.	Patients may be totally dependent on the pacemaker for their rhythm and cardiac output, and the loss of time incurred to change the battery may result in life-threatening consequences.
Monitor for muscle twitching or hiccoughs.	May indicate lead has dislodged and migrated to chest wall or diaphragm after perforation of heart.
Monitor for sudden complaints of chest pain, and auscultate for pericardial friction rub or muffled heart tones. Observe for JVD and pulsus paradoxus.	May indicate perforation of the pericardial sac, and impending cardiac tamponade.
Monitor for dizziness, syncope, weakness, pronounced fatigue, edema, chest pain, palpitations, pulsations in neck veins, or dyspnea.	During ventricular pacing, AV synchrony may cease and cause a sudden decrease in cardiac output. May indicate "pacemaker syndrome" or failure of the pacer to function which results in decreased perfusion.
Limit movement of the extremity involved near insertion site.	Prevents accidental disconnection and dislodgment of lead wires.
If pacemaker is used concurrently with pulmonary artery catheter, obtain wedge pressure only as physician orders.	Inflation of pulmonary artery catheter balloon for capillary wedge pressures may dislodge pacer lead wires and cause pacemaker malfunction.

INTERVENTIONS	RATIONALES
Monitor patient for low blood sugar levels, use of glucocorticoids or sympathomimetics, mineralocorticoids, or anesthetics.	May impair the pacemaker stimulation thresholds.
Protect patient from microwave ovens, radar, diathermy, electrocautery, TENS units, and so forth.	Environmental electromagnetic interference may impair demand pacemaker function by disrupting the electrical stimulus.
If the patient experiences cardiopulmonary arrest, the pacemaker should be turned off and disconnected from the patient for ventricular fibrillation. After defibrillation, the pacemaker should be reconnected, turned on, and output should be raised to 20 mA, rate above 60.	Disconnection prior to DC countershock prevents pacer damage and potential of diversion of electrical current.
Instruct patient on need for pacemaker, procedures involved, expected outcomes, etc.	Provides knowledge, decreases fear and anxiety, and provides baseline for further instruction.
Instruct patient/family in checking pulse rate every day for 1 month, then every week, and to notify physician if rate varies more than 5 beats/minute.	Provides patient with some control over situation. Assists in promoting a sense of security. Allows for prompt recognition of deviations from preset rate and potential pacemaker failure.
Instruct patient/family on activity limitations: avoid excessive bending, stretching, lifting more than 5 pounds, strenuous activities, or contact sports.	Full range of motion can be recovered in approximately 2 months after fibrosis stabilizes the pacemaker lead. Excessive activity may cause lead dislodgment.
Instruct patient to avoid shoulder-strap purses, suspenders, or firing rifle resting over generator site.	May promote irritation over implanted generator site.
Instruct patient to wear a medic-alert bracelet with information about the type of pacemaker and rate.	Provides information about the patient, his condition, and pacemaker should he be incapacitated and cannot speak for himself.
Instruct patient to notify physician if radiation therapy is needed and to wear a lead shield.	Therapy can cause failure of the silicone chip in the pacer with repeated radiation.
Instruct patient to avoid electromagnetic fields, magnetic resonance imaging, radio transmitters, arc welding equipment, large running motors, or large ungrounded power tools. If patient notices dizziness or palpitations, he should try to move	May affect the function of the pacemaker and alter the programmed settings. Sometimes these magnetic fields will affect the pacemaker function only if direct contact is made and once distance is placed between the patient and the equipment,

(continues)

(continued)

INTERVENTIONS	RATIONALES
away from the area, and if symptoms persist, to seek medical attention. Late model microwave ovens are no longer thought to be a threat due to tighter seals preventing leakage of energy.	normal function of the pacemaker resumes. If programmed settings are altered the pacer will require reprogramming. Hyperbaric oxygen chambers may also affect pacer function.

NIC: *Circulatory Care: Manual Assist Device*

Discharge or Maintenance Evaluation

- Patient will be free of dysrhythmias and able to maintain cardiac output within normal limits.
- Patient will be able to recall accurately all instructions given.
- Patient will be able to recall and adhere to all activity restrictions.
- Permanent pacemaker function will be without complication, with no lead dislodgment or competitive rhythms noted.

IMPAIRED SKIN INTEGRITY

Related to: insertion of temporary or permanent pacemaker, alteration in activity

Defining Characteristics: disruption of skin tissue, insertion sites

Outcome Criteria

✔ Patient will have healed wound sites without signs/symptoms of infection.

NOC: *Wound Healing*

INTERVENTIONS	RATIONALES
Inspect pacemaker insertion site for erythema, edema, warmth, drainage, or tenderness.	Prompt detection of problems promotes prompt treatment.
Change dressing daily, or per hospital protocol, using sterile technique.	Allows for observation of site and detection of inflammation or infection. Sterile technique is recommended due to the close proximity of the portal to the heart increasing the potential for systemic infection.

INTERVENTIONS	RATIONALES
Pacemaker lead wires should be coiled and taped securely to patient; pulse generator should be secured to avoid pulling.	Avoids potential for accidentally disconnecting pacemaker from generator, or dislodging leads from heart.
Instruct patient/family on wound care to pacer site; to avoid taking showers for 2 weeks after pacer insertion.	Promotes compliance with care to decrease potential for infection. Moisture can promote bacterial growth.
Instruct patient/family to observe for and report to physician the following symptoms: redness, drainage, temperature greater than 100 degrees, pain or tenderness tosite, or swelling at site.	Provides for prompt recognition of complications and facilitates prompt treatment.
Instruct patient to avoid constrictive clothing until site has healed.	May cause discomfort at incision site from pressure and rubbing against skin.
Instruct patient on need for pacemaker removal/replacement.	Pulse generators may require removal for battery replacement, fracture of lead wires, pacemaker failure, and so forth.

NIC: *Wound Care*

Discharge or Maintenance Evaluation

- Patient will have well-healed incision with no signs/symptoms of infection.
- Patient will be able to recall accurately all instructions given.
- Patient will be able to demonstrate appropriate wound care prior to discharge.

RISK FOR INJURY

Related to: pacemaker failure, hemothorax or pneumothorax after insertion, bleeding, lead migration, heart perforation

Defining Characteristics: decreased cardiac output, hemorrhage, diaphoresis, hypotension, restlessness, dyspnea, cyanosis, chest pain, muscle twitching, hiccoughs, muffled heart sounds, jugular vein distention, pulsus paradoxus

Outcome Criteria

✔ Patient will be free of any complications that may be associated with pacemaker insertion.

NOC: *Risk Control*

INTERVENTIONS	RATIONALES
Monitor for bleeding at pacer site. Apply pressure dressings as warranted.	Bleeding at incisional site may occur based on the patient's coagulation status. Pressure dressings or manual pressure may be required to control bleeding.
Monitor for pulse presence at site distal to pacer insertion.	Hemorrhage may promote tissue edema and compression to arterial blood flow resulting in diminished or absent pulses.
Monitor for hypotension, diaphoresis, dyspnea, and restlessness.	May indicate puncture of the subclavian vasculature and potential hemothorax.
Monitor for dyspnea, chest pain, pallor, cyanosis, absent or diminished breath sounds, tracheal deviation, and feeling of impending doom.	May indicate puncture of the lung and pneumothorax.
Monitor for muscle twitching and hiccoughs. Notify physician.	May indicate perforation of the heart with pacing to the chest wall or diaphragm.
Observe for signs/symptoms of cardiac tamponade—pericardial friction rub, pulsus paradoxus, muffled heart tones, JVD.	May indicate perforation of the pericardial sac and impending cardiac tamponade.
Instruct patient to notify nurse for chest pain, shortness of breath, hiccoughs, or bleeding.	May indicate potential complications from pacemaker insertion. Allows for prompt notification for timely intervention.

NIC: *Surgical Precautions*

Discharge or Maintenance Evaluation

- Patient will have no complications associated with pacemaker insertion.
- Patient will have clear breath sounds, with no inadequacy of oxygenation.
- Patient will be free of infection or hemorrhage.

IMPAIRED PHYSICAL MOBILITY

Related to: newly implanted pacemaker, pain, limb immobilization

Defining Characteristics: inability to move as desired, imposed restrictions on activity, decreased muscle strength and coordination, limited range of motion

Outcome Criteria

✔ Patient will regain optimal mobility within limitations of disease process, and will have increased strength and function of limbs.

NOC: *Mobility Level*

INTERVENTIONS	RATIONALES
Evaluate patient's perception of degree of immobility.	Psychological and physical immobility are interrelated. Psychological immobility is used as a defense mechanism when patients have no control over their body, and this can lead to disproportionate fear and concern. Changes in body image promote psychological immobility and may result in emotional handicaps.
Maintain bedrest for 24–48 hours after permanent pacer inserted if hospital protocol dictates.	Provides time for stabilization of leads and decreases potential for dislodgment.
Immobilize extremity proximal to pacer insertion site with arm board, sling, and so forth.	Prevents potential for dislodgment of lead because of movement.
Provide ROM to unaffected extremity as warranted.	ROM prevents stiffness of shoulders and joint immobility.
Encourage extension/dorsiflexion exercises to feet every 1–2 hours.	Promotes venous return, prevents venous stasis, and decreases potential for thrombophlebitis.
Monitor for progression and improvement in stiffness/pain.	Physical therapy may be required if immobility results are severe.
Apply trapeze bar to bed.	Allows for easier movement by allowing patient to assist with movement in bed.
Reposition every 2 hours and prn.	Prevents potential for immobility hazards such as pressure areas and atelectasis.
Encourage deep breathing exercises every 1–2 hours; avoid forceful coughing.	Facilitates lung expansion and decreases potential for atelectasis. Coughing may dislodge pacemaker lead.
Instruct patient in range of motion exercises 5 days after permanent pacer insertion to affected extremity.	Promotes gradual increase of activity. Stretching should be avoided until lead wire has been secured in heart by fibrotic changes.

NIC: *Exercise Therapy: Muscle Control*

Discharge or Maintenance Evaluation

- Patient will regain optimal mobility of all joints with no signs or symptoms of complications.
- Patient will be able to demonstrate and recall instructions regarding deep breathing and range of motion exercises.

▧ DISTURBED BODY IMAGE

Related to: presence of pulse generator, loss of control of heart function, disease process

Defining Characteristics: fear of rejection, fear of reaction from others, negative feelings about body, refusal to participate in care, refusal to look at wound

Outcome Criteria

✔ Patient will accept change in body image and deal constructively with situation.

NOC: *Self-Esteem*

INTERVENTIONS	RATIONALES
Evaluate level of patient's knowledge about disease process, treatment, and anxiety.	May identify extent of problem and interventions that will be required.
Evaluate the extent of loss to the patient/family, and what it means to them.	Depending on the time frame for patient teaching prior to the insertion of the pacemaker, the patient may not have received adequate information, and may have difficulty dealing with changes in his body appearance as well as generalized health condition and loss of control.
Evaluate stage of grieving.	Provides recognition of appropriate versus inappropriate behavior. Prolonged grief may require further care.
Observe for withdrawal, manipulation, noninvolvement with care, or increased dependency.	May suggest problems with adjustment to health condition, grief response to the loss of

INTERVENTIONS	RATIONALES
Set limits on dysfunctional behavior and help patient to seek positive behaviors that will assist with recovery.	function, or worry about others accepting patient's new body status. Patients may deal with crises in the same manner as previously dealt and may need redirection in behaviors to facilitate recovery and acceptance.
Provide positive reinforcement during care and with instruction and setting goals. Do not give false reassurance.	Promotes trust and establishes rapport with patient as well as provides an opportunity to plan for the future based on reality of situation.
Provide opportunity for patient to take active role in wound care.	Promotes self-esteem and facilitates feelings of control of body and health.
Provide reassurance that pacemaker will not alter sexual activity.	Promotes knowledge and decreases fear.
Discuss potential for mood changes, anger, grief, and so forth after discharge, and to seek help if persisting for lengthy time.	Facilitates identification that feelings are not unusual and must be recognized in order to effectively deal with them.
Identify support groups for patient/family to contact.	Provides ongoing support for patient and family and allows for ventilation of feelings.
Consult counselor/therapist as warranted.	May require further interventions to resolve emotional or psychological problems.

NIC: *Body Image Enhancement*

Discharge or Maintenance Evaluation

- Patient will be able to effectively deal with body image disturbances in present situation.
- Patient will be able to talk with family, therapist, or others about emotional or psychological problems.
- Patient will be able to problem-solve and identify short- and long-term goals within reasonable expectations of clinical situation.

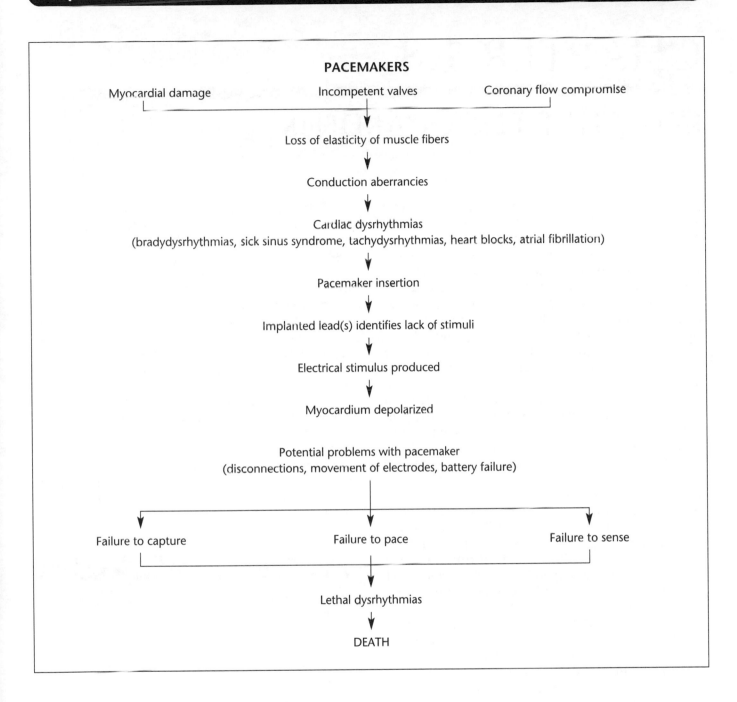

PACEMAKERS

Myocardial damage   Incompetent valves   Coronary flow compromise

Loss of elasticity of muscle fibers

Conduction aberrancies

Cardiac dysrhythmias
(bradydysrhythmias, sick sinus syndrome, tachydysrhythmias, heart blocks, atrial fibrillation)

Pacemaker insertion

Implanted lead(s) identifies lack of stimuli

Electrical stimulus produced

Myocardium depolarized

Potential problems with pacemaker
(disconnections, movement of electrodes, battery failure)

Failure to capture   Failure to pace   Failure to sense

Lethal dysrhythmias

DEATH

CHAPTER 1.8

INFECTIVE ENDOCARDITIS

Bacterial endocarditis is now referred to as infective endocarditis (IE) because of the presence of other organisms besides bacteria being the causative agent. It is an infection of the cardiac valves, inner lining of the heart, the chordae tendineae, the mural endothelium, and the septum that is characterized as a systemic illness. Endocarditis may be misdiagnosed as other infections in the early stages if signs and symptoms of cardiac involvement are not present. Common complaints range from fever with temperature less than 102 degrees, chills, arthralgia, lethargy, and anorexia. Acute endocarditis may result in death within a matter of hours if not treated. Antimicrobial therapy can decrease mortality to 15%, but heart failure secondary to valvular scarring and damage can occur after the infection is resolved.

Almost any organism can cause endocarditis but the most common ones noted have been *Staphylococcus aureus*, *Streptococcus viridans*, *Enterococci faecalis*, gram-negative rods, viruses, *Staphylococcus epidermidis*, *Streptococcus pneumoniae*, *Pseudomonas aeruginosa*, *Candida albicans*, and *Aspergillus fumigatus*.

Endocarditis may be subdivided into the acute and subacute classes, depending on the virulence of the organism involved and the length of duration. Acute infective endocarditis (AIE) has less than one month duration whereas subacute infective endocarditis (SIE) is usually greater than one month in duration. SIE usually involves congenitally-deformed or damaged heart valves, and AIE usually involves normal heart valves. Trauma in many forms can occur to the epithelial layer of the valves/endocardium causing injury and deposits of platelets and fibrin to adhere to this surface. This is known as nonbacterial thrombotic endocarditis (NBTE). After this stage, the heart is then set up for vegetation to colonize from bacteria from other areas of the body during transient episodes of bacteremia. As these organisms grow, more platelets and fibrin adhere and eventually, valves are destroyed, vegetation breaks off and embolizes to other areas of the body, and a systemic immune response occurs.

Patients who are at risk for endocarditis include those with rheumatic heart disease, open-heart surgery, congenital heart defects, prosthetic valve replacements, mitral valve prolapse, cardiomyopathy, inflammatory gastrointestinal disease, previous infectious endocarditis, dental procedures, gynecologic surgery or procedures, genitourinary surgery or procedures, invasive tests or lines, infected peripheral or central venous lines, IUDs, AV shunts or fistulas, skin abnormalities in pre-existing cardiac disease, immunosuppressive therapy, and IV drug use.

Patients who have had prosthetic valves placed and who develop endocarditis are divided into early (occurring less than two months postoperatively) and late (occurring greater than two months postoperatively) classes, and develop chills, fever, leukocytosis, and/or a new murmur. Mortality is higher in early prosthetic valve endocarditis and is a serious problem.

MEDICAL CARE

Antimicrobials: penicillin is the treatment of choice for *Streptococcus viridans*, with cephalothin or vancomycin being alternate choices; penicillin plus gentamicin is the treatment of choice for *Steptococcus faecalis*; synthetic penicillins, such as oxacillin or nafcillin, cephalothin and/or gentamicin are used in *Staphylococcus epidermidis*

Laboratory: a series of blood cultures is done to isolate the causative organism and determine sensitivity to antimicrobial agents; CBC is used to assess for anemia that may occur in up to 70% of patients, to monitor leukocyte levels associated with splenomegaly; sedimentation rate may be increased because of immune processes; RA factor increased; or other abnormalities associated with specific organ dysfunction may occur, and to assess platelet counts; immune titers show antigen–antibody response

Electrocardiography: shows alterations in conduction, dysrhythmias, or ischemia

Echocardiography: used to establish diagnosis, to determine underlying cardiac disease, to estimate myocardial contractility, to demonstrate early mitral valve closure and aortic insufficiency, and to assess the amount of valvular dysfunction and complications like ruptured chordae tendineae or valve cusps, abscesses, or presence of prosthetic valves

Radiology: chest X-ray used to show pulmonary infiltration or pleural effusions

Nuclear cardiologic testing: Technetium-99 scans and Gallium-67 imaging used to evaluate the extent of the infective process and to evaluate potential as a surgical candidate

Surgery: valve replacement is necessary if patient develops intractable congestive heart failure with hemodynamic compromise, persistent bacteremia despite antimicrobial treatment, prosthetic valve endocarditis, major systemic emboli, gram negative or fungal infection; drainage of abscesses or empyema; repair of peripheral or cerebral mycotic aneurysms

Prophylaxis: prophylactic antibiotic therapy must be prescribed prior to dental procedures, urethral or gynecologic procedures, or surgery

COMMON NURSING DIAGNOSES

DECREASED CARDIAC OUTPUT (see MI)

Related to: complications with infected heart valves, potential for cardiac tamponade because of effusion, damaged myocardium, decreased contractility, dysrhythmias, conduction defects, alteration in preload, alteration in afterload, vasoconstriction, myocardial ischemia, ventricular hypertrophy, and fluid volume excess

Defining Characteristics: decreased blood pressure, tachycardia, pulsus paradoxus greater than 10 mm Hg, distended neck veins, increased central venous pressure, dysrhythmias, decreased QRS voltage or electrical alternans, diminished heart sounds, dyspnea, friction rub, cardiac output less than 4 L/min, cardiac index less than 2.5 L/min/m², change in mental status, change or new cardiac murmur, arterial emboli, decreased urine output, cyanosis, cold, clammy skin

ANXIETY (see MI)

Related to: change in health status, fear of death, threat to body image, threat to role functioning, pain

Defining Characteristics: restlessness, insomnia, anorexia, increased respirations, increased heart rate, increased blood pressure, difficulty concentrating, dry mouth, poor eye contact, decreased energy, irritability, crying, feelings of helplessness

DEFICIENT KNOWLEDGE (see MI)

Related to: new disease, lack of understanding, lack of understanding of medical condition, lack of recall

Defining Characteristics: questions regarding problems, inadequate follow-up on instructions given, misconceptions, lack of improvement of previous regimen, development of preventable complications

ADDITIONAL NURSING DIAGNOSES

INEFFECTIVE TISSUE PERFUSION: CARDIOPULMONARY, CEREBRAL, RENAL, GASTROINTESTINAL, AND PERIPHERAL

Related to: valvular vegetation emboli, platelet–fibrin emboli, and immunologic responses causing allergic vasculitis

Defining Characteristics: petechiae, arthritis, arthralgia, myalgias, decreased peripheral pulses, Janeway's lesions, Roth's spots, Osler's nodes, lower back pain, abdominal pain, splinter hemorrhages to subungual areas, hematuria, oliguria, anuria, chest pain, shortness of breath, dyspnea, confusion, weakness, convulsions, coma, hemiplegia, aphasia, hemiparesis, cardiac tamponade, pericardial friction rub, murmur, dysrhythmias, conduction defects, cold, clammy skin, cyanosis, mental status changes, hypotension, tachycardia, decreased urinary output, increased BUN

Outcome Criteria

✔ Patient will achieve and maintain adequate tissue perfusion to all body systems.

✔ Patient will have adequate circulation to all extremities. System embolization will resolve with minimal to no long-term complications.

NOC: *Tissue Perfusion*

INTERVENTIONS	RATIONALES
Determine mental status and level of consciousness. Observe for headache, numbness, tingling, ataxia, sudden blindness, hemiparesis, paralysis, aphasia, convulsions, or coma, and notify physician.	Symptoms may indicate embolization to cerebrum which may require emergency treatment.
Monitor ECG for conduction abnormalities, especially prolonged PR interval, new left bundle branch block, new right bundle branch block with or without left anterior hemiblock. Treat as indicated per protocol.	Because of the close proximity of aortic valve cusps to the conduction system, bacterial invasion and proliferation may extend the infection process into the myocardium and cause dysrhythmias. Extension of the infection from the mitral valve to the Bundle of His and AV node may result in junctional tachycardia, Mobitz I, second degree or third degree AV blocks.
Observe for sudden shortness of breath, tachypnea, pleurisy-type pain, pallor or cyanosis. Administer oxygen as ordered.	Arterial emboli may affect the heart and other vital organs. Venous congestion may result in thrombus formation in deep veins and cause embolization to lungs, or embolization of vegetation thrombi may result in pulmonary embolus. Supplemental oxygen may be required to compensate for decreased perfusion and to help alleviate hypoxia and hypoxemia.
Evaluate chest pain, tachycardia, decreased blood pressure. Auscultate heart sounds for new or changed murmurs, pericardial friction rubs, abnormal lung sounds (crackles, rales), or muffled heart tones.	Arterial emboli may affect the heart and cause myocardial infarction. New murmurs may occur as a result of valve scarring and distortion, valve aneurysm, septal rupture, papillary muscle rupture, or myocardial abscess rupture. Rupture into the pericardial sac can cause cardiac tamponade, in which heart tones will be muffled. Pericardial friction rubs may indicate pericarditis. Abnormal lung sounds may indicate impending congestive heart failure.
Observe extremities for swelling, erythema, tenderness, pain, positive Homans' sign, and/or positive Pratt's sign. Observe for decreased peripheral pulses, pallor, coldness, cyanosis.	Bedrest promotes venous stasis which can increase the risk of thromboembolus formation. Actual vegetation emboli can migrate and occlude peripheral arteries, leading to tissue ischemia and necrosis.

INTERVENTIONS	RATIONALES
Monitor for complaints of abdominal pain to left upper abdomen with radiation to left shoulder, abdominal rigidity, tenderness, nausea, or vomiting.	May indicate embolization to spleen. Vegetative emboli may occlude mesenteric artery and cause bowel infarction. Splenomegaly may be caused by antigen stimulation and allergic vasculitis.
Test all stools and gastrointestinal drainage for occult blood.	Bacteremia can lead to hemorrhage and prompt identification of occult bleeding allows for timely treatment and reversal of coagulopathy.
Observe urine for hematuria, oliguria, anuria, complaints of flank or back pain.	Allergic vasculitis from endocarditis can result in focal, acute, or chronic glomerulonephritis and progress to renal insufficiency, renal failure, and uremia.
Observe for petechiae on mucous membranes, conjunctiva, neck, trunk, wrists, and ankles. Observe for splinter hemorrhages in subungual areas, Osler's nodes to distal fingers and toes, sides of fingers, palms or thighs, and for Janeway's lesions to the palms, soles of feet, arms and legs.	Petechiae is one of the classic symptoms of endocarditis as a result of allergic vasculitis. Petechiae are usually 1–2 mm in diameter, flat, red with white or gray centers, nontender, and groups fade within a few days. Petechiae may be noted in other diagnoses and they should be ruled out. Hemorrhages to the subungual areas may be seen in early infective endocarditis but may be seen in trauma, with hemo- or peritoneal dialysis, or in mitral stenosis. Osler's nodes are nodules that range from 1–10 mm in diameter, red with white centers, overtly tender, and are usually a late sign of endocarditis, typically found in subacute endocarditis infections. Janeway's lesions are nontender, reddened or pink macular lesions, 1–5 mm in diameter, and usually change to tan and fade within 2 weeks. These are usually an early sign of endocarditis.
Evaluate complaints of arthritis, arthralgia, and severe lower back pain. Medicate as needed.	Pain may occur in endocarditis because of localized immune responses or in decreased perfusion.
Monitor blood culture and sensitivity reports.	Usually 3–6 blood cultures are done in a series to assess for sustained bacteremia because microorganisms are continually

INTERVENTIONS	RATIONALES
	released into the system In endocarditis. The series prevents the possibility of false readings. Cultures determine the specific organism responsible for the bacteremia, and sensitivity results enable the choice of antimicrobials to be suited to the specific infection.
Administer antimicrobials as ordered.	Antimicrobials should not be started until culture series is completed in subacute IE, but with acute IE, empiric antimicrobials are given until cultures are available. In some instances, early negative results may indicate only that the culture could not be grown because of low levels of bacteria or an unusual organism being present. Obtaining cultures after antibiotics or antimicrobials have been started do not give accurate information.
Instruct patient in signs/symptoms to report to physician.	Promotes knowledge and compliance with regimen. Prompt recognition of potential complications allows for immediate attention and treatment.
Instruct patient/family in monitoring temperature, and to notify physician if increases above physician-set parameters.	May indicate impending or present infective process.
Instruct patient/family regarding community resources, drug rehabilitation centers, and so forth, as needed.	If patient relies on recreational drugs, or abuses medications, drug treatment centers may be accessed to prevent further risk factors for developing infection.
Instruct patient in need for antimicrobial prophylaxis prior to dental procedures or surgeries.	Prophylactic treatment will be required to ensure latent microorganisms do not reactivate and cause recurrence of IE.

NIC: *Shock Management*

Discharge or Maintenance Evaluation

- Patient will be free of infection.
- Patient will have adequate tissue perfusion to all body systems.
- Patient will be mentally lucid, with no confusion or neurological deficits.

- Patient will have adequate urinary output with no hematuria, and renal function studies will be within normal limits.
- Patient will be able to recall accurately the information instructed.

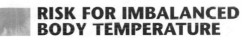

RISK FOR IMBALANCED BODY TEMPERATURE

Related to: bacteremia, allergic vasculitis, arterial occlusion/infarction, abscess

Defining Characteristics: body temperature greater or less than normal range, flushed warm skin, chills, increased heart rate, increased respiratory rate

Outcome Criteria

✔ Patient will maintain body temperature within normal limits.

✔ Patient will have negative blood cultures.

NOC: *Thermoregulation*

NOC: *Risk Control*

INTERVENTIONS	RATIONALES
Monitor temperature every 2–4 hours and prn. Observe for chills and diaphoresis.	Endocarditis usually results in temperatures less than 102 degrees; temperatures greater than this indicate an acute infective process. Chills frequently precede a temperature spike. Recurrence of fever may indicate failure of or inappropriate antimicrobial regimen, presence of separate nosocomial infection, abscess, embolism, or thrombophlebitis.
Monitor environment temperature and limit or add blankets as warranted. Change linens as needed.	Room temperature may be altered to assist with maintenance of normal body temperature.
Monitor I&O; provide adequate fluids.	Diaphoresis and increased metabolic rate from temperature elevations increase fluid loss and may cause dehydration.
Give tepid sponge baths prn.	May assist in lowering temperature by means of evaporation. Using cooler water or alcohol may cause chilling and thus increase body temperature.

(continues)

(continued)

INTERVENTIONS	RATIONALES
Place on cooling blanket as warranted.	Cooling blankets are usually only used for severe fever greater than 104 degrees when risk of brain damage or seizures is imminent.
Administer antipyretic medications as warranted.	Reduces fever by action on the hypothalamus. Low grade temperatures may be beneficial to the body's immune system and ability to retard the growth of organisms.
Obtain series of blood cultures as ordered.	A series of cultures are more effective because bacteria and other microorganisms are continually released into the system and this prevents potential false readings. Cultures determine specific organisms and allow for appropriate antimicrobial treatment to be utilized.
Administer antimicrobials as ordered.	Allows for eradication of causative organism and resultant improvement of patient's condition.
Instruct patient/family on procedures for decreasing temperature.	Provides knowledge, reduces fear, and enhances compliance.
Instruct patient/family to take temperature frequently and to notify physician for elevations immediately.	Temperature elevations indicate infection and prompt notification will allow for prompt treatment.
Instruct on medications, effects, side effects, contraindications, symptoms to report.	Promotes knowledge and compliance.

NIC: *Temperature Regulation*

Discharge or Maintenance Evaluation

- Patient will be normothermic with no overt signs/symptoms of infection.
- Blood cultures will be negative.
- Intake and output will be equivalent with no signs or symptoms of dehydration.

RISK FOR INFECTION

Related to: inhibition of antibodies because of immune system action, inflammatory processes caused by vegetation growth, predisposition to bacteremia, septic emboli, myocardial abscess, occlusion of arteries leading to necrosis of body systems, invasive procedures and lines, dental procedures, nosocomial infections, lack of recognition of infection, lack of prophylactic treatment, super-infection, or drug fever

Defining Characteristics: elevated temperature, elevated WBC count, positive blood cultures, reddened, draining IV sites

Outcome Criteria

✔ Patient will be free of infection, afebrile, with no other symptoms of infection or infective process noted.

NOC: *Risk Control*

INTERVENTIONS	RATIONALES
Monitor temperature trends.	Decreases in body temperature below 96 degrees may indicate advanced shock states and is a critical indicator of decreased tissue perfusion and lack of the body's ability to muster enough defense to raise the temperature. Temperatures greater than 101 degrees are due to the effect of endotoxins on the hypothalamus and of pyrogen-released endorphins.
Monitor for signs/symptoms of deterioration of patient and failure to improve within a timely manner.	May indicate ineffective antimicrobial therapy or abundance of resistant organisms.
Observe mouth for patches of white plaque and perineal areas for vaginal drainage or itching, and notify physician.	Thrush or yeast infections may occur as a secondary infection when normal flora is killed by massive antibiotic therapy.
Inspect wounds, IV sites, catheter sites, invasive devices and lines, changes in drainage or body fluids.	May indicate local secondary infection or inflammation.
Maintain aseptic or sterile technique as warranted.	Reduces the risk of opportunistic infection and chances of cross-contamination.
Obtain urine, blood, sputum, wound, and invasive line/catheter specimens for culture and sensitivity and gram stain as warranted.	Assists with identification of source of infection, causative organism, and antimicrobial of choice to enable prompt and effective treatment.

INTERVENTIONS	RATIONALES
Reposition patient every 2 hours; encourage coughing and deep breathing.	Frequent changes in position and breathing exercises enhance pulmonary status and may help to prevent pneumonia.
Administer antimicrobials as ordered	Antimicrobials may be started prior to receiving final culture reports based on the likelihood of the infective organism. Specific antimicrobials are determined by the culture information.
Instruct patient to cover mouth and nose during coughing/sneezing. Instruct in handwashing and disposal of contaminated materials.	Prevents spread of infection from airborne organisms. Good handwashing reduces spread of infection. Infection control procedures limit contamination and spread of infective materials.
Instruct patient in good dental hygiene to use soft toothbrush; to avoid water pick and toothpicks; to obtain regular dental exams.	Avoids trauma to gums which may promote reinfection. Water pick and toothpicks may cause bleeding and promote infection.
Instruct patient to take temperature every day for 1 month post discharge.	Temperature elevations may indicate infection/reinfection.

INTERVENTIONS	RATIONALES
Prepare patient for surgery as warranted.	Surgery may be required to remove necrotic tissue or limbs and to remove purulent material in order to enhance healing. Surgery may be required to replace damaged heart valves caused by vegetative infection.
Instruct patient in obtaining prophylactic antimicrobial therapy prior to procedures.	Prophylaxis will be required for any invasive procedure because of likelihood of reinfection.

NIC: *Infection Protection*

Discharge or Maintenance Evaluation

- Patient will have normal temperature and vital signs.
- Patient will exhibit no overt symptoms or signs of infection.
- Patient will be able to recall instructions accurately.
- Patient will seek prophylactic antibiotic therapy prior to any procedure and will have no evidence of reinfection.

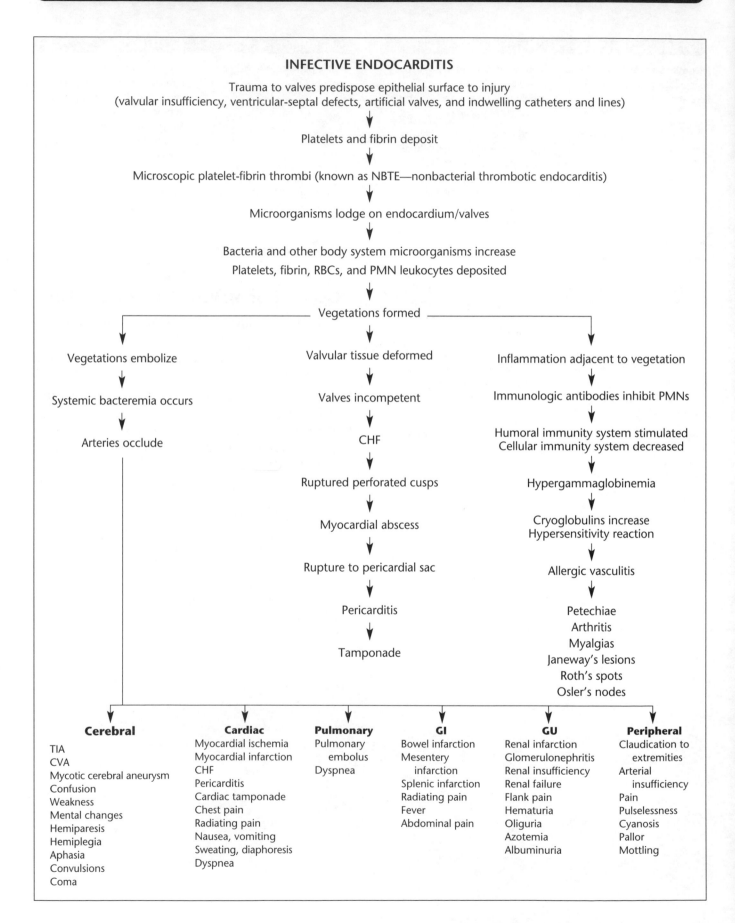

INFECTIVE ENDOCARDITIS

Trauma to valves predispose epithelial surface to injury
(valvular insufficiency, ventricular-septal defects, artificial valves, and indwelling catheters and lines)

↓

Platelets and fibrin deposit

↓

Microscopic platelet-fibrin thrombi (known as NBTE—nonbacterial thrombotic endocarditis)

↓

Microorganisms lodge on endocardium/valves

↓

Bacteria and other body system microorganisms increase
Platelets, fibrin, RBCs, and PMN leukocytes deposited

↓

Vegetations formed

Vegetations embolize	Valvular tissue deformed	Inflammation adjacent to vegetation
↓	↓	↓
Systemic bacteremia occurs	Valves incompetent	Immunologic antibodies inhibit PMNs
↓	↓	↓
Arteries occlude	CHF	Humoral immunity system stimulated Cellular immunity system decreased
	↓	↓
	Ruptured perforated cusps	Hypergammaglobinemia
	↓	↓
	Myocardial abscess	Cryoglobulins increase Hypersensitivity reaction
	↓	↓
	Rupture to pericardial sac	Allergic vasculitis
	↓	↓
	Pericarditis	Petechiae
	↓	Arthritis
	Tamponade	Myalgias
		Janeway's lesions
		Roth's spots
		Osler's nodes

Cerebral	**Cardiac**	**Pulmonary**	**GI**	**GU**	**Peripheral**
TIA	Myocardial ischemia	Pulmonary	Bowel infarction	Renal infarction	Claudication to
CVA	Myocardial infarction	embolus	Mesentery	Glomerulonephritis	extremities
Mycotic cerebral aneurysm	CHF	Dyspnea	infarction	Renal insufficiency	Arterial
Confusion	Pericarditis		Splenic infarction	Renal failure	insufficiency
Weakness	Cardiac tamponade		Radiating pain	Flank pain	Pain
Mental changes	Chest pain		Fever	Hematuria	Pulselessness
Hemiparesis	Radiating pain		Abdominal pain	Oliguria	Cyanosis
Hemiplegia	Nausea, vomiting			Azotemia	Pallor
Aphasia	Sweating, diaphoresis			Albuminuria	Mottling
Convulsions	Dyspnea				
Coma					

CHAPTER 1.9

HYPERTENSION

Essential hypertension, which is an elevated blood pressure of unknown origin, and secondary hypertension, which is an elevated blood pressure resulting from a known cause, will cause inflammation and necrosis in the arterioles which then result in decreased blood flow to vital body organs, and place stress on the heart and vessels. Uncontrolled hypertension is associated with permanent damage to body systems.

Blood pressure is considered to be hypertension if the systolic pressure is greater than 140 mm Hg or the diastolic pressure is greater than 90 mm Hg, and is classified based on the severity from a high normal to malignant hypertension. Hypertensive crisis is defined as a sustained increase in diastolic blood pressure above 120 mm Hg, which is high enough to cause irreversible damage to organs and tissue death and requires emergent reduction within an hour. Malignant hypertension is also associated with rapid vascular injury, papilledema of the optic disc, and retinal hemorrhages.

Hypertension may result from several origins—adrenal (as in pheochromocytoma, Cushing's disease, brain tumor, etc.), renal (as in pyelonephritis), cardiovascular (as in atherosclerosis or coarctation of the aorta, etc.), or unknown, which accounts for the majority of all known hypertension.

Untreated, hypertension will result in death because of cerebrovascular accident, congestive heart failure, intracerebral hemorrhage, kidney failure, or dissecting aneurysms.

Systolic blood pressure is the pressure that the heart produces to force blood from the left side of the heart to the aorta and to major arteries. Diastolic blood pressure is the pressure required to permit filling of the ventricles before the next systole cycle. The pulse pressure, which is the value of the difference between the systolic and diastolic pressures, may be used to indicate perfusion problems. It indicates the function of stroke volume and arterial capacitance and should be 30 to 40 mm Hg nor-mally. A change in pulse pressure may signal impending shock or heart failure, among other complications. The mean arterial pressure, or MAP (or MABP) is the average pressure attempting to push the blood through the circulatory system and should be greater than 60 mm Hg in order to adequately perfuse organs.

Elevated blood pressure may occur as a result of emotional stress with as much as 40 mm Hg increase, and may also result from ventilatory insufficiency, post-seizures, electroconvulsive therapy, intracerebral injury, CNS disorders because of the massive stimulation of catecholamines, coronary artery bypass surgery, myocardial infarction, heart failure, renal dysfunction, eclampsia/toxemia, endocrine disorders, some drugs, tumors, or burns.

Risk factors include: ages between 30 and 70 years of age, race (black), use of birth control pills, obesity, familial history, smoking, stress, diabetes mellitus, hyperlipidemia, and sedentary lifestyle.

Treatment is aimed at lowering blood pressure by use of antihypertensive medications, diuretics to increase urinary output, and by eliminating factors that promote the elevation of blood pressure. A "stepped care" regimen is used most often, with step one involving the use of thiazide diuretics and calcium ion antagonists; step two involves the supplemental use of beta-adrenergic blockers; step three includes vasodilators; and step four involves guanethidine.

MEDICAL CARE

Diuretics: chlorothiazide (Diuril), spironolactone (Aldactone), chlorthalidone (Hygroton), hydrochlorothiazide (Esidrix, HydroDiuril), triamterene (Dyrenium), metolazone (Zaroxolyn, Diulo), ethacrynic acid (Edecrin), furosemide (Lasix) used to promote diuresis and block reabsorption of sodium and water in the kidney

Calcium ion antagonists: verapamil (Calan), diltiazem (Cardizem), nifedipine (Procardia), nitrendipine used to produce vasodilation on vascular smooth muscle

Adrenergic inhibitors: reserpine, methyldopa (Aldomet), propranolol (Inderal), prazosin hydrochloride (Minipress) used to impair synthesis of norepinephrine, suppression of sympathetic outflow by central alpha-adrenergic stimulation, or blocking of preganglionic to postganglionic autonomic transmission

ACE Inhibitors: enalapril (Vasotec), captopril (Capoten), fosinoril (Monopril), lisinopril (Prinivil, Zestril), quinapril (Accupril), or ramipril (Altace) may be used for afterload reduction; these drugs inhibit angiotensin-converting enzyme and prevent the conversion of angiotensin I to angiotensin II, and are able to decrease the workload on the left ventricle to improve cardiac output; contraindicated in hyperkalemic and shock states

Vasodilators: diazoxide (Hyperstat), amyl nitrate (Amyl nitrate), cyclandelate (Cyclan, Cyclospasmol), dipyridamole (Persantine), hydralazine (Apresoline), isosorbide dinitrate (Isorbid, Isordil, Sorbitrate), minoxidil (Loniten), nitroprusside (Nitropress, Sodium nitroprusside, Nipride), nitroglycerine (Minitran, Deponit, Nitro-Bid, Nitrocine, Nitrol, Tridil), and/or tolazoline (Priscoline) used to relax vascular smooth muscle, decrease preload and afterload, decrease oxygen demand, decrease systemic vascular resistance, and increase venous capacitance

Electrolytes: potassium chloride (KCl, K Dur, K tabs) used to replace vital electrolytes lost through diuresis

Electrocardiography: used to monitor for changes in rate and rhythm, conduction abnormalities, left ventricular hypertrophy, ischemia, electrolyte abnormalities, drug toxicity, and presence of dysrhythmias

Laboratory: cholesterol levels and lipid profile used to determine cholesterol and triglyceride levels and their pertinence to atherosclerosis; electrolyte profiles used to monitor for hypokalemia and hypernatremia which may be prevalent because of diuretic therapy; CBC used to identify potential hematocrit reduction seen in renal failure, and polycythemia seen in renal dysfunction; glucose levels used to identify potential causes of hypertension; BUN and creatinine levels used to identify renal dysfunction; urinalysis used to identify proteinuria for possible indication of renal disease and hematuria for possible indication of nephrosclerosis; thyroid profile used to identify hyperthyroidism which may lead to

vasoconstriction and hypertension; aldosterone level used to identify primary aldosteronism; urine VMA to identify elevation of catecholamine metabolites which may indicate pheochromocytoma

Radiographic testing: chest X-ray used to identify cardiomegaly or pulmonary infiltrates; IVP may be used to identify presence of kidney disease; renal arteriogram may be used to show renal artery stenosis or other causes of hypertension

CT Scans: used to show edema of the brain that may occur with hypertensive crisis

COMMON NURSING DIAGNOSES

ANXIETY (see MI)

Related to: diagnosis, change in health status, fear of death, threat to body image, threat to role functioning, pain

Defining Characteristics: restlessness, insomnia, anorexia, increased respirations, increased heart rate, increased blood pressure, difficulty concentrating, dry mouth, poor eye contact, decreased energy, irritability, crying, feelings of helplessness

ADDITIONAL NURSING DIAGNOSES

DECREASED CARDIAC OUTPUT

Related to: malignant hypertension, vasoconstriction, increased preload, increased afterload, ventricular hypertrophy, ischemia

Defining Characteristics: elevated blood pressure, decreased cardiac output, decreased stroke volume, increased peripheral vascular resistance, increased systemic vascular resistance

Outcome Criteria

✔ Patient will have no elevation in blood pressure above normal limits and will maintain blood pressure within acceptable limits.

✔ Patient will maintain adequate cardiac output and cardiac index.

NOC: *Vital Sign Status*

NOC: *Cardiac Pump Effectiveness*

INTERVENTIONS	RATIONALES
Monitor blood pressure every 1–2 hours, or every 5 minutes during active titration of vaso-active drugs. Measure pressure in both arms using appropriate size of cuff. When possible, obtain pressures lying, sitting, and standing.	Changes in blood pressure may indicate changes in patient status requiring prompt attention. Comparing pressures in both sides provides information as to amount of vascular involvement. Blood pressure may vary depending on body position and postural hypotension may result in syncope
Monitor ECG for dysrhythmias, conduction defects, and for heart rate and rhythm changes. Treat as indicated.	Decreases in cardiac output may result in changes in cardiac perfusion causing dysrhythmias.
Observe skin for color, temperature, capillary refill time, and diaphoresis.	Peripheral vasoconstriction may result in pale, cool, clammy skin, with prolonged capillary refill time due to cardiac dysfunction and decreased cardiac output.
Auscultate lungs for adventitious breath sounds.	Crackles (rales) or wheezing may indicate pulmonary congestion caused by cardiac failure as a result of increased blood pressure.
Auscultate heart tones.	Hypertensive patients often have S_4 gallops caused by atrial hypertrophy. Ventricular hypertrophy may result in S_3 gallops.
Administer thiazide, loop, or potassium-sparing diuretics as ordered.	Thiazides are used to reduce blood pressure in patients with normal renal function and these limit fluid retention. Loop diuretics inhibit reabsorption of sodium and chloride and are used in patients who have renal dysfunction. Potassium-sparing diuretics are used in conjunction with thiazides to decrease the amount of potassium lost.
Administer sympathetic inhibitors as ordered.	These drugs reduce blood pressure by decreasing peripheral resistance, reducing cardiac output, inhibiting sympathetic activity, and suppressing the release of renin which is a potent vasoconstrictor.
Administer vasodilators as ordered.	May be used in severe hypertension to increase coronary blood flow and decrease afterload to improve cardiac output.
Administer anti-adrenergic drugs as ordered.	Prevents blood vessels from constricting and increasing blood pressure.

INTERVENTIONS	RATIONALES
Instruct patient/family on fluid and diet requirements and restrictions of sodium.	Restrictions can assist with decrease in fluid retention and hypertension, thereby improving cardiac output.
Instruct patient/family on medications, effects, side effects, contraindications, signs to report.	Promotes knowledge and compliance with drug regimen. Prompt recognition of potential problems allows for timely intervention and management.
Prepare patient for surgery if warranted.	Pheochromocytoma may require surgical intervention for removal of the tumor in order to correct hypertension.

NIC: *Emergency Care*

Discharge or Maintenance Evaluation

- Patient will be normotensive, with adequate cardiac output and index.
- Medications will be taken as ordered with no side effects.
- Patient will have stable heart rate, rhythm, and heart tones, with no adventitious breath sounds.
- Patient will be able to verbalize instructions accurately.

INEFFECTIVE TISSUE PERFUSION: CARDIOPULMONARY, CEREBRAL, RENAL, GASTROINTESTINAL, AND PERIPHERAL

Related to: increased catecholamine stimulation, increased blood pressure, decreased cardiac output, decreased baroreceptor sensitivity, changes in cerebrospinal fluid pressure, angiotensin and aldosterone stimulation, sodium intake, environmental factors, genetic factors, strain on arterial wall, atherosclerosis

Defining Characteristics: increased blood pressure, retinopathy, retinal hemorrhage, headache, epistaxis, tachycardia, rales, S_3 or S_4 gallops, restlessness, bruits to femorals, carotids, abdominal aorta, and anteriorly over renal vasculature, blurred vision, chest pain, shortness of breath, optic disc papilledema, seizures, coma, nystagmus, mental changes, nausea, vomiting, oliguria, azotemia

Outcome Criteria

✔ Patient will achieve and maintain adequate tissue perfusion to all body systems.

✔ Patient will have blood pressure within desired parameters.

NOC: *Tissue Perfusion*

INTERVENTIONS	RATIONALES
Maintain at least one IV line; two preferably.	Allows for venous access and administration of fluids and rapid-acting medications to decrease blood pressure.
Monitor VS q 1 hour and prn, or every 5 minutes during active titration of vasoactive drugs. Arterial line placement is preferred.	Allows for prompt assessment of patient's response to therapy.
Administer vasoactive drugs and titrate as ordered to maintain pressures at set parameters for patient.	Nitroprusside is the drug of choice for cerebral hemorrhage, hypertensive encephalopathy, or dissecting aortic aneurysm. Nitroglycerin (NTG) is the drug of choice for angina, ischemia, adrenergic crises, or left ventricular failure. Phentolamine is the drug of choice for overdoses of alpha-adrenergic agents and pheochromocytoma; and labetalol is utilized for adrenergic crises. These drugs have rapid action and may decrease the blood pressure too rapidly, resulting in complications.
Observe for complaints of blurred vision, tinnitus, confusion, or seizure activity.	May indicate cyanide toxicity from nitroprusside or increasing intracranial pressure.
Administer diuretics as ordered. Monitor I&O status.	May help to decrease fluid excess that contributes to increases in blood pressure. I&O will give an indication of fluid balance or imbalance, thus allowing for changes in treatment regimen when required.
Monitor for sudden onset of chest pain.	May indicate dissecting aortic aneurysm.
Monitor ECG for changes in rate, rhythm, dysrhythmias, and conduction defects. Treat as indicated.	Decreased perfusion may result in dysrhythmias caused by decrease in oxygen. T wave inversion may indicate that the decrease in blood pressure is

INTERVENTIONS	RATIONALES
	being done too rapidly and causing tissue ischemia.
Monitor hemodynamic parameters closely and titrate vasoactive drugs as warranted.	Provides immediate information regarding efficacy of medication and status of hypertension.
Observe for shift of point of maximal impulse (PMI) to left.	Shift occurs in cardiac enlargement.
Auscultate over peripheral arteries for bruits.	Atherosclerosis may cause bruits by obstructing blood flow.
Observe extremities for swelling, erythema, tenderness, pain, positive Homans' sign, positive Pratt's sign. Observe for decreased peripheral pulses, pallor, coldness, cyanosis.	Bedrest promotes venous stasis which can increase the risk of thromboembolus formation. Actual emboli can migrate and occlude peripheral arteries, leading to tissue ischemia and necrosis. If treatment is too rapid and aggressive in decreasing the blood pressure, tissue perfusion will be impaired and ischemia can result.
Instruct patient in signs/symptoms to report to physician, such as headache upon rising, increased blood pressure, chest pain, shortness of breath, increased heart rate, weight gain of >2 lb/day or 5 lb/wk, edema, visual changes, nosebleeds, dizziness, syncope, muscle cramps, nausea/vomiting, impotence or decreased libido.	Promotes knowledge and compliance with treatment. Promotes prompt detection and facilitates prompt intervention.

NIC: *Circulatory Precautions*

Discharge or Maintenance Evaluation

■ Blood pressure will be within set parameters for the patient.

■ Patient will have adequate tissue perfusion to all body systems.

■ Patient will be mentally lucid, with no confusion or neurologic deficits.

■ Patient will have adequate urinary output with no hematuria, and renal function studies will be within normal limits.

■ Patient will be able to recall accurately the information instructed.

RISK FOR DEFICIENT FLUID VOLUME

Related to: rebound hypotension, use of diuretics, use of vasoactive drugs, loss of fluids, electrolyte imbalances

Defining Characteristics: decreased blood pressure, changes in mental status, decreased urinary output, concentrated urine, dry mucous membranes, dry skin, poor skin turgor, dry mouth, weight loss, thirst, weakness, increased hematocrit, increased blood pressure, decreased pulse pressure and volume, decreased venous filling, abnormal electrolytes

Outcome Criteria

✔ Patient will achieve and maintain adequate fluid hydration.

✔ Urinary output will be adequate and electrolytes will be within normal limits.

✔ Vital signs will be within normal limits for patient.

NOC: *Fluid Balance*

INTERVENTIONS	RATIONALES
Monitor VS at least q 1–2 hrs and prn.	Hypotension, shortness of breath, or tachycardia may indicate electrolyte or fluid imbalance.
Adjust IV antihypertensives as ordered, and observe for patient response.	Too rapid decreases in blood pressure may result in decreased perfusion, fluid shifting, and hypotensive crisis.
Measure I&O q 1 hour and notify physician if <30 cc/hr.	Low urinary output and increased specific gravity may indicate hypovolemia and require further treatment.
Administer IV fluids as ordered.	Additional fluid may be required to achieve and maintain fluid balance and help facilitate fluid movement into intravascular space.
Weigh patient daily at same time, with same scale, if possible.	Weight loss or gain >2 lbs/day is a good indication of fluid status. The use of the same scale provides more consistent data.
Test urine specific gravity q 8 hours prn.	Increases in specific gravity may indicate dehydration.
Measure abdominal girth q 8 hours and notify physician of significant changes.	Changes may indicate presence of ascites or third space shifting.
Observe skin turgor and appearance of mucous membranes.	Provides indication of hydration status.

INTERVENTIONS	RATIONALES
Monitor lab values, especially electrolytes.	Fluid loss may cause significant electrolyte imbalances, which may lead to further complications.
Instruct patient/family in medications, effects, side effects, IV fluid use and reason, and reasons for fluid losses.	Involves patient in care, promotes knowledge, and decreases fear.
Instruct patient to weigh daily and keep log of I&O as needed, and when to notify physician.	Provides patient with method to monitor fluid balance and status.
Instruct patient to sit and stand up slowly.	Helps to avoid orthostatic hypotension and potential syncopal episodes.

NIC: *Fluid Monitoring*

Discharge or Maintenance Evaluation

■ Patient will have vital signs within set parameters.

■ Electrolytes and specific gravity will be within normal limits.

■ Patient will have normal skin turgor, moist mucous membranes, and urinary output will be adequate.

■ Patient/family will be able to accurately verbalize information.

DEFICIENT KNOWLEDGE

Related to: new diagnosis, lack of understanding, lack of understanding of medical condition, lack of recall

Defining characteristics: questions regarding problems, inadequate follow-up on instructions given, misconceptions, lack of improvement of previous regimen, development of preventable complications

Outcome Criteria

✔ Patient will be able to verbalize and demonstrate understanding of information given regarding condition, medications, and treatment regimen.

NOC: *Knowledge: Disease Process*

INTERVENTIONS	RATIONALES
Determine patient's baseline of knowledge regarding disease process, normal physiology, and function of the heart.	Provides information regarding patient's understanding of condition as well as a baseline from which to base teaching.
Monitor patient's readiness to learn and determine best methods to use for learning. Attempt to incorporate family/ significant other in learning process. Reinstruct/reinforce information as needed.	Promotes optimal learning environment when patient shows willingness to learn. Family members may assist with helping the patient to make informed choices regarding his treatment. Anxiety or large volumes of instruction may impede comprehension and limit learning.
Provide time for individual interaction with patient.	Promotes relationship between patient and nurse, and establishes trust.
Instruct patient on procedures that may be performed.	Provides knowledge and promotes the ability to make informed choices.
Instruct patient in medications, dose, effects, side effects, contra-indications, and signs/symptoms to report to physician.	Promotes understanding that side effects are common and may subside over time, and facilitates compliance.
Instruct in dietary needs and restrictions, such as limiting caffeine and sodium, or increasing potassium and calcium.	Patient may need to increase dietary potassium if placed on diuretics; caffeine may need to be limited because of the direct stimulant effect on the heart; sodium should be limited because of the potential for fluid retention. Additional calcium has been shown to lower blood pressure. Excessive intake of fat and cholesterol are additional risk factors in hypertension. Low fat diets can decrease BP through prostaglandin balance.
Instruct on hypertension, effects on the blood vessels, heart, brain, and kidneys. Instruct on normal values for BP.	Promotes understanding of the disease process and enhances compliance with treatment.
Instruct on maintaining medication regimen to keep blood pressure well controlled, and in keeping medical appointments.	Assist patient to understand need for life-long compliance to reduce incidence of CVA, MI, cardiac and renal dysfunction. Lack of compliance is the major reason for failure of antihypertensive therapy.

INTERVENTIONS	RATIONALES
Instruct on ways to modify risk factors, such as smoking, obesity, high fat diets, stressful lifestyle, and so forth.	Risk factors contribute to disease and complications associated with hypertension, as well as exacerbate symptoms. Nicotine increases catecholamine release and increases heart rate, blood pressure, and myocardial oxygen demand.
Instruct in self-monitoring for blood pressure; technique to be used post discharge.	Provides reinforcement and the ability to monitor response to medical regimen.
Instruct to take diuretics in A.M.	Decreases incidence of nocturia.
Instruct to weigh daily at same time on same scale.	Monitors effectiveness of diuretics and for fluid retention.
Instruct on leg exercises and position changes.	Decreases venous pooling that can be potentiated by vasodilators and prolonged time in one position.
Instruct to avoid hot baths, saunas, hot tubs, and alcohol intake.	These promote vasodilation and when combined with diuretics, may increase chance of orthostatic hypotension and syncope.
Instruct to avoid over-the-counter medications unless prescribed by physician.	Some drugs contain sympathetic stimulants that can increase blood pressure or may cause drug interactions.
Instruct to rise slowly, allowing time between position changes.	Assists body to equilibrate and adjust in order to decrease the risk of syncope.
Provide printed materials when possible for patient/family to review.	Provides references for patient and family to refer to once discharged, and can enhance the understanding of verbally-given instructions.
Demonstrate and instruct on technique for checking pulse rate and regularity. Instruct in situations where immediate action must be taken.	Self-monitoring promotes self-independence and can provide timely intervention for abnormalities or complications. Heart rates that exceed set parameters may require further medical alteration in medications or regimen.
Have patient demonstrate all skills that will be necessary for post-discharge.	Provides information that patient has gained a full understanding of instruction and is able to demonstrate correct information.

NIC: *Teaching: Disease Process*

Discharge or Maintenance Evaluation

■ Patient will be able to verbalize understanding of condition, treatment regimen, and signs/symptoms to report.

■ Patient will be able to correctly perform all tasks prior to discharge.

■ Patient will be able to verbalize understanding of cardiac disease, risk factors, dietary restrictions, and lifestyle adaptations.

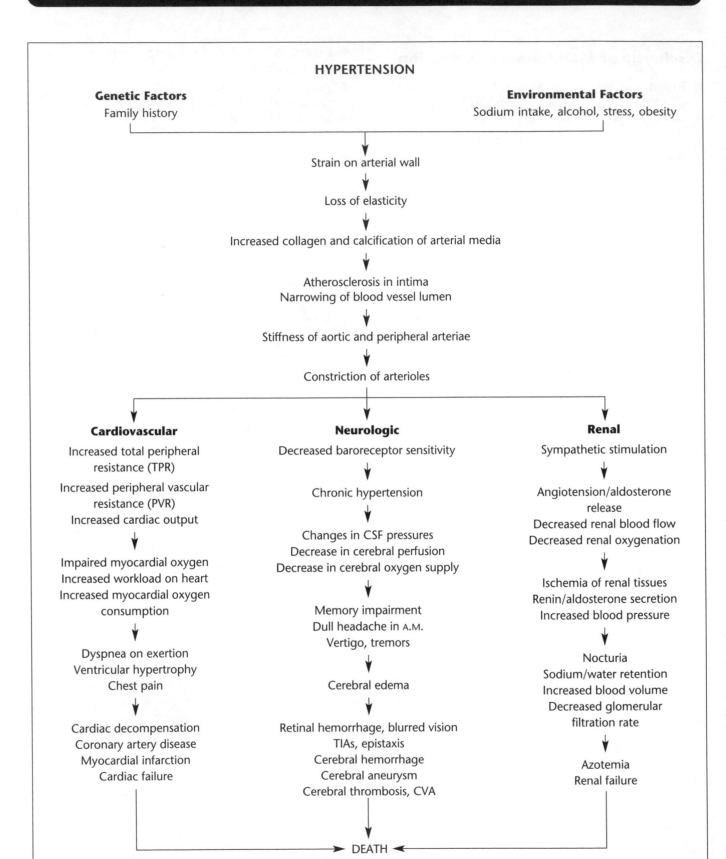

HYPERTENSION

Genetic Factors
Family history

Environmental Factors
Sodium intake, alcohol, stress, obesity

Strain on arterial wall

Loss of elasticity

Increased collagen and calcification of arterial media

Atherosclerosis in intima
Narrowing of blood vessel lumen

Stiffness of aortic and peripheral arteriae

Constriction of arterioles

Cardiovascular

Increased total peripheral
resistance (TPR)

Increased peripheral vascular
resistance (PVR)
Increased cardiac output

Impaired myocardial oxygen
Increased workload on heart
Increased myocardial oxygen
consumption

Dyspnea on exertion
Ventricular hypertrophy
Chest pain

Cardiac decompensation
Coronary artery disease
Myocardial infarction
Cardiac failure

Neurologic

Decreased baroreceptor sensitivity

Chronic hypertension

Changes in CSF pressures
Decrease in cerebral perfusion
Decrease in cerebral oxygen supply

Memory impairment
Dull headache in A.M.
Vertigo, tremors

Cerebral edema

Retinal hemorrhage, blurred vision
TIAs, epistaxis
Cerebral hemorrhage
Cerebral aneurysm
Cerebral thrombosis, CVA

Renal

Sympathetic stimulation

Angiotension/aldosterone
release
Decreased renal blood flow
Decreased renal oxygenation

Ischemia of renal tissues
Renin/aldosterone secretion
Increased blood pressure

Nocturia
Sodium/water retention
Increased blood volume
Decreased glomerular
filtration rate

Azotemia
Renal failure

→ DEATH ←

CHAPTER 1.10

THROMBOPHLEBITIS

Thrombophlebitis occurs when a clot forms in a vein secondary to inflammation or when the vein is partially occluded from some disease process. As a general rule, two out of the following three factors occur prior to the formation of a thrombus—blood stasis, injury to the vessel, and/or altered blood coagulation.

Deep vein thrombosis, or DVT, pertains to clots that are formed in the deep veins and may result in complications such as pulmonary embolus and postphlebotic syndrome, or chronic venous insufficiency. This can be a residual effect of thrombophlebitis in which the veins are partially occluded or valves in the vessels have been damaged. This chronic insufficiency may cause increased venous pressure and fluid accumulation in the interstitial tissues, which results in chronic edema, tissue fibrosis, and induration.

DVT may be asymptomatic, but usually produces side effects such as fever, pain, edema, cyanosis or pallor to the involved extremity, and malaise.

Superficial vein thrombophlebitis causes may include trauma, infection, chemical irritations, frequent IVs, and recreational drug abuse.

The goals in treatment of thrombophlebitis are to control thrombotic development, relieve pain, improve blood flow, and prevent complications.

MEDICAL CARE

Venography: used to visualize the vascular system and locate any impairment in blood flow

Plethysmography: a noninvasive measurement of changes in calf volume that corresponds to changing blood volume as a result of impairment in blood flow

^{125}I Fibrinogen uptake test: a radioactive scan performed after radioactive fibrinogen is injected, which concentrates in the area of clot formation; not sensitive to thrombi high on the iliofemoral region or with inactive thrombi

Anticoagulants: used to prolong clotting time to prevent further clot formation

Thrombolytics: streptokinase (Streptase, Kabikinase) and urokinase (Abbokinase) may be used if thrombophlebitis progresses to pulmonary movement of the clot; these drugs are fibrinolytic activators and enhance the conversion of plasminogen to plasmin; unfractionated or low-molecular-weight heparin (LMWH) may be used prophylactically or therapeutically, but may cause heparin-induced thrombopenia and thrombosis (HITT syndrome)

Surgical intervention: may be required to insert embolism filter to prevent further pulmonary emboli, pulmonary embolectomy, or interruption of the inferior vena cava; morbidity with these procedures may be as high as 15%

COMMON NURSING DIAGNOSES

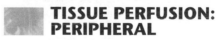

ACUTE PAIN (see AORTIC ANEURYSM)

Related to: inflammation, impaired blood flow, intermittent claudication, venous stasis, lactic acid in tissues, surgical procedures, fever

Defining Characteristics: complaints of pain, tenderness to touch, aching, burning, restlessness, facial grimacing, guarding of extremity

ADDITIONAL NURSING DIAGNOSES

TISSUE PERFUSION: PERIPHERAL

Related to: impaired blood flow, venous stasis, venous obstruction

Defining Characteristics: pain, tissue edema, decreased peripheral pulses, prolonged capillary refill time, pallor, cyanosis, erythema, paresthesia, necrosis

Outcome Criteria

✔ Patient will have improved peripheral perfusion, with palpable and equal pulses, normal skin color, temperature, and sensation, and have no evidence of edema.

NOC: *Tissue Perfusion: Peripheral*

INTERVENTIONS	RATIONALES
Observe lower extremities for edema, color, and temperature. Measure calf circumference every shift. Monitor for capillary refill time.	Findings may help to differentiate between superficial thrombophlebitis and deep vein thrombosis. Measurements can facilitate early recognition of edema and changes. Edema, redness, and warmth are indicative of superficial phlebitis whereas DVT usually is exhibited by cool, pale skin. DVT may prolong capillary refill time.
Observe extremity for prominence of veins, knots, bumps, or stretched skin.	Superficial veins may become distended because of backflow through veins. Evidence of thrombophlebitis to superficial veins may be visible or easily palpable.
Maintain bedrest.	Activity limitation may minimize the potential for dislodgment of the clot.
Elevate legs while in bed or sitting in chair.	Reduces swelling and increases venous return. Some experts believe that elevation may actually enhance the release of thrombi.
Observe for positive Homan's sign (pain in calf upon dorsiflexion of foot).	Homan's sign may or may not be present consistently and should not be used as a sole indicator of thrombophlebitis.
Perform active or passive ROM exercises while at bedrest.	Promote increased venous blood return and decrease venous stasis.
Apply TED hose after acute phase is over. Remove for at least 1 hour every shift.	Assists to minimize postphlebotic syndrome and increases blood flow to deep veins. Removal allows time for compression of veins to be relaxed.
Apply warm moist soaks as ordered.	Promotes vasodilation and may improve venous return and decrease in edema.
Administer anticoagulants as ordered.	Heparin is used initially because of its action on thrombin formation and the removal of the

INTERVENTIONS	RATIONALES
	intrinsic pathway to prevent further clot formation. Coumadin is usually used for long-term therapy. Low-molecular-weight heparin (LMWH) is frequently used, either prophylactically or therapeutically, but has the potential for inducing heparin-induced thrombopenia and thrombosis (HITT syndrome) in which the heparin directly interacts with platelets and causes a decrease in their amount because of antibody-dependent platelet activation, which in turn, may lead to further thromboemboli being formed. If patient is suspected of developing HITT, the heparin should be stopped and replaced by an alternative anticoagulant. Direct thrombin-inhibitors (recombinant hirudins) are usually considered to be practical and effective because they have no immunological properties. Hirudins, such as Refludan, can induce a prolonged anticoagulation action up to a week in duration with patients who have concurrent renal failure because the kidneys clear the drug, so continued monitoring of PTT levels must be performed to maintain efficacy.
Monitor laboratory studies for PT, PTT, APTT, and CBC.	Monitors efficacy of anticoagulant therapy and potential for clot formation due to hemoconcentration/dehydration.
Instruct on avoidance of rubbing or massaging extremity involved.	May promote risk of dislodging clot and causing embolization.
Avoid crossing legs, prolonged positions with legs dangling, or knees bent.	Positions tend to restrict circulation and increase venous stasis, and increase edema.
Instruct in deep breathing exercises.	Promotes emptying of large veins by increasing negative pressure in the thorax.
Instruct on maintaining fluid intake of at least 2 L/day.	Dehydration promotes increased viscosity of blood, and increases venous stasis.
Prepare patient for surgery if warranted.	Surgical intervention may be required if circulation is severely compromised. Recurrent

INTERVENTIONS	RATIONALES
	episodes of thrombi may require a vena caval umbrella to filter out thrombi going to lungs.
Instruct on lying in a slightly reversed Trendelenburg's position.	Promotes blood flow to dependent extremities; preferable to have extremities full of blood as opposed to empty.

NIC: *Circulatory Precautions*

Discharge or Maintenance Evaluation

- Patient will have palpable pulses of equal strength to all extremities.
- Skin will be within normal limits of coloration, temperature, and sensation.
- Patient will be able to recall all instructions accurately.
- Patient will have no complications from anticoagulation therapy.

RISK FOR IMPAIRED SKIN INTEGRITY

Related to: clot formation, edema, venous stasis, bedrest, surgery, pressure, altered circulation and blood flow, altered metabolic states

Defining Characteristics: skin surface disruptions, incisions, ulcerations, wounds that do not heal, edema, skin induration, cyanosis, mottling, pallor, cold extremities, pulselessness to involved extremity, necrosis

Outcome Criteria

- ✔ Patient will have no evidence of impairment to skin tissues.
- ✔ Patient will have surgical wound approximated and well-healed with no evidence of infection.

NOC: *Wound Healing: Primary Intention*

INTERVENTIONS	RATIONALES
Monitor extremities for presence of ulcers, wounds, symptoms of decreased circulation (redness, edema, mottling, pallor, cyanosis, pulselessness).	Provides prompt assessment and treatment for impaired tissues.

INTERVENTIONS	RATIONALES
If surgery is required, change dressing using aseptic or sterile technique as warranted. Leave wound open to air as soon as is feasible, or apply light dressing.	Prevents drainage accumulations from excoriating skin, provides assessment to monitor for changes in wound appearance and deterioration/improvement, and prevents wound from contamination. Allowing air to reach wound facilitates drying and promotes the healing process. Sutures may be abrasive to skin or get caught on garments and irritation may be reduced with a light gauze dressing.
Cleanse wound as ordered with each dressing change.	Various agents can be used to remove exudate or necrotic material from wound to promote healing. Any packing of the wound should be done using sterile technique to reduce the risk of contamination.
Monitor wound for skin integrity to incision and surrounding tissues, noting increases and changes in characteristics of drainage.	Prompt recognition of problems with healing may prevent exacerbation of wound. Increased drainage or malodorous drainage may indicate infection and delayed wound healing.
Monitor any drainage tubes for amounts and character of drainage. Use ostomy bags over tubes when drainage is massive.	Provides indication of decreasing or increasing wound drainage and assessment of healing process. Collection of drainage in bags facilitates more accurate measurement of fluid loss and prevents excoriation of skin from copious drainage.
Apply skin prep, moisture barrier, or benzoin to skin prior to tape application. Use hypoallergenic tape or Montgomery straps to secure dressings.	Provides protection to skin and reduces potential for skin trauma. Reduces potential for skin/wound disruption when frequent dressing changes are required.
Instruct to avoid scratching, hitting or bumping legs, or other injurious activities.	Injuries may damage tissues that may deteriorate into ulcer formation.
Instruct on signs/symptoms of infection to wound/skin and to report to nurse/physician.	Provides prompt notification to enhance prompt treatment.
Instruct on cleansing incision area post discharge.	Reduces skin surface contaminants and prevents infection.

NIC: *Skin Surveillance*
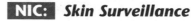

Discharge or Maintenance Evaluation

- Patient will have approximated, healed surgical wound with no drainage, erythema, or edema to site.
- Patient will be able to recall instructions accurately.
- Patient will be compliant with avoiding injurious activities, and will seek medical help when injury occurs.

DEFICIENT KNOWLEDGE

Related to: new diagnosis, lack of understanding, lack of understanding of medical condition, lack of recall

Defining Characteristics: questions regarding problems, inadequate follow-up on instructions given, misconceptions, lack of improvement of previous regimen, development of preventable complications

Outcome Criteria

✔ Patient will be able to verbalize and demonstrate understanding of information given regarding condition, medications, and treatment regimen.

NOC: *Knowledge: Disease Process*

NOC: *Knowledge: Health Promotion*

INTERVENTIONS	RATIONALES
Determine patient's baseline of knowledge regarding disease process, normal physiology, and function.	Provides information regarding patient's understanding of condition as well as a baseline from which to base teaching.
Monitor patient's readiness to learn and determine best methods to use for learning. Attempt to incorporate family/significant other in learning process. Reinstruct/reinforce information as needed.	Promotes optimal learning environment when patient shows willingness to learn. Family members may assist with helping the patient to make informed choices regarding his treatment. Anxiety or large volumes of instruction may impede comprehension and limit learning.
Provide time for individual inter-action with patient.	Promotes relationship between patient and nurse, and establishes trust.
Instruct patient on procedures that may be performed.	Provides knowledge and promotes the ability to make informed choices.

INTERVENTIONS	RATIONALES
Instruct on signs/symptoms of possible complications, such as pulmonary emboli, venous insufficiency, and venous stasis ulcers.	Provides knowledge and assists patient to understand health care needs.
Instruct on care to lower extremities and to notify physician for development of any lesion.	Chronic venous stasis may occur and promotes risk of infection and/or ulcer formation.
Instruct patient in medications, dose, effects, side effects, contraindications, and signs/symptoms to report to physician.	Promotes understanding that side effects are common and may subside over time, and facilitates compliance.
Instruct on leg exercises and position changes. Assist with setting up activity program post-discharge.	Decreases venous pooling that can be potentiated by vasodilators and prolonged time in one position. Exercise may assist in developing collateral circulation and enhances venous return.
Instruct to rise slowly, allowing time between position changes.	Assist body to equilibrate and adjust in order to decrease the risk of syncope.
Instruct to balance rest with activity.	Rest decreases oxygen demands of compromised tissue and decreases potential for embolization of thrombus. Balancing rest with graduated activity prevents exhaustion and impairment of tissue perfusion.
Instruct on proper application of TED stockings.	Improper application may cause a tourniquet-like effect and impede circulation.
Avoid valsalva-type maneuvers. Provide increased fiber to diet and administer stool softeners as warranted.	Increases venous pressure in the leg which increases potential for thrombophlebitis.
Instruct on anticoagulation therapy—dosage, effects, side effects, when to administer, other medications to avoid.	Promotes compliance with medical regimen and decreases potential for improper dosage and adverse drug interactions. Aspirin and salicylates decrease prothrombin activity, vitamin K increases prothrombin activity, antibiotics may interfere with vitamin K synthesis, and barbiturates can potentiate anticoagulant effect.
Instruct on importance of keeping physician appointments for followup laboratory studies.	Promotes compliance with treatment and decreases potential for non-therapeutic levels of anticoagulation therapy.
Provide printed materials when possible for patient/family to review.	Provides references for patient and family to refer to once discharged, and can enhance the

INTERVENTIONS	RATIONALES
	understanding of verbally-given instructions.
Have patient demonstrate all skills that will be necessary for post-discharge.	Provides information that patient has gained a full understanding of instruction and is able to demonstrate correct information.

NIC: *Teaching: Disease Process*

Discharge or Maintenance Evaluation

- Patient will be able to verbalize understanding of condition, treatment regimen, and signs/symptoms to report.
- Patient will be able to correctly perform all tasks prior to discharge.
- Patient will be able to verbalize understanding of safety precautions, correct dosage and administration of all medications, and activity limitations.

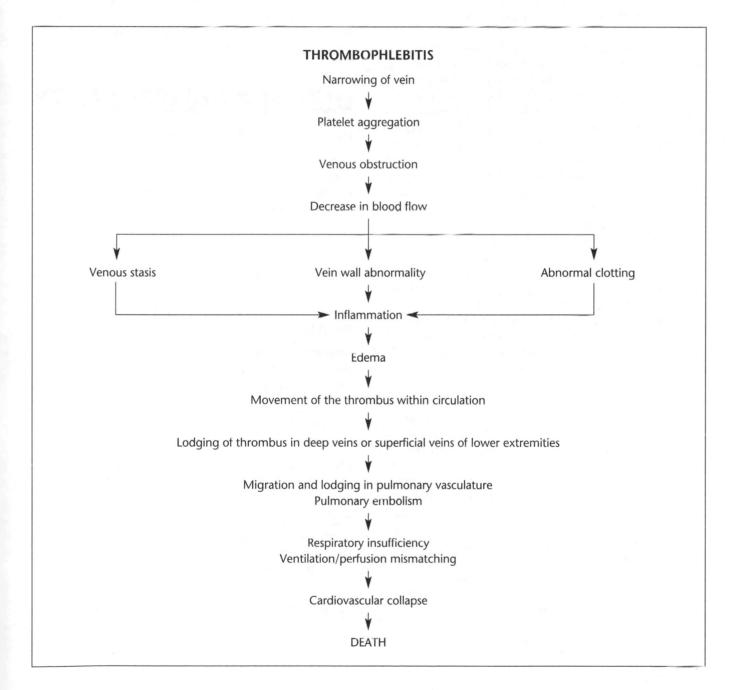

THROMBOPHLEBITIS

Narrowing of vein
↓
Platelet aggregation
↓
Venous obstruction
↓
Decrease in blood flow
↓

Venous stasis   Vein wall abnormality   Abnormal clotting
↓
→ Inflammation ←
↓
Edema
↓
Movement of the thrombus within circulation
↓
Lodging of thrombus in deep veins or superficial veins of lower extremities
↓
Migration and lodging in pulmonary vasculature
Pulmonary embolism
↓
Respiratory insufficiency
Ventilation/perfusion mismatching
↓
Cardiovascular collapse
↓
DEATH

CHAPTER 1.11

AORTIC ANEURYSM

An aneurysm is a localized dilation of an artery that may occur as a congenital anomaly or as a result of atherosclerosis and high blood pressure. There are three types of aneurysms found—saccular in which the vessel distention protrudes from one side; fusiform in which the distention involves the entire circumference of the vessel; and dissecting in which a tear occurs in the intimal layer of the artery and with pressure, blood splits the wall, producing a hematoma that separates the medial layers of the aortic wall. In dissecting aneurysms, generally the separation of the layers does not completely encircle the lumen but may run the entire length of the vessel.

Factors that may precipitate aneurysm formation include atherosclerosis, hypertension, syphilis, Marfan's syndrome, cystic medial necrosis, trauma, congenital abnormalities, and pregnancy.

Aneurysms that result from Marfan's syndrome usually involve the first portion of the aorta, and result in aortic insufficiency. Syphilitic aneurysms usually occur in the ascending thoracic aorta.

Abdominal aortic aneurysms (AAA) usually involve that part of the aorta between the renal and iliac arteries, and thoracic aortic aneurysms (TAA) occur mainly in the ascending, transverse or descending aorta with a prevalence toward men between 60 and 70 years of age. Mycotic aneurysms occur as a result of weakness in the vessel from an infective process, such as endocarditis, and usually involve the peripheral arteries, but have been known to affect the aorta.

AAA as a result of atherosclerosis may be asymptomatic until they become large enough to palpate, large enough to cause pressure and pain, or until leaking or rupture occurs. Frequently, rupture of the AAA leads to vascular collapse and shock, and ultimately, death, if not treated.

The goal for treatment is to remove or repair the aneurysm and restore vascular circulation. Aneurysms are generally monitored until their size reaches 5–6 cm or greater, and then surgical intervention is indicated to prevent complications such as rupture, stroke, or organ ischemia. Grafts are made from numerous materials and percutaneous stenting procedures are used to help establish blood flow.

MEDICAL CARE

Oxygen: used to increase available oxygen supply

Electrocardiography: used to monitor heart rhythm and rate for changes associated with decreases in perfusion, dysrhythmias, and for signs of left ventricular hypertrophy

Chest X-ray: used to observe for increase in aortic diameter, right tracheal deviation, and pleural effusions

Abdominal X-ray: used to visualize aneurysm

CT scans: used to visualize vessel wall thickness, lumen size, length of the aneurysm, and any mural thrombi

Angioaortography: used to visualize lumen, extent of disease, extent of collateral circulation, arteriovenous fistulas, extent of dissection, and double lumens

Ultrasound: used to visualize the vessels and aneurysm non-invasively, amount of blood flow, and velocity of blood flow

MRI: used to visualize the extent and origin of aneurysm dissection, as well as the size of the aneurysm

TEE: used to identify presence of dissection in the aortic root, proximal ascending aorta, or descending thoracic aorta, to evaluate pericardial effusions and aortic insufficiency

Laboratory: CBC used to monitor for decreases in hemoglobin and hematocrit and for increases in leukocytes; BUN and creatinine used to monitor for renal dysfunction; urinalysis used to monitor hematuria and proteinuria to detect renal compromise

Surgery: necessary to replace aneurysm with dacron graft and/or repair the aneurysm

COMMON NURSING DIAGNOSES

RISK FOR IMPAIRED SKIN INTEGRITY (see THROMBOPHLEBITIS)

Related to: surgery, edema, bedrest, pressure, altered circulation and blood flow, altered metabolic states

Defining Characteristics: skin surface disruptions, incisions, ulcerations, wounds that do not heal

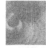

DEFICIENT KNOWLEDGE (see MI)

Related to: disease process, surgery, lack of understanding, lack of understanding of medical condition, lack of recall

Defining Characteristics: questions regarding problems, inadequate follow-up on instructions given, misconceptions, lack of improvement of previous regimen, development of preventable complications

ADDITIONAL NURSING DIAGNOSES

INEFFECTIVE TISSUE PERFUSION: CARDIOPULMONARY, CEREBRAL, GASTROINTESTINAL, PERIPHERAL, RENAL

Related to: arterial occlusion, aneurysm, dissecting aneurysm, or operative complications

Defining Characteristics: pulsating mass, bruits, thrills, abdominal pain, low back pain, nausea/vomiting, syncope, chest pain, cough, hoarseness, weak voice, dysphagia, dyspnea, shortness of breath, pallor, loss of pulses, paresthesias, paralysis, syncope, numbness, aphasia, arm pain, "ripping" or "tearing" sensations, severe and sudden sharp abdominal pain radiating to back, hips, or pelvis, sudden sharp chest pain radiating to jaw, neck, back, and abdomen, bruits, cardiac murmur, hypertension, hypotension

Outcome Criteria

✔ Patient will achieve and maintain hemodynamic stability, with all body systems adequately perfused, and in the absence of pain.

✔ Patient will have no operative complications.

NOC: *Tissue Perfusion*

NOC: *Circulation Status*

INTERVENTIONS	RATIONALES
Monitor blood pressure in upper and lower extremities bilaterally.	Normally systolic BP in thigh is greater than in the arm, but is reversed much of the time with abdominal aneurysms. Pressure differences >20 mm Hg in the upper extremities may indicate aneurysm dissection, or occlusion of the subclavian, innominate, brachial, and/or axillary arteries.
Monitor vital signs and hemodynamic parameters. Maintain blood pressure at physician-ordered parameters.	Hypertension may exacerbate bleeding due to pressure on suture lines, and hypotension may not provide enough blood flow to keep graft open. Hypotension, tachycardia, and decreased hemodynamic pressures may indicate hypovolemia or hemorrhage.
Monitor pulses in both wrists as well as in both legs.	Pulse differences may be noted between wrists and between legs if the aneurysm interferes with circulation to that particular extremity.
Observe for the 5 Ps—pain to extremity, pallor, pulselessness, paresthesia, and paralysis. Notify physician.	These may be associated with thrombosis of an abdominal aortic aneurysm.
Monitor for pain, especially onset of sudden sharp pain with radiation, and notify physician.	Abrupt severe tearing pain in chest radiating to shoulders, neck, back, and abdomen is indicative of aortic dissection and requires prompt intervention. Low back pain may indicate impending rupture.
Administer analgesics as ordered.	Relieves pain, decreases myocardial oxygen consumption and

(continues)

(continued)

INTERVENTIONS	RATIONALES
	demand, and assists to improve perfusion.
Observe for dysphagia.	Aneurysm may exert pressure on esophagus.
Observe for voice weakness, hoarseness, paroxysmal cough, or dyspnea.	Aneurysm may exert pressure on laryngeal nerve or on the trachea.
Auscultate for bruits over arteries; observe and palpate gently for thrill over abdomen. Auscultate for cardiac murmurs.	Indicates diminished blood flow indicative of aneurysm. A large aneurysm will have a palpable mass and thrill. An aortic murmur will be present if the aneurysm involves the aortic ring.
Administer antihypertensives as ordered to maintain BP within acceptable parameters.	Hypertension may exacerbate decreased tissue perfusion and compromise cardiovascular status.
Prepare patient for surgery as indicated.	Surgical intervention may be mandatory if circulation is compromised.
Auscultate lung fields for adventitious breath sounds. Assist patient with cough, deep breathing exercises, incentive spirometry.	Bedrest promotes atelectasis and decreased lung expansion which may lead to pneumonia.
Monitor oxygen saturation by oximetry. Administer oxygen as ordered.	Maintenance of adequate oxygenation necessary for adequate tissue perfusion.
Monitor peripheral pulses every hour for 24 hours, then every 4 hours, for color, temperature, capillary refill, and presence of pulses post-op. Notify physician if absent.	Pulselessness indicates decreased or no blood flow. Occlusion of peripheral arteries leads to ischemia and necrosis.
Measure circumference of abdomen or legs and notify physician of significant changes.	Significant differences between extremities or from day to day may indicate hemorrhage.
Monitor ECG for changes and dysrhythmias.	Decreases in tissue perfusion may cause cardiac decompensation, MIs, and dysrhythmias.
Monitor I&O every hour and notify physician if <30 cc/hr.	Surgical procedures may result in decreased renal blood flow due to length of cross clamp time during aneurysm repair.
Do not elevate head of bed >30–45 degrees.	Higher flexion may cause flexion at femoral artery site and may impede blood flow.

Auscultate abdomen for bowel sounds. Monitor NG aspirate for amount and characteristics.	Most major thoracoabdominal surgical patients develop an ileus and require decompression of bowel with nasogastric tube.
Monitor patient for diarrheal stools and notify physician.	May indicate bowel ischemia caused by the length of surgical procedure and decreased perfusion to gut.
Observe for mental changes, confusion, restlessness, and headache.	May be caused by repair of ascending and thoracic aortic aneurysms or to decreased cerebral perfusion.
Instruct patient/family on disease process, need for surgery, postoperative care.	Reduces anxiety and promotes knowledge and compliance.

NIC: *Circulatory Care*

Discharge or Maintenance Evaluation

- Patient will have stable vital signs and hemodynamic pressures.
- Patient will be pain free.
- Patient will be alert, oriented, and able to verbalize instructions accurately.
- Patient will have adequate perfusion to all body systems.
- Lung fields will be clear and patient eupneic.

ACUTE PAIN

Related to: pressure exerted on various structures by aneurysm, infringement on nerves, surgical procedures

Defining Characteristics: pain to abdomen, lower back, hips, scrotum, chest, shoulders, neck, and back; nausea/vomiting, increases in blood pressure, increased heart rate, facial grimacing, moaning, shortness of breath, decreased blood pressure

Outcome Criteria

✔ Patient will be free of pain, with no associated deviations of vital signs.

NOC: *Pain Level*

INTERVENTIONS	RATIONALES
Monitor vital signs, and notify physician for unstable vital signs that do not change with analgesia.	Pain may increase heart rate, increase blood pressure or decrease blood pressure, but instability may occur from a variety of other causes.
Assess for dull abdominal pain, lower backache, lower back pain.	May indicate impending rupture of abdominal aortic aneurysm.
Assess for sudden severe pain to abdomen that may radiate to back, hips, or scrotum, and is associated with nausea, vomiting, and hypotension.	May indicate aortic dissection or rupture of AAA and requires immediate surgical intervention. MI should also be ruled out.
Assess for sudden tearing-type of pain to chest that may radiate to shoulders, neck, and back.	May indicate thoracic aortic aneurysm.
Observe for difficulty in swallowing or talking. Assess for voice hoarseness or cough. Observe for shortness of breath.	May indicate that aneurysm is placing pressure against esophagus, laryngeal nerve, or trachea.
Assess for pain to extremities, with mottling/cyanosis/pallor, pulselessness, or paralysis.	May indicate claudication of peripheral arteries as a result of enlarged aneurysm placing pressure on vasculature. Paralysis may indicate acute thrombosis of the AAA.
Assess for complaints of pain that are vague or involve unrelated areas of body.	May be an early sign of impending complications, such as thrombophlebitis or ulcer.
Administer analgesics as ordered. Medicate prior to painful procedures as warranted.	Provides pain relief/reduction, decreases anxiety, and reduces the workload on the heart and vasculature. Comfort and cooperation with painful procedures may be enhanced by prior medication administration.
Maintain bedrest with position of comfort.	Reduces oxygen consumption and demand.
Maintain relaxing environment to promote calmness.	Reduces competing stimuli which reduces anxiety and assists with pain relief.

INTERVENTIONS	RATIONALES
Provide back rubs, repositioning every 2 hours and prn, and encourage diversionary activity.	Promotes relaxation and may redirect attention from pain. Analgesics may be reduced in dosage and frequency by minimizing pain level.
Instruct in relaxation techniques, deep breathing, guided imagery, visualization, and so forth.	Helps to decrease pain and anxiety and provides distraction from pain.
Instruct in activity alterations and limitations.	Decreases myocardial oxygen demand and workload.
Instruct patient/family in medication effects, side effects, contraindications, and symptoms to report.	Promotes knowledge and compliance with therapeutic regimen. Alleviates fear.
Instruct patient to request pain medication when pain becomes noticeable and not to wait until pain is severe.	Pain promotes muscle tension, and may impair circulatory status and impair healing process.
Instruct patient in methods of splinting abdomen when coughing or deep breathing.	Supports surgical incision to allow patient to expand lungs to prevent atelectasis, and minimizes pain level.
Instruct patient in using pillows to maintain body alignment and support extremities.	Promotes comfort and reduces muscle tension and strain.

NIC: *Pain Management*

Discharge or Maintenance Evaluation

- Patient will report pain being absent or relieved with medication administration.
- Medication will be administered prior to pain becoming severe.
- Patient will be able to recall instructions on medications accurately.
- Activity will be modified in such a way as to prevent increased pain.

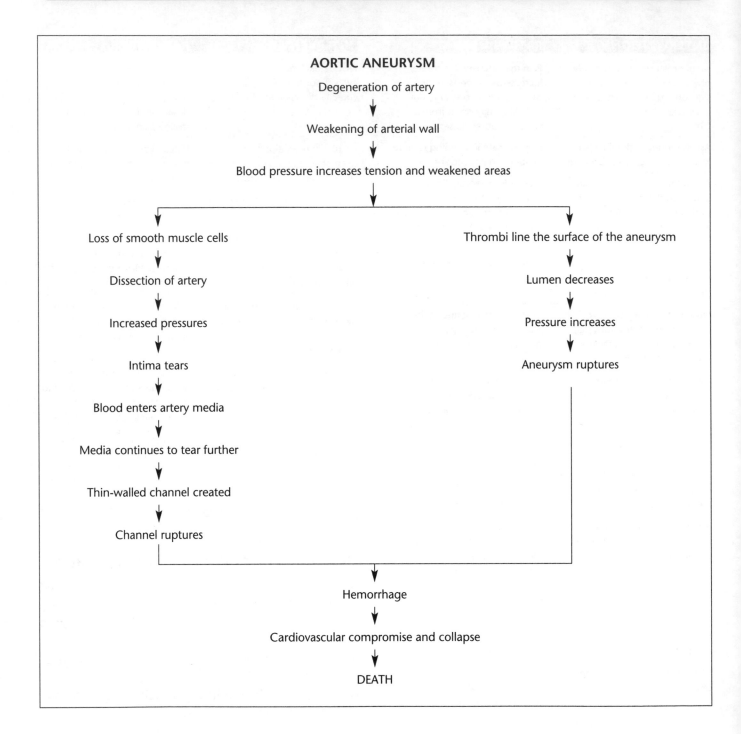

UNIT 2

RESPIRATORY SYSTEM

CHAPTER 2.1

MECHANICAL VENTILATION

Mechanical ventilation is used as an artificial adjunct to maintain and optimize ventilation and oxygenation in those patients that are unable to do so on their own for whatever the reason. It is utilized when other adjuncts are ineffective to regulate oxygen and carbon dioxide levels and provide for an adequate acid–base balance.

Major types of ventilators include negative external pressure and positive pressure ventilators. The external type is very rarely seen today, such as the "iron lung" used for the treatment of polio and the chest ventilator used for home treatment of neuromuscular diseases. These ventilators apply pressure against the thorax that is less than room air, in order to accomplish ventilation by changes in lung pressures. There are no requirements for artificial airways and they are fairly easy to use. The patient must remain in or under the unit and, as such, activity is limited, and the negative pressure exerted may result in venous pooling and decreased cardiac output.

Positive pressure ventilators are further subclassified according to the factor that initiates the inspiratory phase, and what factor causes the inspiratory phase to cease. Pressure-cycled ventilators use oxygen or compressed air valves to deliver a gas volume until a preset pressure limit is achieved. As the lung compliance and airway resistance changes, inspired tidal volumes, alveolar ventilation and FIO_2 changes also. The alarm systems for this ventilator are sometimes inadequate and the ventilator cannot compensate for leaks that may occur in the system.

Volume-cycled ventilators, currently the most common found in intensive care settings, deliver a preset gas volume to the patient regardless of airway resistance or compliance. Most have safety features to limit excessive airway pressures, and FIO_2 and exhaled tidal volumes are more accurate.

High-frequency ventilation is used when other methods have not been successful in oxygenation and ventilation of the patient. It uses lower tidal volumes and increased respiratory rates to decrease the incidence of barotrauma and cardiac decompensa-

tion. Frequencies range from 60–200 times/min, and in high-frequency oscillation, movement of air to and from the airway is performed at 600–3000 cycles/min.

Differential lung ventilation (DLV) provides for each lung to be ventilated independently by use of a double lumen endobronchial tube that has the distal tip inserted into the left main stem bronchus. Two ventilators are used with settings on each based on the degree of lung injury involved to the particular lung being ventilated.

Pressure support ventilation (PSV) is a type of ventilatory support in which every breath is triggered by the patient with the application of different amounts of positive pressure. This is utilized during the weaning process and to decrease the work of breathing for the patient.

Continuous positive airway pressure (CPAP) is used to increase end-expiratory pressures above atmospheric pressure in an attempt to increase oxygenation and lung volume. This helps to decrease the work of breathing and to open previously closed alveoli.

PEEP, or positive end-expiratory pressure, is used to improve oxygen exchange in persistent hypoxemia when increases in FIO_2 have not improved the situation. PEEP produces an increased functional residual capacity (FRC) which increases the available lung alveoli surface for oxygenation by maintaining the alveoli in an open position. High levels of PEEP may contribute to the incidence of barotrauma and hemodynamic compromise, and are most effective when maintained for lengthy periods of time. To this end, a special PEEP ambu bag must be used to maintain the pressure in order to maintain the beneficial effects.

MEDICAL CARE

Laboratory: CBC, transferrin, albumin, prealbumin, electrolytes used to monitor infection, imbalance, and nutritional status; cultures done to identify infective organism and specify antimicrobial agent required for eradication of infection

Intubation: artificial airway is required for mechanical ventilation

Arterial blood gases: used to determine levels of oxygen, carbon dioxide, and pH to identify acid–base disturbances, hypoxemia, and to monitor for changes in respiratory status

Respiratory treatments: used to instill varied agents into the lungs to reduce spasm, increase hydration and liquification of secretions, and to facilitate removal of secretions

Ventilatory management: ventilator settings are changed periodically based on patient condition and arterial blood gas analysis to ensure optimum ventilation and oxygenation

Tracheostomy: performed when nasal or oral intubation is impossible, or after significant time of nasal/oral intubation on a ventilator-dependent patient

COMMON NURSING DIAGNOSES

DECREASED CARDIAC OUTPUT (see ARDS)

Related to: decreased venous return to the heart, decreased transmural pressures, increased peripheral vascular resistance

Defining Characteristics: heart rate changes, decreased urinary output, decreased blood pressure, decreased preload, decreased afterload, dysrhythmias

RISK FOR IMBALANCED FLUID VOLUME (see ARDS)

Related to: overhydration with airway humidification, decreased urinary output caused by ADH effects, dehydration caused by decreased enteral/parenteral intake, overdiuresis

Defining Characteristics: weight gain, intake greater than output, decreased vital capacity, increased A-a gradient, decreased lung compliance, increased dead space/tidal volume ratios, decreased hematocrit, decreased sodium, increased bronchial secretions, fever, decreased skin turgor, intake less than output, weight loss, thick secretions

ADDITIONAL NURSING DIAGNOSES

IMPAIRED SPONTANEOUS VENTILATION

Related to: inability to adequately breathe independently

Defining Characteristics: apnea, dyspnea, tachypnea, hypermetabolic states, use of accessory muscles, decreased oxygen saturation, increased carbon dioxide levels, decreased tidal volumes, increased restlessness, tachycardia, confusion, mental status changes, dysrhythmias

Outcome Criteria

✔ Patient will have respiratory rate within set limitations of baseline.

✔ Patient will have arterial blood gases within normal limits.

✔ Patient will be able to maintain spontaneous respiration with minimal oxygen supplementation.

NOC: *Respiratory Status: Ventilation*

INTERVENTIONS	RATIONALES
Monitor VS q 15 minutes until stable, then q 1–2 hours. Notify physician of significant changes.	Tachypnea and tachycardia may be early signs of impending respiratory distress.
Observe patient for changes in respiratory status, noting presence of nasal flaring, cyanosis, increased work of breathing, or decrease in oxygen saturation/oximetry.	The symptoms represent signs of respiratory distress and patient may require respiratory assistance.
Administer oxygen supplementation with oxygen concentration as low as possible to ensure SaO_2 90% or above.	Supplemental oxygen with concentrations as low as possible to achieve the desired results helps to prevent oxygen toxicity, which can cause physiologic changes in lung tissue.
Place in semi-Fowler's or high Fowler's position.	Increases patient comfort, eases breathing, and facilitates chest expansion.
Monitor ABGs and notify physician of abnormalities.	Decreasing oxygenation will require revision of oxygen therapy.
Monitor lab work, such as hemoglobin and hematocrit, electrolytes, and so forth.	Decreases in hemoglobin and hematocrit reflect a decrease in the oxygen-carrying capability of

(continues)

(continued)

INTERVENTIONS	RATIONALES
	the blood. Abnormal electrolytes may result in cardiac dysrhythmias, which increase the workload on the cardiac and pulmonary systems.
Anticipate and prepare for intubation and placement on mechanical ventilation.	If patient is unable to compensate with an FIO_2 of 100% on non-rebreather, the patient will require placement on mechanical ventilator to maintain adequate oxygenation and perfusion.
Instruct patient/family, if time warrants, for placement on mechanical ventilation.	Provides knowledge and decreases fear. Emergent nature of the problem may negate the ability to do pre-procedure teaching but should be done as soon as possible.
Instruct patient/family regarding weaning procedures.	Progressive, but slow weaning helps the patient to adjust to the increase in work of breathing.
Instruct patient/family in potential use of restraints as needed.	Restraints may be required if patient is confused or tries to pull at airway.

NIC: *Ventilation Assistance*

Discharge or Maintenance Evaluation

- Patient will have normal spontaneous breathing pattern after the mechanical ventilation is no longer required.
- Arterial blood gases will be within baseline parameters for the patient.
- Patient will be able to increase activity with minimal oxygen supplementation.

INEFFECTIVE AIRWAY CLEARANCE

Related to: thick tenacious secretions, airway obstruction, edema of bronchioles, inability to cough or to cough effectively, presence of artificial airway

Defining Characteristics: adventitious breath sounds, dyspnea, tachypnea, shallow respirations, cough with or without productivity, cyanosis, fever, anxiety, restlessness

Outcome Criteria

✔ Patient will maintain patency of airway, have clear breath sounds, and will be able to effectively clear secretions.

NOC: *Respiratory Status: Airway Patency*

INTERVENTIONS	RATIONALES
Monitor airway for patency and provide artificial airways as warranted. Prepare for mechanical ventilation.	Artificial airways will be required if patient cannot maintain patency. Oropharyngeal airways hold tongue anteriorly but may precipitate vomiting if length is not accurately measured. Nasopharyngeal airways are more easily tolerated in conscious patients but may cause nosebleeds and may easily become occluded. Esophageal obturator airways are useful only in emergency situations and must be replaced as quickly as possible. These are easier to insert than endotracheal tubes, but stimulate vomiting and cannot be used in conscious patients. The trachea may accidentally be intubated and the esophagus may be perforated. Endotracheal intubation requires advanced training and skill, and may be accidentally placed in the esophagus, develop leaks that may decrease oxygenation, and over time, may necrotize tissues. Artificial airways may become occluded by mucus, blood, or other secretions; endotracheal tubes may become twisted or compressed, or severe spasms may occlude airway.
Monitor tube placement for migration; place marking on tube and note length and position at least every 8 hours; tube should be adequately secured to maintain placement.	Tube migration may occur with coughing, re-taping, or accidentally, with the potential for improper placement resulting in hypoxia. Comparison of previous placement guidelines will provide prompt recognition of differences and changes, and facilitate prompt intervention.

INTERVENTIONS	RATIONALES
Prepare for placement on mechanical ventilation as warranted.	If routine medical therapeutics are not effective in controlling the spasms, hypoxemia, and hypoxia, respiratory failure will ensue, and mechanical ventilation will be required to assure adequate oxygenation and perfusion.
Auscultate lung fields for presence of breath sounds, changes in character, and presence to all lobes; observe for symmetric chest expansion.	Proper tube placement will result in equal bilateral breath sounds and symmetric chest expansion. Adventitious breath sounds, such as rhonchi and wheezes, may indicate airflow has been obstructed by occlusion of the tube or migration into an inappropriate position. Absence of breath sounds to left lung fields may indicate intubation of the right mainstem bronchus.
Suction patient every 2–4 hours and prn, being sure to hyperoxygenate patient prior to, during, and after procedure; limit active suctioning to 15 seconds or less at a time.	Patients who are intubated frequently have ineffective cough reflexes or are sedated and have some muscular involvement that may impair coughing, and suctioning is required to remove their secretions. Suctioning time should be minimized and hyperoxygenation performed to reduce the potential for hypoxia.
Position patient in high-Fowler's or semi-Fowler's position.	Promotes maximal lung expansion.
Turn patient every 2 hours and prn.	Repositioning promotes drainage of pulmonary secretions and enhances ventilation to decrease potential for atelectasis.
Administer bronchodilators as ordered.	Promotes relaxation of bronchial smooth muscle to decrease spasm, dilates airways to improve ventilation, and maximizes air exchange.
Instruct on splinting abdomen with pillow during cough efforts.	Promotes increased expiratory pressure and helps to decrease discomfort.
Perform chest percussion and postural drainage as warranted.	Mobilizes secretions and facilitates ventilation of all lung fields.
Instruct patient/family regarding need and procedure for suctioning.	Removes mucoid secretions that may impair breathing by blocking passages with thick, tenacious mucus. Information regarding procedure will facilitate compliance.

INTERVENTIONS	RATIONALES
Instruct patient to notify nurse if he experiences shortness of breath or air hunger.	May indicate bronchial tubes are blocked with mucus, leading to hypoxia and hypoxemia.
Instruct patient/family regarding medications, effects, side effects, and symptoms of adverse effects to report to nurse or physician.	Promotes prompt identification of potential adverse reaction to facilitate timely intervention.

NIC: *Airway Suctioning*

Discharge or Maintenance Evaluation

- Patient will maintain patent airway and be able to cough and clear own secretions.
- Patient will have clear breath sounds with no adventitious sounds or airway compromise.
- Patient will not have any aspiration complications.
- Patient will be able to adequately perform coughing.

IMPAIRED GAS EXCHANGE

Related to: barotrauma, atelectasis, bronchospasm, mucus production, edema, inflammation to bronchial tree, hypoxemia, hypercapnia, fatigue

Defining Characteristics: dyspnea, tachypnea, hypoxia, hypoxemia, hypercapnia, confusion, restlessness, cyanosis, inability to move secretions, tachycardia, dysrhythmias, abnormal ABGs, decreased oxygen saturation by oximetry

Outcome Criteria

✔ Patient will have arterial blood gases within normal range for patient, with no signs of ventilation/perfusion mismatching.

NOC: *Respiratory Status: Ventilation*

INTERVENTIONS	RATIONALES
Monitor pulse oximetry for oxygen saturation and notify physician if <90.	Oximetry readings of 90 correlate with PaO_2 of 60. Levels below 60 do not allow for adequate perfusion to tissues and vital organs. Oximetry uses light waves to identify differences between saturation and reduced hemoglobin of the tissues and may be inaccurate in low blood flow states.

(continues)

(continued)

INTERVENTIONS	RATIONALES
Monitor transcutaneous oxygen tension if available.	Measures the oxygen concentration of the skin, but may cause burns if monitor site is not rotated frequently. Skin, blood flow and temperature may affect these readings.
Provide oxygen as ordered.	Provides supplemental oxygen to benefit patient. Low flow oxygen delivery systems use some room air and may be inadequate for patient's needs if their tidal volume is low, respiratory rate is high, or if ventilation status is unstable. Low flow systems should be used in patients with COPD so as to not depress their respiratory drive. High levels of oxygen may cause severe damage to tissues, oxygen toxicity, increases in A-a gradients, microatelectasis, and ARDS.
Monitor for changes in mental status, restlessness, anxiety, headache, confusion, dysrhythmias, hypotension, tachycardia, and cyanosis.	May indicate impending or present hypoxia and hypoxemia.
Monitor ABGs for changes and/or trends.	Provides information on measured levels of oxygen and carbon dioxide as well as acid–base balance. Promotes prompt intervention for deteriorating airway status. PaO_2 alone does not reflect tissue oxygenation; ventilation must be adequate to provide gas exchange.
Monitor for signs/symptoms of oxygen toxicity (nausea, vomiting, dyspnea, coughing, retrosternal pain, extremity paresthesias, pronounced fatigue, or restlessness).	Oxygen toxicity may result when oxygen concentrations are greater than 40% for lengthy durations of time, usually 8 to 24 hours, and may cause actual physiologic changes in the lungs. Progressive respiratory distress, cyanosis, and asphyxia are late signs of toxicity. Oxygen concentrations should be maintained as low as possible in order to maintain adequate PaO_2.
Limit PEEP (positive end-expiratory pressures) to 5–20 cm H_2O. Use PEEP ambu bag or in-line suctioning apparatus when suctioning patient.	PEEP is used to improve oxygen exchange in persistent hypoxemia despite increasing levels of oxygen by producing an increased functional residual capacity

INTERVENTIONS	RATIONALES
	which then increases the available lung alveoli surface for oxygenation. Peep may predispose the patient to barotrauma with elevated levels. Ambu bags that are capable of maintaining PEEP levels are required because short intervals without PEEP minimize the beneficial effects of PEEP.
Prepare patient for placement on mechanical ventilation as warranted.	May be necessary to maintain adequate oxygenation and acid–base balance.
Assist with respiratory therapists measurements of oxygen analyzing, lung compliance, vital capacity, and A-a gradients.	Provides information to facilitate early detection of oxygen toxicity.

NIC: *Respiratory Monitoring*

Discharge or Maintenance Evaluation

- Patient will have arterial blood gases within normal limits for patient.
- Patient will be eupneic with adequate oxygenation and no signs/symptoms of oxygen toxicity.

INEFFECTIVE BREATHING PATTERN

Related to: fatigue, dyspnea, secretions, inadequate oxygenation, respiratory muscle weakness, respiratory center depression, decreased lung expansion, placement on mechanical ventilation

Defining Characteristics: dyspnea, tachypnea, bradypnea, apnea, cough, nasal flaring, cyanosis, shallow respirations, pursed-lip breathing, changes in inspiratory/expiratory ratio, use of accessory muscles, diminished chest expansion, barrel chest, abnormal arterial blood gases, fremitus, anxiety, decreased oxygen saturation

Outcome Criteria

✔ Patient will be eupneic, with adequate oxygenation, and will maintain adequate ABGs within normal limits.

NOC: *Respiratory Status: Ventilation*

INTERVENTIONS	RATIONALES
Prepare patient for placement on mechanical ventilation and intubation procedures.	Promotes knowledge and reduces fear. May promote cooperation.
Assist with intubation of patient; auscultate all lung fields for breath sounds.	Placement of an artificial airway (endotracheal tube [ETT] or tracheostomy) is required for mechanical ventilation support. Nasotracheal intubation may be preferred to prevent oral discomfort and necrosis, but is associated with a high incidence of sinus disease.
Hyperoxygenate patient and auscultate for bilateral breath sounds and observe for bilateral symmetric chest expansion.	Prolonged difficulty in placement of the tube may result in hypoxia. If symmetric chest expansion is not observed, or if breath sounds cannot be heard bilaterally, this may indicate improper placement of the tube into the right main bronchus or esophagus, and correction of this problem must be addressed promptly.
Utilize low pressure endotracheal tubes for intubation.	High pressure cuffed tubes may promote tracheal necrosis or result in a tracheal fistula.
Maintain airway; secure tube with tape or other securing device.	Artificial airways may become occluded by mucous or other secretory fluids, may develop a cuff leak resulting in inability to maintain pressures sufficient for ventilation, or may migrate to a position whereby adequate oxygenation is impaired. Tubes should be adequately secured to prevent movement, loss of airway, and tracheal damage.
Obtain chest X-ray after ETT is inserted.	Radiographic confirmation of tube placement is mandatory; the tube should be 2–3 cm above the carina.
If ETT is placed orally, daily changes from side to side of mouth should be routinely performed. Perform oral care 4 hrs. and prn.	Prevents tissue necrosis from pressure of tube against teeth, lips, and other tissues. Oral tubes promote saliva formation, cause nausea and vomiting if movement of tube stimulates retching, and prevents the patient from closing his mouth without biting down on the tube.
Suction patient as needed, making sure to hyperoxygenate	Suctioning is required to remove secretions because the patient is

INTERVENTIONS	RATIONALES
before, during, and after procedure.	unable to do so on his own. Effective coughing is decreased because of the inability to increase intrathoracic pressure when the glottis is restricted from air. Suctioning places patient at risk for inadequate oxygenation and decreased perfusion. Hyperoxygenation helps to limit this sudden decrease in available oxygen. Mucus production is usually increased with placement of ETT because of ciliary movement being impaired and the body's response to the foreign tube. Pulmonary toilette is controversial but may be helpful to liquefy secretions to facilitate easier removal.
Restrain patient as warranted only as a last resort, and as per hospital protocol.	Prevents accidental extubation in sedated or confused patients.
Monitor ventilator settings at least every 2–4 hours and prn; FIO$_2$ should be analyzed periodically to ensure correct amount is being maintained; tidal volume should ideally be 10–15 cc/Kg body weight; airway pressures (peak inspiratory pressure and plateau pressure) should be noted for identification of trends; inspiratory and expiratory ratio; sigh volume and rate.	Ventilator settings are adjusted based on the disease process and patient's condition to maintain optimal oxygenation and ventilation while the patient is unable to do so on his own. Oxygen percentages may not be completely accurate and analysis must be performed to ensure proper amounts are being delivered. Exhaled tidal volumes should be monitored and changes may indicate changes in lung compliance or problems with delivering specific volumes. Increases in airway pressures may indicate bronchospasm, presence of mucoid and other secretions, obstruction of the airway, pneumothorax, or ARDS with high pressure levels and disconnection of tubing, inadequate cuff pressure or nonsynchronous breathing with low pressure levels. I:E ratio should be 1:2 but may be altered to improve gas exchange. Sighs, when used, are commonly 1½ times the volume of a normal breath, 2–6 times per hour to facilitate expansion of alveoli to

(continues)

(continued)

INTERVENTIONS	RATIONALES
	reduce the potential for atelectasis. Ventilator settings may be inadvertently changed, or because of forgetfulness, increased oxygenation used for suctioning procedure may not be turned down to ordered amounts. This may result in oxygen toxicity or inadequate ventilation.
Observe for temperature of ventilator circuitry; drain tubing away from the patient as warranted.	Intubation bypasses the body's natural warming/humidifying action, and requires increased temperature and moisturizing of the delivered oxygen. The temperature of the ventilator circuitry (and the delivered oxygen) should be maintained at approximately body temperature to avoid hyperthermic reactions. Temperature increases and humidification promote condensation of water in tubing which may restrict adequate volume delivery. Drainage of fluid toward the patient or toward the reservoir may promote bacterial infestations.
Monitor airway cuff for leakage, noting amount of air volume in cuff and cuff pressures at least every 4–8 hours and prn.	Proper cuff inflation is done with the least amount of air to ensure a minimal leak with maintenance of adequate ventilatory pressures and tidal volumes. Cuff pressures should be less than 25 cm H_2O to prevent tracheal necrosis. Increasing volumes of air required to maintain ventilatory pressures, or increasing cuff pressures may indicate cuff leak and will require replacement of airway to maintain oxygenation.
Auscultate for adventitious breath sounds, subcutaneous emphysema, or localized wheezing.	May indicate migration of airway tube. Movement from trachea into tissue may cause mediastinal or subcutaneous emphysema and/or pneumothorax. Intubation of the bronchus may result in decreased unilateral chest expansion with decreased breath sounds, and localized wheezing. Movement of the tube to the level of the carina may result in excessive coughing, diminished breath sounds, and inability to

INTERVENTIONS	RATIONALES
	insert suction catheter. Adventitious breath sounds may indicate worsening respiratory status, atelectasis, pneumonia, or other conditions that require medical attention.
Monitor ventilatory pressure wave forms and notify physician of significant abnormalities.	Airway pressure tracing can identify asynchronous respiratory status between patient and ventilator, patient's effort and work of breathing, and auto-PEEP identification in order to promptly correct disadvantageous situations.
Monitor ABGs for trends, and change ventilator settings as ordered.	Maintains adequate oxygenation and acid–base balance.
Observe breathing patterns and note if patient has spontaneous breaths in addition to ventilatory breaths.	Increased or decreased ventilation may be experienced by ventilator patients who may try to compensate by competing with ventilatory breaths. Tachypnea may result in respiratory alkalosis; bradypnea may result in acidosis with increased $PaCO_2$.
Observe patient for nonsynchronous respirations with ventilator ("fighting the ventilator"). Administer sedation or sedation/neuromuscular blockade, as ordered.	Asynchrony with the ventilator decreases alveolar ventilation, increases intrathoracic pressures, and decreases venous return and cardiac output. Pavulon and other drugs, such as neuromax, paralyzes all muscles in body to facilitate synchrony with ventilation support. Patients may be completely alert when paralyzed, so sedation is MANDATORY prior to administration of these drugs. Often, a sedation cocktail of narcotics and/or benzodiazepines may be titrated with better results to achieve adequate sedation.
Prepare patient for placement of tracheostomy as warranted.	Prolonged ventilatory support via nasal or oral endotracheal tube may lead to necrosis of tissues because of pressure exerted by the tube. Tracheostomy is more comfortable for the patient, decreases the airway resistance, and may reduce the amount of dead space.

INTERVENTIONS	RATIONALES
Observe for pulsation of tracheostomy with neck vein pulsation and notify physician.	May indicate close proximity to innominate vessels that may lead to necrosis and erosion into vessels and result in hemorrhage.
Assess for cuff leakage and change/notify physician for change of airway	Cuffs which have leaks that enable a patient to have the ability to speak, in which air may be felt at the nose and/or mouth, changing pressures with ventilation, and/or decreased exhaled volumes require change in order to maintain adequate oxygenation and ventilation.
Obtain chest X-rays every day and prn while patient is intubated.	Facilitates recognition of tube migration, atelectatic changes, presence of pneumothorax, or other significant changes.
Insure that neostigmine bromide or edrophonium chloride is available.	These reverse effects of neuromuscular blocking agent.
Instruct patient/family in regard to all procedures, placement on ventilator, what to expect, and methods to use to communicate.	Provides knowledge to facilitate compliance and decrease anxiety.
Instruct patient/family regarding equipment and alarms. Ensure that patient understands that he will not be able to speak, but will have nurse available at all times.	Reduces anxiety and fear of being left alone without method of calling for help.
Instruct patient/family that medications may need to be administered that will decrease patient's consciousness level temporarily.	Patient may be anxious and "fight the ventilator" requiring sedation to achieve adequate ventilation.

NIC: *Ventilation Assistance*

Discharge or Maintenance Evaluation

- Patient will be able to maintain own airway and expectorate sputum.
- Patient will have arterial blood gases within normal limits of patient disease process.
- Patient will be eupneic with no adventitious breath sounds.
- Patient will have artificial airway intact with no signs/symptoms of complications.

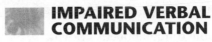

IMPAIRED VERBAL COMMUNICATION

Related to: intubation, artificial airway, muscular paralysis

Defining Characteristics: inability to speak, inability to communicate needs, inability to make sounds

Outcome Criteria

✔ Patient will achieve a method to communicate his needs.

NOC: *Communication: Expressive Ability*

INTERVENTIONS	RATIONALES
Evaluate patient's ability to communicate by other means.	Patient may be fluent in sign language, or able to communicate in writing to make needs known.
Ensure that call light is placed within easy reach of patient at all times, and that the light system is flagged to denote patient's impairment.	Provides patient with concrete evidence that he may call for assistance and that the nurse will be available to meet his needs. Flagging system ensures that personnel not familiar with the patient will be alerted to his inability to speak.
Make eye contact with patient at all times; ask questions that may be answered by nodding of the head; provide paper and writing utensils, magic slate, or communication board for communication.	Communication may be possible if patient is able to nod head yes or no, or blink eyes in sequence. Writing may be illegible due to disease process or sedation, and may frustrate and fatigue patient.
Instruct patient in using tongue to make clicking noise, or in tapping table or side rails to gain nurse's attention as a secondary means of calling for assistance.	Provides alternate method to communicate with nurse and helps to allay fear of abandonment.
Instruct family members in talking with patient to provide information about issues of concern to patient, and help them to deal with the awkwardness of a one-sided conversation.	Promotes understanding for the family and assists in incorporating family into the patient's care to maintain contact with reality.

NIC: *Communication Enhancement: Speech Deficit*

Discharge or Maintenance Evaluation

- Patient will be able to make needs known.
- Patient will develop an adequate alternative means of communication and be able to utilize communication to make needs known.
- Patient's family will be able to recognize their own contribution to the patient's recovery.

ANXIETY

Related to: ventilatory support, threat of death, change in health status, change in environment, life-threatening crises

Defining Characteristics: fear, restlessness, muscle tension, apprehension, helplessness, communication of uncertainty, sense of impending doom, worry

Outcome Criteria

✔ Patient will have decreased anxiety and be able to function at acceptable levels with anxiety-producing stimuli.

NOC: *Anxiety Control*

INTERVENTIONS	RATIONALES
Evaluate patient's perception of crisis or threat to self.	Identifies problem base and facilitates plan for intervention.
Monitor for changes in vital signs, restlessness, or facial tension.	May indicate patient's level of response to stressors and level of anxiety.
Encourage patient to express fears and concerns and provide information pertinent to those concerns. Do not give false reassurance.	Promotes verbalization of concerns, and allows time for identification of fears to progressively begin work on emotional barriers. False reassurance tends to minimize patient's feelings resulting in impaired trust and increased anxiety.
Provide support and encouragement to family members and assist them in dealing with their own fears/concerns.	Family's anxiety may be communicated to the patient and result in increased anxiety levels.
Discuss safety precautions involved with ventilatory support; emergency power source, emergency oxygen and equipment, alarm systems, and so forth.	Provides concrete answers to help decrease anxiety and fear of the unknown, and to relay emergency plans for patient.
Ensure that patient's call light is placed within easy reach at all	Provides reassurance that nurses will be available to assist with

INTERVENTIONS	RATIONALES
times, and that alternative methods of summoning assistance have been discussed.	patient's needs, and decreases anxiety.
Administer antianxiety medications as ordered.	Helps to reduce anxiety to a manageable level when other techniques have failed.
Instruct in use of relaxation techniques and guided imagery.	Promotes reduction in stress and anxiety, and provides opportunity for patient to control his situation.
Consult psychiatrist, psychologist, or counselor as warranted.	Patient may require further intervention for dealing with emotional problems.

NIC: *Anxiety Reduction*

Discharge or Maintenance Evaluation

- Patient will be able to notify nurse of concerns and fears and be able to rationally deal with them in appropriate ways.
- Patient will be able to function with anxiety reduced at a manageable level.
- Patient will be able to utilize methods to reduce anxiety.

INEFFECTIVE COPING

Related to: placement on ventilator support, change in health status, change in ability to communicate, sensory overload, change in environment, fear of death, physical limitations, inadequate support system, inadequate coping mechanisms, threat to self, pain

Defining Characteristics: inability to meet role expectations, inability to meet basic needs, worry, apprehension, fear, inability to problem solve, hostility, aggression, inappropriate defense mechanisms, low self-esteem, insomnia, depression, destructive behaviors, vacillation when choices are required, delayed decision making, muscle tension, headaches, pain

Outcome Criteria

✔ Patient will be able to recognize problems with coping and be able to problem-solve adequately.

NOC: *Coping*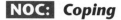

INTERVENTIONS	RATIONALES
Evaluate patient's/family's coping skills and ability to Identify problems.	Provides baseline information to establish interventions best suited to the patient/family/ situation. Coping abilities that the patient has utilized previously may be used in the current crisis to provide a sense of control.
Discuss concerns and fears of loss of control with patient, and provide feedback.	Identifies needs for intervention and helps to establish a trusting relationship.
Monitor for dependence on others, inability to make decisions, inability to involve self in care, or inability to express concerns/questions.	May indicate patient's need to depend on others to allow time to regain ability for coping with crises, and promotes feeling of safety. Patient may be afraid to make any decision in which his tenuous condition could be compromised.
Provide opportunities for patient to make decisions regarding his care, when feasible.	Provides opportunity to gain some sense of control of his life, decreasing anxiety, and assisting in coping skills.
Discuss current problems and assist with problem-solving to find solutions.	Identifies actual problems and assists patient/family to find real solutions to facilitate increasing self-control and self-esteem.
Discuss feelings of blame, either on self, or on others.	Blaming oneself or others prolongs inability to cope and increases feelings of hopelessness.
Remain nonjudgmental of choices patient/family may make. Adopt a non-threatened attitude when anger and hostility are expressed. Set limits on unacceptable behaviors.	Anger and hostile feelings may promote resolution of stages of grief and loss, and should be regarded as an important step in that process. Limits must be set to prevent destructive behavior that will impair patient's self-esteem.
Discuss feelings of anger at God, religious alienation, lack of meaning to life, and so forth.	Spiritual beliefs are questioned when threats of death occur, and may affect patient's ability to cope with and problem-solve during crises.
Assess rapport of family members with patient. Involve the family members in the care of the patient, when feasible.	Actions of the family may be helpful, but the patient may perceive these as being over-protective or smothering. Helping with patient's care may enhance the family's feelings of importance and control of the situation.

INTERVENTIONS	RATIONALES
Provide information to the patient and family regarding other agencies and personnel who may assist them with their crisis.	Identifies opportunities for other resources that may be available, and provides means of control over situation.

NIC: *Behavior Management*

Discharge or Maintenance Evaluation

- Patient/family will be able to recognize ineffective coping behavior and regain emotional equilibrium.
- Patient/family will be able to adequately problem-solve during crises.
- Patient/family will be able to recognize options and resources for use posthospitalization.
- Patient/family will be able to make appropriate, informed decisions and be satisfied with choices.

RISK FOR INFECTION

Related to: intubation, disease process, immunosuppression, compromised defense mechanisms

Defining Characteristics: increased temperature, chills, elevated white blood cell count, purulent sputum

Outcome Criteria

✔ Patient will have no evidence of infective process.

NOC: *Risk Control*

INTERVENTIONS	RATIONALES
Evaluate risk factors that would predispose patient to infection.	Intubation and prolonged mechanical ventilation predispose patient to nosocomial infection. Age, nutritional status, chronic disease progression and invasive procedures and lines also predispose patient to infection. Patient is also at risk for sinus infections with prolonged intubation, especially if he has concurrent NG tube placement.
Provide oral hygiene q 4 hrs and prn.	Freshens mouth, decreases bacterial formation, and moistens mucous membranes to provide comfort.

(continues)

(continued)

INTERVENTIONS	RATIONALES
Monitor sputum for changes in characteristics and color; culture sputum as warranted.	Purulent, malodorous sputum indicates infection. Cultures may be required to identify causative organism and to prescribe appropriate anti-microbials.
Monitor tracheostomy site for redness, foul odor, or purulent drainage; culture site as warranted.	Purulent drainage indicates infection. Cultures may be required to identify causative organism and to prescribe appropriate antimicrobials.
Maintain good handwashing technique and isolation pre-cautions when warranted.	Handwashing is the most impor-tant step in preventing nosoco-mial infection. Patients may require isolation based on their diagnosis to prevent transmis-sion of infection to or from the patient.
Screen visitors who are ill themselves.	Patients are already immuno-compromised and at risk for development of infection.
Maintain sterile technique for all dressing changes and suctioning.	Reduces spread of infection.
Administer antimicrobials as ordered.	Required to treat infective organism.
Instruct patient/family in proper handwashing and disposal of contaminated secretions, tissues, etc.	Reduces risk of transmission of infection to others.
Instruct family to avoid visiting if they have upper respiratory infections.	Patient is already immuno-compromised and is at risk for infection.
Instruct patient/family on meds: effects, side effects, contra-indications, and foods/drugs to avoid.	Provides knowledge and enhances cooperation with treatment.

NIC: *Infection Protection*

Discharge or Maintenance Evaluation

- Patient will be free of fever, chills, purulent drainage, or other indicators of infective process.
- Patient will be able to recall information accu-rately regarding antimicrobials and infection con-trol procedures.
- Patient/family will be able to recognize risk factors and avoid further compromise of patient.

IMPAIRED ORAL MUCOUS MEMBRANE

Related to: oral intubation, increased or decreased saliva, inability to swallow, antibiotic-induced fungal infection

Defining Characteristics: oral pain or discomfort, stomatitis, oral lesions, thrush

Outcome Criteria

✔ Patient will be free of oral pain and mucous membranes will remain intact.

NOC: *Oral Health*

INTERVENTIONS	RATIONALES
Observe mouth for missing, loose, or chipped teeth; bleeding, sores, lesions, necrotic areas, or reddened areas.	Teeth may be chipped or knocked out during intubation process and loose teeth may pose a potential for aspiration. Identifi-cation of lesions or other prob-lems may facilitate prompt intervention.
Move oral endotracheal tube to other side of mouth at least daily and prn.	Decreases potential for pressure and ultimately, ulceration of lips or mucous membranes.
Provide oral care at least every 4 hours and prn.	Promotes cleanliness, reduces odor, and reduces potential environment for bacterial invasion.
Swab mouth with mouthwash or other cleansing solution every 4–8 hours and prn.	Removes transient bacteria, reduces odor, and helps to stimulate circulation to oral membranes. Mouthwash solu-tion may tend to dry mucous membranes.
Apply lip balm every 2–4 hours and prn.	Prevents drying and cracking of lips.
Suction patient's oral cavity frequently if patient is unable to handle secretions.	Removes excessive saliva and mucus which may facilitate bacterial growth.
Observe for white patches on tongue and mucous membranes, and notify physician.	May indicate presence of fungal infection (thrush) which will require antifungal solution, such as Nystatin.
Instruct patient on antifungals as warranted.	Provides knowledge.

INTERVENTIONS	RATIONALES
Instruct patient in utilizing oral suction equipment when feasible, if patient has copious oral secretions.	Provides a sense of control to the patient, and facilitates removal of excessive secretions.

NIC: *Oral Health Maintenance*

Discharge or Maintenance Evaluation

- Patient will have intact oral mucous membranes, with no evidence of infection.
- Patient will be able to recall instructions accurately.
- Patient will be able to adequately remove secretions by use of suction equipment.
- Patient will be compliant with performance of oral care.

IMBALANCED NUTRITION: LESS THAN BODY REQUIREMENTS

Related to: intubation, inability to swallow, inability to take in food, increased metabolism caused by disease process, surgery, decreased level of consciousness

Defining Characteristics: actual inadequate caloric intake, altered taste, altered smell sensation, weight loss, anorexia, absent bowel sounds, decreased peristalsis, muscle mass loss, decreased muscle tone, changes in bowel habits, nausea, vomiting, abdominal distention

Outcome Criteria

✔ Patient will have adequate nutritional intake with no weight or muscle mass loss.

NOC: *Nutritional Status*

INTERVENTIONS	RATIONALES
Evaluate ability to eat.	Some patients with tracheostomies are able to eat, while those patients who are endotracheally intubated must be kept NPO because of the positioning of the epiglottis, and will require enteral or parenteral alimentation.
Weigh every day.	Continued weight loss will result in catabolic metabolism and impaired respiratory function.

INTERVENTIONS	RATIONALES
Observe for muscle wasting.	May indicate muscle stores depletion which can impair respiratory muscle function.
Observe for nausea, vomiting, abdominal distention and palpability, and stool characteristics.	Ventilator patients may develop GI dysfunction from analgesics/sedatives, bed rest, trapped air, and stress, which may result in ileus formation.
Test stools and gastric contents for guaiac.	Stressors of ventilation and presence in ICU may predispose patient to the formation of a stress ulcer resulting in GI bleeding.
Obtain calorie count and assessment of metabolic demands based on disease process.	Establishes imbalances between actual nutritional intake and metabolic needs.
Monitor lab work as warranted; electrolytes, BUN, creatinine, albumin and prealbumin, glucose levels.	Evaluates need for and/or adequacy of nutritional support.
Administer enteral solutions at continual rate by infusion pump as warranted.	Bolus feedings may result in dumping syndrome. Continuous infusion feedings are generally better tolerated and have better absorption. Enteral feeding formulas vary depending on the nutritional needs of the patient. The use of enteral formulas require a functioning GI system.
Determine patency of enteral feeding tubes at least every 8 hours. Flush with 20–30 cc of water every 8 hours, before and after medication administration via the tube, and prn.	Oral or nasal tubes may migrate with coughing, resulting in improper placement and potential for aspiration. Flushing of tube maintains patency.
Aspirate gastric residuals every 4–8 hours, and decrease or hold feedings per hospital protocol.	Increasing residuals may indicate decreased or absent peristalsis and lack of absorption of required nutrients which may require another form of nutritional support.
Use food coloring to tint feedings per hospital protocol. Do not use red coloring.	Helps to identify aspiration of feedings when suctioned. Be aware that the food coloring may cause false readings on occult blood tests on stools. Red coloring should be avoided because of similarity of blood color and this may impair ability to differentiate bleeding problems. Some facilities avoid the

(continues)

(continued)

INTERVENTIONS	RATIONALES
	use of food coloring because of potential contamination and increased risk of bacteria.
Instill warm cranberry juice, carbonated cola, or mixture of monosodium glutamate and water in enteral tube for signs of occlusion.	Helps to dissolve clogged particulate matter to maintain patency of tube.
Administer antidiarrheal medications as warranted.	Osmolality imbalances may result in diarrhea requiring antidiarrheals for control. Changing strengths or types of feedings may be helpful.
Administer cholinergic drugs, such as metoclopramide or neostigmine as ordered.	Medication helps to stimulate gastric motility and may be helpful to increase absorption.
Administer parenteral alimentation fluids as warranted via infusion pump.	Provides complete nutritional support without dependence on GI function for absorption. Additives are based upon lab work and patient requirements. Increases in protein and nitrogen may be prescribed for increased metabolic demands of the patient.
Administer intralipids as ordered, if not admixed with TPN solution.	Provides additional caloric benefits as well as a source of essential fatty acids. Lipids may be utilized for respiratory failure to help decrease CO_2 retention.
Change solution at least every 24 hours, as well as tubing, per hospital protocol.	Some additives may be unstable after 24 hours, and prolonged infusion with same solution may promote bacterial growth.
Monitor lab work per hospital protocol; general chemistry, renal profile, CBC, urine or blood glucose levels.	Requirements for electrolyte replacement or alteration in formula may be changed based on this information. High dextrose content in TPN solutions may require additions of insulin to meet metabolic demands if pancreatic disease, hepatic disease, or diabetes are present.
Do not stop TPN abruptly; taper over several days/hours per protocol.	Rebound hypoglycemia may result if dextrose concentrations are abruptly changed.
Insert nasogastric feeding tube as warranted, utilizing small weighted tube. Obtain chest X-ray or KUB post-procedure.	Smaller lumen tube is less irritating to nasal mucosa, and decreases the incidence of gastroesophageal reflux. Radiographic confirmation of placement is

INTERVENTIONS	RATIONALES
	necessary due to the potential for aspiration when patients may have impaired gag reflex.
Maintain elevation of the head of the bed at least 30 degrees at all times.	Helps prevent potential aspiration.
Assist with placement of central venous catheter for TPN administration. Obtain chest X-ray post-procedure.	Centrally-placed intravenous lines may enable higher concentrations of amino acids to be utilized. Radiographic confirmation of placement, as well as ruling out hemo- or pneumothorax post-procedure, is mandatory.
Instruct patient/family in need for supplemental nutritional support, procedures to be performed, and tests that will be required.	Promotes knowledge, decreases fear of the unknown, and facilitates cooperation with procedures. Provides opportunity for patient to make informed choices.

NIC: *Feeding*

Discharge or Maintenance Evaluation

- Patient will maintain baseline weight with no loss of muscle mass.

- Patient will maintain adequate nutritional status with use of nutritional support, and will experience no complications from support.

- Patient will show no signs of malnutritional status.

- Patient will be able to recall information accurately.

- Patient will maintain a normal nitrogen balance and immunity will not be compromised.

DYSFUNCTIONAL VENTILATORY WEANING RESPONSE

Related to: fever, pain, muscle fatigue, sedation, anemia, electrolyte imbalance, sleep deprivation, poor nutrition, cardiovascular lability, psychological instability

Defining Characteristics: inability to wean, lack or inadequacy of spontaneous respirations, negative inspiratory force or pressure <-20 cm H_2O, $PaO_2 <60$ mm Hg on $FIO_2 >50\%$, $PaCO_2 >40$ mm Hg, tidal volume <5 cc/kg, vital capacity <10 cc/kg, minute ventilation >10 L/min

Outcome Criteria

✔ Patient will be able to be weaned from ventilatory support successfully with arterial blood gases within normal limits.

NOC: *Respiratory Status: Ventilation*

INTERVENTIONS	RATIONALES
Monitor vital signs.	Temperature elevations increase metabolism and oxygen demand. Unstable heart rate and rhythm result in increased workload on the heart, increased oxygen consumption and demand. Process of weaning will increase workload and may compromise an already-stressed body and should not be attempted until these factors have been corrected. Once weaning process has begun, significant changes in heart rate and rhythm, respiratory rate, and blood pressure may indicate a need to slow or discontinue weaning because of respiratory compromise.
Monitor ECG for dysrhythmias and treat as warranted.	Ventilatory support decreases venous return to the heart, increases PVR and SVR. Hypoxemia and pH imbalances may result in dysrhythmias from cardiac compromise.
Monitor nutritional status. Evaluate lab work: CBC, transferrin, albumin, prealbumin, electrolytes, and so forth.	Protein, carbohydrate and fat concentrations can alter the ability to maintain oxygenation. Increased fat concentration prior to weaning may assist in decreasing potential for CO_2 retention and decrease in respiratory drive. Lab work may be used to verify adequacy of nutritive state. Calcium imbalances can decrease the function of the diaphragm, and phosphorus may affect 2, 3-DPG and ATP function, affect respiratory muscle function and red cell membrane stability.
Stay with patient until stable, once weaning process has	Respiratory deterioration may occur rapidly and physical pres-

INTERVENTIONS	RATIONALES
begun. Observe for use of accessory muscles, nonsynchronous respiratory pattern, or skin color changes.	sence is required to observe patient to facilitate prompt intervention. May indicate deterioration in respiratory status, resulting in inability to wean.
Monitor oxygen saturation per oximetry and notify physician if reading less than 90% per pulse oximetry, or sustained reading less than 60% per mixed venous oxygen oximetry; obtain ABGs per protocol.	Oximetry provides identification of tissue oxygen desaturation which usually coincides with decreases in arterial blood gases. Oximetry does not give indication of increased CO_2 levels and these must be verified with ABGs.
Attempt to wean only during the day and after the patient has had a restful sleep period. Avoid activity during weaning. Current evidence suggests weaning may be done whenever patient is physiologically ready and respiratory status is stable, but many facilities prefer to wean patients during the day only.	Crises that may occur with respiratory deterioration and failure to wean may be handled more efficiently when sufficient medical personnel are available, usually during the day. Fatigue may predispose patient to failure because of the need for stamina to withstand the effort of spontaneous breathing. Activity increases oxygen demand and consumption.
Evaluate patient's emotional status and ability to cope with weaning.	Weaning process may result in anxiety because of fear of failure to wean and/or ability to breathe spontaneously.
Prior to attempt, assess weaning parameters to ensure patient meets requirements for successful weaning: NIF >−20 cm H_2O, vital capacity >10–15 cc/kg, PaO_2 >60 mm Hg on FIO_2 <40%, resting minute ventilation <10 L/min, $PaCO_2$ <40 mm Hg, tidal volume >5 cc/kg.	Attainment of parameters facilitate best chance for successful weaning and ensures that neuromuscular control is adequate for maintenance of spontaneous ventilation. If carbon dioxide retention is chronic, pH is more indicative of weaning readiness.
Assess patient for resolution of disease process, absence of inspiratory muscle fatigue, absence of fever, absence of hemodynamic instability, absence of sedative agents or respiratory suppressants, presence of spontaneous respirations, pulmonary shunt <20%, and adequate hemoglobin and hematocrit.	Factors may promote respiratory insufficiency and compromise which may result in unsuccessful weaning.
Suction patient and perform chest physiotherapy, percussion and postural drainage as warranted prior to disconnection from ventilator.	Removes secretions that may compromise weaning process and promotes improved pulmonary conditions.

(continues)

(continued)

INTERVENTIONS	RATIONALES
Utilize T-bar/T-piece adaptor as ordered. (Usually on T-bar for 10–30 minutes per hour initially.)	Provides oxygen via endotracheal tube or tracheostomy with patient spontaneously breathing.
Utilize SIMV/IMV mode on ventilator as ordered. (Usually IMV rate decreased by 1–2 breaths/minute every 15–30 minutes during weaning phase.)	Provides ventilatory support to patient with gradually decreasing ventilator breaths and increase of spontaneous breaths. Facilitates gradually increasing respiratory workload. If weaning is not tolerated, may increase $PaCO_2$ and decrease pH.
Utilize PS (pressure support) as ordered. (Usually 3–5 initially and may increase to 20, with gradual lowering as IMV/SIMV rate lowered.)	Assists patient to overcome airway resistance and support spontaneous breathing by increasing respiratory muscle function.
Utilize CPAP (continuous positive airway pressure) as ordered. (Usually 2–5 cm H_2O.)	Patient exhales against continuous positive pressure to prevent atelectasis and improve arterial oxygen tension.
Monitor for physician-set parameters or respiratory rate >30, increasing PA pressures, heart rate >110 with new or increased ectopic activity, blood pressure >20 mm Hg from baseline, SaO_2 <90%, tidal volumes <250 cc; if significant changes occur, place back on ventilator as per protocol.	Alterations in vital signs and hemodynamic may result from insufficient ventilation and respiratory compromise and indicates intolerance of attempts to wean.
Gradually increase time off ventilator with each successful attempt. Once patient is able to tolerate 1–2 hours off of ventilator at a time, weaning may be advanced more rapidly.	The patient's progress will increase as fatigue decreases, respiratory muscle function improves, and patient is emotionally ready to wean.
Determine patient's emotional status and ability to cope with weaning process.	Weaning may result in excessive anxiety due to fear of failure and/or the ability to breathe spontaneously.
Extubate patient when he is able to maintain an airway and his spontaneous respirations are able to maintain oxygenation and ventilatory status per protocol. Intubation equipment should be available post-extubation per protocol.	Emergency equipment should be easily available in case reintubation is required due to bronchospasm, laryngospasm, or respiratory deterioration.
To extubate, increase oxygen and suction secretions from trachea, nose and mouth.	Removes secretions that may potentially be aspirated upon removal of tube.

INTERVENTIONS	RATIONALES
Deflate cuff and remove tube at the peak of the inspiratory effort.	Promotes full inflation of the lungs so that patient will exhale or cough as tube is removed to prevent aspiration of any secretions that may be remaining after suctioning.
Administer humidified oxygen at prescribed amount.	Provides moisture and oxygen to increase available oxygen, helps to reduce swelling, and facilitates liquification of secretions for easier removal.
Monitor for dyspnea, bronchospasm, laryngospasm, or stridor. Encourage deep breaths and coughing.	May indicate partial obstruction of airway. Deep breathing helps to expand lungs and facilitates movement of secretions.
Monitor for persistent hoarseness and sore throat.	Transient hoarseness and sore throat is normal postextubation but persistent symptoms may indicate vocal cord paralysis or glottis edema.
Instruct on weaning process and procedures based on physician protocol.	Decreases fear and anxiety, promotes cooperation, and increases potential for successful weaning attempt.

NIC: *Endotracheal Extubation*

Discharge or Maintenance Evaluation

- Patient will be able to maintain adequate ventilatory status during weaning process.
- Patient will be able to be weaned successfully from mechanical ventilator and be able to maintain spontaneous respirations and adequate oxygenation.
- Patient will exhibit no signs or symptoms of complications from weaning or extubation process.

DEFICIENT KNOWLEDGE

Related to: placement on ventilator, change in health status, situational crisis, lack of information, misinterpretation of information, stress, inability to recall information, lack of understanding, new procedures

Defining Characteristics: verbalized questions regarding care, inadequate follow-up on instructions given, misconceptions, lack of improvement, development of preventable complications, anxiety

Outcome Criteria

✔ Patient will be able to verbalize and demonstrate understanding of information given regarding condition, treatment regimen, and medications.

NOC: *Knowledge: Treatment Regimen*

INTERVENTIONS	RATIONALES
Determine patient's baseline of knowledge regarding disease process, normal physiology and function of body systems, and medical treatment regimens.	Provides information regarding patient's understanding of condition as well as a baseline from which to plan teaching.
Monitor patient's readiness to learn and determine best methods to use for teaching. Attempt to incorporate family members in learning process. Reinstruct/reinforce information as needed.	Patient's physical condition may not facilitate participation in learning, with cognition affected by high stress levels or disease process. Family members may be fearful of equipment and environment which may hamper their ability to learn. Instructions may require repetitive teaching because of competition with other stimuli.
Provide time for individual interaction with patient.	Promotes relationship between patient and nurse, and establishes trust.
Instruct patient/family on specific disease process that has required ventilatory support, procedures that may be required, diagnostic tests to be performed, and plans for weaning off ventilator.	Provides knowledge to enable patient to make informed choices, and provides knowledge base on which to build for further teaching.
Instruct patient/family on medications pertinent to patient's care.	Provides knowledge and facilitates compliance with regimen.
Discuss potential for ventilator dependence and alterations that may be required in lifestyle. Encourage setting of short- and long-term goals.	Unsuccessful weaning attempts may foster depression and attitude of "giving up." Practical solutions and trouble-shooting problems that may arise, as well as participation in setting of realistic goals may enhance self-worth and self-control.
Instruct family on ventilatory support procedures—function of	Reduces fear, enables the family to have sense of security about

INTERVENTIONS	RATIONALES
all equipment, how to trouble-shoot problems, and personnel to contact in case of an emergency.	problems that may arise, and assures them that medical assistance can be easily obtained in an emergency.
Instruct family on procedures for suctioning, tracheostomy care, and administration of breathing treatments as ordered.	Promotes knowledge, enhances proper technique for care, and decreases fear.
Instruct family on infection control techniques.	Decreases potential for infection and/or spread of biohazardous materials.
Instruct patient/family on signs/symptoms to notify physician or medical personnel.	Promotes prompt recognition of potentially dangerous problems to facilitate prompt intervention.
Have patient/family perform return demonstration of all tasks instructed.	Provides assurances that care is able to be performed with proper technique, and allows for correction of erroneous methods.
Ensure that prior to discharge, all equipment required will be set up in home.	Reduces anxiety with discharge.
Instruct patient/family on all safety concerns; back-up power and equipment.	Promotes sense of security that emergency situations can be handled.

NIC: *Anxiety Reduction*

Discharge or Maintenance Evaluation

- Patient/family will be able to accurately recall instructions.
- Patient/family will be able to demonstrate all tasks with appropriate proper methods.
- Patient/family will be able to recall emergency numbers, and signs/symptoms for which to notify medical personnel, and can accurately demonstrate backup power and equipment.
- Patient/family will be able to follow infection control procedures.
- Patient/family will be able to problem-solve and set realistic goals.

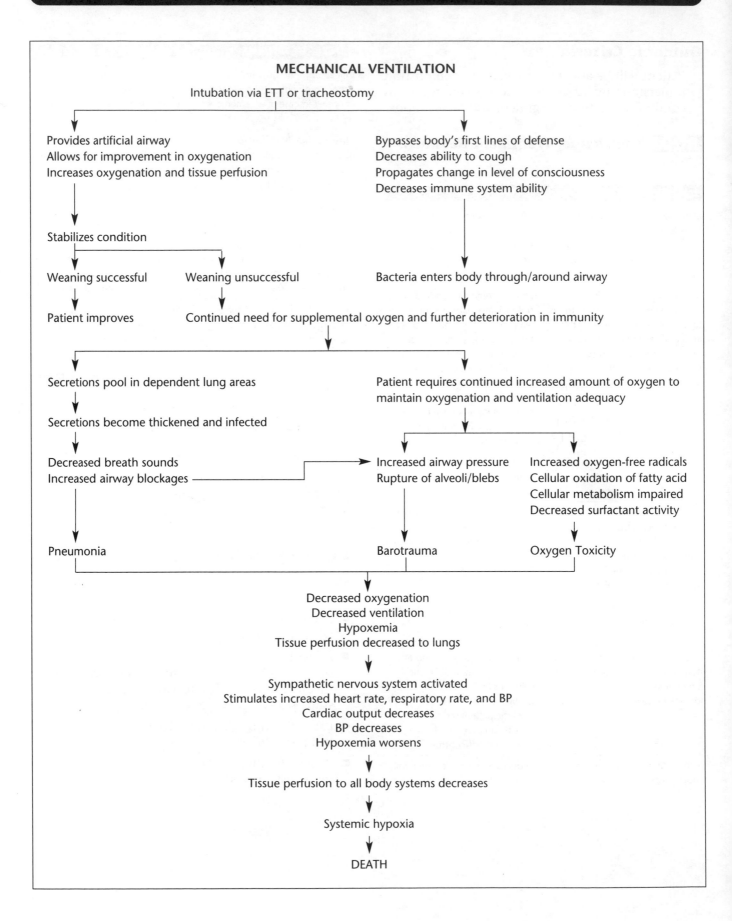

MECHANICAL VENTILATION

Intubation via ETT or tracheostomy

Provides artificial airway
Allows for improvement in oxygenation
Increases oxygenation and tissue perfusion

Bypasses body's first lines of defense
Decreases ability to cough
Propagates change in level of consciousness
Decreases immune system ability

Stabilizes condition

Weaning successful

Weaning unsuccessful

Bacteria enters body through/around airway

Patient improves

Continued need for supplemental oxygen and further deterioration in immunity

Secretions pool in dependent lung areas

Secretions become thickened and infected

Patient requires continued increased amount of oxygen to maintain oxygenation and ventilation adequacy

Decreased breath sounds
Increased airway blockages

Increased airway pressure
Rupture of alveoli/blebs

Increased oxygen-free radicals
Cellular oxidation of fatty acid
Cellular metabolism impaired
Decreased surfactant activity

Pneumonia

Barotrauma

Oxygen Toxicity

Decreased oxygenation
Decreased ventilation
Hypoxemia
Tissue perfusion decreased to lungs

Sympathetic nervous system activated
Stimulates increased heart rate, respiratory rate, and BP
Cardiac output decreases
BP decreases
Hypoxemia worsens

Tissue perfusion to all body systems decreases

Systemic hypoxia

DEATH

CHAPTER 2.2

ADULT RESPIRATORY DISTRESS SYNDROME

Adult respiratory distress syndrome (ARDS) is also known as shock lung, wet lung, white lung, or acute respiratory distress syndrome, and occurs frequently after an acute or traumatic injury or illness involving the respiratory system. The body responds to the injury with life-threatening respiratory failure and hypoxemia.

ARDS is usually noted 12–24 hours after the initial insult or 5–10 days after sepsis occurs. Dyspnea with hyperventilation and hypoxemia are usually the first clinical symptoms. Adventitious breath sounds frequently are not present initially.

Some of the most common precipitating factors are trauma, aspiration, pneumonia, near-drowning, toxic gas inhalation, sepsis, shock, DIC, oxygen toxicity, coronary artery bypass, pancreatitis, fat or amniotic embolism, radiation, head injury, heroin use, massive hemorrhage, smoke inhalation, drug overdose, or uremia. Mortality is high (60–70%) despite treatment and often, patients who do survive, may have chronic residual lung disease. In some cases, patients may have normal pulmonary function after recovery.

The latent phase of ARDS begins when the pulmonary capillary and alveolar endothelium become injured. The insult causes complement to be activated, as well as granulocytes, platelets, and the coagulation cascade. Free oxygen radicals, arachidonic acid metabolites, and proteases are released into the system. Humoral substances, such as serotonin, histamine and bradykinin, are released. This results in red blood cell and high plasma protein leakage into the interstitial spaces, because of increased capillary permeability and increased pulmonary hydrostatic pressure. Initially, there may be little evidence of respiratory problems, and chest X-rays may be normal or show minimal diffuse haziness. The fluid leakage increases and lymphatic flow increases with the acute phases with widespread damage to pulmonary capillary membranes and inflammation. Increases in intra-alveolar edema leads to capillary congestion and collagen formation. Surfactant production and activity decreases, which causes decreased functional residual capacity, increased pulmonary shunting with widening A-a gradients, decreased pulmonary compliance, and ventilation/perfusion mismatching results. Chest X-rays will then show the "ground glass" appearance and finally a complete white-out of the lung.

The chronic phase occurs when the endothelium thickens; Type I cells, which are the gas-exchange pneumocytes, are replaced by Type II cells, which are responsible for producing surfactant, and along with fibrin, fluid and other cellular material form a hyaline membrane in place of the normal alveoli.

The goals of treatment are to improve ventilation and perfusion, to treat the underlying disease process that caused the lung injury, and to prevent progression of potentially fatal complications. Oxygen therapy with high levels of oxygen, mechanical ventilatory support with PEEP, and fluid and drug management are required.

MEDICAL CARE

Laboratory: cultures to identify causative organisms when bacterial infection is present and to identify proper antimicrobial agent; C5A levels increase with disease process; fibrin split products increase; platelets decrease; lactic acid levels increase

Chest X-ray: used to evaluate lung fields; early X-rays may be normal or have diffuse infiltrates; later X-rays will show bilateral "ground glass" appearance or complete whiting-out of lung fields; assists with differentiation between ARDS and cardiogenic pulmonary edema since heart size is normal in ARDS

Oxygen: used to correct hypoxia and hypoxemia

Arterial blood gases: to identify acid–base problems, hypocapnia, and hypoxemia, and to evaluate progress of disease process and effectiveness of oxygen therapy; hypoxemia is the hallmark symptom of ARDS caused by intrapulmonary shunting, and is refractory to oxygen therapy; respiratory alkalosis occurs in the early phase caused by hyperventilation; hypercapnia is rarely seen initially and is often a very ominous and fatal sign when present

Ventilation: to provide adequate oxygenation and ventilation in patients who are unable to maintain even minimal levels

Pulmonary function studies: used to evaluate lung compliance and volumes which are normally decreased; physiologic dead space is increased and alveolar ventilation is compromised

COMMON NURSING DIAGNOSES

INEFFECTIVE BREATHING PATTERN (see MECHANICAL VENTILATION)

Related to: decreased lung compliance, pulmonary edema, increased lung density, decreased surfactant, hypoxemia

Defining Characteristics: use of accessory muscles, dyspnea, tachypnea, bradypnea, abnormal ABGs, altered chest expansion, nasal flaring, orthopnea, PaO$_2$ <60 mm Hg or S$_a$O$_2$ <90% with FIO$_2$ >0.50, respiratory alkalosis, hypercapnia, confusion, hypoxemia, pale, dusky skin, restlessness, tachycardia

INEFFECTIVE AIRWAY CLEARANCE (see MECHANICAL VENTILATION)

Related to: interstitial edema, increased airway resistance, decreased lung compliance, pulmonary secretions

Defining Characteristics: dyspnea, tachypnea, cyanosis, use of accessory muscles, cough with or without production, anxiety, restlessness, feelings of impending doom

ANXIETY (see MECHANICAL VENTILATION)

Related to: health crisis, effects of hypoxemia, fear of death, change in health status, change in environment, dyspnea

Defining Characteristics: apprehension, restlessness, fear, verbalized concern, trembling, worry, impaired attention, forgetfulness, preoccupation, fidgeting

DEFICIENT KNOWLEDGE (see MECHANICAL VENTILATION)

Related to: new disease, lack of information, inability to process information, lack of recall, threat to self

Defining Characteristics: verbalized concerns and questions

ADDITIONAL NURSING DIAGNOSES

IMPAIRED GAS EXCHANGE

Related to: intra-alveolar edema, atelectasis, ventilation/perfusion mismatching, decreased arterial PO$_2$, decreased amount and activity of surfactant, alveolar hypoventilation, formation of hyaline membranes, alveolar collapse, decreased diffusing capacity, shunting

Defining Characteristics: tachypnea, cyanosis, use of accessory muscles, tachycardia, restlessness, mental changes, abnormal arterial blood gases, intrapulmonary shunting increased, A-a gradient changes, hypoxemia, increased dead space

Outcome Criteria

✔ Patient will have arterial blood gases within normal range for patient, with no signs of ventilation/perfusion mismatching.

NOC: *Respiratory Status: Gas Exchange*

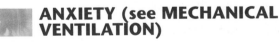

INTERVENTIONS	RATIONALES
Provide oxygen as ordered.	Provides supplemental oxygen to benefit patient. Low-flow oxygen delivery systems use some room air and may be inadequate for patient's need if their tidal volume is low, respiratory rate is high, or if ventilation status is unstable. Low-flow systems should be used in patients with COPD so as to not depress their respiratory drive. High levels of oxygen may cause severe damage to tissues, oxygen toxicity, increases in A-a gradients, microatelectasis, and ARDS.

INTERVENTIONS	RATIONALES
Monitor pulse oximetry for oxygen saturation and notify physician if <90%.	Oximetry readings of 90 correlate with P$_a$O$_2$ readings of 60. Levels below this do not allow for adequate perfusion to tissues and vital organs. Oximetry uses light waves to identify differences between saturation and reduced hemoglobin of the tissues and may be inaccurate in low blood flow states.
Monitor ABGs for changes and trends.	Provides information on measured levels of oxygen and carbon dioxide, as well as acid–base balance. Promotes prompt intervention for deteriorating airway status. P$_a$O$_2$ alone does not reflect tissue oxygenation; ventilation must be adequate to provide gas exchange. If P$_a$CO$_2$ continues to go upward despite increased patient respiratory efforts, endotracheal intubation and mechanical ventilation may be required.
Monitor I&O q 1 hour, and notify physician if urinary output <30 cc/hr.	May indicate impending or present pulmonary edema.
Monitor patient for changes in mental status, restlessness, anxiety, confusion, or headache.	May indicate impending or present hypoxia and hypoxemia that has caused reduced neurologic tissue perfusion.
Monitor ECG for changes in cardiac rhythm, dysrhythmias, or conduction defects.	Hypoxic states can result in cardiac tissue perfusion problems leading to life-threatening dysrhythmias that require emergent treatment.
Monitor patient for signs and symptoms of oxygen toxicity (nausea, vomiting, dyspnea, coughing, retrosternal pain, extremity paresthesias, pronounced fatigue, or restlessness).	Oxygen toxicity may result when the oxygen concentrations are greater than 40% for lengthy durations of time, usually 8 to 24 hours, and may cause actual physiologic changes in the lungs. Progressive respiratory distress, cyanosis, and asphyxia are late signs of toxicity.
Reposition patient at least every 2 hours and prn.	Assists in mobilizing secretions and allows for aeration of all lung fields.
Reposition patient into a prone position for at least 6 hours out of every 24 hours, ensuring that	Studies have shown that "proning" a patient can rapidly improve oxygenation and gas

INTERVENTIONS	RATIONALES
body alignment and invasive lines and tubes are maintained in position, as warranted. Ensure that at least 4 persons are available for this maneuver.	exchange approximately 70% of the time, while preventing potential complications, especially if patient requires mechanical ventilation and PEEP. The mechanisms that are thought to be responsible for this include re-expansion of gravity-induced atelectasis by the change in chest wall mechanics, increasing end-expiratory lung volumes, improvement in ventilation/perfusion matching, and correction of venous stasis. This positioning technique requires a minimum of 4 persons to reduce adverse effects and to adequately support an intensive care patient.
If patient is placed in prone position, assess for pressure areas to thorax, cheeks, breast, knees and iliac crest.	Prone positioning may result in weight-bearing sites to be disposed to pressure sores.
If "proning" is done, ensure that all IV access lines, indwelling catheters, tubes, endotracheal tubes and other lines remain patent.	Vigilant surveillance for accidental extubation or removal of tubes/lines will result in decreased adverse responses to this therapy. The patient may require more sedation due to anxiety.
Instruct patient/family in use of mechanical ventilation as warranted.	Hypoxia and hypoxemia may necessitate supportive oxygenation with the use of mechanical ventilation, and knowledge will decrease apprehension and increase compliance.
Instruct patient/family regarding the use of prone positioning, explaining the benefits, and that patient may require additional medication for sedation. Explain potential complications, such as facial edema and pressure areas.	Complete explanations regarding this unusual technique will facilitate compliance and decrease apprehension that the patient will not be able to breathe. Ensuring that the patient and family are aware of benefits and risks will help to facilitate compliance, and will assist family in helping with patient's care.

NIC: *Ventilation Assistance*

Discharge or Maintenance Evaluation

- Patient will have arterial blood gases within normal limits for patient.

- Patient will be eupneic with adequate oxygenation and no signs or symptoms of oxygen toxicity.
- Patient will be able to tolerate six hours of prone positioning to improve oxygenation and will exhibit no adverse effects.
- Patient will exhibit improved oxygenation while in prone position and for hours thereafter.
- Patient/family will be able to verbalize understanding of all instructions and procedures.
- Patient will be able to have improved gas exchange and be extubated with spontaneous respirations.

DECREASED CARDIAC OUTPUT

Related to: increased positive airway pressures, sepsis, dysrhythmias, increased intrapulmonary edema, left ventricular failure

Defining Characteristics: tachycardia, cardiac output <4 L/min, cardiac index <2.5 L/min/m^2, cold, clammy skin, decreased blood pressure, use of accessory muscles, altered mental status, dysrhythmias, S$_3$ or S$_4$ gallops, chest pain, crackles (rales), decreased peripheral pulses, increased pulmonary artery pressures, jugular vein distention, oliguria, weight gain

Outcome Criteria

✔ Patient will be hemodynamically stable.
✔ Patient will have stable vital signs with no dyspnea or adventitious breath sounds to auscultation.

NOC: *Vital Sign Status*

NOC: *Circulation Status*

INTERVENTIONS	RATIONALES
Monitor vital signs every 1–2 hours, and prn.	Mechanical ventilation and the use of PEEP increase the intrathoracic pressures which results in compression of the large vessels in the chest and this causes decreased venous return to the heart and decreased blood pressure.
Obtain PA pressures every hour, cardiac output/index every 4 hours, and calculate other hemodynamic values.	PA pressures will be elevated but wedge pressure will be normal. This is the classic marker to differentiate between

INTERVENTIONS	RATIONALES
	cardiogenic and non-cardiogenic pulmonary edema. Most ARDS patients have adequate cardiac function at least initially, unless decreases in CO/CI are caused by PEEP.
Monitor for mental changes, decreased peripheral pulses, cold or clammy skin.	May indicate decreased cardiac output and decreased perfusion.
Auscultate lung fields and heart tones at least q 2–4 hours and prn.	Extra cardiac sounds may indicate cardiac decompensation. Adventitious breath sounds may indicate increased pulmonary congestion leading to decreased cardiac output and decreased perfusion.
Administer oxygen as ordered. Monitor oxygen saturation by oximetry and notify physician for significant decreases.	Supplemental oxygen increases the available oxygen to the myocardium. Decreases in oxygen saturation may be the initial symptom of a change in patient's status and worsening perfusion.
Monitor I&O q 1–2 hours, and notify physician if urinary output <30 cc/hr.	Oliguria without a notable decrease in fluid intake may indicate decreased renal perfusion and decreased cardiac output.
Monitor cardiac rhythm and treat dysrhythmias per protocol.	Prompt treatment of potentially life-threatening dysrhythmias prevents further decrease in cardiac output and perfusion.
Instruct patient in planning activities with interspersed rest periods.	Avoids fatiguing patient and allows the heart time to compensate for the increased workload during activity and increased oxygen demand.
Instruct patient in stress reduction techniques.	Reduces anxiety and allows patient to have a sense of control over situation and himself.
Instruct patient/family in all procedures.	Reduces anxiety and promotes understanding and compliance. Enables family members to understand and decreases their fear.
Instruct patient/family in signs/symptoms to report, such as shortness of breath, chest pain, and so forth.	Involves patient and family in planning care and allows for prompt identification of complications which can lead to timely intervention.

NIC: *Hemodynamic Regulation*

Discharge or Maintenance Evaluation

- Patient will have adequate perfusion and cardiac output/index within normal limits for physiologic condition.
- Patient will have no mental status changes or peripheral perfusion impairment.

EXCESS FLUID VOLUME

Related to: interstitial edema, increased pulmonary fluid with normal intravascular volume, transfusions, resuscitative fluids

Defining Characteristics: edema, dyspnea, orthopnea, rales, wheezing

Outcome Criteria

✔ Patient will be hemodynamically stable, with no signs of pulmonary edema.

NOC: *Fluid Balance*

INTERVENTIONS	RATIONALES
Monitor for peripheral or dependent edema, or distended neck veins.	May indicate fluid excess that results in venous congestion and leads to respiratory failure.
Auscultate lung fields for adventitious breath sounds.	Bronchovesicular sounds heard over entire lung fields result when lung density increases. Crackles and rhonchi may be auscultated in pulmonary edema.
Monitor intake and output every hour. Notify physician if urine less than 30 cc/hr.	Identifies fluid imbalances.
Weigh every day.	Weight gains of >2 lbs/day or 5 lbs/week indicate fluid retention.
Monitor for vocal fremitus.	May be present because of increased lung density resulting from pulmonary edema.
Monitor vital signs.	Tachycardia and elevated blood pressure may result from fluid excess and heart failure.
Restrict fluids as warranted.	May be required to help with fluid balance regulation.
Monitor IV fluids and rate carefully.	Excess IV and oral fluid can exacerbate patient's condition.
Instruct patient in fluid and dietary restrictions.	Fluid restriction may be required to compensate for the patient's fluid overload and to avoid

INTERVENTIONS	RATIONALES
	exacerbation of his condition. Avoidance of sodium- and potassium-rich foods may be required to prevent increased fluid retention.

NIC: *Fluid Management*

Discharge or Maintenance Evaluation

- Patient will have no edema or weight gain.
- Patient will be eupneic with no adventitious breath sounds to auscultation.

RISK FOR DEFICIENT FLUID VOLUME

Related to: respiratory status, fluid shifts, diuretics, hemorrhage, hypermetabolic state

Defining Characteristics: decreased blood pressure, oliguria, anuria, low pulmonary artery wedge pressures, changes in mental status, dry mucous membranes, increased temperature, tachycardia, decrease pulse volume, tachypnea, weight loss, thirst, weakness, increased urinary concentration

Outcome Criteria

✔ Patient will achieve and maintain a normal and balanced fluid volume status and be hemodynamically stable.

NOC: *Fluid Balance*

INTERVENTIONS	RATIONALES
Monitor vital signs every 1–2 hours, and prn.	Tachycardia, hypotension and decreases in pulse quality may indicate fluid shifting has resulted in volume depletion. Temperature elevations with diaphoresis may result in increased insensible fluid loss.
Monitor intake and output every hour, and notify physician of significant fluid imbalances.	Continuing negative balances may result in volume depletion.
Weigh daily.	Changes in weight from day to day may correlate to fluid shifts that may occur.

(continues)

(continued)

INTERVENTIONS	RATIONALES
Observe skin turgor and hydration status.	Decreases in skin turgor, tenting of skin, and dry mucous membranes may indicate fluid volume deficits.
Administer IV fluids as ordered.	Replaces fluids and maintains circulating volume.
Monitor lab work for sodium and potassium levels.	Diuretic therapy may result in hypokalemia and hyponatremia.
Avoid overheating patient.	Prevents vasodilatation and decreased circulating blood volume.
Monitor urinary specific gravity q 8 hours and prn.	Increased specific gravity may indicate dehydration.
Instruct patient in rising slowly, sitting on edge of bed prior to standing.	Helps to prevent orthostatic hypotension and syncope that may result from position changes during compromised circulatory perfusion.
Instruct patient/family in reasons for fluid loss and how to monitor for fluid volume balance at home.	Involves the patient and family in care and promotes understanding of disease process. Promotes compliance that can help identify problems to ensure timely intervention.

NIC: *Fluid Management*

Discharge or Maintenance Evaluation

- Patient will achieve normal fluid balance.
- Patient will be hemodynamically stable, with no weight change.
- Patient will have urine output within normal limits.

INEFFECTIVE INDIVIDUAL COPING

Related to: situational crisis of disease process, inability to cope with stress, hypoxemia

Defining Characteristics: apprehension, use of defense mechanisms, emotional extremes, feelings of being overwhelmed, anxiety, helplessness, disorganized thoughts, inability to make decisions, inability to concentrate, focusing on crisis only, increased tension

Outcome Criteria

✔ Patient will be able to handle new situations or will be able to obtain needed resources to assist him.

✔ Patient will be able to utilize coping mechanisms.
✔ Patient will be able to realistically identify the crisis.

NOC: *Coping*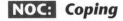

INTERVENTIONS	RATIONALES
Assist patient to verbalize feelings and ideas.	Allows opportunity for patient to explore feelings with the security of not being abandoned.
Assist patient to discuss perceptions of crisis, identify and clarify problems, and help to correct distorted information.	Allows for objectively identifying misperceptions and time to reinstruct in correct information. Listening to patient helps him to grasp situation and cope effectively.
Assist patient with development of coping strategies, alternative behaviors to ineffective ones previously identified by patient, use of support systems, fostering self-esteem, and so forth.	Assists patient to handle situation with acceptable methods.
Assist patient to perform constructive actions, as condition allows, that can be met with success.	Enhances self-esteem and establishes sense of control.
Assign same nurse to the patient as much as is possible.	Fosters continuity of care and helps to develop a therapeutic and trusting relationship.
Reduce unnecessary environmental stimuli.	Helps patient to avoid sensory overload and to be able to effectively hear and understand what is being said.
Instruct patient regarding all treatments and procedures. Answer all questions honestly. Use terminology that patient can understand.	Helps to decrease fear and allows patient to gain some self-control.
Encourage patient's decision-making, when feasible.	Increases self-worth, self-esteem, and helps patient to achieve control over current situation.
Involve community resources, counselors, social workers, and so forth, as needed.	Patient may require additional support systems to assist with coping. Counselors may be required if patient has a high crisis potential and this will help to increase objectivity.

NIC: *Learning Facilitation*

Discharge or Maintenance Evaluation

- Patient will be able to discuss recent situation crisis event and related emotions.

- Patient will be able to utilize coping skills to identify problem and take action appropriately.

- Patient will be able to request and accept assistance from family and/or community resources.

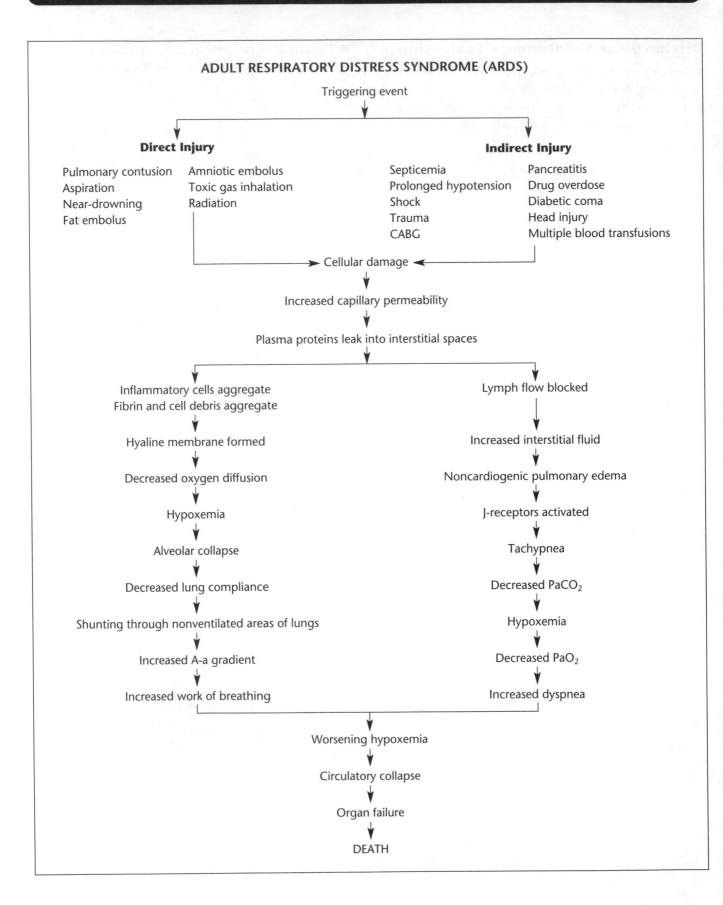

ADULT RESPIRATORY DISTRESS SYNDROME (ARDS)

Triggering event

Direct Injury

Pulmonary contusion   Amniotic embolus
Aspiration   Toxic gas inhalation
Near-drowning   Radiation
Fat embolus

Indirect Injury

Septicemia   Pancreatitis
Prolonged hypotension   Drug overdose
Shock   Diabetic coma
Trauma   Head injury
CABG   Multiple blood transfusions

Cellular damage

Increased capillary permeability

Plasma proteins leak into interstitial spaces

Inflammatory cells aggregate
Fibrin and cell debris aggregate

Hyaline membrane formed

Decreased oxygen diffusion

Hypoxemia

Alveolar collapse

Decreased lung compliance

Shunting through nonventilated areas of lungs

Increased A-a gradient

Increased work of breathing

Lymph flow blocked

Increased interstitial fluid

Noncardiogenic pulmonary edema

J-receptors activated

Tachypnea

Decreased $PaCO_2$

Hypoxemia

Decreased PaO_2

Increased dyspnea

Worsening hypoxemia

Circulatory collapse

Organ failure

DEATH

CHAPTER 2.3

PNEUMONIA

Pneumonia is an acute infection of the lung's terminal alveolar spaces and/or the interstitial tissues which results in gas exchange problems. The major challenge is identification of the source of the infection. Pneumonia ranks as the sixth most common cause of death in the United States.

When the infection is limited to a portion of the lung, it is known as segmental or lobular pneumonia; when the alveoli adjacent to the bronchioles are involved, it is known as bronchopneumonia, and when the entire lobe of the lung is involved, it is known as lobar pneumonia.

Pneumonia may be caused by bacteria, viruses, mycoplasma, rickettsias, or fungi. The causative organism gains entry by aspiration of oropharyngeal or gastric contents, inhalation of respiratory droplets, from others who are infected, by way of the bloodstream, or directly with surgery or trauma.

Viral types are more common in some areas, but identification of causative organisms may be difficult with limited technology.

Patients who develop bacterial pneumonia usually are immunosuppressed or compromised by a chronic disease, or have had a recent viral illness. The most common type of bacterial pneumonia is pneumococcal pneumonia, in which the *Streptococcus pneumoniae* organism reaches the lungs via the respiratory passageways and result in the collapse of alveoli. The inflammatory response that this generates causes protein-rich fluid to migrate into the alveolar spaces and provides culture media for the organism to proliferate and spread.

Frequently pneumonia is predisposed by upper respiratory infections, chronic illness, cancer, surgery, atelectasis, chronic obstructive pulmonary disease, asthma, cystic fibrosis, bronchiectasis, influenza, malnutrition, smoking, alcoholism, immunosuppressive therapy, aspiration, sickle cell disease, head injury or coma.

Aspiration pneumonia occurs after aspiration of gastric or oropharyngeal contents, or other chemical irritants into the trachea and lungs. Stomach acid damages the respiratory endothelium and may result in noncardiogenic pulmonary edema, hemorrhage, destruction of surfactant-producing cells, and hypoxemia. The pH of the aspirated material determines the severity of the injury with pH less than 2.5 causing severe damage. Morbidity is high even with treatment.

In pneumonia's early stages, pulmonary vessels dilate and erythrocytes spread into the alveoli and cause a reddish, liver-like appearance, or red hepatization, in the lung consolidation area. Polymorphonuclear cells then enter the alveolar spaces and the consolidation increases to a gray hepatization. The leukocytes trap bacteria against the alveolar walls or other leukocytes so that more organisms are found in the increasing margins of the consolidation. The macrophage reaction occurs when mononuclear cells advance into the alveoli and phagocytize the exudate debris.

Diagnosis may be assisted with the observation of sputum characteristics, with bacterial pneumonia having mucopurulent sputum, viral and mycoplasmic pneumonias having more watery secretions, pneumococcal pneumonia having rust-colored sputum, and klebsiellal pneumonia noting dark red mucoid secretions.

The initial signs/symptoms are sudden onset of shaking chills, fever, purulent sputum, pleuritic chest pain that is worsened with respiration or coughing, tachycardia, tachypnea, and use of accessory muscles.

Staphylococcal pneumonia is frequently noted after influenza or in hospitalized patients with a nosocomial superinfection following surgery, trauma, or immunosuppression. Pleural pain, dyspnea, cyanosis, and productive coughing with copious pink secretions are common symptoms. Streptococcal pneumonia occurs rarely with the exception as a complication after measles or influenza. Klebsiellal pneumonia is virulent and necrotizing, and is usually seen with alcoholic or severely debilitated patients. Pneumonia that is caused by *Hemophilus influenzae* occurs after viral upper respiratory infections, or concurrently with bronchopneumonia, bronchitis, and bronchiolitis. Sputum is usually yellow or green, and patients have fever, cough, cyanosis, and arthralgias. Viral pneumonia may be caused by influenza, adenoviruses, respiratory syncytial virus, rhinoviruses, cytomegalovirus, herpes simplex virus, and childhood diseases; it is usually milder. Symptoms include headache, anorexia, and occasionally mucopurulent sputum that is bloody.

MEDICAL CARE

Laboratory: white blood cell count may be normal or low but usually is elevated with polymorphonuclear neutrophils; leukocyte counts frequently increase in lobar pneumonia, are normal with atypical pneumonia, and are normal or decreased in the elderly, immunocompromised patients, and with viral infections; cultures of sputum, blood, and CSF may be obtained to identify the causative organism and antimicrobial agent best suited for eradication; electrolytes may show decreased sodium and chloride levels; serology and cold agglutinins may be done for identification of viral titers; sedimentation rate is usually elevated

Pulmonary function studies: used to evaluate ventilation/perfusion problems; volumes may be decreased due to alveolar collapse; airway pressures may be increased; lung compliance may be decreased

Arterial blood gases: to evaluate adequacy of oxygen and respiratory therapies, as well as to identify acid–base imbalances and acidotic/alkalotic states; hypoxemia and hypocapnia seen in lobar pneumonia

Chest X-ray: used to demonstrate small effusions and abscesses, pulmonary consolidations, and empyema; may be clear with mycoplasma pneumonia

Oxygen: used to supplement room air, and to treat hypoxemia that may occur

Antimicrobials: used in the treatment after culture results are obtained to eradicate the infective organism

Thoracentesis: used to remove fluid if pleural fluid is present; assists in the diagnosis of pleural empyema

Surgery: may be required for open lung biopsy or treatment of effusions and empyema; bronchoscopy with bronchial brushings may be indicated for progressive pneumonias that are unresponsive to medical treatment

Nerve blocks: intercostal blocks may be required to control pleuritic pain

COMMON NURSING DIAGNOSES

IMPAIRED GAS EXCHANGE (see MECHANICAL VENTILATION)

Related to: inflammation, infection, ventilation/perfusion mismatching, fever, changes in oxyhemoglobin dissociation curve

Defining Characteristics: dyspnea, tachycardia, cyanosis, hypoxia, hypoxemia, abnormal arterial blood gases, hypercepnia, mental changes

ACUTE PAIN (see MI)

Related to: inflammation, dyspnea, fever, coughing

Defining Characteristics: pleuritic chest pain worsened with respiration or cough, muscle aches, joint pain, restlessness, communication of pain/discomfort

IMBALANCED NUTRITION: LESS THAN BODY REQUIREMENTS (see MECHANICAL VENTILATION)

Related to: increased metabolic demands, fever, infection, abnormal taste sensation, anorexia, abdominal distention, nausea, vomiting

Defining Characteristics: actual inadequate food intake, altered taste, altered smell sensation, weight loss, anorexia, nausea, vomiting, abdominal distention, decreased muscle mass and tone

RISK FOR DEFICIENT FLUID VOLUME (see ARDS)

Related to: fluid loss from fever, diaphoresis, or vomiting, decreased fluid intake

Defining Characteristics: decreased blood pressure, oliguria, anuria, low pulmonary artery wedge pressures

EXCESS FLUID VOLUME (see ARDS)

Related to: inflammatory response, pulmonary edema

Defining Characteristics: rales, crackles, wheezing, pink frothy sputum, abnormal arterial blood gases

ADDITIONAL NURSING DIAGNOSES

INEFFECTIVE AIRWAY CLEARANCE

Related to: infection, inflammation, edema, increased secretions, fatigue

Defining Characteristics: adventitious breath sounds, use of accessory muscles, cyanosis, dyspnea, cough with or without production

Outcome Criteria

✔ Patient will maintain patency of airway, have clear breath sounds, and will be able to effectively clear secretions.

NOC: *Respiratory Status: Airway Patency*

INTERVENTIONS	RATIONALES
Monitor respiratory status for changes, increased work of breathing, use of accessory muscles, and nasal flaring.	Tachypnea and hyperpnea are frequently noted with pneumonia.
Observe for symmetric chest expansion.	Unilateral pneumonia will result in asymmetrical chest movement due to decreased lung compliance on the affected side and because of pleuritic pain.
Observe for cyanosis and/or mental status changes.	May indicate impending or present hypoxemia.
Assess vocal fremitus.	Increased fremitus is noted over consolidated areas in pneumonia. Decreased or absent fremitus may indicate that a foreign body is obstructing a large bronchus.
Percuss chest for changes.	Percussion may be dull over consolidated areas or in areas of atelectasis.
Auscultate lung fields.	Fine crackles or bronchial breath sounds are noted in lobar pneumonia; in other types of pneumonia, bronchial sounds are rarely heard. Wheezes may

INTERVENTIONS	RATIONALES
	indicate aspiration of a solid object. Inspiratory stridor may indicate the presence of an obstruction to a large bronchus.
Assess for bronchophony.	Bronchophony is increased when lung consolidation is present.
Assist with, or perform chest physiotherapy.	Helps to mobilize secretions so that patient may be able to more easily expectorate them.
Administer antimicrobial therapy as ordered.	Controls infection by elimination of causative organism.
Administer IV fluids as ordered.	Helps to maintain hydration and fluid status, as well as helps to thin viscous secretions to allow for easier expectoration.
Utilize appropriate isolation technique, as warranted.	May be required dependent on type of pneumonia to prevent spread of infection.
Assist with bronchoscopy as warranted.	May be required to remove mucus plugs and prevent or improve atelectasis.
Assist with thoracentesis as warranted.	May be required to drain purulent fluid.
Instruct patient/family in disease process.	Promotes knowledge and increases compliance.
Instruct patient/family regarding any isolation precautions.	Helps to prevent the spread of infection to or from the patient.
Instruct patient/family regarding handwashing procedures.	Handwashing is the single most important factor in helping to avoid spread of disease.
Instruct patient/family to notify nurse/physician of sputum color changes, increased work of breathing, or abrupt onset of chest pain.	May signal worsening of condition that requires immediate medical intervention to prevent further complications.

NIC: *Airway Management*

Discharge or Maintenance Evaluation

■ Patient will maintain patent airway.

■ Patient will be eupneic with no adventitious breath sounds to auscultation.

■ Patient will have normal CBC, with no signs or symptoms of infection.

■ Patient will be able to expectorate sputum and cough effectively.

■ Patient/family will be able to accurately verbalize understanding of hand washing and isolation techniques, and will prevent spread of infection.

DEFICIENT KNOWLEDGE

Related to: hypoxemia, lack of information, competing stimuli, misinterpretation of information, disease process

Defining Characteristics: request for information, failure to improve, development of preventable complications, noncompliance

Outcome Criteria

✔ Patient will be able to verbalize and demonstrate understanding of information.

NOC: *Knowledge: Disease Process*

INTERVENTIONS	RATIONALES
Instruct patient/family on need for vaccines for influenza and pneumonia.	Influenza increases the chance of secondary pneumonia infection; vaccinations help to prevent the occurrence and spread of infective process.

INTERVENTIONS	RATIONALES
Instruct patient/family in continued need for coughing and deep breathing.	Patient is at risk for recurrence of pneumonia for 6–8 weeks following discharge.
Instruct patient/family in importance of continuing with follow-up medical care.	Helps prevent complications and recurrence of pneumonia.
Instruct in need to quit or avoid smoking.	Smoking destroys the action of the cilia and impairs the lungs' first line of defense against infection.

NIC: *Teaching: Disease Process*

Discharge or Maintenance Evaluation

■ Patient will be able to accurately verbalize understanding of all instructions.

■ Patient will be compliant in avoiding smoking.

■ Patient will not have preventable complications from illness.

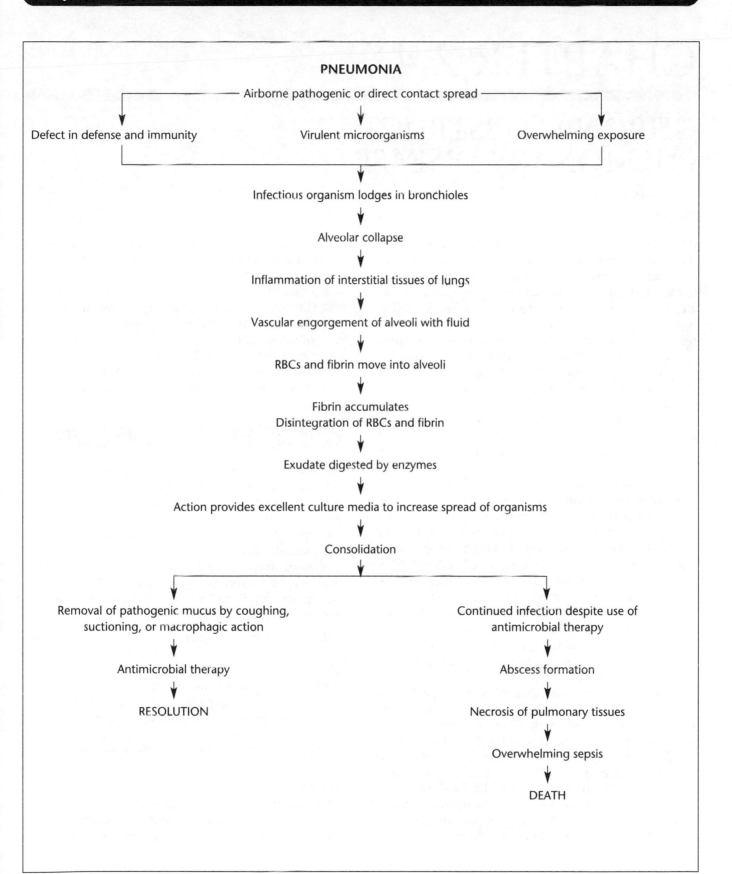

PNEUMONIA

— Airborne pathogenic or direct contact spread —

Defect in defense and immunity   Virulent microorganisms   Overwhelming exposure

Infectious organism lodges in bronchioles

Alveolar collapse

Inflammation of interstitial tissues of lungs

Vascular engorgement of alveoli with fluid

RBCs and fibrin move into alveoli

Fibrin accumulates
Disintegration of RBCs and fibrin

Exudate digested by enzymes

Action provides excellent culture media to increase spread of organisms

Consolidation

Removal of pathogenic mucus by coughing, suctioning, or macrophagic action   Continued infection despite use of antimicrobial therapy

Antimicrobial therapy   Abscess formation

RESOLUTION   Necrosis of pulmonary tissues

Overwhelming sepsis

DEATH

CHAPTER 2.4

CHRONIC OBSTRUCTIVE PULMONARY DISEASE

Chronic obstructive pulmonary disease (COPD) is an irreversible condition in which airways become obstructed and resistance to airflow is increased during expiration when airways collapse. COPD is usually further subdivided into other diseases such as bronchitis and emphysema, and actually COPD refers to these often simultaneous disease entities. COPD is also known as chronic obstructive lung disease (COLD), chronic airflow obstruction or chronic airway obstruction (CAO), and chronic airflow limitation (CAL).

Emphysematous changes include enlarging of the air spaces distally to the terminal bronchioles, and concurrent changes in alveolar walls. Capillary numbers decrease in the remaining walls and may sclerose. Gas exchange is decreased because of the reduction in available alveolar surfaces as well as decreased perfusion to nonventilated areas. Ventilation/perfusion mismatching occurs and functional residual capacity is increased. The anteroposterior diameter of the chest is often enlarged because of the loss of elasticity and increased air trapping in the airway supportive structures. These type A patients are often called "pink puffers" because of the increased response to hypoxemia. Symptoms include dyspnea and increase in breathing effort, which result in a well-oxygenated, or pink, patient who displays overt dyspnea, or puffing.

Bronchitis is usually associated with prolonged exposure to lung irritants, which results in inflammatory changes and thickening of bronchial walls, and increases in mucus production. The patient exhibits a chronic productive cough caused in part by the increase in size of mucus glands, decrease in cilia, and to the increase in bronchial wall thickness with obstruction to airflow. Exacerbations are usually caused by infection. These type B patients are often called "blue bloaters" because their response to hypoxemia is reduced, with increasing $PaCO_2$ levels and cyanosis. These patients frequently have chronic hypoxemia with bouts of cor pulmonale, or right-sided heart failure, resulting in peripheral edema.

The most common precipitating factors for COPD include cigarette smoking, air or environmental pollution, allergic response, autoimmunity, and genetic predisposition. Treatment is aimed at avoidance of respiratory allergens and irritants, controlling bronchospasms, and improving airway clearance.

MEDICAL CARE

Laboratory: cultures used to identify causative organisms and determine appropriate antimicrobial therapy; CBC used to identify presence of infection with elevated white blood cell count, and to monitor for increases in RBCs and hematocrit as the body tries to compensate for oxygen transport requirements; alpha$_1$-antitrypsin levels used to identify deficiency that may be present if patient has heredity predisposition; theophylline levels used to monitor for therapeutic levels and/or toxicity

Pulmonary function studies: used to evaluate pulmonary status and function, and to identify airway obstruction, increased residual volume, total lung capacity, compliance, decreased vital capacity, diffusing capacity, and expiratory volumes with emphysema patients; increased residual volume, decreased vital capacity and forced expiratory volumes with normal static compliance and diffusion capacity with bronchitis patients

Chest X-ray: used to identify hyperinflation of lungs, flattened diaphragm, or pulmonary hypertension; used to identify barotrauma that may occur, increased anteroposterior chest diameter, large retrosternal air spaces, or secondary cardiovascular complications with right-sided heart failure

Electrocardiography: used to identify dysrhythmias associated with this disease: tall P waves in inferior leads, vertical QRS axis, atrial dysrhythmias, right ventricular hypertrophy, sinus tachycardia, and right axis deviation

Oxygen: used to improve hypoxemia; liter flow should be low in order to maintain the patient's respiratory drive; PaO_2 may be acceptable at 55–60 mm Hg to avoid hypoventilation and maintain function

IV fluids: used to maintain hydration and for administration of medical therapeutics

Bronchodilators: xanthines and sympathomimetics are used to relieve bronchospasms and help to promote clearance of mucoid secretions

Antimicrobials: used to treat respiratory infections

Arterial blood gases: used to identify acid–base disturbances, presence of hypoxemia and hypercapnia, and to evaluate responses to therapies

Chest physiotherapy: percussion and postural drainage are used to facilitate mobilization of secretions and promote clearance of airways

Corticosteroids: used to decrease secretions and reduce inflammation in the lungs; use of steroids is controversial

Psychological treatment: use of anti-anxiety agents to decrease fear and anxiety related to dyspnea, without sedation to depress the respiratory drive; psychotherapy may be required to enable patients to cope with their ongoing disease process

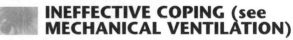

COMMON NURSING DIAGNOSES

INEFFECTIVE AIRWAY CLEARANCE (see MECHANICAL VENTILATION)

Related to: secretions, bronchospasm, fatigue, increased work of breathing, increased mucus production, infection, cough

Defining Characteristics: dyspnea, tachypnea, bradypnea, bronchospasms, increased work of breathing, use of accessory muscles, increased mucus produc-

tion, cough with or without productivity, adventitious breath sounds, fever

INEFFECTIVE BREATHING PATTERN (see MECHANICAL VENTILATION)

Related to: respiratory muscle fatigue, pain, increased lung compliance, decreased lung expansion, fear, obstruction, decreased elasticity/recoil

Defining Characteristics: dyspnea, tachypnea, use of accessory muscles, cough with or without productivity, adventitious breath sounds, prolongation of expiratory time, increased mucus production, abnormal arterial blood gases, fremitus, pursed-lip breathing, nasal flaring, 3-point positioning, increased anteroposterior chest diameter, altered chest excursion

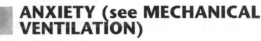

IMPAIRED GAS EXCHANGE (see MECHANICAL VENTILATION)

Related to: obstruction of airways, bronchospasm, air-trapping, right-to-left shunting, ventilation/perfusion mismatching, inability to move secretions, hypoventilation

Defining Characteristics: hypoxemia, hypercapnia, mental changes, confusion, restlessness, dyspnea, vital sign changes, inability to tolerate activity, respiratory acidosis, hypoxia, inability to mobilize secretions, tachycardia, dysrhythmias, anxiety

ANXIETY (see MECHANICAL VENTILATION)

Related to: threat of death, change in health status, life-threatening crises, exacerbations of disease

Defining Characteristics: fear, restlessness, muscle tension, helplessness, communication of uncertainty and apprehension, feeling of suffocation

INEFFECTIVE COPING (see MECHANICAL VENTILATION)

Related to: changes in lifestyle and health status, sensory overload, fear of death, physical limitations, inadequate support system, inadequate coping mechanisms, continual dyspnea

Defining Characteristics: inability to meet role expectations, inability to meet basic needs, constant worry, apprehension, fear, inability to problem-solve, anger, hostility, aggression, inappropriate defense mechanisms, low self-esteem, insomnia, depression, destructive behaviors, vacillation when choices are required, delayed decision-making, muscle tension, fatigue

IMPAIRED SPONTANEOUS VENTILATION (see MECHANICAL VENTILATION)

Related to: ventilatory capacity and ventilatory demand imbalances

Defining Characteristics: ineffective breathing pattern, dyspnea, apnea, tachypnea, use of accessory muscles, abnormal arterial blood gases, mental status changes, increased work of breathing, cyanosis, decreased oxygen saturation

IMBALANCED NUTRITION: LESS THAN BODY REQUIREMENTS (see MECHANICAL VENTILATION)

Related to: dyspnea, inability to take in sufficient food, increased metabolism caused by disease process, decreased level of consciousness, fatigue, increased sputum, medication side effects

Defining Characteristics: actual inadequate food intake, altered taste, altered smell sensation, weight loss, anorexia, absent bowel sounds, decreased peristalsis, muscle mass loss, changes in bowel habits, abdominal distention, nausea, vomiting

INEFFECTIVE COPING (see ARDS)

Related to: situational crisis of disease process, inability to cope with stress, hypoxemia

Defining Characteristics: apprehension, use of defense mechanisms, emotional extremes, feelings of being overwhelmed, anxiety, helplessness, disorganized thoughts, inability to make decisions, inability to concentrate, focusing on crisis only, increased tension

ADDITIONAL NURSING DIAGNOSES

ACTIVITY INTOLERANCE

Related to: oxygen supply/demand imbalance, fatigue, weakness, increased effort and work of breathing, inadequate rest, hypoxia, hypoxemia

Defining Characteristics: dyspnea, decreased oxygen saturation levels with movement or activity, increased heart rate and blood pressure with movement or activity, feelings of tiredness and weakness, decreased oxygen saturations, dysrhythmias

Outcome Criteria

✔ Patient will be able to tolerate minimal activity without respiratory compromise.

NOC: *Activity Tolerance*

INTERVENTIONS	RATIONALES
Monitor for patient's response to activity changes.	Identifies patient's ability to compensate for increases in activity and provides baseline date from which to plan care.
Monitor vital signs before, during, and after increased activity levels.	Increases in heart rate greater than 10/minute or respiratory rate greater than 32 may indicate that patient has reached his maximal activity limit and further activity may result in circulatory/ respiratory dysfunction.
Plan activities to ensure patient obtains adequate amounts of rest and sleep.	Decreases potential for dyspnea and provides rest to prevent excessive fatigue.
Assist patient with activities as warranted.	Conserves energy and decreases oxygen consumption and dyspnea.
Increase activity gradually and encourage patient participation.	Gradual increases facilitate increased tolerance to activity by balancing oxygen supply and demand, and patient cooperation may facilitate feelings of self-worth and adequacy.
Administer inhalers as ordered prior to activities.	Helps prevent dyspnea by performing activities at peak time of medication effects.
Instruct on techniques to save energy expenditure: shower stools, arm and leg rests, gathering required articles and placement within reach, and so forth.	Helps to decrease energy expenditure and fatigue, which may result in increased dyspnea.
Provide patient with exercise regimen protocol.	Promotes independence and self-worth; increases tolerance to exercises.
Instruct on breathing exercises to be performed with activity.	Promotes effective respiratory patterns during exertion.

NIC: *Body Mechanics Promotion*

Discharge or Maintenance Evaluation

■ Patient will be able to tolerate activity without excessive dyspnea or hemodynamic instability.

■ Patient will be able to perform ADLs within limits of disease process.

■ Patient will be able to recall information accurately, and will be able to utilize relaxation and breathing techniques effectively.

■ Patient will be compliant with prescribed exercise regimens.

RISK FOR INFECTION

Related to: chronic disease process, inability to move secretions, decreased cilia function, immunosuppression, poor nutrition, invasive procedures

Defining Characteristics: increased temperature, chills, elevated white blood cell count, inability to move secretions, tachycardia, sepsis

Outcome Criteria

✔ Patient will avoid infective process by maintaining immune status and expectorating secretions, or if infection is present, the patient will improve with the administration of antimicrobials and use of techniques to facilitate recovery.

NOC: *Risk Control*

INTERVENTIONS	RATIONALES
Monitor for increased dyspnea, sputum color and character changes, cough, and temperature elevation.	Yellow or green sputum, with increased viscosity usually indicates infection. Prompt recognition facilitates prompt treatment.
Obtain sputum and other specimens for culture and sensitivity as ordered.	Identifies the causative organism and provides information regarding appropriate antimicrobial agent required.
Administer antimicrobials as ordered.	Controls and clears the infection and any secondary infections in the bronchial tree. Improvement should be noted within 24–48 hours after antimicrobial agent has begun.
Monitor for abrupt changes in other body systems; cardiac abnormalities and alteration in heart sounds, increasing pain, changes in mental status, recur-	May indicate presence of secondary infection or resistance to ordered antimicrobials. Super-infections, systemic bacteremia, inflammatory cardiac conditions,

INTERVENTIONS	RATIONALES
ring temperature elevations.	meningitis or encephalitis may occur.
Provide adequate rest time for patient.	Helps to facilitate healing and natural immunity.
Monitor VS q 2–4 hours and prn. Notify physician of significant abnormalities.	Sustained temperature increases may indicate the onset of infection complications, or superinfection if patient is on antimicrobial therapy.
Wash hands prior to and after caring for patient. Use gloves when providing direct care.	Minimizes risk of infection. Gloves provide protection from pathogens and help to avoid cross-contamination.
Maintain strict aseptic technique when suctioning lower airway or inserting invasive lines or catheters.	Avoids introducing or spreading pathogens.
Encourage coughing and deep breathing exercises at least q 2–4 hours.	Assists with prevention of pulmonary complications and helps remove secretions that could be medium for pathogenic growth.
Use appropriate isolation techniques when required.	Protects patient from pathogens in environment, protects caregivers, and prevents cross-contamination with other pathogens.
Instruct patient/family in proper handwashing technique.	Handwashing is the single most important way to avoid spreading germs. Provides knowledge to patient and family to assist with prevention of pathogenic spread or cross-contamination.
Instruct patient/family in signs and symptoms of infection, such as increased temperature, drainage, redness to insertion sites, and so forth.	Allows for prompt identification of problem and assists with timely treatment.

NIC: *Infection Protection*

Discharge or Maintenance Evaluation

■ Patient will exhibit no signs/symptoms of infection.

■ Patient will be afebrile with normal WBC and differentials.

■ Patient/family will be able to accurately observe handwashing and isolation procedures effectively, and no cross-contamination will occur.

▨ DEFICIENT KNOWLEDGE

Related to: hypoxemia, lack of information, lack of recall of information, cognitive limitations, disease process

Defining Characteristics: request for information, statement of misconception, statement of concerns, development of preventable complications, inaccurate follow-through with instructions

Outcome Criteria

✔ Patient will be able to recall information accurately and will follow through with all instructions.

NOC: *Knowledge: Disease Process*

INTERVENTIONS	RATIONALES
Assess knowledge of COPD disease process, medications, and treatments.	Identifies level of knowledge and provides baseline from which to plan teaching.
Instruct patient/family on medication effects, side effects, contraindications, and signs/symptoms to report.	Promotes knowledge and compliance with treatment regimen.
Instruct patient/family in proper technique for using and cleaning inhalers.	Proper technique, including appropriate time intervals between puffs, facilitates effective delivery and therapeutic effect.
Instruct patient/family on need to avoid smoking and other respiratory irritants.	May initiate and exacerbate bronchial irritation which can result in increased mucus production and airway obstruction.
Instruct patient/family on effective coughing techniques; postural drainage, chest physiotherapy, and so forth.	Effective coughing reduces fatigue and facilitates removal of secretions. Percussion and postural drainage help to mobilize tenacious secretions.
Instruct patient/family to drink 10–12 glasses of water per day unless contraindicated.	Maintains hydration and promotes easier mobilization of secretions.
Instruct patient/family on use of supplemental oxygen at low flow rates, and reasons to avoid increasing flow indiscriminately.	COPD patients will rarely require more than 2–3 L/min to maintain their optimum oxygenation levels. Increasing flow rates will increase their PaO_2 but may decrease their respiratory drive and may result in drowsiness, confusion, and coma.
Instruct patient/family on oxygen safety: avoiding flammable	Promotes physical and environmental safety.

INTERVENTIONS	RATIONALES
objects, use of vaseline or other petroleum products, and ambulation with tubing.	
Instruct patient/family on avoiding sedative or antianxiety drugs as warranted.	Sedatives may result in respiratory depression and impair cough reflexes.
Instruct patient/family on avoiding people with infections; encourage patient to obtain influenza and pneumonia vaccinations as warranted.	Prevents exposure to other infections, and decreases potential for incidence of upper respiratory infections.
Instruct patient/family on activity limitations, methods to conserve energy and promote rest, pursed-lip breathing, and so forth.	Helps decrease fatigue, optimizes activity level within range of disease process, and reduces dyspnea and oxygen consumption.
Instruct patient/family on signs/symptoms to notify physician: increased temperature, change in sputum color or character, increasing dyspnea.	Provides for prompt recognition of infection to facilitate prompt intervention prior to respiratory failure.
Instruct patient/family to continue with follow-up medical care.	Provides for monitoring of progression of disease, presence of complications, or exacerbations, and facilitates changes in medical regimen to concur with current medical condition.
Provide patient/family with information regarding support groups, such as the American Lung Association, and so forth.	Support groups may be required to provide emotional assistance and respite for caregiver(s).
Assist patient/family to set realistic goals for long- and short-term.	Provides a plan for patient and facilitates self-involvement with realistic goals and methods to meet them. Fosters independence and reduces anxiety.

NIC: *Teaching: Individual*

Discharge or Maintenance Evaluation

■ Patient will be able to recall information regarding disease process and treatment regimen.

■ Patient will be able to recall accurately the signs/symptoms for which to notify physician, the effects and side effects of medications, and proper procedure for using inhalers.

■ Patient will be able to demonstrate accurately proper cough techniques, pursed-lip breathing, and proper positioning to facilitate breathing.

■ Patient/family will be able to access support systems effectively.

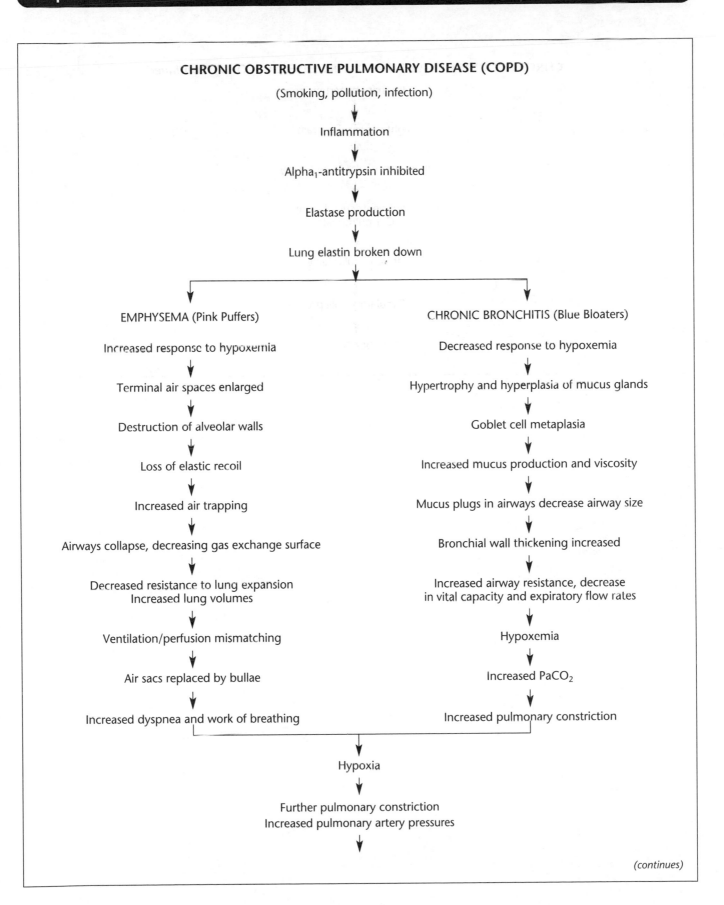

CHRONIC OBSTRUCTIVE PULMONARY DISEASE (COPD)

(Smoking, pollution, infection)

↓

Inflammation

↓

Alpha$_1$-antitrypsin inhibited

↓

Elastase production

↓

Lung elastin broken down

↓

EMPHYSEMA (Pink Puffers)

Increased response to hypoxemia

↓

Terminal air spaces enlarged

↓

Destruction of alveolar walls

↓

Loss of elastic recoil

↓

Increased air trapping

↓

Airways collapse, decreasing gas exchange surface

↓

Decreased resistance to lung expansion
Increased lung volumes

↓

Ventilation/perfusion mismatching

↓

Air sacs replaced by bullae

↓

Increased dyspnea and work of breathing

CHRONIC BRONCHITIS (Blue Bloaters)

Decreased response to hypoxemia

↓

Hypertrophy and hyperplasia of mucus glands

↓

Goblet cell metaplasia

↓

Increased mucus production and viscosity

↓

Mucus plugs in airways decrease airway size

↓

Bronchial wall thickening increased

↓

Increased airway resistance, decrease
in vital capacity and expiratory flow rates

↓

Hypoxemia

↓

Increased PaCO$_2$

↓

Increased pulmonary constriction

↓

Hypoxia

↓

Further pulmonary constriction
Increased pulmonary artery pressures

↓

(continues)

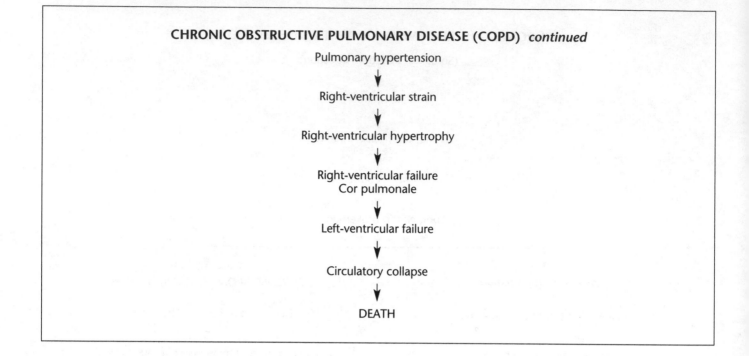

CHRONIC OBSTRUCTIVE PULMONARY DISEASE (COPD) *continued*

Pulmonary hypertension

↓

Right-ventricular strain

↓

Right-ventricular hypertrophy

↓

Right-ventricular failure
Cor pulmonale

↓

Left-ventricular failure

↓

Circulatory collapse

↓

DEATH

CHAPTER 2.5

STATUS ASTHMATICUS

Status asthmaticus is a critical emergency that requires prompt intervention to avoid acute and possibly fatal, respiratory failure. In this condition, the asthmatic attacks are unresponsive to medical therapeutics, with severe bronchospasms creating decreased oxygenation and perfusion.

During an acute asthmatic attack, the individual may demonstrate varying degrees of respiratory distress depending on the duration of the attack, and the severity of spasm. The underlying cause of asthma is still as yet unknown, but is thought to be caused by imbalances in adrenergic and cholinergic control of the airways, and their response to the allergens, infections, or emotional factors with which they come in contact. Intrinsic asthma occurs when the triggering factors are irritation, infection, or emotions, and extrinsic asthma occurs when precipitated by allergic or complement-mediated factors. Asthma may be drug-induced by aspirin, indomethacin, tartrazine, propranolol, and timolol.

In asthma, the airways are narrowed because of the bronchial muscle spasms, edema, inflammation of the bronchioles, and thick, tenacious mucus production. The narrowing leads to areas of obstruction and these become hypoventilated and hypoperfused. Eventually a ventilation/perfusion mismatch occurs and may lead to hypoxemia and an increasing A-a gradient. When $PaCO_2$ rises to the point of respiratory acidosis, the patient is then considered to be in respiratory failure.

The most common causes of status asthmaticus are allergen exposure, noncompliance with medication regime, idiosyncratic drug reactions, and respiratory infection exposure. Environmental factors, such as excessively hot, cold, or dusty areas, may initiate status asthmaticus because of the effect they have on the air that is breathed.

Wheezing may occur not only with asthma, but with chronic obstructive pulmonary disease, congestive heart failure, pulmonary embolism, and tuberculosis, and these diagnoses should be ruled out.

Patients who have status asthmaticus suffer pronounced fatigue because of the continuous efforts of breathing, and they easily become dehydrated because of the hyperpnea. The patient usually has dyspnea, tachypnea, wheezing, tachycardia, pulsus paradoxus, and severe anxiety. The goals of treatment include ventilatory support, maintenance of adequate airway, and the prevention of respiratory failure or barotrauma.

MEDICAL CARE

Laboratory: CBC and sputum specimens usually show eosinophilia; elevated WBC; positive sputum cultures

Chest X-ray: used to observe for infiltrates or hyperinflation to the lungs; may be used to visualize pneumothorax, hemothorax, or pneumomediastinum; chest X-ray offers little to confirm status asthmaticus but can be of value to rule out other causes

Arterial blood gases: to identify problems with oxygenation and acid–base balance; initially $PaCO_2$ may be low normal or decreased with an elevated pH and decreased PaO_2; with severe asthmatic attacks a progression to normal or increased $PaCO_2$ may indicate impending respiratory failure

Spirometry: to provide information about severity of an attack, and to assess for improvement with therapy; FEV_1 is the forced expiratory volume for 1 second and is usually <1500 cc during an asthmatic attack and will increase 500 cc or more if treatment is successful; peak expiratory flow rates (PEFR) are decreased and may be <60 L/minute initially, but will increase to 50% or more of predicted values after one hour if treatment is successful

Oxygen: to provide supplemental available oxygen

Bronchodilators: albuterol (Proventil, Ventolin), aminophylline (Aminophylline, Phyllocontin),

127

epinephrine (Adrenaline Chloride, Epi-Pen, Vaponefrin, Bronkaid), ipratropium bromide (Atrovent), isoproterenol (Isuprel, Isuprel Mistometer), levalbuterol hydrochloride (Xopenex), metoproterenol sulfate (Alupent, Metaproterenol), oxtriphylline (Choledyl SA), Pirbuterol acetate (Maxair), salmeterol xinafoate (Serevent), terbutaline (Brethaire, Brethine, Bricanyl), or theophylline (Aerolate, Elixophyllin, Theolair, Theostat, Theochron) used to relax bronchial smooth muscle to dilate the bronchial tree to facilitate air exchange; many inhibit the enzyme that breaks down cAMP to help relax pulmonary blood vessels; some are beta-adrenergic agents

Corticosteroids: dexamethasone (Decadron, Cortastat), hydrocortisone (Cortef, Solu-Cortef, Cortenema), or methylprednisolone (Medrol, Depo-Medrol, Solu-Medrol) among others are used to decrease the inflammatory response and edema; most act by suppression of the immune response by stabilization of the leukocytic lysosomal membranes

Antimicrobials: used when infective process is documented; usually bacterial infection is not a common precipitating factor

Mechanical ventilation: may be necessary when respiratory failure is present and hypoxemia persists despite medical therapy

IPPB: used to assist the patient with deep inspiration to facilitate more productive coughing of thick mucus and to deliver medication by an aerosol route

COMMON NURSING DIAGNOSES

IMPAIRED GAS EXCHANGE (see MECHANICAL VENTILATION)

Related to: bronchospasm, inflammation to bronchi, hypoxemia, fatigue, secretions

Defining Characteristics: dyspnea, tachypnea, hypoxia, hypoxemia, hypercapnia, restlessness, anxiety, abnormal ABGs, dysrhythmias, decreased oxygen saturation

ANXIETY (see MECHANICAL VENTILATION)

Related to: dyspnea, change in health status, threat of death

Defining Characteristics: fear, restlessness, muscle tension, apprehension, helplessness, sense of impending doom, tachycardia, tachypnea

ADDITIONAL NURSING DIAGNOSES

INEFFECTIVE AIRWAY CLEARANCE

Related to: airway obstruction, edema of bronchioles, inability to cough or to cough effectively, excessive mucus production

Defining Characteristics: adventitious breath sounds, dyspnea, tachypnea, shallow respirations, cough with or without productivity, cyanosis, anxiety, restlessness, wheezing, chest tightness

Outcome Criteria

✔ Patient will maintain patency of airway and will be able to effectively clear secretions.

✔ Patient will have clear breath sounds without wheezing or dyspnea.

NOC: *Respiratory Status: Airway Patency*

INTERVENTIONS	RATIONALES
Monitor VS q 1–2 hours and prn. Observe for pulsus paradoxus. Notify physician for significant abnormalities.	Pulse rates >110/min with pulsus >12 mm Hg with concurrent tachypnea >30/min indicates severe respiratory distress.
Observe respiratory status, patient's ability to maintain airway, work of breathing, nasal flaring, pursed-lip breathing, and prolonged expiratory phase.	Presence of these symptoms may indicate impending respiratory failure.
Auscultate lung fields q 1–4 hours and prn. Notify physician for significant changes.	Expiratory wheezing or rhonchi may be heard as secretions and air move through the narrowed airways. Decreased breath sounds throughout the lung fields is a critical sign because it means the patient cannot move enough air to be heard by the clinician, and oxygenation and perfusion are severely compromised.
Monitor arterial blood gases, and notify physician for significant abnormalities.	May indicate impending respiratory distress and failure.
Administer bronchodilators as ordered.	Nebulizers are usually the first line treatment for asthma. Aminophylline is frequently prescribed to relax bronchial smooth muscle and mediates histamine release and cAMP

INTERVENTIONS	RATIONALES
	degradation, which facilitates improved air flow.
Monitor lab levels for attainment and maintenance of therapeutic levels. Observe patient for anorexia, nausea, vomiting, abdominal pain, nervousness, restlessness, and tachycardia.	Therapeutic levels of Aminophylline range between 10–20 mcg/ml. Symptoms may indicate theophylline toxicity, which will require titration of the drug dosage.
Administer sympathomimetics as ordered.	Epinephrine is usually given SQ every 20–30 minutes for 3 doses as needed to relieve broncho-constriction. Terbutaline is usually not the first drug of choice in acute situations because of the delayed onset of action, but is frequently used after the patient shows improvement.
Assist/administer inhalation therapy as ordered.	Nebulizers and intermittent positive pressure breathing treatments may be used in mild to moderate episodes but should not be used during acute attacks because of the potential for bronchospasm in response to the aerosol agent.
Administer IV fluids as ordered.	Helps to maintain hydration to allow for thinning of secretions.
Administer humidified oxygen as ordered. Monitor oxygen saturation by oximetry and notify physician if <90%.	Humidification of oxygen helps to keep secretions thinned to allow for easy expectoration. Oxygen saturation levels <90% correspond to arterial blood gas readings of PaO$_2$ 60 mm Hg or less, which compromises perfusion and oxygenation of tissues.
Assess vocal and rhonchal fremitus.	Vocal fremitus may be decreased because of hyperinflation of the lungs and rhonchal fremitus may be present if secretions are copious.
Have emergency equipment on hand, including crash cart, tracheostomy tray, and so forth.	Severe bronchospasm with asthmaticus can result in cardiopulmonary compromise and arrest requiring emergent treat-

INTERVENTIONS	RATIONALES
	ment to sustain life. Intubation may not be possible utilizing endotracheal tubes and patient may require emergent tracheostomy to provide a patent airway.
Monitor for side effects, such as tachycardias, tremors, nausea, vomiting, or bronchospasm.	May occur as adverse reactions from medications. May require change in specific drug used.
Instruct patient in avoidance of allergens, emotional stressors, and medication changes without physician's knowledge.	The presence of allergens, emotional stress, and nonsanctioned changes of medication or noncompliance with medication regime may result in asthmatic attacks.
Instruct patient/family in correct medication administration, correct dosages, times, and appropriate MDI usage technique.	Noncompliance or changes in schedules of medications can result in asthma exacerbations.
Instruct in dietary limitations as warranted.	Some foods and food preservatives are known allergens and can provoke asthma attacks.

NIC: *Airway Management*

Discharge or Maintenance Evaluation

- Patient will maintain patent airway and be able to cough and clear own secretions.
- Patient will have clear breath sounds with no adventitious sounds or airway compromise.
- Patient will have adequate oxygenation.

INEFFECTIVE COPING (see ARDS)

Related to: situational crisis of disease process, inability to cope with stress, hypoxemia

Defining Characteristics: apprehension, use of defense mechanisms, emotional extremes, feelings of being overwhelmed, anxiety, helplessness, disorganized thoughts, inability to make decisions, inability to concentrate, focusing on crisis only, increased tension

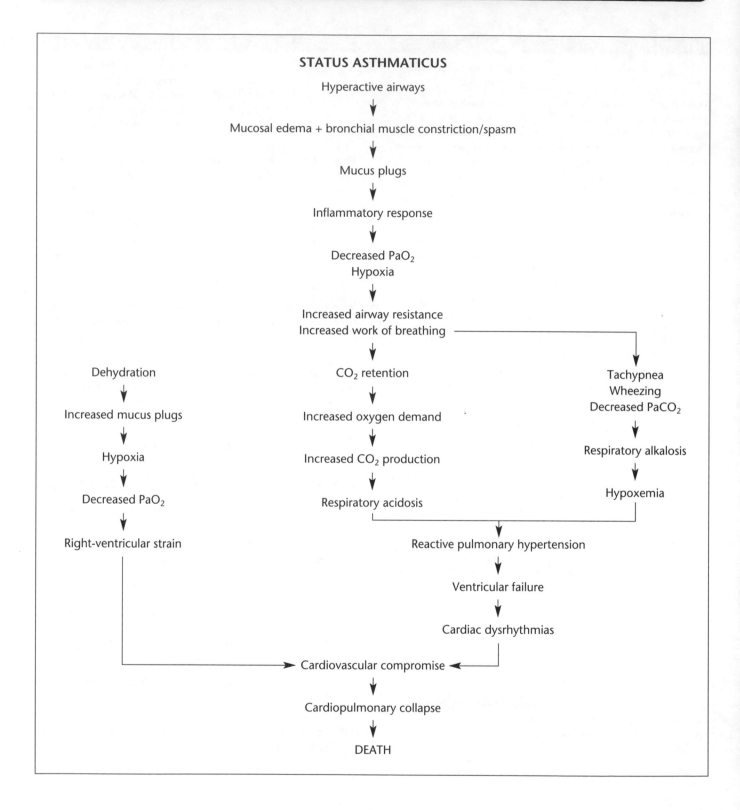

STATUS ASTHMATICUS

Hyperactive airways

↓

Mucosal edema + bronchial muscle constriction/spasm

↓

Mucus plugs

↓

Inflammatory response

↓

Decreased PaO_2
Hypoxia

↓

Increased airway resistance
Increased work of breathing

↓

| Dehydration | CO₂ retention | Tachypnea Wheezing Decreased PaCO₂ |

Dehydration

↓

Increased mucus plugs

↓

Hypoxia

↓

Decreased PaO_2

↓

Right-ventricular strain

CO_2 retention

↓

Increased oxygen demand

↓

Increased CO_2 production

↓

Respiratory acidosis

Tachypnea
Wheezing
Decreased $PaCO_2$

↓

Respiratory alkalosis

↓

Hypoxemia

Reactive pulmonary hypertension

↓

Ventricular failure

↓

Cardiac dysrhythmias

Cardiovascular compromise

↓

Cardiopulmonary collapse

↓

DEATH

CHAPTER 2.6

PULMONARY EMBOLISM

A pulmonary embolus (PE) usually results after a deep vein thrombus partially or totally dislodges from the pelvis, thigh, or calf. The clot then lodges in one or more of the pulmonary arteries and obstructs forward blood flow and oxygen supply to the lung parenchyma. Pressure is backed up and results in increased pulmonary artery pressures and vascular resistance, right ventricular failure, tachycardia, and shock. Alveolar dead space is increased which results in ventilation/perfusion mismatching and decreased PaO_2. The embolus releases chemicals that decrease surfactant and increase bronchoconstriction. Hyperventilation caused by carbon dioxide retention results in decreased $PaCO_2$. Fat embolism, septic embolism, or amniotic fluid embolism are rarely causes of PE and when they are, usually occlude smaller arterioles or capillaries. A pulmonary embolus is classified as being massive when more than half the pulmonary artery circulation is occluded.

Infarction of the pulmonary circulation occurs less than 10% of the time and usually results when the patient has an underlying chronic cardiac or pulmonary disease. Pulmonary infarcts may be reabsorbed and fibrosis may cause scar tissue formation. Usually collateral pulmonary circulation maintains lung tissue viability to alveolar structures.

The main risk factors that may predispose pulmonary embolism formation are acute myocardial infarction, congestive heart failure, shock states, diabetes mellitus, venous disease of the lower extremities, previous pulmonary embolism, immobility, cardiac disease, pregnancy, malignancy, fractures, estrogen contraceptives, obesity, burns, blood dyscrasias, surgery, and trauma. Thrombus formation occurs with blood flow stasis, coagulopathy alterations, and damage to the endothelium of the vessel walls, and these three factors are known as Virchow's triad.

The most common signs/symptoms are dyspnea, chest pain, and cough with hemoptysis. Other symptoms may be present, such as lightheadedness, diaphoresis, cyanosis, pleural friction rubs, S_2 split, tachypnea, tachycardia, anxiety, mental changes, gallops, dysrhythmias, rales, and hypotension, but are dependent on the size of the embolus, presence of infarction, or complications.

MEDICAL CARE

Laboratory: PTT done daily to monitor heparin therapy; LDH may be elevated in pulmonary embolus, but other diagnoses must be ruled out; fibrin split products usually increase consistently with PE; CBC may show increased hematocrit caused by hemoconcentration, and increased RBCs

Chest X-ray: used to rule out other pulmonary diseases; shows atelectasis, elevated diaphragm and pleural effusions, prominence of pulmonary artery, and occasionally, a wedge-shaped infiltrate commonly seen in pulmonary embolism

Nuclear radiographic testing: lung scans are used to show perfusion defects beyond occluded vasculature; xenon ventilation scans are used to differentiate between pulmonary embolism and COPD, and together with perfusion scans, will reveal ventilation/perfusion mismatches

Pulmonary angiography: used as a definitive test when other tests do not ensure the diagnosis in high-risk patients; identifies intra-arterial filling defects and obstruction of pulmonary artery branches

Electrocardiography: used to reveal right axis deviation, right-sided heart strain, right bundle branch block, tall peaked P waves, ST segment depression and T wave inversion, as well as supraventricular tachydysrhythmias; in massive PE, ECG may show P pulmonale, right axis deviation, or incomplete or new right bundle branch block

Phlebography: used to identify deep vein thrombosis in legs

Oxygen: to provide supplemental oxygen to maintain oxygenation

Pulmonary artery catheterization: used to enable hemodynamic monitoring and to assess response to therapies

Arterial blood gases: used to assess for hypoxemia and acid–base imbalances; may indicate respiratory alkalosis as a result of hyperventilation and hypoxemia; A-a gradient increased

Thoracentesis: may be used to rule out empyema if pleural effusion is noted on chest X-ray

Beta-blockers: drugs such as acebutolol (Sectral), atenolol (Tenormin), betaxolol hydrochloride (Kerlone), bisoprolol fumarate (Zebeta), carteolol hydrochloride (Cartrol), carvedilol (Coreg), esmolol (Brevibloc), metoprolol (Toprol XL, Betaloc, Lopressor), labetalol hydrochloride (Normodyne, Trandate), nadolol (Corgard), pindolol (Visken), propranolol (Inderal), sotalol hydrochloride (Betapace), and timolol (Blocadren) used in pulmonary hypertension to dilate the pulmonary vasculature to increase tissue perfusion

Cardiac glycosides: digoxin used only if absolutely mandatory during the acute hypoxemia phase because of the potential for lethal dysrhythmias or cardiac failure

Analgesics: used to alleviate pain and discomfort

Anticoagulants: heparin is used initially in the treatment of PE, with change to coumadin/warfarin PO for 3–6 months

Thrombolytics: streptokinase or urokinase used to enhance conversion of plasminogen to plasmin to prevent venous thrombus

Antiplatelet drugs: aspirin and dipyridamole used to prevent venous thromboembolism

Surgery: embolectomy may be performed to remove the clot; umbrella filter may be placed or surgical interruption of the inferior vena cava may be performed to prevent migration of clots into the pulmonary vasculature

COMMON NURSING DIAGNOSES

IMPAIRED GAS EXCHANGE (see MECHANICAL VENTILATION)

Related to: atelectasis, airway obstruction, alveolar collapse, pulmonary edema, increased secretions, active bleeding, altered blood flow to lung, shunting

Defining Characteristics: dyspnea, restlessness, anxiety, apprehension, cyanosis, arterial blood gas changes, hypoxemia, hypoxia, hypercapnia, decreased oxygen saturation

DECREASED CARDIAC OUTPUT (see HEART FAILURE)

Related to: occlusion of pulmonary vasculature, dysrhythmias, cardiogenic shock, heart failure

Defining Characteristics: elevated blood pressure, elevated mean arterial blood pressure, elevated systemic vascular resistance greater than 1400 dyne-seconds/cm^5, cardiac output less than 4 L/min or cardiac index less than 2.5 L/min/m^2, cold, pale extremities, ECG changes, hypotension, S_2 split sounds, S_3 or S_4 gallops, dyspnea, crackles (rales), chest pain, decreased urinary output, orthopnea, jugular vein distention, edema, confusion, restlessness

INEFFECTIVE COPING (see ARDS)

Related to: situational crisis of disease process, inability to cope with stress, hypoxemia

Defining Characteristics: apprehension, use of defense mechanisms, emotional extremes, feelings of being overwhelmed, anxiety, helplessness, disorganized thoughts, inability to make decisions, inability to concentrate, focusing on crisis only, increased tension

ADDITIONAL NURSING DIAGNOSES

INEFFECTIVE BREATHING PATTERN

Related to: increase in alveolar dead space, physiologic lung changes caused by embolism, bleeding, increased secretions, decreased lung expansion, inflammation

Defining Characteristics: dyspnea, use of accessory muscles, shallow respirations, tachypnea, increased work of breathing, decreased chest expansion on involved side, cough with or without productivity, adventitious breath sounds

Outcome Criteria

✔ Patient will be eupneic with clear lung fields and arterial blood gases within normal limits.

NOC: *Respiratory Status: Ventilation*

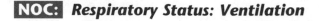

INTERVENTIONS	RATIONALES
Monitor respiratory status for changes in rate and depth, use of accessory muscles, increased work of breathing, nasal flaring, and symmetrical chest expansion.	In PE, respiratory rate is usually increased. The effort of breathing is increased and dyspnea is often the first sign of PE. Depending on the severity and location of the PE, depth of respirations may vary. Chest expansion may be decreased on the affected side due to atelectasis or pain.
Provide supplemental oxygen via nasal cannula or mask.	Provides oxygen and may decrease work of breathing.
Monitor for presence of cough and character of sputum.	Bloody secretions may result from pulmonary infarction or abnormal anticoagulation. A dry cough may result with alveolar congestion.
Auscultate lung fields for adventitious breath sounds and/or rubs.	Breath sounds may be diminished or absent if airway is obstructed due to bleeding, clotting, or collapse. Rhonchi or wheezing may result in conjunction with obstruction.
Auscultate heart sounds.	Splitting of S_2 may occur with pulmonary embolus.
Encourage deep breathing and effective coughing exercises.	Improves lung expansion and helps to remove secretions which may be increased with PE.
Prepare patient/family for placement on mechanical ventilation.	May be required if respiratory distress is severe.
Instruct on avoiding shallow respirations and splinting.	Eupnea decreases potential for atelectasis and improves venous return.
Prepare patient/family for bronchoscopy as warranted.	May be required to remove mucus plugs and/or clots in order to clear airways.
Instruct and prepare patient/family for surgical procedures.	Umbrella filter or ligation of the inferior vena cava may be required to prevent further clot migration.

NIC: *Embolus Precautions*

Discharge or Maintenance Evaluation

- Patient will be able to maintain his own respirations without mechanical assistance.

- Patient will be eupneic, with no adventitious lung or heart sounds.

- Patient will be able to recall all information accurately.

INEFFECTIVE TISSUE PERFUSION: CARDIOPULMONARY, PERIPHERAL, CEREBRAL

Related to: impaired blood flow, alveolar perfusion and gas exchange impairment, occlusion of the pulmonary artery, migration of embolus, hypoxemia, increased cardiac workload

Defining Characteristics: dyspnea, chest pain, tachycardia, dysrhythmias, productive cough, hemoptysis, edema, cyanosis, syncope, jugular vein distention, weak pulses, hypotension, use of accessory muscles, abnormal arterial blood gases, skin temperature changes, skin color changes, capillary refill >3 seconds, claudication, bruits, weakness, mental status changes, behavior changes, convulsions, loss of consciousness, restlessness, hemiplegia, coma

Outcome Criteria

✔ Patient will be hemodynamically stable, eupneic, with no alterations in perfusion to any body system.

NOC: *Tissue Perfusion: Cardiac, Pulmonary, Peripheral, Cerebral*

INTERVENTIONS	RATIONALES
Monitor vital signs and notify physician for significant changes.	Hypoxemia will result in increased heart rate as the body tries to compensate for the decrease in perfusion.
Monitor ECG for rhythm disturbances and treat as indicated.	Hypoxemia, right-sided heart strain, and electrolyte imbalances may induce dysrhythmias.
Auscultate for S_3 or S_4 heart sounds.	Increases in heart workload may result in heart strain and failure as perfusion decreases, and may result in gallop rhythm.
Monitor for presence of peripheral pulses and notify physician for significant changes.	Presence of deep vein thrombus may occlude the circulation and result in diminished or absent pulses.
Assess for Homan's and Pratt's signs.	Presence of these signs may or may not be related to PE.
Assess skin color, temperature and capillary refill.	Impairment of blood flow may induce pallor or cyanosis to the skin or mucous membranes. Cool, clammy skin or mottling may indicate peripheral vasoconstriction or shock.

(continues)

(continued)

INTERVENTIONS	RATIONALES
Monitor for restlessness or changes in mental status or level of consciousness.	May indicate occlusion, impaired cerebral blood flow, hypoxia, or development of stroke.
Prepare patient for insertion of pulmonary artery catheter.	May be required to monitor hemodynamic status and assess response to therapy.
Prepare patient for surgery as warranted.	Surgical intervention may be required if patient develops recurrent emboli in spite of treatment, or if anticoagulant therapy cannot be given. Ligation of the vena cava or insertion of an umbrella filter may be necessary.
Instruct patient/family on thrombolytic agents as warranted.	Streptokinase, urokinase, or alteplase (t-PA) may be required

INTERVENTIONS	RATIONALES
	if the pulmonary embolus is massive and compromises hemodynamic stability.

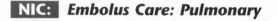 **NIC:** *Embolus Care: Pulmonary*

Discharge or Maintenance Evaluation

- Patient will have adequate tissue perfusion to all body systems.
- Patient will have stable hemodynamic parameters and vital signs will be within normal limits.
- Oxygenation will be optimal as evident by pulse oximetry greater than 90% and adequate ABGs.

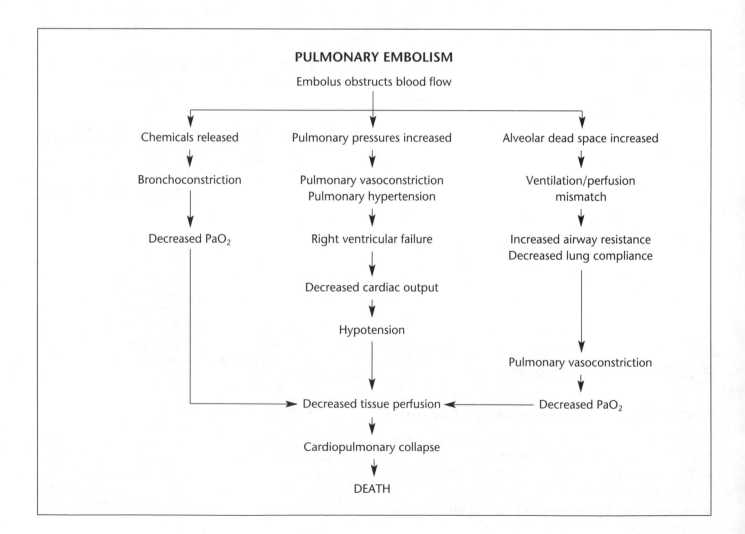

PULMONARY EMBOLISM

CHAPTER 2.7

PNEUMOTHORAX

A pneumothorax occurs when free air accumulates in the pleural cavity between the visceral and parietal areas, and causes a portion or the complete lung to collapse. Pressure in the pleural space is normally less than that of atmospheric pressure but following a penetration injury, air can enter the cavity from the outside, changing the pressure within the lung cavity and causing it to collapse. Air can also migrate to the area when the esophagus is perforated or a bronchus ruptures, leaking air into the mediastinum (pneumomediastinum). Barotrauma related to mechanical ventilatory support using high levels of PEEP leads to alveoli rupture and collapse. Gas formation from gas-forming organisms can also result in pneumothorax.

Pneumothorax may occur spontaneously in cases where a subpleural bleb or emphysematous bulla ruptures because of chronic obstructive pulmonary disease, tuberculosis, cancer, or infection and this is the most common reason in otherwise healthy individuals.

A pneumothorax may result spontaneously or with trauma, such as a penetrating chest wound, gunshot wound, knife wound, or after a procedure such as insertion of a centrally placed venous catheter line. Some symptoms of pneumothorax include abrupt onset of pleuritic chest pain, shortness of breath, decreased or absent breath sounds, tachycardia, tachypnea, hyperresonant percussion, shock, and hypotension.

A tension pneumothorax is a life-threatening emergency and occurs when air is permitted into the pleural cavity but not allowed to escape, resulting in increased intrathoracic pressure and complete collapse of the lung. It compromises the opposite lung because of increasing pleural pressures and causes a mediastinal shift which interferes with ventilation and venous return. Severe shortness of breath, hypotension, and shock ensues, and emergent treatment of a needle thoracentesis must be performed to relieve the pressure until a chest tube can be placed.

A hemothorax occurs when the lung collapse caused by accumulation of blood. Blood accumulations usually occur from the pulmonary vasculature, the intercostal and internal mammary arteries, the mediastinum, the spleen, or the liver. A hemothorax not only results in cardiopulmonary effects, but also may involve problems with hemorrhagic shock. The rate at which shock may occur depends on the source and rapidity of bleeding.

The severity of a pneumothorax, no matter what the origin, relates to the degree of collapse. A small partial pneumothorax may resolve by itself when the air is reabsorbed. In cases where collapse is more than 20–30%, a closed, water-seal drainage system and insertion of a chest tube via a lateral intercostal space is required. In cases where rapid re-expansion is desired, 15–25 cm H_2O suction may be added to the drain system.

MEDICAL CARE

Laboratory: hemoglobin and hematocrit may be decreased with blood loss

Chest X-ray: used to evaluate air or fluid accumulations, collapse of lungs, or mediastinal shifts; a visceral pleural line may be visualized

Arterial blood gases: vary depending on the severity of the pneumothorax; oxygen saturation usually decreases, PaO_2 is usually normal or decreased, and $PaCO_2$ is occasionally increased

Chest tube: placement required to facilitate re-expansion of the collapsed lung and to permit drainage of fluid from lung if collapse is significant

Thoracentesis: needle thoracentesis is required for the immediate management of a tension pneumothorax to relieve the pressure in the pleura by removing air and/or fluid

Surgery: thoracotomy with excision or oversewing of the bullae may be required if the patient develops two or more pneumothorax on one side

NURSING DIAGNOSES

INEFFECTIVE BREATHING PATTERN

Related to: air and/or fluid accumulations, pain, decreased lung expansion, lung collapse

Defining Characteristics: dyspnea, tachypnea, use of accessory muscles, nasal flaring, decreased chest expansion, cyanosis, abnormal arterial blood gases, hypotension, tachycardia

Outcome Criteria

✔ Patient will be eupneic, with adequate oxygenation, and will maintain adequate ABGs.

NOC: *Respiratory Status: Ventilation*

INTERVENTIONS	RATIONALES
Monitor respiratory status for increase in rate, decrease in depth, dyspnea, or cyanosis.	Physiologic changes that result from the lung collapse may cause respiratory distress and may lead to hypoxia.
Auscultate breath sounds.	Breath sounds may be absent in areas where atelectasis occurs, and may be decreased with partially collapsed lung fields.
Observe for symmetric chest expansion.	Moderate to severe pneumothorax will result in asymmetrical chest expansion until the lung is fully re-expanded.
Observe for position of trachea.	Tracheal deviation away from the affected lung occurs in tension pneumothorax.
Listen for sucking sounds with inspiration; if present, apply occlusive dressing over wound while patient performs Valsalva's maneuver.	Indicates an open pneumothorax which impairs ventilation. During inspiration air moves into the pleural space and collapses lung; with expiration, air moves out of the pleural space. Application of a dressing seals the chest wall defect, while the Valsalva maneuver helps to expand the lung.
Observe for paradoxical movements of the chest during respiration; if present, stabilize the flail area with a sandbag or pressure dressing, and turn to the affected side.	May indicate flail chest and impaired ventilation. Procedures help to stabilize the area to facilitate improved respiratory exchange.

INTERVENTIONS	RATIONALES
Place patient in semi-sitting position.	Promotes lung expansion and improves ventilatory efforts.
Prepare patient for and assist with insertion of chest tube.	Intercostal tube placement is required when a pneumothorax is greater than 20–30% in order to facilitate re-expansion of the lung. Instruction, when feasible, reduces patient anxiety and improves cooperation.
Once chest tube is inserted, ensure that connections are tightened and taped securely per hospital protocol.	Prevents air leaks and disconnections at the connector sites.
Monitor water-seal drainage bottles to ensure fluid level is above drain tube.	Fluid must be maintained above the end of the tube to prevent air from being sucked into lung and resulting in further collapse.
Maintain prescribed level of suction to drainage system.	Usually 15–25 cm H_2O pressure suction is sufficient to maintain intrapleural negative pressure and facilitate fluid drainage and re-expansion of the lung.
Observe the water-seal drainage system for bubbling.	Bubbling should occur during expiration and demonstrates that the pneumothorax is vented through the system. Bubbling should diminish and finally cease as the lung re-expands. If no bubbling is present in system, this may indicate either complete re-expansion of the lung or obstruction in the chest tube/drainage system.
Monitor drainage system for continuous bubbling and ascertain if the problem is patient- or system-centered. Clamp chest tube near the patient's chest to assess for air leak.	Continuous bubbling may result from a large pneumothorax or from air leaks in the drainage system. When the tube is clamped as described and bubbling ceases, the problem is patient-centered with potential air leak at the insertion site or within the patient. If the bubbling continues, the leak is within the drainage system.
If patient has insertion site air leak, apply vaseline–impregnated gauze around site, and reassess the problem.	Provides a seal and corrects the air leak problem.

INTERVENTIONS	RATIONALES
If patient has drainage system air leak, ascertain the location by clamping the tube downward toward the system by increments. Secure connections.	Determines the location of the problem and corrects air leaks at the connectors.
Observe for fluid tidaling.	Fluctuation of the fluid within the tubing, or tidaling, demonstrates pressure changes during inspiration and expiration, and is normally 2–10 cm during inspiration. Increases may occur during coughing or forceful expiration but continuous increases in tidaling may indicate a large pneumothorax or airway obstruction.
Monitor fluid drainage for character and amount, and notify physician if drainage is greater than 100 cc/hr for more than 2 hours.	Provides for prompt detection of hemorrhage and prompt intervention. Some drainage systems have the potential for autotransfusion, and this should be done per hospital policy.
Strip chest tubes gently, if at all, per hospital protocol.	Some facilities and physicians avoid milking, or stripping, of the tubes because of the potential for suction to draw lung tissue into the orifice of the tube and damage the tissue, as well as rupturing of small blood vessels. The procedure changes intrathoracic pressure which may result in chest pain or coughing. Stripping may be required to maintain drainage when large blood clots or fibrin strands are present or if the drainage is viscid or purulent.
Place chest drainage system below the level of the chest, and coil tubing carefully to avoid kinking.	Promotes drainage of air and fluid, and prevents kinking and occlusion of tubing.
Obtain chest X-rays daily.	Identifies the presence of pneumothorax and resolution or deterioration.
If chest tube is accidentally removed, apply vaseline-impregnated gauze and pressure dressing, and notify physician.	Provides a seal over chest wound to prevent pneumothorax from recurring or worsening. Prompt treatment may prevent cardiopulmonary impairment.

INTERVENTIONS	RATIONALES
If chest tube becomes accidentally disconnected from tubing, reconnect as cleanly and quickly as possible.	Disconnection may result in atmospheric air entering the pleural space and worsening or causing pneumothorax.
Observe dressing over chest tube insertion site for drainage and notify physician for significant drainage.	Excessive drainage on dressing may indicate malposition of the chest tube, infection, or other problem.
Assure that chest tube clamps (2 for each tube) are present in patient's room and are taken with patient when transported out of unit.	Provides for emergencies which may require clamping of the tube.
Assist with removal of chest tube as warranted, and apply vaseline-impregnated gauze and dry sterile dressing over site, and change per hospital protocol.	Once lung is re-expanded and fluid drainage has ceased, chest tubes are removed. Gauze provides a seal over the open wound to prevent recurrence of pneumothorax.
Monitor patient for changes in respiratory status, oxygenation, chest pain, dyspnea, or presence of subcutaneous emphysema.	May indicate recurrent pneumothorax and requires prompt intervention and reinsertion of intercostal tube.
Instruct patient/family on function of chest tube/drainage system.	Provides knowledge and decreases patient anxiety.
Instruct patient to avoid pulling or lying on tubing.	Prevents obstruction of tube and facilitates drainage.
Instruct patient/family on signs/symptoms to report to nurse: dyspnea, chest pain, changes in sounds of bubbling from drainage system.	Promotes prompt recognition of problems that may require prompt intervention.

NIC: *Tube Care: Chest*

Discharge or Maintenance Evaluation

- Patient will be eupneic with no adventitious breath sounds.
- Patient will have symmetric chest expansion and midline tracheal placement with no episodes of dyspnea.
- Patient will achieve and maintain re-expansion of lung with no recurrence or complications.

PNEUMOTHORAX

Air enters pleural cavity

↓

Pleural pressure increased above atmospheric pressure

↓

Lung collapses

↓

High pressure gradient between alveolus and adjacent vascular sheet

↓

Decreased PaO_2
Increased $PaCO_2$

↓

Air moves along pulmonary vessels to mediastinum

↓

Mediastinal shifting

↓

Interference with ventilation and venous return

↓

Increased pulmonary pressures
Low PCWP, high CVP

↓

Shock

↓

Cardiovascular collapse

↓

DEATH

UNIT 3

NEUROLOGIC SYSTEM

CHAPTER 3.1

CEREBROVASCULAR ACCIDENT

A cerebrovascular accident (CVA), or stroke, occurs when a sudden decrease in cerebral blood circulation as a result of thrombosis, embolus, or hemorrhage leads to hypoxia of brain tissues, causing swelling and death. When circulation is impaired or interrupted, an area of the brain becomes infarcted and this changes membrane permeability, resulting in increased edema and intracranial pressure (ICP). The clinical symptoms may vary depending on the area and extent of the injury.

Thrombosis of small arteries in the white matter of the brain account for the most common cause of strokes. A history of hypertension, diabetes mellitus, cardiac disease, vascular disease, or atherosclerosis may lead to thrombosis, which causes ischemia to the brain supplied by the vessel involved.

Embolism is the second most common cause of CVA, and happens when a blood vessel is suddenly occluded with blood, air, tumor, fat, or septic particulate. The embolus migrates to the cerebral arteries and obstructs circulation causing edema and necrosis.

When hemorrhage occurs, it is usually the sudden result of ruptured aneurysms, tumors, or AV malformations, or involves problems with hypertension or bleeding dyscrasias. The cerebral bleeding decreases the blood supply and compresses neurons, leading to a loss in function and death of neuronal tissue. Hypertensive intracranial hemorrhage occurs most often in the basal ganglia, cerebellum, or the brain stem, but can affect other more superficial areas of the brain. Hemorrhage can account for as much as 25% of all strokes.

Patients who have strokes frequently have had prior events, such as TIAs (transient ischemic attacks) with reversible focal neurologic deficits lasting less than 24 hours, or RINDs (reversible ischemic neurologic deficits) lasting greater than 24 hours but leaving little, if any, residual neurologic impairment.

In addition to the disease processes discussed earlier, cardiac dysrhythmias, alcohol use, cocaine or other recreational drug use, smoking, and the use of oral contraceptives may predispose patients to strokes.

Strokes may cause temporary or permanent losses of motor function, thought processes, memory, speech, or sensory function. Difficulty with swallowing and speaking, hemiplegia, and visual field defects are also related complications of this disease. Treatment is aimed at supporting vital functions, ensuring adequate cerebral perfusion, and prevention of major complications or permanent disability.

MEDICAL CARE

CT scans: used to identify thrombosis or hemorrhagic stroke, tumors, or hydrocephalus; may not reveal changes until 24 hours later; ischemic infarctions show up as decreased areas of absorption, whereas hemorrhage appears as increased absorption and can be seen immediately after the event

Skull X-rays: may show calcifications of the carotids in the presence of cerebral thrombosis, or partial calcification of an aneurysm in subarachnoid hemorrhage; pineal gland may shift to the opposite side if mass is expanding

Brain scans: used to identify ischemic areas caused by CVA but usually are not discernible until up to 2 weeks after injury

Angiography: used to identify site and degree of occlusion or rupture of vessel, assess collateral blood circulation, presence of AV malformations, and vessels in spasm

MRI: used to identify areas of infarction, hemorrhage, AV malformations, and edema

Ultrasound: may be used to gather information regarding flow velocity in the major circulation

Lumbar puncture: performed to evaluate ICP and to identify infection; bloody CSF may indicate a hemorrhagic stroke, and clear fluid with normal pressure may be noted in cerebral thrombosis, embolism, and with TIAs; protein may be elevated if thrombosis results from inflammation; contraindicated if ICP increased

EEG: may be used to help localize area of injury based on brain waves

Laboratory: CBC used to identify blood loss or infection; RBCs and protein in cerebrospinal fluid will increase with cerebral hemorrhage; coagulation profiles used to assess adequacy of clotting; serum osmolality used to evaluate oncotic pressures and permeability; electrolytes, glucose levels, and urinalysis performed to identify other problems and imbalances that may be responsible

Surgery: endarterectomy may be required to remove the occlusion, or microvascular bypass may be performed to bypass the occluded area, such as the carotid artery, aneurysm, or AV malformation

Corticosteroids: dexamethasone (Decadron, Cortastat), hydrocortisone (Cortef, Solu-Cortef, Cortenema), or methylprednisolone (Medrol, Depo-Medrol, Solu-Medrol) used to decrease cerebral edema

Anticonvulsants: drugs such as carbamazepine (Atretol, Carbatrol, Tegretol), clonazepam (Klonopin), ethosuximide (Zarontin), fosphenytoin sodium (Cerebryx), gabapentin (Neurontin), lamotrigine (Lamictal), levetiracetam (Keppra), oxcarbazepine (Trileptal), phenobarbital (Barbita, Solfoton, Luminal), phenytoin (Dilantin, Phenytex), primadone (Mysoline), tiagabine hydrochloride (Gabitril), topiramate (Topamax), valproic acid or valproate (Depacon, Depakene, Depakote), or zonisamide (Zonegran) used in the treatment and prophylaxis of seizure activity; method of action dependent on drug utilized—some increase cerebral levels of GABA, some help to stabilize neuronal membranes and synchronization, and some act upon sodium, potassium, or calcium ion concentrations within the neuronal cells

Analgesics: used for discomfort and pain; aspirin and aspirin-containing products are contraindicated with hemorrhage

Tissue plasminogen activator (tPA, TPA): use is controversial because of risks of uncontrolled bleeding

COMMON NURSING DIAGNOSES

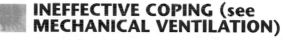

IMPAIRED PHYSICAL MOBILITY (see HEAD INJURIES)

Related to: weakness, paralysis, paresthesias, impaired cognition

Defining Characteristics: inability to move at will, muscle incoordination, decreased range of motion, decreased muscle strength

INEFFECTIVE COPING (see MECHANICAL VENTILATION)

Related to: stroke, situational crisis, loss of control, loss of independence

Defining Characteristics: inability to meet basic needs, inadequate problem solving, inability to meet role expectations, inappropriate use of defense mechanisms, verbal manipulation, irritability, fatigue, lack of goals, poor concentration, sleep disturbances, statements demonstrating inability to cope

ADDITIONAL NURSING DIAGNOSES

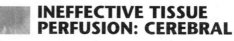

INEFFECTIVE TISSUE PERFUSION: CEREBRAL

Related to: increased intracranial pressure, occlusion, hemorrhage, interruption of cerebral blood flow, vasospasm, edema

Defining Characteristics: changes in level of consciousness, mental changes, personality changes, memory loss, restlessness, combativeness, vital sign changes, motor function impairment, sensory impairment

Outcome Criteria

✔ Patient will have improved or normal cerebral perfusion with no mental status changes or complications.

NOC: *Neurologic Status: Consciousness*

NOC: *Tissue Perfusion: Cerebral*

INTERVENTIONS	RATIONALES
Measure blood pressure in both arms.	Cerebral injury may cause variations in blood pressure readings. Hypotension may result from circulatory collapse, and increased ICP may result from edema or clot formation. Differences in readings between arms may indicate a subclavian artery blockage. Cerebral blood flow (CBF) is dependent on blood pressure, so if blood pressure drops, CBF decreases and cerebral ischemia occurs.
Maintain head of bed in elevated position with head in a neutral position.	Helps to improve venous drainage, reduces arterial pressure, and may improve cerebral perfusion. Rotation, or flexion or extension of the head can result in compression of jugular veins, causing venous engorgement and inhibiting venous return.
Provide calm, quiet environment with adequate rest periods between activities.	Bedrest may be required to prevent rebleeding after initial hemorrhage. Activity may increase ICP.
Observe patient for complaints of increasing headache, blurred vision, photophobia, nausea/vomiting, nuchal rigidity, or seizure activity.	May indicate a change in neurologic status or increasing intracranial pressure (ICP). Seizure activity may be related to cerebral anoxia or trauma. Vomiting may be a result of brain stem compression. Nuchal rigidity indicates meningeal irritation potentially caused by subarachnoid hemorrhage or meningitis.
Assess pupillary size and reflexes and accommodation to light.	Dilated pupils, unequal pupils, or nonreactive pupillary response may all indicate increasing ICP.
Administer anticoagulants as ordered.	May be warranted to improve blood flow to cerebral tissues and to prevent further clotting and embolus formation. These are contraindicated in hypertension due to the potential for hemorrhage.
Administer antihypertensives as ordered.	Hypertension may be transient when occurring during the CVA, but chronic hypertension will require judicious treatment to prevent further tissue ischemia and damage.

INTERVENTIONS	RATIONALES
Administer vasodilators as ordered.	Helps to improve collateral circulation and to reduce the incidence of vasospasm.
Instruct patient on use of stool softeners and avoidance of straining at stool.	Valsalva maneuvers increase ICP, decrease venous return causing venous engorgement, and may result in rebleeding. Stool softeners help to prevent straining.
Prepare patient for surgery as warranted.	May be required to treat problem and prevent further complications.
Instruct/prepare patient/family for ICP monitoring.	ICP monitoring may be required to observe for fluctuations in pressure to ensure prompt identification of potential complications and allow for timely intervention.

NIC: *Cerebral Perfusion Promotion*

Discharge or Maintenance Evaluation

- Patient will maintain or improve his level of consciousness and be oriented in all spheres.
- Patient will have normal intracranial pressures.
- Vital signs will be stable, with blood pressure adequate to meet cerebral perfusion pressure needs.

IMPAIRED VERBAL COMMUNICATION

Related to: cerebral circulation impairment, weakness, loss of muscle control, neuromuscular impairment

Defining Characteristics: inability to speak, inability to identify objects, inability to comprehend language, inability to write, inability to choose and use appropriate words, dysarthria, stuttering, slurring

Outcome Criteria

✔ Patient will be able to communicate normally or will be able to make needs known by some form of communication.
✔ Patient will be able to answer questions appropriately.

NOC: *Communication: Expressive Ability*

INTERVENTIONS	RATIONALES
Evaluate patient's ability to speak or understand language.	Provides a baseline from which to begin planning intervention. Determination of specific areas of brain injury involvement will preclude what type of assistance will be required.
Assess whether patient suffers from aphasia or dysarthria.	Aphasic patients have difficulty using and interpreting language, comprehending words, and inability to speak or make signs. Dysarthric patients can understand language but have problems forming or pronouncing words as a result of weakness or paralysis of the oral muscles.
Evaluate patient's response to simple commands.	Inability to follow simple commands may indicate receptive aphasia
Evaluate patient's ability to name objects.	Inability to do so indicates expressive aphasia.
Evaluate patient's ability to write simple sentences or his name.	May indicate patient's disability with receptive and expressive aphasia.
Avoid talking down to patient or making patronizing comments.	Intellect frequently remains unimpaired after injury.
When asking questions, use yes or no type questions initially, and progress as patient is able.	Provides for method of communication without necessity of response to large volumes of information. As patient progresses, the intricacy of questions may increase.
Provide a method of communication for patient, such as a writing board, or communication board to which a patient may point.	Allows for communication of needs and allays anxiety.
Consult with speech therapy.	May be required to identify cognition, function, and plan interventions for recovery.
Assist patient/family to identify and use methods for communication.	Provides method for patient to communicate his needs.

NIC: *Communication Enhancement: Speech Deficit*

Discharge or Maintenance Evaluation

- Patient will be able to communicate effectively.
- Patient will be able to understand communication problem and access resources to meet needs.

DISTURBED SENSORY PERCEPTION: VISUAL, KINESTHETIC, GUSTATORY, TACTILE, OLFACTORY

Related to: neurological trauma/deficit, stress, altered reception, transmission, or integration of stimuli

Defining Characteristics: behavior changes, disorientation to time, place, self, and situation, diminished concentration, inability to focus, alteration in thought processes, decreased sensation, paresthesias, paralysis, altered ability to taste and smell, inability to recognize objects, muscle incoordination, muscle weakness, inappropriate communication, altered communication, change in response to stimuli, hallucinations, change in auditory or visual acuity, restlessness, loss of appetite, weight loss, decreased sensitivity to pain

Outcome Criteria

✔ Patient will achieve and maintain alertness and orientation with acceptable behavior and motor/sensory function.

NOC: *Cognitive Orientation*

INTERVENTIONS	RATIONALES
Assess patient's perceptions and reorient as necessary.	May help decrease distortions of thought and identify reality.
Assess for visual field defects, visual disturbances, or problems with depth perception.	Visual distortion may prevent patient from having realistic perception of his environment.
Assist patient by placing objects in his field of vision.	Allows for recognition of people and objects, and decreases confusion.
Limit amount of stimuli. Avoid excess noise or equipment.	May create sensory overload and confusion.
Observe patient for nonuse of extremities. Test for sensation awareness and ability to discern position of body.	May create self-care deficiencies. Loss of sensation or inability to recognize objects may impair return to level of functioning. Sensory impairment affects balance and positioning.
Evaluate environment for safety hazards, such as temperature extremes.	Promotes safety and decreases potential for injury.
Instruct patient to observe feet when standing or ambulating,	Visual and tactile stimulation helps to retrain movement and

(continues)

(continued)

INTERVENTIONS	RATIONALES
and to make a conscious effort to reposition body parts. Assist with sensory stimulation to nonuse side.	to experience sensations.
Assist patient/family in obtaining community resources for post-discharge care.	Allows for further assistance and helps patient to regain as much return of function as possible.
Instruct patient in weighing every week.	Detects weight loss and assists with detection of possible malnutrition.
Instruct in dietary changes.	Changes in diet may help compensate for the lack of taste, smell, and appetite.
Instruct family in inspection of skin daily.	Allows for prompt detection of skin breakdown and helps to integrate family into plan of care.
Instruct patient/family in exercise program using active and passive range of motion exercises.	Helps to maintain range of motion of joints and prevent muscle degeneration.

NIC: *Cognitive Stimulation*

Discharge or Maintenance Evaluation

- Patient will be alert and oriented to all phases.
- Patient will be able to understand changes in functional ability and residual neurologic deficits.
- Patient will be able to compensate for dysfunctional abilities.

IMPAIRED SWALLOWING

Related to: neuromuscular impairment

Defining Characteristics: inability to swallow effectively, choking, aspiration, food refusal, nausea, vomiting, lack of tongue action, abnormal swallowing study, incomplete lip closure, inability to clear oral cavity, coughing, lack of chewing, drooling, regurgitation, repetitive swallowing, heartburn, reflux

Outcome Criteria

✔ Patient will be able to swallow effectively with no incidence of aspiration.

NOC: *Swallowing Status*

INTERVENTIONS	RATIONALES
Evaluate patient's ability to swallow, extent of any paralysis, ability to maintain airway.	Provides baseline information from which to plan interventions for care.
Maintain head position and support, head of bed elevated at least 30 degrees or more during and after feeding.	Helps to prevent aspiration and facilitates ability to swallow.
Place food in the unaffected side of mouth.	Allows for sensory stimulation and taste, and may assist to trigger swallowing reflexes.
Provide foods that are soft and require little, if any, chewing, or provide thickened liquids.	These types of foods are easier to control and decrease potential for choking or aspiration.
Assist with stimulation of tongue, cheeks, or lips as warranted.	May help to retrain oral muscles and facilitate adequate tongue movement and swallowing.
Monitor intake and output, and caloric intake.	Insufficient nutrient intake orally may result in the need for alternative types of nutritional support.
Administer tube feedings/TPN as warranted/ordered.	May be required if oral intake is insufficient.
Instruct patient to use straw for drinking liquids. Maintain swallowing precautions identified by speech therapists.	Helps to strengthen facial and oral muscles to decrease potential for choking.
Encourage family to bring patient's favorite foods.	Familiar foods may increase oral intake.

NIC: *Swallowing Therapy*

Discharge or Maintenance Evaluation

- Patient will be able to eat and swallow normally.
- Patient will be able to ingest an adequate amount of nutrients without danger of aspiration.
- Patient will be able to follow instructions and strengthen muscles used for eating/swallowing.

DRESSING/GROOMING SELF-CARE DEFICIT

Related to: weakness, decreased muscle strength, muscle incoordination, paralysis, paresthesia, pain, functional impairment

Defining Characteristics: inability to perform ADLs, inability to maintain personal hygiene, inability to dress/undress self

Outcome Criteria

✔ Patient will be able to meet self-care needs within own ability level.

NOC: *Self-Care: Dressing, Grooming*

INTERVENTIONS	RATIONALES
Evaluate level of neurologic impairment and patient's abilities to perform ADLs.	Provides baseline from which to plan care for patient needs.
Assist patient with ADLs as needed and encourage patient to perform tasks he may be capable of doing.	Assistance may reduce levels of frustration but patient will have more self-esteem with tasks he may complete.
Alter plans of care keeping in mind patient's visual, motor, or sensory deficits.	Assists patient with safety concerns and allows for some degree of independence.
Utilize self-help devices and instruct patient in their use.	Allows patient to perform tasks and improves his self-esteem.
Consult physical/occupational therapist.	May be required to assist with development of therapy plan and to identify methods for patient to compensate for neurologic deficits.

NIC: *Self-Care Assistance: Dressing/Grooming*

Discharge or Maintenance Evaluation

■ Patient will be able to perform self-care activities by himself or with the assistance of a caregiver.

■ Patient will be able to understand and identify methods to facilitate meeting self-care needs.

■ Patient will be able to access community resources to meet continuing needs.

FEEDING SELF-CARE DEFICIT

Related to: weakness, decreased muscle strength, muscle incoordination, paralysis, paresthesias, pain, functional impairment, inability to feed oneself

Defining Characteristics: inability to swallow food, inability to prepare food, inability to chew food, inability to use utensils or assistive devices, inability to pick up food or glass, inability to take in sufficient food for nutritional balance

Outcome Criteria

✔ Patient will be able to consume adequate amounts of food to maintain weight.

✔ Patient will be able to use assistive devices/utensils for feeding.

✔ Patient and family will be able to adequately complete feeding program on a daily basis.

NOC: *Self-Care: Feeding*

INTERVENTIONS	RATIONALES
Evaluate level of neurologic impairment and patient's abilities to perform eating tasks.	Provides baseline from which to plan care for patient needs.
Assist patient with feeding or self-feeding tasks as needed. Encourage patient to perform tasks he may be capable of doing.	Assistance may reduce levels of frustration at first. As patient improves, self-feeding attempts and success will promote self-esteem and fosters independence.
Utilize self-help utensils and devices and instruct patient in their use.	Allows patient to perform tasks and improves self-esteem.
Ascertain which foods are best handled by the patient—liquids, soft foods, finger foods, and so forth.	Easily handled foods allow patient to feed self more easily and fosters independence.
Place patient in high Fowler's position for meals and have patient remain upright for at least 30 minutes after meal.	Helps to reduce swallowing difficulty, aids with digestion, and helps to prevent aspiration.
Auscultate breath sounds at least every 4 hours and prn. Notify physician of adventitious breath sounds or significant changes.	Changes in breath sounds, such as crackles, rhonchi, or wheezing may indicate patient has aspirated food or fluid into lungs.
Weigh patient daily and notify physician of weight loss >2 lbs/day.	Helps to ensure that diet is adequate and patient is receiving appropriate nutrition to maintain weight and hydration.
Suction and emergency equipment should be easily available at bedside.	Patient may require suctioning of foods or fluids if aspiration is imminent.
Allow sufficient time for patient to eat. Cut food into small pieces and feed patient slowly, making sure each bite is swallowed.	Cutting food into small pieces helps reduce the potential for choking or aspiration and assists with chewing, swallowing and digestion. Hurrying patient to

(continues)

(continued)

INTERVENTIONS	RATIONALES
	finish meal causes undue stress and reduces digestion caused by increased intestinal spasms.
Instruct patient/family in feeding techniques and use of adaptive equipment.	Promotes knowledge, involves family in patient's care, and encourages compliance.
Instruct patient/family in community resources, support groups, home health care, and so forth.	Patient may require these resources postdischarge to reinforce planned activities and to assist patient in meeting needs.

NIC: *Self-Care Assistance: Feeding*

Discharge or Maintenance Evaluation

■ Patient will be able to meet self-care needs with use of adaptive equipment or staff members.

■ Patient will be able to maintain weight and adequate nutrition.

■ Patient will be able to receive help from family members for feeding assistance.

■ Patient/family will be able to contact available community resources as needed

TOILETING SELF-CARE DEFICIT

Related to: weakness, decreased muscle strength, muscle incoordination, paralysis, paresthesias, pain, functional impairment, inability to complete own toileting activity

Defining Characteristics: inability to carry out toilet hygiene, inability to flush toilet, inability to sit on or rise from toilet, inability to manipulate clothing for toileting, inability to get to toilet, impaired transfer ability, impaired mobility, pain

Outcome Criteria

✔ Patient will be able to have toileting needs met.

✔ Patient will be able to maintain continence.

✔ Patient/family will be able to perform toileting program.

NOC: *Self-Care: Toileting*

INTERVENTIONS	RATIONALES
Evaluate level of neurologic impairment and patient's ability to perform toileting skills.	Provides baseline from which to plan care for patient needs.
Establish a bowel regime, using stool softeners, suppositories, and so forth.	Medications may be helpful when establishing a bowel regime and to regulate function. Retraining allows the patient to gain independence and fosters self-esteem.
Measure I&O q 2–4 hr. Notify physician of significant imbalances.	Provides information regarding hydration status, and can identify potential fluid imbalances.
Use assistive devices for toileting, such as external catheters, offering bedpan or urinal frequently during the day, and so forth. Assist with toileting as needed, but allow patient independence as warranted.	Assistance helps to maintain patient's self-esteem. Allowing patient to perform autonomously as much as possibe helps promote independence.
Plan and perform urinary and bowel care programs as needed.	Provides for elimination and assists to identify potential problems with patient's status and to correct them.
Instruct patient/family in toileting routines. Provide written instructions as needed. Have family demonstrate routines.	Provides knowledge, provides reminders for postdischarge care to refer back to, and return demonstrations help to identify potential areas of problems or incorrect understanding.
Obtain and use community resources, support groups, home health care, etc., as needed.	Further resources may be required for post discharge care.

NIC: *Self-Care: Toileting*

Discharge or Maintenance Evaluation

■ Patient will be able to have his self-care needs met by staff members or family.

■ Patient will maintain continence.

■ Patient and family will be able to demonstrate correct use of assistive devices and toileting program.

DISTURBED THOUGHT PROCESSES

Related to: confusion, short-term memory loss, inability to process thoughts accurately

Defining Characteristics: inappropriate thinking, disorientation, memory deficit, easy distractibility, egocentricity, decreased problem solving ability, noncompliance with instructions, inability to complete tasks, poor judgment, short attention span, inaccurate interpretation of environment

Outcome Criteria

✔ Patient will be oriented in all spheres.

✔ Patient will be able to respond coherently and appropriately.

NOC: *Cognitive Orientation*

INTERVENTIONS	RATIONALES
Assess orientation and reorient to person, place, time, and surroundings frequently. Provide calendar, clock, TV, and so forth.	Helps to maintain orientation and awareness of self and surroundings.
Provide simple instructions and reinforce prn.	Provides opportunity for patient to succeed and to increase self-esteem.
Place patient near nurse's station. Use restraints and side rails as needed/ordered	Protects patient from injury. Patient may be unable to understand and consider his own safety needs and may have a distorted sense of risks.

INTERVENTIONS	RATIONALES
Provide structured environment with daily routines.	Provides continuity of care.
Provide frequent rest periods and decrease sensory stimuli.	Fatigue and sensory overload increases confusion.
Instruct family to assist with reorientation as needed.	Involves family in care. Patient may be more trusting of family members.
Assist family members to develop coping skills to deal with patient.	Family will need these skills to deal with the patient's new neurologic impairment and potential for deterioration in condition.
Instruct family in community resources, including support groups, therapy, home health, and so forth.	Patient may require continuing care postdischarge and may require support services available through community agencies.

NIC: *Reality Orientation*

Discharge or Maintenance Evaluation

■ Patient will be oriented to person, place, and time.

■ Patient will have no evidence of injury or risk of injury.

■ Patient and family demonstrate appropriate interventions and care.

■ Family can demonstrate appropriate reorientation skills and are able to utilize community resources.

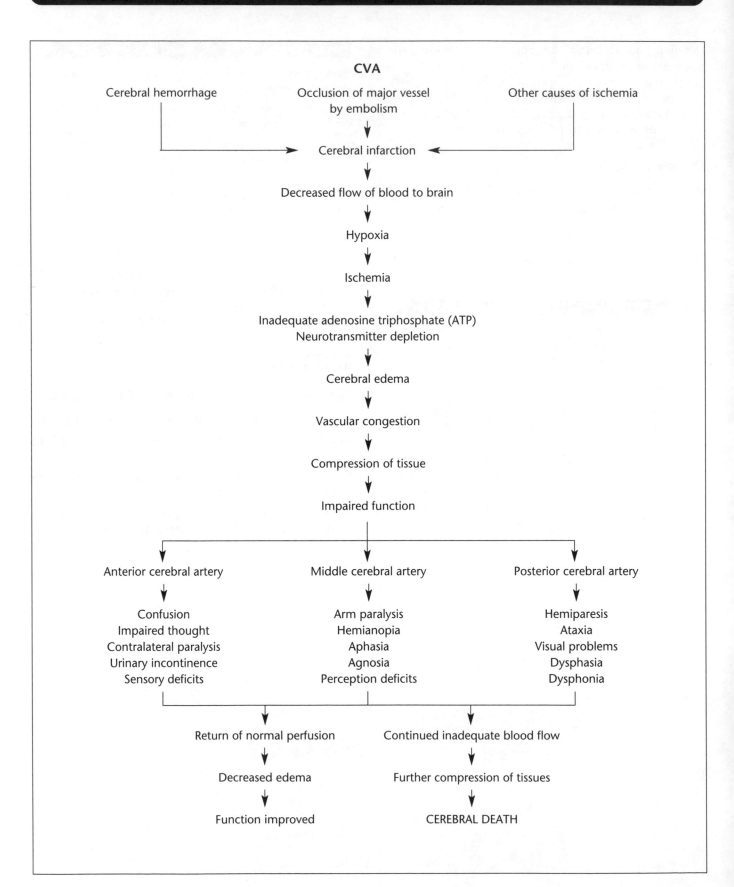

CHAPTER 3.2

HEAD INJURIES

Head injuries, both open and closed, are usually the result of some type of trauma, and include skull fractures, concussions, lacerations, contusions, and cerebral hemorrhages. The injury can be the result of a direct blow to the head, or may involve acceleration/deceleration injuries. Acceleration, or coup, injuries occur when the brain is forced against the cranium. Deceleration, or contrecoup, injuries occur after the initial impact when the brain is rotated or thrown in the opposite direction of the force.

Closed head injuries (CHI) result when a blunt trauma to the head causes a neurologic deficit or loss of consciousness from bruising, hemorrhage, or laceration of brain tissues. This type of injury may be further categorized into mild concussion, classic concussion, diffuse injury with loss of consciousness greater than 24 hours, and diffuse shearing and disruption of brain structures.

A mild concussion occurs when forces on the brain stretch nerve fibers and result in impaired conduction of nerve responses. Neurologic dysfunction is temporary with no residual effects. In a classic concussion, the loss of consciousness is usually less than 24 hours in length and the patient experiences disorientation and a degree of retrograde amnesia when consciousness is regained. Some patients may experience residual personality changes or impairment in memory recall. Patients may exhibit a focal deficit caused by an injury that occurs to a specific area.

With diffuse closed head injuries, the loss of consciousness is greater than 24 hours and the coma may last up to weeks. The patient can exhibit restlessness, withdrawal from painful or noxious stimuli, or purposeful movement. Disorientation and amnesia occur with the return of consciousness, and personality changes are permanent because of the widespread cerebrum disruption.

When injury to the axons and neurons in the hemispheres, brain stem, and diencephalon occur and result in diffuse shearing of white matter with concurrent cerebral edema, dysfunction results in coma. More than half of these patients die, and those who do survive, have severe residual dysfunction. Contusions of the brain stem result in coma, as well as cranial nerve dysfunction and cardiopulmonary instability.

Skull fractures are normally classified as linear, basilar, or depressed. If a linear skull fracture does not puncture the dura mater, the fracture will heal without treatment. If the dura is torn, there is an increased chance that the middle meningeal artery is also punctured, and this will cause an epidural hematoma.

A basilar skull fracture can occur in the anterior or posterior fossa, and classic symptoms include cerebrospinal fluid leakage from the nose or ears, or ecchymoses over the mastoid projection or around the eyes. With basilar fractures, there exists a high risk for cranial nerve injury and dysfunction, infection, and residual neurologic impairment.

Depressed skull fractures that are not depressed more than the thickness of the skull are usually not treated. A depression 5 millimeters or more in depth will require surgery in order to relieve the compression on structures. If the dura mater is punctured, the possibility of bone fragments entering the brain tissue is increased, as is the potential for infection.

Lacerations of the scalp may occur with head injury or skull fractures, and will potentiate the danger of infection.

Intracranial hematomas result after trauma to the head, and frequently occur in conjunction with scalp lacerations, skull fractures, contusions, or penetrating wounds to the head. Subdural hematomas (SDH) usually are caused by venous bleeding, most often from the superior sagittal sinus, and involves the area between the dura mater and the arachnoid space. It may be acute, happening within 24–48 hours of injury, subacute, within 3–20 days of injury, or chronic, greater than 20 days from injury, depending on the time elapsed from injury to the onset of symptoms. SDH may occur spontaneously if the patient has a blood dyscrasia or clotting problem.

Epidural hematomas (EDH) are usually caused by arterial bleeding, generally from the middle meningeal artery, and involve the area above the outer dura mater and below the skull. These occur frequently when skull fractures cross the middle meningeal artery, or transverse or superior sagittal sinus, and the bleeding causes the dura to be pulled away from the skull. A posterior fossa EDH is usually caused by a venous bleed and may result in delayed symptoms because of the slow oozing. With EDH, the patient may have a brief episode of unconsciousness, followed by a varying length of lucid behavior prior to neurologic deterioration and increased intracranial pressure.

Intracerebral hemorrhage into the brain may occur hours or days after a closed head injury, and many result after rupture of an aneurysm, AV malformation, tumor, or vessel that has been weakened from hypertension. If the hemorrhage occurs in the internal capsule of the brain, paralysis will ensue. Symptoms vary depending on site, size, cerebral edema, and blood accumulation rate.

Head injuries can result in varying severity from absence of neurologic dysfunction to death, and each injury must be considered potentially critical. The severity of the head injury is based on the level of consciousness determined by the Glasgow Coma Scale (GCS). A mild head injury will have a 13–15 GCS, moderate head injury, 9–12 GCS, and a severe head injury, 3–8 GCS. These patients in the latter group are comatose with no eye opening, no verbal response, and inability to follow commands. Cervical spine injury evaluation may be required depending on the mechanisms of the closed head injury.

MEDICAL CARE

CT scans: used to identify cerebral edema, lesions, hemorrhage, ventricle size, tissue shifts, infarctions, or basilar skull fracture; brain swelling and edema may not be apparent until after 24 hours after injury

X-rays: skull X-rays may be used to identify fractures or midline shifts, or presence of bone fragments, and to evaluate healing or resolution; cervical spine X-rays are always done with patients who have moderate to severe head injuries to exclude fractures or dislocations of spine; if patient is involved in trauma, such as a MVA or fall, thoracic and lumbar spine X-rays are done to rule out problems

Transcranial Doppler: used to identify vasospasm and flow velocity

MRI: used to reveal disruption of axonal pathways and white matter shearing

Angiography: cerebral angiograms may be used to identify circulatory anomalies, shifting of structures, hemorrhage, or edema

Lumbar puncture: may be contraindicated in suspected or known intracranial hypertension

Laboratory: electrolyte imbalances may increase ICP or alter mental status; CBC to evaluate blood loss and hydration status; drug toxicology studies to identify drugs that may be responsible for consciousness level changes; anticonvulsant drug levels to monitor therapeutic maintenance levels

Arterial blood gases: used to evaluate hypoxemia and acid–base imbalances that can increase ICP; intracranial hematomas may result in respiratory alkalosis, or metabolic acidosis if patient is also in shock

Diuretics: furosemide (Lasix, Furosemide, Luramide), bumetanide (Bumex), chlorothiazide (Diuril), hydrochlorothiazide (Esidrex, Hydrochlorthiazide, HydroDiuril, Thiuretic), chlorthalidone (Chlorthalidone, Hygroton, Hylidone, Thalitone), indapamide (Lozol), metolazone (Diulo, Zaroxolyn), ethacrynic acid (Edecrin), torsemide (Demadex), acetazolamide (Acetazolamide, Diamox), methazolamide (Neptazane), amiloride (Amiloride, Midamor), spironolactone (Aldactone), triamterene (Dyrenium), mannitol (Mannitol, Osmitrol), and urea (Ureaphil) may be used to draw water from the brain cells in order to decrease cerebral edema and ICP

Corticosteroids: dexamethasone (Decadron, Cortastat), hydrocortisone (Cortef, Solu-Cortef, Cortenema), or methylprednisolone (Medrol, Depo-Medrol, Solu-Medrol) among others are used to decrease the inflammatory response and edema; most act by suppression of the immune response by stabilization of the leukocytic lysosomal membranes

Anticonvulsants: drugs such as carbamazepine (Atretol, Carbatrol, Tegretol), clonazepam (Klonopin), ethosuximide (Zarontin), fosphenytoin sodium (Cerebryx), gabapentin (Neurontin), lamotrigine (Lamictal), levetiracetam (Keppra), oxcarbazepine (Trileptal), Phenobarbital (Barbita, Solfoton, Luminal), phenytoin (Dilantin, Phenytex), primadone (Mysoline), tiagabine hydrochloride (Gabitril), topiramate (Topamax), valproic acid or valproate (Depacon, Depakene, Depakote), or zonisamide (Zonegran) used in the treatment and prophylaxis of seizure activity; method of action dependent on drug utilized—some increase cerebral levels of GABA, some help to stabilize neuronal membranes and synchronization, and some act upon sodium, potassium, or calcium ion concentrations within the neuronal cells

COMMON NURSING DIAGNOSES

IMBALANCED NUTRITION: LESS THAN BODY REQUIREMENTS (see MECHANICAL VENTILATION)

Related to: inability to take in sufficient nutrients, inability to chew or swallow, decreased level of consciousness, intubation, increased metabolism

Defining Characteristics: weight loss, muscle wasting, catabolism

IMPAIRED GAS EXCHANGE (see MECHANICAL VENTILATION)

Related to: altered oxygen-carrying capability, altered oxygen supply

Defining Characteristics: dyspnea, nasal flaring, tachycardia, pale, dusky skin, confusion, diaphoresis, hypoxia, hypoxemia, irritability, restlessness, abnormal arterial blood gases

ADDITIONAL NURSING DIAGNOSES

INEFFECTIVE TISSUE PERFUSION: CEREBRAL

Related to: hemorrhage, hematoma, lesions, cerebral edema, metabolic changes, hypoxia, hypovolemia, cardiac dysrhythmias, increased ICP

Defining Characteristics: disorientation, confusion, changes in mental status, combativeness, inability to focus on topic, amnesia, memory loss, restlessness, inability to follow commands, increased intracranial pressure above 20 mm Hg consistently, decrease in cerebral perfusion pressure below 70 mm Hg, vital sign changes, impaired motor function, impaired sensory function

Outcome Criteria

✔ Patient will achieve and maintain consciousness, and will have normal cognition and motor function.

NOC: *Neurologic Status: Consciousness*

INTERVENTIONS	RATIONALES
Assess patient for cause of impairment, problem with perfusion, and potential for increased ICP.	Establishes plan of care and identifies appropriate choices for intervention. Depending on patient's condition/problem, surgical intervention may be required.
Evaluate neurologic status every hour initially, then every 1–2 hours, and notify physician for pertinent changes. Assess GCS.	Establishes a baseline from which to gauge changes or trends. Alterations in level of consciousness and behavior, as well as other symptoms may be helpful to determine area of damage.
Assess patient's arousal or lack of arousal to verbal and noxious stimuli.	Establishes level of consciousness which is the single most important measure of the patient's status. Extensive damage involving the cerebral cortex may result in delayed responses to commands, drowsiness and inability to stay awake unless stimulated, or disorientation. Lack of response to stimuli may indicate that damage has occurred to the midbrain, pons, and/or medulla. If a minimal amount of damage has occurred in the cerebral cortex, the patient may be uncooperative or drowsy.
Assess patient's best verbal response to questions and whether words/sentences are appropriate.	Identifies speech ability and orientation levels.
Assess ability to follow simple commands, noting purposeful and nonpurposeful movements bilaterally.	Identifies ability to respond to stimuli when patient is unable to open eyes or cannot speak. Purposeful movement, such as holding up two fingers or squeezing and releasing hands when instructed to do so, can help identify awareness and the ability to respond appropriately. Abnormal posturing may indicate diffuse cortical damage, and the

(continues)

(continued)

INTERVENTIONS	RATIONALES	INTERVENTIONS	RATIONALES
	absence of any movement to one side of the body usually indicates damage has been done to the motor tracts of the opposite side of the cerebral hemisphere.	Obtain CSF sample as ordered and as per hospital protocol.	May be required for diagnostic testing or to relieve pressure.
Observe pupils bilaterally, noting equality, size, and reaction to light. Notify physician of significant changes.	Compression of the brain stem and impairment of the second and third cranial nerves will alter pupillary response.	Monitor vital signs; observe for widening pulse pressure, blood pressure changes, bradycardia, tachycardia, apnea, Cheyne–Stokes respiration, or fever.	Autoregulation may be impaired after cerebral vascular injury. Temperature elevation may increase cerebral blood flow and volume, which can increase ICP. Widening pulse pressure may indicate increasing intracranial pressure, especially when consciousness level is deteriorating concurrently. Hypotension from hypovolemia may occur when patient has associated multiple trauma. Cardiac dysrhythmias may result from brain stem pressure or injury, or may be seen in cardiac disease. Increasing ICP or compression of brain structures may result in loss of spontaneous respiration and may require mechanical ventilation. Damage to the hypothalamus may result in hyperthermia which can result in increased ICP.
Observe position of eyes, noting any deviation laterally or vertically. Observe for presence of doll's eyes reflex.	Loss of doll's eyes, or the oculocephalic reflex, indicates impairment in the function of the brain stem. Positions and movement of the eyes may indicate which area of the brain has been involved. Problems with abduction of the eyes may be an early indication of increased intracranial pressure.		
Observe for presence of blink reflex.	Loss of blinking reflex may indicate injury to the pons and medulla.		
Monitor intracranial pressure at least hourly, or use continuous monitoring per hospital policy.	Provides immediate information about changes in pressure of the cerebrospinal fluid and blood to facilitate detection of life-threatening increases that can lead to brain deterioration. ICP fluctuates continuously and maintained increases longer than 10–15 minutes should be reported. Normal ventricular pressure is less than 10 mm Hg, and readings of 20 mm Hg and above are considered dangerously elevated. Pressures can be elevated with any Valsalva-type maneuvers, such as suctioning, turning, or coughing.	Monitor ECG for rhythm and rate changes and treat per hospital protocol.	Bradycardia is frequently seen with brain stem injury. Dysrhythmias may become life-threatening and require emergent intervention.
		Assess for presence of cough and gag reflexes.	Injuries to the medulla will result in impairment of these reflexes and may cause further complications.
		Observe for restlessness, moaning, or nonverbal changes in behavior.	May indicate presence of discomfort or pain and this may increase ICP.
Monitor ICP waves.	Plateau, or A waves, have rapid increases and decreases of pressure ranging from 15–50 mm Hg, last from 2–15 minutes, and are usually noted in cerebral dysfunction caused by shifting of the brain. B waves last from 30 seconds to 2 minutes, and are usually less significant unless they occur in runs, which may precede changes to A waves. C waves are small and normally occur at the rate of 6/minute, and relate to variances in arterial blood pressure.	Observe for presence of seizure activity and provide appropriate safety precautions. Administer anticonvulsants as ordered.	Cerebral injury and irritation, hypoxemia, hypoxia, and increased ICP may result in seizures. Seizure activity increases metabolic demands which can also increase ICP.
		Observe for nuchal rigidity.	May be present when meninges are irritated, if dura mater has been punctured or if infection develops.
		Elevate head of bed 15–30 degrees as indicated.	Reduces intracranial pressure and cerebral congestion and edema.
		Support head and neck in a neutral midline position utilizing pillows, sand bags, or towels.	Movement of the head to either side can compress jugular veins inhibiting venous drainage and can result in increased ICP.

INTERVENTIONS	RATIONALES
Limit suctioning to only when needed.	Suctioning procedures can increase intrathoracic, intra-abdominal, and intracranial pressures.
Administer oxygen as warranted.	Reduces hypoxemia which may result in increased ICP.
If patient requires mechanical ventilation, monitor hyperventilatory status.	Hyperventilation results in respiratory alkalosis, which results in cerebral vasoconstriction and decreases in ICP.
Administer sedation and neuromuscular paralyzing agents as ordered and warranted.	Paralyzing drugs may be ordered to prevent sudden rises in ICP caused by coughing, suctioning, or other muscular activities, but should *never* be given without sedation of patient.
Monitor pulse oximetry and notify physician if levels remain below 90%.	Indicates respiratory insufficiency and impending/present hypoxia.
Monitor ABGs as warranted.	Identifies acid–base imbalances and presence of hypoxemia. Elevations in $PaCO_2$ will cause vasodilation in the cerebral vasculature with a resultant increase in ICP.
Monitor intake and output hourly. Notify physician if urine output <30 cc/hr or >200 cc/hr.	Reflects amounts of total body water which influences tissue perfusion. Cerebral injury may result in inappropriate ADH or diabetes insipidus, and may lead to hypovolemia.
Provide calm, quiet environment without extraneous stimuli, and provide rest periods between care activities. Use restraints only when absolutely necessary.	Helps to reduce ICP. Use of restraints may be required to ensure the patient's safety, but may cause irritation and fighting against the restraints which can increase ICP.
Administer osmotic diuretics as ordered.	Drugs remove water from areas in the brain that maintain an intact blood–brain barrier, and helps to reduce ICP. Mannitol is usually the drug of choice and is given as a bolus to decrease elevated ICP by also decreasing the viscosity of the blood, thereby assisting with improvement in the microcirculation.
Administer IV fluids and/or blood products as ordered.	Crystalloid solutions and colloids may be required to maintain cerebral perfusion pressure above 70 mm Hg.

INTERVENTIONS	RATIONALES
Administer barbiturates as ordered.	Barbiturates may be required as a last effort to lower increased ICP by suppressing metabolism, inhibiting free radical-mediated peroxidation, and changes in the vascular tone. Usually barbiturates are not utilized until ICP is above 30 mm Hg for at least 30–45 minutes with CPP less than 70 mm Hg. The patient should be adequately hydrated prior to instigating barbiturate therapy.
Instruct patient to avoid coughing, straining, or any Valsalva-like maneuvers.	Activities increase ICP by increasing intrathoracic and intra-abdominal pressures.
Prepare patient/family for placement on mechanical ventilation as warranted.	Injury to certain areas of the brain may result in insufficient respiratory status and may require intubation and mechanical ventilation to maintain life support.
Prepare patient/family for surgical procedures.	Craniotomy or burr holes may be necessary to remove bone fragments, remove a hematoma, stop hemorrhage, remove necrotic tissue, or elevate a depressed skull fracture.

NIC: *Cerebral Perfusion Promotion*

Discharge or Maintenance Evaluation

- Patient will be alert, oriented in all phases, with no speech or motor impairment.
- Patient will have no sensory impairment.
- Patient will have stable vital signs and no increase in ICP.

INEFFECTIVE BREATHING PATTERN

Related to: respiratory center injury, obstruction, structural shifting, surgical intervention, decreased level of consciousness, metabolic imbalance, inadequate airway

Defining Characteristics: dyspnea, Cheyne-Stokes respirations, bradypnea, apnea, hypoxia, hypoxemia, abnormal arterial blood gases pH <7.35, $PaCO_2$ <30 mm Hg or >45 mm Hg, changes in alveolar minute ventilation, tachypnea, shallow respirations, altered level of responsiveness, nasal flaring, ICP >20 mm Hg

Outcome Criteria

✔ Patient will maintain a patent airway with no evidence of respiratory insufficiency.

✔ Patient will have arterial blood gases within normal limits.

✔ ICP will remain <20 mm Hg.

NOC: *Respiratory Status: Ventilation*

INTERVENTIONS	RATIONALES
Observe respiratory status for rate, depth, rhythm, irregularity, chest expansion and symmetry, and apnea.	Changes from patient's baseline may indicate pulmonary complications or involvement or brain injured areas. Respiratory insufficiency may require mechanical ventilation.
Maintain patency of airway.	Depending on location of injury, patient may not be able to maintain his own airway or ventilation and may require artificial means of doing so.
Auscultate breath sounds for changes and presence of adventitious lung sounds.	May indicate hypoventilation, obstruction, atelectasis, or infection which may impair cerebral oxygenation.
Observe for presence of gag, cough, and swallow reflexes.	Lack of these reflexes may impair the patient's ability to handle his secretions and may require an artificial airway. Nasopharyngeal airways are preferred to avoid stimulation of the gag reflex which can increase ICP.
Administer oxygen as warranted. Monitor oximetry.	Provides supplemental oxygen to reduce hypoxia and prevent desaturation.
Elevate head of bed as warranted.	Promotes chest expansion and ventilation.
Avoid suctioning unless mandatory, and observe for changes in sputum color, consistency, or odor.	Suctioning may cause hypoxia and decreases cerebral perfusion, while increasing ICP. Changes in sputum characteristics may indicate impending or presence of infection.
Instruct patient in deep breathing exercises.	Reduces potential for atelectasis and/or pneumonia.

INTERVENTIONS	RATIONALES
Avoid chest physiotherapy during acute phases.	CPT is contraindicated with patients with increased ICP because this potentiates the increase.
Prepare patient/family for intubation/mechanical ventilation as warranted.	As time and condition permits, instruction may be given. Provides knowledge and decreases fear in patients who are awake.

NIC: *Airway Management*

Discharge or Maintenance Evaluation

■ Patient will maintain his own airway and be able to sustain spontaneous respiration.

■ Patient will be able to handle secretions and dispose of them adequately.

■ Arterial blood gases will be within normal limits for the patient.

■ Patient will be able to recall information accurately and be able to demonstrate appropriate deep breathing.

DISTURBED THOUGHT PROCESSES

Related to: head injury, psychological problems, medications

Defining Characteristics: memory deficit, diminished attention span, inability to focus, disorientation to time, place, person, or situation, poor recall, distractibility, personality changes, inappropriate behavior, inability to problem-solve

Outcome Criteria

✔ Patient will be oriented in all phases and will be able to recall data.

NOC: *Concentration*

INTERVENTIONS	RATIONALES
Evaluate orientation status with regard to time, place, person, circumstance, and recent events.	Provides a baseline on which to begin and plan intervention.
Observe patient for ability to concentrate and attention span.	Ability to concentrate may be diminished because of injury and this further potentiates anxiety for the patient.

INTERVENTIONS	RATIONALES
Assist family members to understand patient's aberrant behavior, personality changes, and other responses.	Head injury recovery includes agitation and hostility, anger, and disorganized thought sequences. Family members may have difficulty dealing with the patient's changed personality and behavior.
Encourage family to discuss news and family occurrences with patient.	Helps to maintain contact with normal events and assists with orientation.
Explain all procedures with clear concise explanations.	Patient may have lost the ability to reason or conceptualize, and may require repeated reinforcement. Retention of information may be decreased and result in further anxiety.
Reduce competing stimuli when conversing with the patient.	Brain injured patients may be overly excitable and become violent with excess stimulation.
Be consistent with staff assignments as much as possible.	Provides continuity of care and allows patient some control in situation.
Remain with patient during episodes of fright or agitation.	Offers support and helps to calm patient to reduce anxiety to prevent loss of control and panic.
Assist patient/family to set realistic goals and instruct in ways to control behavior.	Helps to maintain a sense of hope for improvement and to facilitate rehabilitation.
Consult rehabilitation counselor for assistance with cognitive training as warranted.	Assists patient with methods to compensate for problems with concentration, memory, judgment, and problem-solving.
Make appropriate referrals to support groups or counseling as warranted.	Additional help may be needed to help with recovery.

NIC: *Cognitive Restructuring*

Discharge or Maintenance Evaluation

- Patient will regain normal mental skills and be oriented in all phases.
- Patient will be able to recognize aberrant behavior and control negative reactions.
- Patient will participate in rehabilitation/counseling for retraining.

RISK FOR INFECTION

Related to: trauma, lacerations, broken skin, open wounds, invasive procedures, surgery, use of steroids, cerebrospinal fluid leakage, nutritional deficiency, invasive lines

Defining Characteristics: fever, tachycardia, elevated white blood cell count, shift to the left on differential, redness to wounds, purulent drainage or sputum, nuchal rigidity, bloody or purulent CSF

Outcome Criteria

✔ Patient will be free of signs/symptoms of wound or intracranial infection.

NOC: *Risk Control*

INTERVENTIONS	RATIONALES
Monitor temperature every 2–4 hours.	Elevation may indicate development of infection.
Observe wounds, incision lines, invasive line sites, or other skin breaks for drainage, redness, or edema.	Prompt identification of developing problems may result in prompt intervention to prevent systemic sepsis.
Observe for CSF leakage from ears and nose, and report to physician.	Indicates a serious complication from head injury and may result in meningitis.
Observe for raccoon's eyes or Battle's sign, and clear or serous drainage from nose or ears. Assess for patient's complaints of sweet or salty taste in mouth.	CSF leakage may occur because of a fracture of the frontal or middle basilar fossae. Battle's sign, or ecchymoses over the mastoid bone, indicates middle fossa basilar skull fracture. Raccoon's eyes, with periorbital edema and ecchymosis, is caused by anterior fossa basilar skull fractures. CSF leakage may produce a sweet or salty taste.
If CSF leak is observed, notify physician. Allow fluid to flow freely. A dry sterile dressing can be placed loosely to absorb drainage. Monitor amount of dressing changes.	Gives indications of amount of CSF drainage.
Use aseptic or sterile technique when changing dressings or providing wound care.	Prevents spread of infection.
Utilize good handwashing practices.	Prevents nosocomial infections.

(continues)

(continued)

INTERVENTIONS	RATIONALES
Monitor urine output for adequacy of amount, color, clarity, and presence of foul odor.	May identify presence of bacterial infection.
Obtain cultures of wound, urine, blood, stool, sputum, or other body fluids/surfaces as warranted, and as per hospital protocol.	Identifies the presence of infection and the causative agent, as well as identification of appropriate antimicrobial agent to treat infection.
Administer antimicrobials as ordered.	May be given prophylactically when trauma, surgery or CSF leakage occurs. Appropriate antimicrobials may be ordered after results of culture and sensitivity are received.
Instruct patient on isolation procedures as warranted. Instruct visitors on avoiding patient if they have upper respiratory or other type of infection.	Isolation may be required based on type of organism grown. Restriction of ill visitors may reduce exposure of an already susceptible patient.
Instruct patient on deep breathing and pulmonary exercises as warranted.	Promotes lung expansion and reduces potential for atelectasis and pneumonia. Postural drainage is contraindicated if patient has increased ICP.

NIC: *Infection Protection*

Discharge or Maintenance Evaluation

- Patient will be normothermic with normal white blood cell count.
- Patient will exhibit no signs/symptoms of infection.
- Wounds will heal without complications.

IMPAIRED PHYSICAL MOBILITY

Related to: trauma, immobilization, mental impairment, decreased strength, paralysis, weakness

Defining Characteristics: inability to move at will, inability to transfer or ambulate, decreased range of motion, decreased muscle strength, muscle incoordination, footdrop, contractures, decreased reflexes

Outcome Criteria

✔ Patient will achieve and maintain an optimal level of motor function.

NOC: *Mobility Level*

INTERVENTIONS	RATIONALES
Evaluate patient's ability and function and injury.	Identifies impairments and allows for identification of appropriate interventions.
Assess patient for degree of immobility.	Provides a baseline on which to base interventions. Patient may only require minimal assistance or be completely dependent on caregivers for all body needs.
Observe skin for redness, warmth, or tenderness.	May indicate pressure is being concentrated in one area and may predispose patient to decubitus formation.
Provide kinetic bed or alternating pressure mattress for patient.	Helps promote circulation and reduces venous stasis and tissue pressure to prevent formation of pressure sores.
Maintain good body alignment and use pillows/rolls to support body. Use high-top tennis shoes and remove/reapply every 4–8 hours.	Prevents further complications and contractures. Use of tennis shoes helps prevent footdrop.
Perform range of motion exercises every 4 hours.	Helps to maintain mobility and function of joints.
Provide skin care every 8 hours and prn. Change wet clothing and linens prn.	Helps to promote circulation and reduces potential for skin breakdown.
Instill artificial tears or lubrication ointment to eyes every 4 hours and prn as ordered.	Prevents eye tissues from drying out. If patient is unable to maintain closed eyes, eye patches or tape may be required.
Instruct patient/family in range of motion exercises and mobility aids.	Helps patient to regain some control and allows family some involvement in reconditioning program.
Instruct patient/family in reasons for impairment and realistic goals for changes in patient's lifestyle as warranted.	Promotes understanding and compliance with treatment regimen.
Consult physical and/or occupational therapy, as warranted.	Assists patient with identifying methods to compensate for impairments and provides for post-discharge care.

NIC: *Exercise Therapy: Muscle Control*

Discharge or Maintenance Evaluation

- Patient will be able to maintain skin integrity with no complications.

- Patient will be able to increase muscle strength and tone and achieve a functional level of muscle function.
- Patient will be able to demonstrate exercise program.
- Patient and family will become involved in recovery programs.

RISK FOR INJURY

Related to: cranial defect, skull fracture, open head wound, cranial nerve damage from depressed fracture, seizure activity

Defining Characteristics: unprotected brain, loose bone chips, neurologic deficits, seizures, unilateral loss of sensation, unilateral loss of movement on face, decreased hearing, decreased gag or swallow reflex, loss of consciousness

Outcome Criteria

✔ Patient will develop no further injury from the initial head injury and cranial defect.

✔ Patient will experience no injuries related to seizures.

NOC: *Risk Control*

INTERVENTIONS	RATIONALES
Position head away from cranial defect.	Protects brain from further depression and injury.
Assess cranial nerve (CN) function and notify physician of abnormalities.	Loss of sensation to one side of face indicates damage to CN V. Loss of movement on one side of face or facial palsy indicates damage from a CN VII injury. Loss or decreased hearing results from a CN VIII injury. Decreased swallow and gag reflexes result from CN IX and X injuries. Tongue injuries may occur with CN V or VII deficits.
Close eye, place 2 x 2 gauze over eye, then tape over gauze to keep eye closed. Instill eye drops or ointment frequently.	Helps protect eye from corneal abrasions and drying out corneal tissues.
Assess patient's ability to handle his secretions by using gelatin instead of liquids.	Swallowing reflexes may be diminished with CN injury that occurs from posterior fossa fractures or hematomas. Patient

INTERVENTIONS	RATIONALES
	may have less difficulty swallowing thickened fluids, such as gelatin, than with thinner liquids, such as water. If coughing and choking occur, patient should not be fed orally because of risk of aspiration.
Observe patient for seizure activity, noting type, duration, and post-ictal phase.	Seizures may occur as a direct result from brain injury or with anoxia or increased ICP. Grand mal seizures (tonic–clonic) involve the whole body and last from 1–5 minutes. Myoclonic seizures usually involve the arms and are of brief nature. Partial seizures are confined to specific body areas and may progress to generalized seizures, and are usually associated with an aura or sensory symptom. Seizures increase ICP and increase metabolic needs of the brain.
Pad side rails.	Protects patient from injury during seizure activity.
Administer anticonvulsants as ordered.	These drugs stop the seizure activity, but can result in dysrhythmias.
Observe for rashes, nystagmus, ataxia, or dysmetria.	May indicate toxic levels of anticonvulsants.
Monitor lab work for therapeutic levels of anticonvulsants.	Subtherapeutic or toxic levels of anticonvulsant drugs create more potential for injury. Therapeutic levels of drugs should be maintained to achieve optimum benefit from the specific drug being utilized.
Instruct patient/family about medications.	Promote knowledge and compliance.
Instruct patient/family to notify nurse if aura or sensory signs, such as numbness and tingling, occur.	May indicate impending seizure activity.
Instruct patient to chew on unaffected side of mouth. Consult speech/occupational therapy for swallowing dysfunction.	Assists with a multidisciplinary approach to improve patient function.
Instruct family in speaking to patient on patient's unaffected side if hearing is impaired.	Patients with CN VIII injury cannot hear if a person is speaking to them on the side that is affected by the injury.

Discharge or Maintenance Evaluation

- Patient will exhibit no evidence of brain injury.
- Patient will have no toxic effects from anti-convulsants.
- Patient will have adequate control of seizures.
- Patient will have no signs of injury.

RISK FOR DEFICIENT FLUID VOLUME

Related to: blood loss from scalp laceration, decreased intake, diabetes insipidus, cerebral salt wasting syndrome

Defining Characteristics: oliguria, weight loss, altered electrolytes, serum osmolality >31 mOsm/L, increased urine specific gravity, decreased blood pressure, rapid, thready pulse, increased temperature, decreased central venous pressure, decreased pulmonary capillary wedge pressures, decreased level of consciousness, urine output >200 cc/hr with specific gravity <1.005

Outcome Criteria

- ✔ Patient will have stable vital signs and neurological status.
- ✔ Patient will have urinary output within range of 30–100 cc/hr.

NOC: *Fluid Balance*

INTERVENTIONS	RATIONALES
Monitor VS q 1 hour and prn.	Increased heart rate and decreased blood pressure may indicate hemorrhage and presence of shock. Close monitoring of vital signs promotes identification of changes in status to allow for interventional care.
Monitor neurological signs q 1 hour initially, then q 1–2 hours. Notify physician of significant changes.	Changes in neurologic status may indicate increasing ICP and potential life-threatening complications.

INTERVENTIONS	RATIONALES
Measure I&O q 1 hour. Notify physician if <30 cc/hr or >200 cc/hr.	Urinary output gives indication of fluid balance; low urinary output may indicate hypovolemia.
Monitor specific gravity of urine q 2–4 hours as ordered.	Increased specific gravity may indicate hypovolemia.
Administer IV fluids and blood products as ordered.	IV fluids may be required to maintain circulating vascular volume. Blood products may be required in the presence of hemorrhage or coagulopathy.
Monitor cardiac rhythm and hemodynamics. Notify physician of changes from set parameters.	Hypovolemia and electrolyte disturbances can result in cardiac dysrhythmias. Changes in hemodynamics may be the first indicator of changes in fluid status.
Assess patient's skin turgor and mucous membrane hydration at least every shift. Notify physician of significant changes.	Poor skin turgor and dry mucous membranes are signs of dehydration.
Administer pitressin as ordered.	May be used if patient develops diabetes insipidus in order to control the massive dehydration that occurs.
Observe lacerations and/or dressings for drainage. Note increases in amounts of drainage. If copious amounts of drainage are present on dressings, weigh dressings and record with other I&O.	The scalp is very vascular and vessels have poor contractility so wounds can result in significant blood loss, which may result in increased potential for hypovolemic shock. Excessive wound drainage can create significant fluid imbalances (a 1 kg dressing equals about 1 L of fluid drainage.)
Monitor lab work, especially hemoglobin and hematocrit, as well as electrolytes.	Increased hematocrit and hemoglobin indicate dehydration. Significant fluid loss may result in electrolyte imbalances.
Instruct patient/family in reasons for maintaining fluid intake.	Encourages patient and family participation in care, fosters patient's sense of control, and provides knowledge.
Instruct patient/family in keeping daily weights, measurement of intake and output, and of identification of signs of dehydration.	Provides knowledge and encourages family and patient participation in care. Allows for prompt identification of potential dehydration and for timely intervention.

NIC: *Fluid Monitoring*

Discharge or Maintenance Evaluation

- Patient will have vital signs within normal limits.
- Hemodynamic parameters will be within normal limits for patient.
- Patient will have balanced fluid intake and output.
- Lab work will be within normal limits for patient.
- Patient/family will be able to verbalize and demonstrate understanding of instructions regarding I&O, weighing patient, and signs of dehydration for which to be observant.

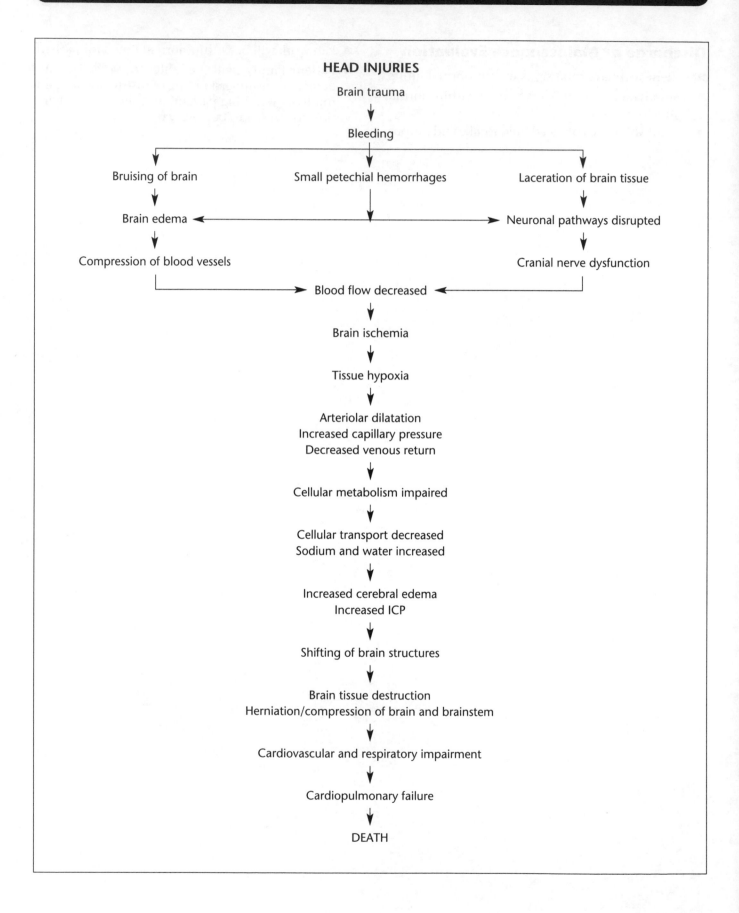

HEAD INJURIES

Brain trauma

↓

Bleeding

Bruising of brain   Small petechial hemorrhages   Laceration of brain tissue

Brain edema ← → Neuronal pathways disrupted

Compression of blood vessels   Cranial nerve dysfunction

→ Blood flow decreased ←

↓

Brain ischemia

↓

Tissue hypoxia

↓

Arteriolar dilatation
Increased capillary pressure
Decreased venous return

↓

Cellular metabolism impaired

↓

Cellular transport decreased
Sodium and water increased

↓

Increased cerebral edema
Increased ICP

↓

Shifting of brain structures

↓

Brain tissue destruction
Herniation/compression of brain and brainstem

↓

Cardiovascular and respiratory impairment

↓

Cardiopulmonary failure

↓

DEATH

HEAD INJURIES

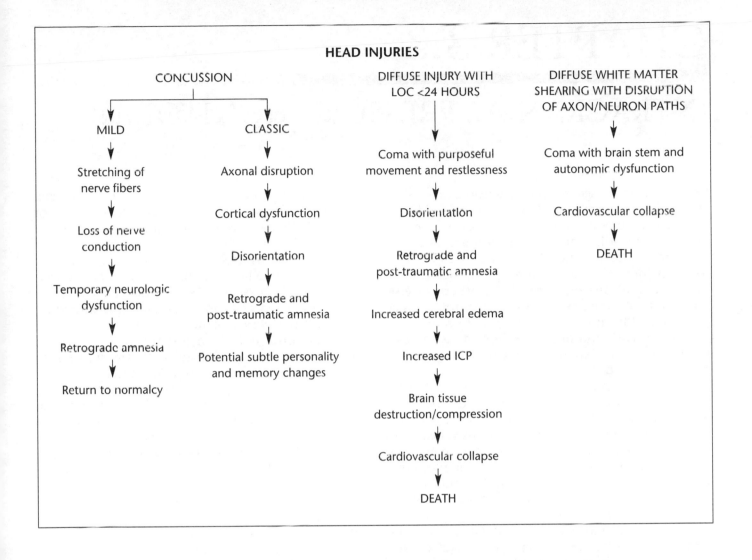

CONCUSSION

MILD

Stretching of
nerve fibers
↓
Loss of nerve
conduction
↓
Temporary neurologic
dysfunction
↓
Retrograde amnesia
↓
Return to normalcy

CLASSIC

Axonal disruption
↓
Cortical dysfunction
↓
Disorientation
↓
Retrograde and
post-traumatic amnesia
↓
Potential subtle personality
and memory changes

DIFFUSE INJURY WITH
LOC <24 HOURS
↓
Coma with purposeful
movement and restlessness
↓
Disorientation
↓
Retrograde and
post-traumatic amnesia
↓
Increased cerebral edema
↓
Increased ICP
↓
Brain tissue
destruction/compression
↓
Cardiovascular collapse
↓
DEATH

DIFFUSE WHITE MATTER
SHEARING WITH DISRUPTION
OF AXON/NEURON PATHS
↓
Coma with brain stem and
autonomic dysfunction
↓
Cardiovascular collapse
↓
DEATH

CHAPTER 3.3

INTRACRANIAL PRESSURE MONITORING

The brain is housed in a nondistensible cavity that is filled to capacity with CSF, interstitial fluid, and intravascular blood, all of which possess very minimal ability for adjustment for increasing intracranial pressure. If the volume of any one of these constituents increases, there is a reciprocal decrease in the volume of one or more of the others, or else intracranial pressure becomes elevated. Intracranial pressure (ICP) is normally between 2–15 mm Hg or 50–200 cm H_2O, and fluctuates depending on positioning, vital signs changes, increased intraabdominal pressure, and stimuli.

There are compensatory mechanisms that assist in decreasing intracranial hypertension. The most easily changed element is intravascular volume that results from compression of the venous system and decreases fluid level. The CSF is another element that can be used to compensate for increasing pressures. CSF can be displaced from the cranial vault to the spinal canal, which increases absorption of CSF by the arachnoid villi, slows production of CSF by the choroid plexus, and decreases ICP. Other compensatory mechanisms may be seen, such as skull expansion in infants whose sutures have not closed, as well as reduction of cerebral blood flow to a small extent, but these are not desirable.

Although autoregulatory mechanisms can control small increases in ICP, rapid or sustained increases suppress these compensatory efforts, and decompensation occurs. As the ICP increases, the cerebral blood flow decreases because of pressure exerted on vessels. This causes brain ischemia and accumulation of lactic acid and carbon dioxide, resulting in hypoxemia and hypercapnia. Cerebral vasodilation ensues that increases blood volume and cerebral edema, which further increases ICP, until a vicious cycle is established. When ischemia increases to a certain level, the medulla causes blood pressure to rise in an effort to compensate for the increasing ICP, but eventually the ICP will equal the MAP and precipitate curtailing of cerebral blood flow, resulting in vascular collapse and brain death.

ICP is increased when brain volume is enlarged by mass lesions, tumors, abscesses, hematomas or cerebral edema. Vasodilation and venous outflow obstructions cause changes in cerebrovascular status caused by hypoventilation, hypercapnia, improper position of the head, or maneuvers that increase intrathoracic pressure. CSF volumes may increase from decreased reabsorption from an obstruction, such as with hydrocephalus.

Monitoring of ICP can be done from several sites. The lumbar or cervical subarachnoid area is simple to access, but potential for herniation exists. The lateral cerebral ventricles (per ventriculostomy) is highly accurate and allows for withdrawal of CSF and measurement of compliance, but infection to this area is catastrophic. Subdural sites are most easily inserted but carry serious infection risks, and an epidural site has less potential for infection, but lacks accuracy.

The three usual types of ICP monitoring are epidural sensor monitoring through a burr hole, subarachnoid screw or bolt monitoring through a twist drill burr hole, and ventricular catheter monitoring. Insertion of these may be performed in surgery or in the intensive care setting, but requires sterile-field maintenance.

It has been discovered that cerebral oxygenation can be measured by the use of a fiberoptic catheter inserted into the dominant internal jugular vein, placed retrograde in the jugular bulb, allowing for sampling of oxygen saturation levels. This measurement, $SjvO_2$, is dependent on blood flow and cerebral metabolism, and is used to correlate the balance between oxygen delivery and oxygen consumption by the brain. A normal measurement ranges between 60 to 90%, with decreases below 50% indicating cerebral ischemia is present. Focal brain ischemia may still be undetectable using this method.

Another method of cerebral oxygenation monitoring that is being considered is brain tissue PO_2 monitoring ($PtiO_2$), in which a microcatheter is inserted into the frontal cerebral white matter of the brain. Generally accepted values for this reading have not been established yet, but no complications were attributed to the PtiO$_2$ catheters during trials, such as intracranial bleeding or infection.

ICP monitoring may be performed on patients with head trauma, ruptured aneurysms, Reye's syndrome, intracranial bleeds, hydrocephalus, or tumors. A ventriculostomy is a cannula placed in the lateral ventricle and connected with a transducer for measurement of pressures of CSF directly, for periodic drainage of CSF, and for withdrawal of fluid for analysis.

Cerebral perfusion pressure (CPP) is the difference between the mean arterial pressure (MAP) and the mean ICP, and indicates the pressure in the cerebral vascular system and approximates the cerebral blood flow. A CPP of 60 mm Hg is the minimum value for perfusion to occur, with normal ranges from 80–100 mm Hg.

Increases in ICP can be manifested by signs such as systolic blood pressure elevations, widening pulse pressure, bradycardia, headache, nausea with projectile vomiting, papilledema, changes in level of consciousness, pupillary changes, respiratory changes, and cerebral posturing.

MEDICAL CARE

Surgery: may be required for traumatic injuries and/or placement of ICP monitoring devices

Arterial blood gases: may be used to identify acid–base imbalances, hypoxemia, and hypercapnia; frequently patients are hyperventilated to keep PaCO$_2$ between 25–28

Osmotics: mannitol used to create osmotic diuresis in an attempt to decrease ICP

Barbiturate therapy: pentothal or nembutal used to place patient in coma to produce burst-suppression on the EEG and to reduce metabolic activity

Paralyzing drug therapy: pancuronium, among other drugs, may be used to decrease metabolic requirements but *must* be used in conjunction with sedatives as drug only paralyzes muscles and does not change level of awareness

Adrenocorticosteroids: decadron has less sodium-retaining properties and is used to assist with decreasing edema

CT scans: used to identify lesions, hemorrhage, ventricular size, structural shifting, ischemic event (may be several days prior to visibility on scan)

Laboratory: electrolytes drawn to evaluate imbalances that may contribute to ICP increases; toxicology screens to identify other drugs that may be responsible for changes in mentation and level of consciousness; serum levels of drugs to assess therapeutic response versus toxicity

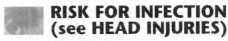

RISK FOR INFECTION (see HEAD INJURIES)

Related to: invasive monitoring, lack of skin integrity, increased metabolic state, intubation, compromised defense mechanisms

Defining Characteristics: increased temperature, chills, elevated white blood cell count, differential shift to the left, drainage, presence of wounds, positive cultures

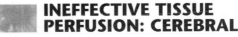

INEFFECTIVE TISSUE PERFUSION: CEREBRAL

Related to: cerebral edema, space-occupying lesions, hemorrhage, substance overdose, hypoxia, hypovolemia, trauma, increased ICP

Defining Characteristics: increased ICP >20 mm Hg for longer than 15 minutes, decreased CPP <70 mm Hg, changes in vital signs, changes in level of consciousness, memory deficit, restlessness, lethargy, coma, stupor, pupillary changes, headache, nausea/vomiting, purposeless movements, papilledema

Outcome Criteria

✔ Patient will have stable vital signs and mentation with no signs or symptoms of increased ICP.

NOC: *Neurologic Status*

INTERVENTIONS	RATIONALES
Monitor for changes in level of consciousness or mentation, speech, or response to commands/questions.	Alterations in levels of consciousness are among the earliest signs of increasing ICP and can facilitate prompt intervention. Progressive deterioration may require emergent care.

(continues)

(continued)

INTERVENTIONS	RATIONALES
Monitor vital signs at least every hour, and prn.	As ICP increases, blood pressure elevates, pulse pressure widens, bradycardia may occur, changing to tachycardia as ICP progressively worsens. Tachypnea is seen as an early sign but slows with increasingly longer periods of apnea. Fever may indicate hypothalamic damage or infection which can increase metabolic demands and further increase ICP. Cushing's reflex (increased systolic blood pressure, widening pulse pressure, and decreased heart rate) may result from ischemia of the vasomotor center in the brain stem.
Perform pupillary checks, noting equality, position, response to light, and nystagmus every 1–2 hours and prn.	Increased ICP or expansion of a clot can cause shifting of the brain against the oculomotor or optic nerve which causes pupillary changes. Early increased ICP may be signified by impairment of abduction of the eyes as a result of injury to the fifth cranial nerve. Absence of the doll's eyes reflex may indicate brain stem dysfunction and poor prognosis. Uncal herniation produces ipsilateral pupillary changes.
Monitor neurologic status utilizing the Glasgow Coma Scale (GCS).	GCS facilitates identification of arousability and level and appropriateness of responses. Motor response to simple commands or purposeful movement with stimuli assist with identification of problem. Abnormal posturing, decerebrate and decorticate, may indicate diffuse cortical damage. Inability to move one side of the body may indicate damage to the opposite side's cerebral hemisphere.
Monitor ECG for changes in heart rate and rhythm, and treat per protocol.	Brain stem pressure or injury may result in rate changes, normally bradycardia, or cardiac dysrhythmias.
Observe for presence of blink, gag, cough, and Babinski reflexes.	Reflex changes may be indicative of injury at the mid brain or brain stem level. Lack of blink reflex indicates damage to the pons and medulla. Cough and gag reflexes that are absent may

INTERVENTIONS	RATIONALES
	indicate damage at medulla and presence of Babinski reflex indicates pyramidal pathway injury.
Observe for nuchal rigidity, tremors, fasciculations, twitching, seizures, irritability, or restlessness.	May indicate meningeal irritation from a break in the dura or the development of an infection. Seizures may occur from an increased ICP, hypoxia, or cerebral irritation.
Elevate head of bed 30–45 degrees as warranted.	Decreases cerebral edema and congestion, thereby decreasing ICP.
Maintain head placement in neutral, or midline, position, using rolled towels or sandbags as warranted.	Moving head from side to side compresses jugular veins and increases ICP.
Avoid excess stimuli in room; allow visitation when warranted.	All stimulation increases ICP and should be limited to necessary tasks only in the presence of intracranial hypertension. Family members may have calming effect on patient and may facilitate decreased ICP.
Avoid suctioning unless mandatory, and when necessary, limit active suctioning to 15 seconds or less.	Minimizes hypoxia and acid–base disturbances. Hyperoxygenation prior to, during, and after procedure may also minimize complications.
Provide continuous monitoring of oximetry.	Provides for prompt recognition of deterioration in patient's ability to maintain saturation which allows for prompt intervention.
Apply oxygen at ordered concentrations; prepare for mechanical ventilation as warranted.	Supplemental oxygen decreases hypoxemia which results in increased ICP. Mechanical ventilation may be required if space-occupying lesions shift and destroy respiratory center enervation.
Administer medications as ordered.	Diuretics and/or mannitol may be used to draw water from cerebral cells to decrease edema and ICP. Steroids may be used to decrease tissue edema and inflammation. Anticonvulsants may be used prophylactically and for the treatment of seizures. Sedatives or analgesics may be used to control restlessness or agitation.
Observe continuous intracranial pressure monitoring for	Increases above 25 mm Hg that are sustained for at least 5 minutes

INTERVENTIONS	RATIONALES
fluctuations that are sustained, and for the presence of A, B, and C waves. Notify physician for wave changes.	may indicate severe intracranial hypertension. A waves, or plateau waves, have elevations from 60–100 mm Hg and then drop sharply, and often coincide with headaches or deterioration. Cellular hypoxia is most likely to occur during A waves, and sustained A waves indicate irreversible brain damage. B waves have elevations up to 50 mm Hg and occur every 1.5–2 minutes in a sawtooth-type pattern. B waves can precede A waves and/or appear in runs, and occur with decreases in compensation. C waves are rapid, rhythmic, and may fluctuate with changes in respiration or blood pressure, and are not of clinical significance.
Measure/obtain the mean ICP every hour and prn; set alarms for sustained elevations above ordered limits.	Provides direct measurement of changes in ICP and cerebral perfusion status.
Calculate CPP and do not allow CCP to fall below 50 mm Hg.	CPP = MAP – MICP; normal CPP is 80–100 mm Hg, and levels below 50 mm Hg decrease cerebral blood flow and perfusion, which frequently precipitates death.
Recalibrate ICP monitoring device to level of foramen of Monro (eye canthus level approximately) every 4 hours and prn suspicious readings or position changes.	Ensures accuracy of readings.
Maintain a sterile set up, with air-free tubing and transducer.	Reduces risk of infection and avoids dampening of waveforms and inaccurate ICP readings.
Assist with removal of specified amounts of CSF through ventriculostomy utilizing sterile technique.	May be required to decrease severe ICP and prevent herniation from structural shifting.
CSF should always be drained against positive pressure.	Incorrect removal technique may result in draining too much fluid or draining the fluid too quickly, which can then cause intracranial hemorrhaging. CSF drainage can result in a loss of the ICP waveform caused by ventricular collapse surrounding the catheter, and may require

INTERVENTIONS	RATIONALES
	allowing a reaccumulation of fluid until the waveform is recognizable. In some instances if the patient has a CSF leak, the ventricular catheter may be left open to drainage and closed every 30–60 minutes for ICP reading checks. This form of drainage may assist the dural tear in healing.
Measure jugular bulb oxygen saturation, if facility has this technology, as per hospital protocol. Notify physician of significant changes.	$SjvO_2$ identifies the balance between oxygen delivery and consumption to the brain and is dependent on cerebral metabolism and blood flow. Anything that increases cerebral metabolism and/or decreases the cerebral oxygen supply will cause a decrease in $SjvO_2$, and anything that causes a decrease in oxygen consumption and/or and increase in the oxygen supply will cause an increase in $SjvO_2$. This allows for identification of hypoperfusion in neurologically impaired patients. A normal reading of $SjvO_2$ can be from 60 to 90%, with decreases below 50% that last for 15 minutes or more, indicating cerebral ischemia, which requires emergent treatment.
If $SjvO_2$ monitoring is utilized, assess for signs/symptoms of infection or vein thrombosis upon removal of the catheter.	Risk of bacteremia related to $SjvO_2$ monitoring is very low, but thrombosis risk is significant. In clinical trials, although patients developed a thrombus, they did not become symptomatic.
If ICP is increasing, ensure that airway is patent, and prepare for placement on mechanical ventilation.	Hyperventilation results in respiratory alkalosis that causes cerebral vasoconstriction, decreases cerebral blood volume, and can decrease ICP. Levels of $PaCO_2$ are usually kept from 25–35 to decrease ICP, but if allowed to go below 25, may adversely affect ICP. Hyperventilation has been found to be associated with a poor short-term outcome with head trauma patients, and has also been shown to increase jugular vein desaturation and impair CBF. If the CBF is low, hyperventilation

(continues)

(continued)

INTERVENTIONS	RATIONALES
	within the first 24 hours should be avoided when possible.
Administer sedatives and narcotics as ordered.	May help to reduce ICP in restless or anxious patients.
Administer neuromuscular blocking agents in conjunction with narcotics, as ordered.	May be required if ICP remains high despite use of other medications, or if patient is fighting against the ventilator. Narcotics should always be given in conjunction because the neuromuscular blockers do nothing to the level of consciousness, and the paralysis can be fearful.
Administer mannitol as ordered for ICP >20 mm Hg. Monitor lab work for serum osmolality prior to mannitol administration and maintain <310 mOsm/kg, and for renal profiles.	Mannitol reduces ICP by osmotic diuresis and decreasing viscosity of the blood, which improves the microcirculation. Frequent dosing of mannitol may affect renal function.
Administer IV fluids as ordered.	CPP should be maintained above 70 mm Hg with crystalloid fluids and/or colloids. CP should be maintained at least at 5–10 mm Hg, with PCWP 10–12 mm Hg. Vasoactive drugs may also be required to maintain hydration and perfusion.
Administer barbiturates as ordered.	Barbiturates act to lower the ICP by suppressing metabolism, inhibiting free radical-mediated lipid peroxidation, and changing the vascular tone. Barbiturates are usually considered as a last resort and are used when ICP remains >30 mm Hg for more than 30 minutes with CPP <70 mm Hg, or when ICP is >40 mm Hg. It requires that the patient be stable hemodynamically and hydration-wise prior to starting

INTERVENTIONS	RATIONALES
	therapy, and complications include hypotension, hypothermia, infections, and pneumonia.
Change ventriculostomy tubing set every 48 hours and prn, and change fluid solution every 24 hours.	Reduces risk of infection.
Maintain clean dressing over site, and change prn using sterile technique. Observe site for signs of infection and notify physician.	Reduces risk for infection. Prompt recognition of infection symptoms allows for prompt intervention.
Instruct patient/family in procedures and medications to be used.	Promotes knowledge, decreases fear, and assists to obtain compliance.
Prepare patient/family for placement on mechanical ventilation as needed.	Patient may require mechanical ventilation because of complications from head injury, hypoxemia, or structural shifts that predispose the patient to ineffective respiration.
Instruct patient/family regarding need for maintenance of sterility regarding ICP monitoring.	Reduces fear and also reduces chances for infection.
Prepare patient/family for use of barbiturate therapy to produce coma.	Used as a last resort, pentobarbital or other drugs are given to produce complete unresponsiveness, to reduce metabolic activity, and decrease ICP.

NIC: *Intracranial Pressure Monitoring*

Discharge or Maintenance Evaluation

- Patient will exhibit no complications due to ICP monitoring.
- Patient will have ICP stabilized and controlled.
- Patient will have appropriate actions taken to control increasing ICP.

CHAPTER 3.4

GUILLAIN–BARRÉ SYNDROME

Guillain–Barré syndrome, also known as infectious polyneuritis, polyradiculoneuritis, and Landry–Guillain–Barré–Strohl syndrome, is an acute neuropathy in which inflammation and swelling of spinal nerve roots create demyelination and degeneration to the nerves beginning distally and ascending symmetrically.

Demyelination causes nerve impulse conduction to be delayed. Both dorsal and ventral nerve roots are involved, so both sensory and motor impairment is noted. The disease progress may cease at any point or continue to complete quadriplegia with cranial motor nerve involvement. Symmetric muscle weakness occurs and moves upward, with associated paresthesias and pain. Dysphagia, facial weakness, and extraocular muscle paralysis occur. Blood pressure and heart rate can be affected with marked fluctuations in response to a dysfunctional autonomic nervous system. After demyelination stops, remyelination begins and frequently complete function is restored in approximately 70% of patients. The recovery phase may last from 4 months to 2 years.

The exact cause of the syndrome is not known but several factors have been known to be associated with Guillain–Barré, such as, viral infections occurring 2–3 weeks prior, vaccinations, surgery, preexisting systemic disease, and autoimmune diseases.

Guillain–Barré syndrome may cause complications of hypertension, bradycardia, respiratory failure, and cardiovascular collapse. When sacral nerve roots are affected, incontinence becomes a problem.

MEDICAL CARE

Lumbar puncture: used in the diagnostic process; initially protein levels are normal for the first 48 hours but then increase as the disease progresses; highest protein level in CSF usually occurs between 10–20 days after initial onset; albumino-cytologic dissociation occurs when protein is elevated with red and white blood cells are normal; ICP may be elevated

Electromyography: helps to differentiate Guillain–Barré from myasthenia gravis; in Guillain–Barré, nerve impulse conduction speed is decreased

Nerve conduction studies: nerve conduction velocity is slowed between 1–2 weeks after initial onset

Plasmapheresis: may be used on an experimental basis to remove circulating antibodies that compromise nerve receptors

Laboratory: white blood cell count is elevated; sedimentation rate is elevated; electrolytes are done to identify hyponatremia that may occur because of problems with volume receptors

COMMON NURSING DIAGNOSES

INEFFECTIVE BREATHING PATTERN (see HEAD INJURIES)

Related to: muscle weakness, inability to swallow, ineffective coughing ability, inability to deep breathe, respiratory muscle paralysis

Defining Characteristics: dyspnea, bradypnea, apnea, tachypnea, deep, labored breathing, shallow, rapid breathing, change in level of responsiveness, ICP greater than 20 mm Hg, nasal flaring, changes in alveolar minute ventilation, hypoxia, hypoxemia, abnormal arterial blood gases, inability to handle secretions

IMPAIRED PHYSICAL MOBILITY (see HEAD INJURIES)

Related to: neuromuscular impairment, paralysis

Defining Characteristics: inability to move at will, inability to turn, transfer, or ambulate, decreased range of motion, muscle weakness, muscle incoordination, decreased reflexes

IMBALANCED NUTRITION: LESS THAN BODY REQUIREMENTS (see MECHANICAL VENTILATION)

Related to: neuromuscular impairment, intubation

Defining Characteristics: weight loss, muscle wasting, catabolism, inability to take in sufficient nutrients, impaired cough/gag/swallow reflexes, inability to chew, facial paralysis, tongue paralysis, ileus, gastric paralysis

IMPAIRED VERBAL COMMUNICATION (see CVA)

Related to: neuromuscular impairment, loss of muscle control, weakness, intubation, alteration of the central nervous system, stress

Defining Characteristics: inability to speak, inability to write, difficulty speaking or writing, difficulty forming words or sentences, apraxia, dyspnea, inability to use facial expressions

DISTURBED SENSORY PERCEPTION: VISUAL, KINESTHETIC, GUSTATORY, TACTILE (see CVA)

Related to: neuromuscular deficits, altered reception of stimuli, altered sensation, inability to communicate, hypoxia

Defining Characteristics: paresthesias, hypersensitivity to stimuli, muscle incoordination, inability to communicate, anxiety, restlessness, inability to concentrate, disorientation to time, place, self, and situation, hallucinations, distorted sounds, behavior changes, diminished concentration, inability to focus, alteration in thought processes, decreased sensation, paralysis, altered ability to taste and smell, inability to recognize objects, muscle weakness, inappropriate communication, changes in auditory or visual acuity

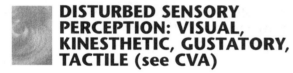

ADDITIONAL NURSING DIAGNOSES

INEFFECTIVE COPING (see ARDS)

Related to: situational crisis of disease process, inability to cope with stress, hypoxemia

Defining Characteristics: apprehension, use of defense mechanisms, emotional extremes, feelings of being overwhelmed, anxiety, helplessness, disorganized thoughts, inability to make decisions, inability to concentrate, focusing on crisis only, increased tension

IMBALANCED NUTRITION: LESS THAN BODY REQUIREMENTS (see MECHANICAL VENTILATION)

Related to: inability to take in sufficient food, increased metabolism caused by disease process, decreased level of consciousness, fatigue, paralysis

Defining Characteristics: actual inadequate food intake, altered taste, altered smell sensation, weight loss, anorexia, absent bowel sounds, decreased peristalsis, muscle mass loss, changes in bowel habits, abdominal distention, nausea, vomiting, inability to chew, absent gag and swallow reflexes, facial paralysis, tongue paralysis, ileus

IMPAIRED SPONTANEOUS VENTILATION (see MECHANICAL VENTILATION)

Related to: inability to adequately breathe independently

Defining Characteristics: apnea, dyspnea, tachypnea, hypermetabolic states, use of accessory muscles, decreased oxygen saturation, increased carbon dioxide levels, decreased tidal volumes, increased restlessness, tachycardia, confusion, mental status changes, dysrhythmias

ACUTE PAIN

Related to: neuromuscular impairment, hyperesthesias

Defining Characteristics: communication of pain or discomfort with minimal stimuli, muscle aches, tenderness, joint pain, flaccidity, spasticity, grimacing

Outcome Criteria

✔ Patient will have no complaints of pain, or pain will be controlled to patient's satisfaction.

NOC: *Pain Control*

INTERVENTIONS	RATIONALES
Monitor for complaints of pain/ discomfort and for nonverbal indications that patient may be in discomfort.	Patient may be unable to verbalize complaints.

INTERVENTIONS	RATIONALES
Administer medications as ordered.	Reduces or alleviates pain. Narcotics may cause respiratory depression.
Apply hot or cold packs as warranted.	Helps to alleviate discomfort and improves muscle and joint stiffness.
Use therapeutic touch, massage, imagery, visualization, or relaxation therapies as warranted.	Helps to refocus attention away from pain and provides for active participation in relieving pain.
Instruct patient to notify nurse when pain first begins.	Alleviation of pain or discomfort at the onset will require less medication to achieve analgesia.
Instruct patient/family regarding comfort measures, such as back rubs, turning and repositioning, therapeutic touch, biofeedback, and so forth.	These measures help to relieve discomfort and promote relaxation.
Instruct patient/family in effects, side effects, and signs to report for medication effects.	Promotes knowledge and assists with prompt identification of adverse effects of medications in order to effect a timely intervention.

NIC: *Pain Management*

Discharge or Maintenance Evaluation

- Patient will have no complaints of pain or paresthesias.
- Patient will be able to communicate pain and requests for analgesics.
- Patient will have pain controlled effectively to his satisfaction.

INEFFECTIVE TISSUE PERFUSION: CARDIOPULMONARY, PERIPHERAL, RENAL

Related to: autonomic nervous system impairment, hypovolemia, electrolyte imbalance, hypoxemia, venous thrombosis

Defining Characteristics: hypotension, hypertension, blood pressure lability, bradycardia, tachycardia, dysrhythmias, altered temperature regulation, decreased urine output, anuria, skin breakdown

Outcome Criteria

✔ Patient will achieve and maintain normal perfusion of all body systems.

NOC: *Tissue Perfusion*

INTERVENTIONS	RATIONALES
Monitor vital signs at rest and with turning. Notify physician of significant changes.	Severe changes with blood pressure may occur as a result of autonomic dysfunction because of the loss of sympathetic outflow to maintain peripheral vascular tone. Postural hypotension may occur as a result of impaired reflexes which normally readjust pressure during changes in position.
Monitor ECG for changes, and treat dysrhythmias per protocol.	Rate changes may occur as a result of vagal stimulation and impairment of the sympathetic innervation of the heart. Hypoxemia or electrolyte imbalances may alter vascular tone and impair venous return.
Monitor temperature of skin and core body. Observe for inability to perspire.	Vasomotor tone changes can impair the ability to perspire and cause temperature regulation problems. The patient's impaired sensation may further promote difficulty with warming and cooling the body.
Measure hemodynamics if pulmonary artery catheter in place, and notify physician for significant changes.	Impairment in vascular tone and venous return can decrease cardiac output.
Observe skin surfaces for redness or breakdown. Place patient on kinetic bed, egg crate mattress, alternating pressure mattress, and so forth, if warranted.	Decreases in sensation as well as circulatory changes may result in impaired perfusion and facilitate skin breakdown or ischemia. Special beds/mattresses help to reduce hazards of immobility.
Observe calves for redness, edema, or positive Homan's or Pratt's signs.	Venous stasis may increase potential for deep vein thrombosis formation, and patient may be unaware of discomfort because of paresthesias.
Provide anti-embolic hose or sequential compression devices to both legs and remove at least once every 8 hours.	Helps to decrease venous stasis and promotes venous return.

(continues)

(continued)

INTERVENTIONS	RATIONALES
Monitor hourly intake and output. Notify physician if urine output is less than 30 cc/hr for 2 hours, or if significant imbalance in I&O occurs.	Circulating volume may be decreased by patient's inability to take in adequate hydration, fluid shifting, and decreases in vascular tone.
Administer IV fluids as ordered.	Fluids help to prevent or correct hypovolemia but impaired vascular tone may result in severe hemodynamic lability based on small increases in circulating volumes.
Administer heparin SQ/IV as ordered, if no contraindications.	May be given prophylactically due to immobilization.

NIC: *Circulatory Care*

Discharge or Maintenance Evaluation

- Patient will be able to maintain adequate perfusion.
- Patient will have stable vital signs and hemodynamic parameters.
- Patient will have regular cardiac rhythm with no dysrhythmias.

URINARY RETENTION

Related to: neuromuscular impairment, immobility

Defining Characteristics: inability to void, inability to completely empty bladder

Outcome Criteria

✔ Patient will be able to empty bladder with no signs/symptoms of infection or retention.

NOC: *Urinary Elimination*

INTERVENTIONS	RATIONALES
Monitor for ability to void. Measure output carefully.	Provides information regarding neuromuscular progression. Progression of disease may predispose patient to retention which may lead to urinary tract infection or other complications.
Observe and palpate for bladder distention.	Bladder may become distended as sphincter reflex is involved in neuromuscular progression.
Insert indwelling catheter as warranted.	May be required to facilitate urinary emptying until disease

INTERVENTIONS	RATIONALES
	process has resolved and bladder control has been achieved.
Observe for concentrated urine, presence of blood or pus, changes in clarity or odor.	May indicate presence of urinary infection.
Instruct patient on need and procedure for catheter placement.	Promotes understanding and facilitates compliance.

NIC: *Urinary Retention Care*

Discharge or Maintenance Evaluation

- Patient will be able to void sufficient amounts without presence of retention or infection.
- Patient will be able to accurately recall information regarding need and procedure for catheter placement.
- Patient will be able to achieve bladder control once disease process has resolved.

RISK FOR CONSTIPATION

Related to: neuromuscular impairment, bed rest, immobility, changes in dietary habits, changes in environment, analgesics

Defining Characteristics: inability to expel all or part of stool, passage of hard stool, frequency less than normal pattern, rectal fullness, abdominal pain/pressure, decreased bowel sounds, decreased peristalsis, weakness, fatigue, appetite impairment

Outcome Criteria

✔ Patient will be able to eliminate soft, formed stool on a normal basis.

NOC: *Bowel Elimination*

INTERVENTIONS	RATIONALES
Evaluate elimination pattern, normal habits, ability to sense urge to defecate, presence of nausea/vomiting, presence of painful hemorrhoids, and history of constipation problems.	Provides baseline information to facilitate appropriate intervention for the patient's plan of care.
Observe for abdominal distention, tenderness, or guarding, nausea, vomiting, and absence of stool.	May indicate present or impending ileus or impaction.

INTERVENTIONS	RATIONALES
Palpate rectum for presence of stool/impaction.	Manual removal of stool may be required, and should be performed gently to avoid vagal stimulation. Other interventions may be necessary to allow for bowel elimination.
Auscultate bowel sounds for presence, pitch, and changes.	Diminished or absent bowel sounds, or presence of high-pitched tinkling sounds may indicate that an ileus has developed.
Administer stool softeners, laxatives, suppositories, or enemas as warranted/ordered.	May be required to stimulate bowel evacuation and to establish a bowel regime until patient is able to regain normal musculature control.
Insert nasogastric tube as ordered. Connect with intermittent suction per hospital policy.	Decompresses abdominal distention that occurs with ileus formation, and helps prevent nausea and vomiting.
Increase fiber in diet/tube feedings as warranted.	Helps to promote elimination by adding bulk and helps to regulate fecal consistency.
Instruct patient on increases in fluid intake, dietary requirements, use of fruits and juices to improve bowel elimination.	Promotes knowledge and can help facilitate improvement in bowel regime.
Instruct patient on need/procedure for nasogastric tube insertion.	Helps to promote understanding of complications that may occur with the loss of peristalsis caused by the disease process.

NIC: *Constipation/Impaction Management*

Discharge or Maintenance Evaluation

- Patient will achieve normal bowel elimination.
- Patient will require no bowel aids to facilitate his normal routine.
- Patient will regain muscle control and be able to evacuate stool.
- Patient will be able to utilize dietary modification to maintain bowel regime.
- Patient will be able to recall information correctly.

FEAR

Related to: disease process, change in health status, paralysis, respiratory failure, change in environment, threat of death

Defining Characteristics: restlessness, apprehension, tension, fearfulness, sympathetic stimulation, changes in vital signs, inability to concentrate or focus, poor attention span, uncertainty of treatment and outcome, insomnia, jitteriness, alarm, terror, panic, nausea, vomiting, diarrhea, muscle tightness, increased perspiration, dry mouth, decreased problem-solving ability

Outcome Criteria

✔ Patient will be able to reduce and/or relieve anxiety with appropriate methods.

NOC: *Fear Control*

INTERVENTIONS	RATIONALES
Evaluate anxiety level frequently. Stay with patient during acute episodes.	Determination of severity of patient's anxiety/fear can help to determine appropriate intervention. Nurse's presence during acute anxiety may foster feelings of reassurance and concern for the patient's well-being.
Maintain consistency with nurse assignments.	Helps to decrease anxiety and builds trust in relationships.
Patient should be placed near nurse's station and within visual contact.	Reassures patient that assistance will be nearby should he be unable to use call bell.
Provide method for patient to summon assistance.	Reduces anxiety and fear of abandonment.
Involve patient and family in plan of care. Allow patient to make as many decisions as warranted.	Helps to foster understanding and facilitates feelings of control and improved self-esteem. Improves cooperation with procedures and care.
Provide time for patient/family to discuss fears and concerns. Offer realistic options and do not give false reassurance.	Discussion of fears provides opportunity for clarification of misperceptions and for realistic methods of dealing with problems.
Administer anti-anxiety medications or sedation as warranted/ordered.	Patient's anxiety may result in alterations in hemodynamic stability and may require medication to initially deal with situational crises. Patient may require medication to facilitate improved ventilation should mechanical ventilation be required.

(continues)

(continued)

INTERVENTIONS	RATIONALES
Instruct patient/family in all treatment, care, and procedures, and answer questions honestly.	Promotes knowledge, reduces fear and anxiety of the unknown, and helps to ensure compliance.
Instruct family regarding specific needs for patient and allow family members to assist with care, when possible.	Provides familiar person for patient and allows for family and patient to provide support and help to cope with fears.
Allow family member to stay with patient when possible during acute episodes of fear.	Reduces fear by providing familiar person to assist with alleviating patient's fear of being alone and defenseless.

NIC: *Anxiety Reduction*

Discharge or Maintenance Evaluation

- Patient will be able to deal with changes in health status effectively.
- Patient will be able to control anxiety and reduce fear to a manageable level.
- Patient will have decreased anxiety and fear.

POWERLESSNESS

Related to: total physical dependency on others, loss of control, lack of environmental control

Defining Characteristics: nonparticipation in care, resentment, anger, passivity, irritability, frustration, expressions of dissatisfaction or doubt, unwillingness to seek information, apathy, depression, verbal expressions of having no control, fear of alienation of caregivers

Outcome Criteria

✔ Patient will be able to identify feelings of powerlessness and will be able to utilize methods to regain control over the situation.

✔ Patient will participate in self-care.

NOC: *Health Beliefs: Perceived Control*

INTERVENTIONS	RATIONALES
Assess patient's knowledge of current situation and disease process.	Allows for baseline information from which to plan patient's care, and facilitates identification of incorrect information that requires re-education.

INTERVENTIONS	RATIONALES
Allow sufficient time spent with the patient to share feelings and ask questions.	Provides time for patient to feel comfortable, establishes trust, and allows for therapeutic learning environment.
Decrease competing stimuli in patient's room.	Excessive sensory stimulation can result in disorientation, delusions, or hallucinations, and prevent information from being understood.
Always remember to place call light, controls for television, phone bedside table, and other necessary items within easy reach for patient. Use adaptive equipment based on patient's inabilities.	Assists with reduction of frustration over inability to reach items or to call for assistance.
Orient patient to environment, allowing patient to select placement of items whenever possible.	Assists with fostering sense of power and control over environment.
Allow patient to make decisions with regard to care, such as timing of procedures, and so forth, whenever possible.	Promotes feelings of importance, and increases feeling of powerfulness. Reduces passivity and apathy while promoting sense of trust with caregiver.
Encourage patient to participate as able with self-care.	Encourages patient to continue to assist in own care and reduces feelings of powerlessness.
Instruct patient/family in measures to help patient gain control over environment, ways to summon assistance, and alternatives to use.	Promotes knowledge, decreases fear of abandonment and of not being able to receive assistance, and promotes trust in caregiver.
Instruct patient/family about all treatments and procedures, and allow for participation in planning care whenever possible.	Increases patient's feelings of powerfulness and decreases fear of the unknown.
Instruct patient/family in disease process, progression, what to expect, and answer all questions honestly.	Promotes understanding and knowledge, which in turn, will result in increased feelings of patient control.

NIC: *Coping Enhancement*

Discharge or Maintenance Evaluation

- Patient will be able to express feelings of lack of power and control.
- Patient will be able to verbalize feelings of regaining control using methods that were given.
- Patient will be able to modify his environment in such a way as to promote feelings of control.
- Patient will participate in self-care as much as possible.

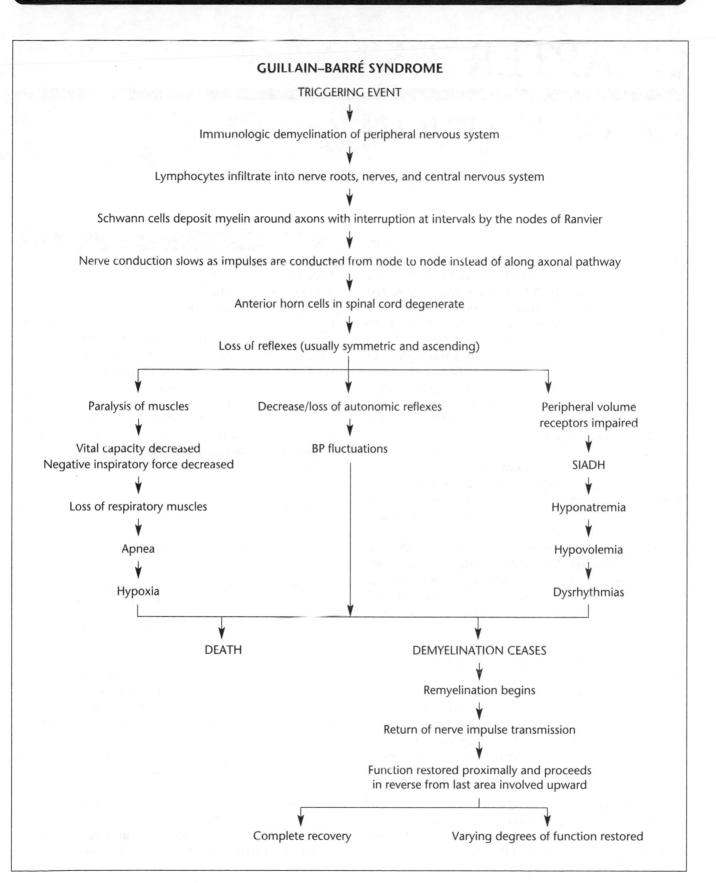

CHAPTER 3.5

STATUS EPILEPTICUS

Seizures occur when uncontrolled electrical impulses from the nerve cells in the cerebral cortex discharge and result in autonomic, sensory, and motor dysfunction. Status epilepticus is a series of repeated seizures, a prolonged seizure, or sequential seizures longer than 30 minutes in which the patient does not regain consciousness. This seizure activity has a high mortality rate of up to 30% as a result of neurologic and brain damage.

There are three types of status epilepticus: convulsive, nonconvulsive, and partial status epilepticus. In the convulsive type, seizure activity may have a focal onset, but has tonic–clonic, grand mal–type seizures without experiencing alertness between motor attacks. Nonconvulsive seizures are noted with a prolonged twilight state and are usually not motor activity. Partial status epilepticus occurs when continuous or repetitive focal seizures occur but consciousness is not altered.

Status epilepticus usually occurs in patients with pre-existing seizure disorders who have a precipitating factor occurrence. These factors can include withdrawal from anticonvulsant medication, alcohol withdrawal, sedative or antidepressant withdrawal, sleep deprivation, meningitis, encephalitis, brain abscesses or tumors, pregnancy, hypoglycemia, hyponatremia, uremia, cerebrovascular disease, cerebral edema, or cerebral trauma.

The initial stage causes sympathetic activity increases with a decrease in the cerebral vascular resistance. After 30 minutes, hypotension occurs with a decrease in cerebral blood flow because of loss of autoregulation. The continuing massive autonomic discharges can cause bronchial secretions and restriction, with increased capillary permeability and pulmonary edema. Dysrhythmias can occur and patients may develop rhabdomyolysis and renal failure. Other complications may occur as a result of the significantly elevated metabolic state.

MEDICAL CARE

Laboratory: electrolytes to identify imbalances that may be precipitating factor or result from prolonged seizure activity; enzymes, especially creatine phosphokinase, elevated after seizure activity; drug screen done to identify potential factor for drug withdrawal; CBC used to identify hemorrhage or infection with shift to the left on differential; drug levels for medications being given for seizures to evaluate therapeutic response and discern toxicity; renal profiles to evaluate renal function; urinalysis to identify hematuria or myoglobinuria, which is common after prolonged seizure activity; decreased glucose levels may be precipitating factor, or may occur after prolonged seizures

CT scans: may be done to identify lesions or precipitating factors

Electroencephalogram: used to identify presence of seizure activity

Arterial blood gases: used to identify hypoxia and acid–base imbalances; usually acidosis seen

Anticonvulsants: drugs such as carbamazepine (Atretol, Carbatrol, Tegretol), clonazepam (Klonopin), ethosuximide (Zarontin), fosphenytoin sodium (Cerebryx), gabapentin (Neurontin), lamotrigine (Lamictal), levetiracetam (Keppra), oxcarbazepine (Trileptal), Phenobarbital (Barbita, Solfoton, Luminal), phenytoin (Dilantin, Phenytex), primadone (Mysoline), tiagabine hydrochloride (Gabitril), topiramate (Topamax), valproic acid or valproate (Depacon, Depakene, Depakote), or zonisamide (Zonegran) used in the treatment and prophylaxis of seizure activity; method of action dependent on drug utilized—some increase cerebral levels of GABA, some help to stabilize neuronal membranes and synchronization, and some act upon sodium, potassium, or calcium ion concentrations within the neuronal cells

COMMON NURSING DIAGNOSES

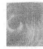

IMPAIRED GAS EXCHANGE (see MECHANICAL VENTILATION)

Related to: altered oxygen supply from repetitive seizures, cognitive impairment, neuromuscular impairment

Defining Characteristics: restlessness, cyanosis, inability to move secretions, tachycardia, dysrhythmias, abnormal arterial blood gases, alkalosis, hypoxia, hypoxemia, decreased oxygen saturation

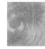

INEFFECTIVE AIRWAY CLEARANCE (see MECHANICAL VENTILATION)

Related to: neuromuscular impairment, cognitive impairment, tracheobronchial obstruction

Defining Characteristics: adventitious breath sounds, dyspnea, tachypnea, shallow respirations, cough with or without productivity, cyanosis, anxiety, restlessness

HYPERTHERMIA (see PHEOCHROMOCYTOMA)

Related to: continued seizure activity, increased metabolic state

Defining Characteristics: fever, persistent tonic–clonic seizure activity, persistent focal seizures, persistent generalized seizures, tachycardia

DEFICIENT FLUID VOLUME (see ARDS)

Related to: excessive loss of fluid, decreased intake

Defining Characteristics: hypotension, tachycardia, fever, weight loss, oliguria, abnormal electrolytes, low filling pressures, decreased mental status, decreased specific gravity, increased serum osmolality

ANTICIPATORY GRIEVING (see AMPUTATION)

Related to: traumatic injury, loss of physical well-being

Defining Characteristics: communications of distress, denial, guilt, fear, sadness, changes in affect, changes in ability and desire for communication, crying, insomnia, lethargy

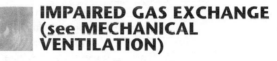

IMPAIRED GAS EXCHANGE (see MECHANICAL VENTILATION)

Related to: seizure activity, altered oxygen-carrying capability, altered oxygen supply

Defining Characteristics: dyspnea, nasal flaring, tachycardia, pale, dusky skin, confusion, diaphoresis, hypoxia, hypoxemia, irritability, restlessness, abnormal arterial blood gases, seizures

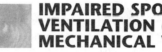

IMPAIRED SPONTANEOUS VENTILATION (see MECHANICAL VENTILATION)

Related to: seizure activity, lowered ventilatory capacity and ventilatory demand imbalances

Defining Characteristics: ineffective breathing pattern, dyspnea, apnea, tachypnea, use of accessory muscles, abnormal arterial blood gases, mental status changes, increased work of breathing, cyanosis, decreased oxygen saturation

ADDITIONAL NURSING DIAGNOSES

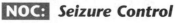 **RISK FOR INJURY**

Related to: seizure activity, increased metabolic demands

Defining Characteristics: respiratory acidosis, metabolic acidosis, hypoxemia, hyperthermia, hypoglycemia, electrolyte imbalances, renal failure, rhabdomyolysis, exhaustion, death

Outcome Criteria

✔ Patient will achieve and maintain seizure-free status.

✔ Patient will have optimal oxygenation and ventilation, without noted complications.

NOC: *Risk Control*

NOC: *Seizure Control*

INTERVENTIONS	RATIONALES
Maintain patent airway and adequate ventilation.	Intubation and placement on mechanical ventilation may be required if seizures cannot be controlled.
Monitor oxygen saturation by oximeter.	Decreases in saturation that cannot be improved with supplemental oxygen may require mechanical ventilation. Seizure activity increases oxygen consumption and demand.
Provide supplemental oxygen as warranted.	May be required to maintain desired levels of oxygen.
Monitor ABGs for imbalances and treat per protocol.	Metabolic increases may lead to lactate formation and acidosis.
Administer medications as ordered to stop the seizures.	Valium may be given IV at 5 mg/min rate to control seizure activity by enhancing neurotransmitter GABA. Cardiovascular and respiratory depression may occur, especially if diazepam is used in conjunction with phenobarbital. Ativan 2–4 mg IV may be given and repeated every 15 minutes as needed for seizure control. Caution should be exercised because respiratory and cardiovascular depression can occur. Phenobarbital IV at 60 mg/min may be given to depress excitation, decrease calcium uptake by nerves, increase neuron threshold for chemical and electrical stimulation, and to strengthen repression of synapses. Dilantin IV at 50 mg/min rate may be given to decrease cellular influx of sodium and calcium and blocking neurotransmission release. Caution must be maintained to avoid giving phenytoin any faster than prescribed rate because of its pH, and the ECG must be monitored for conduction changes or dysrhythmias while administering drug. Patients who have heart block or Stokes–Adams syndrome should only have this drug utilized with extreme caution. If these drugs are able to halt the seizure activity, pentobarbital may be required. Pentobarbital should

INTERVENTIONS	RATIONALES
	be given with a loading dose of 5–10 mg/kg over 1 hour, then 5 mg/kg per hour three times, then a maintenance drip at 1–3 mg/kg per hour IV.
Maintain patient in seizure-free status.	Once seizures have stopped, anticonvulsant drugs must be continued to prevent recurrence of seizure activity.
Monitor ECG for dysrhythmias and treat per protocol.	Electrolyte imbalances, too-rapid administration of medications, and hypoxia may contribute to appearance of cardiac dysrhythmias that may require interventional care.
Monitor intake and output every 1–2 hours and prn.	Identifies imbalances with fluid status and fluid shifting.
Monitor lab work for changes and trends.	Electrolytes may fluctuate because of cellular movement of ions. Myoglobin may be present in urine as a result of prolonged seizure activity and can lead to renal failure. Drug levels may rise to toxic levels and should be evaluated for therapeutic effectiveness. Severe imbalances of glucose, sodium, potassium, calcium, phosphorus, magnesium or BUN may precipitate or maintain seizure activity. CBC and differential may be helpful to expose disorders that could occur with seizure activity, such as lead poisoning, leukemia, or sickle cell anemia. Cultures should be done to ascertain if sepsis might be a causative factor. Toxic drug screening may be helpful when looking for recreational drug use or lead poisoning.
Identify and treat underlying cause of seizures.	Identification may lead to timely intervention and treatment. The nurse should be cognizant and assess for potential causes, such as signs of head trauma, drug abuse needle tracks, or metabolic or intracranial pathology, which can result in seizure activity.
Maintain IV access and administer IV fluids as ordered.	IV access is mandatory in case emergency drugs are required

INTERVENTIONS	RATIONALES
	for complications that might ensue. Phenytoin can result in precipitation or crystallization with glucose solutions. Fluids may be required to treat myoglobinuria and renal failure, maintain hydration status, and to administer supplemental electrolytes as needed.
Use padding on side rails.	Provides protection against injury from hitting rails during seizure activity.
Instruct patient/family in disease process and methods for reduction of seizures.	Promotes knowledge and facilitates compliance.
Instruct patient/family in drug regimen, effects, side effects, contraindications, and precautions.	Promotes knowledge and helps prevent lack of cooperation with medication regime with resultant seizure breakthrough activity. Presence of side effects may indicate the need for changes in doses or medication type. Interactions with other drugs may produce adverse reactions, such as potentiated anticoagulation effect when dilantin and coumadin are concurrently taken.
Instruct patient/family in oral care.	Prevents gingival hypertrophy that may occur while taking dilantin.
Instruct patient/family on use of medical alert bracelet.	May hasten emergency treatment in critical situations.
Instruct patient/family on methods to promote safety with activities, such as, driving, using mechanical equipment, swimming, or hobbies.	May facilitate prevention of injury to self or other if seizures occur without warning.
Instruct patient/family on contact people, community resource groups, counselors, as warranted.	May provide opportunities for long-term support and sharing ideas with others who have similar problems.

NIC: *Seizure Precautions*

Discharge or Maintenance Evaluation

- Patient/family will be able to verbalize understanding of all instructions and comply with medical regimen.
- Patient will remain free of seizures and injury.

- Patient will be able to effectively access community resources for help and support.
- Patient will exhibit no signs of complications.

SITUATIONAL LOW SELF-ESTEEM

Related to: perception of loss of control, ashamed of medical condition

Defining Characteristics: fear of rejection, concerns about changes in lifestyle, negative feelings about self, change in perception of role, changes in responsibilities, lack of participation in therapy or care, passiveness, inability to accept positive reinforcement, little eye contact, brief responses to questions

Outcome Criteria

✔ Patient will be able to participate in own care and have positive perceptions of self.

NOC: *Self-Esteem*

INTERVENTIONS	RATIONALES
Encourage patient to initiate self-care or request assistance.	Participation in care facilitates feelings of normalcy.
Discuss patient's perceptions of illness and potential reactions of others to his disease.	Provides opportunities to establish patient's knowledge base, clear up any misconceptions, and opportunity to problem-solve responses to future seizures.
Discuss previous success episodes and patient's strengths.	Concentrating on the positive experiences may help to reduce self-consciousness and allow patient to begin to accept condition.
Assess patient's mental status every shift and prn.	Anxiety that results from self-rejection may become so severe that the patient may become disoriented or develop psychotic symptoms.
Encourage patient involvement with decisions.	Low self-esteem may result in feelings of ambivalence and procrastination.
Give patient positive feedback for behavior that shows constructive self-appraisal.	Provides patient with approval and increases ability to cope effectively with stressful situations.
Obtain permission from patient to enter his personal space.	As the patient's self-esteem decreases, the significance of personal space increases. Asking

(continues)

(continued)

INTERVENTIONS	RATIONALES
	permission provides patient with a sense of control and improves self-esteem.
Discuss concerns with family members, allowing ample time for members to discuss problems and attitudes.	Negative feelings from patient's family may affect his sense of self-esteem.
Consult with counselors, ministerial support, or resource groups.	Provides opportunity for patient to deal with stigma of disease and overcome feelings of inferiority.

NIC: *Self-Modification Assistance*

Discharge or Maintenance Evaluation

- Patient will be able to identify ways to cope with negative feelings.
- Patient/family will be able to discuss concerns and effect realistic problem-solving plans.
- Patient will become more accepting of self, with increased self-esteem.
- Patient will be able to effectively access community resources to gain help and support.

STATUS EPILEPTICUS

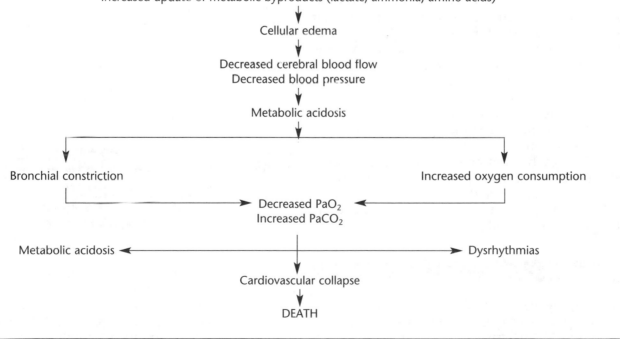

Pre-existing seizure disorder (tumors, trauma, encephalopathy)

Seizure activity
Rapid succession of action potentials in cells

Increased sympathetic activity

Increased metabolic demand
Increased temperature, pulse, and blood pressure

Decreased ATP
Sodium–potassium ATP pump failure

Decreased cerebral vascular resistance
Increased cerebral vascular dilation

Increased cerebral metabolic rate

Increased oxygen utilization
Increased glucose utilization
Increased glycolysis

Prolonged seizure state (>30 minutes)

Blood flow becomes pressure dependent
Cerebrovascular autoregulation mechanisms fail

Increased update of metabolic byproducts (lactate, ammonia, amino acids)

Cellular edema

Decreased cerebral blood flow
Decreased blood pressure

Metabolic acidosis

Bronchial constriction   Increased oxygen consumption

Decreased PaO$_2$
Increased PaCO$_2$

Metabolic acidosis   Dysrhythmias

Cardiovascular collapse

DEATH

CHAPTER 3.6

MENINGITIS

Meningitis is an acute infection of the pia and arachnoid membrane that surrounds the brain and the spinal cord caused by any type of microorganism. Bacterial meningitis is frequently caused by *Streptococcus pneumoniae, Haemophilus influenzae, Neisseria meningitidis, Staphylococcus aureus, Staphylococcus epidermidis, Escherichia coli, Serratia, Klebsiella, Citrobacter, Pseudomonas, Proteus, Acinetobacter,* and *Mycobacterium tuberculosis.* Enterovirus, herpesvirus, arbovirus, and the mumps virus can cause viral meningitis.

Organisms are able to thrive because of opportune access during surgery, with invasive monitoring and lines, penetrating injuries, skull fractures, dural tears, otitis media, sinusitis, dental abscesses, septicemia, or with septic emboli. Once the organism begins multiplying, neutrophils infiltrate into the subarachnoid space and form an exudate. The body's defenses attempt to control the invading pathogens by walling off the exudate and effectively creating two layers. If appropriate medical treatment is begun early, the outer and inner layers will disappear, but if the infection persists for several weeks, the inner layer forms a permanent fibrin structure over the meninges. This meningeal covering causes adhesions between the pia and the arachnoid membranes and results in congestion and increased ICP.

One of the major complications of meningitis is residual cranial nerve dysfunction, such as deafness, blindness, tinnitus, or vertigo. Sometimes these symptoms resolve, but cerebral edema may occur and cause seizures, nerve palsy, bradycardia, hypertension, coma, and even death.

The main goal of treatment is to eliminate the causative organism and prevent complications.

MEDICAL CARE

Laboratory: white blood cell count elevation to identify infection; cultures to identify the causative organism; CSF analysis to identify infection, with protein increased in most cases and higher in bacterial meningitis than in viral meningitis, low glucose in most cases of bacterial meningitis but may be normal with viral; clarity may be normal with viral meningitis, or turbid and purulent in bacterial meningitis; cells are predominantly lymphocytes with viral meningitis and polymorphonuclear leukocytes in bacterial meningitis; urinalysis may show albumin and red and white blood cells; glucose levels elevated in meningitis, LDH elevated with bacterial meningitis, ESR elevated; electrolytes done with either hyponatremia or hypernatremia noted

Radiography: skull and spine X-rays used to identify sinus infections, fractures, or osteomyelitis; chest X-rays may be used to identify respiratory infections, abscesses, lesions, or granulomas

CT scan: will usually be normal in uncomplicated cases of meningitis, but can show diffuse enhancement in some types or show hydrocephalus

Lumbar puncture: treatment of choice to identify presence of meningitis, help identify type of meningitis, and identify causative organism

Electroencephalogram: may be performed to show slow wave activity

Antimicrobials: used to eradicate the causative organism

COMMON NURSING DIAGNOSES

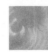

INEFFECTIVE TISSUE PERFUSION: CEREBRAL (see ICP MONITORING)

Related to: increased intracranial pressure

Defining Characteristics: increased ICP, changes in vital signs, changes in level of consciousness, memory deficit, restlessness, lethargy, coma, stupor, pupillary changes, headache, pain in neck or back, nausea/vomiting, purposeless movements, papilledema

ACUTE PAIN
(see GUILLAIN-BARRÉ)

Related to: meningeal irritation, infectious organisms, circulating toxins, invasive lines, bedrest

Defining Characteristics: headache, muscle spasms, backache, photophobia, crying, moaning, restlessness, communication of pain, muscle tension, facial grimacing, pallor, neck pain, crying, changes in time perception, withdrawal from contact, guarding, unwillingness to move in bed, increases in pulse rate, blood pressure and respirations

HYPERTHERMIA
(see PHEOCHROMOCYTOMA)

Related to: infection process

Defining Characteristics: fever, tachycardia, tachypnea, warm, flushed skin, seizures

ADDITIONAL NURSING DIAGNOSES

 # RISK FOR INJURY

Related to: infection, shock, seizures

Defining Characteristics: presence of infection, elevated white blood cell count, differential shift to the left, positive cultures, hypotension, tachycardia, tremors, fasiculations, seizures, hypoxemia, acid–base disturbances

Outcome Criteria

✔ Patient will be free of infection with stable vital signs.

NOC: *Risk Control*

INTERVENTIONS	RATIONALES
Assist with lumbar puncture.	Identifies presence of infection and can differentiate between types of meningitis. CSF with low white cell counts, less protein elevation, and glucose levels approximately half that of the blood

INTERVENTIONS	RATIONALES
	glucose level may be indicative of viral meningitis. CSF that has an elevated initial pressure, high protein, low glucose, cloudy color, and high white cell count indicates bacterial meningitis.
Administer antimicrobials as ordered, as soon as possible.	Aqueous penicillin G is usually the drug of choice, but culture results may indicate a different agent needed to eradicate the organism. Antimicrobials are usually given in larger doses at closer intervals in order to facilitate penetration across the blood–brain barrier.
Observe appropriate isolation techniques up to 48 hours after antimicrobial regimen has begun.	Prevents spread of infection. After antimicrobial therapy has been instituted for 2 days, the patient is not considered infectious.
Administer anticonvulsants as ordered.	May be required for control of new seizure activity due to meningeal irritation.
Pad side rails of bed.	Decreases risk of injury if patient should have seizure and hit side rails.
Instruct patient/family regarding use of isolation.	Facilitates compliance with procedure and promotes knowledge.
Instruct patient/family in signs/symptoms to observe for, and instruct to notify nurse or physician if patient develops increased temperature, changes in behavior or mental status, drainage from wound site, and so forth.	Promotes knowledge, involves family in patient care, and assists in identification of potential problems to optimize timely intervention.

NIC: *Infection Protection*

Discharge or Maintenance Evaluation

■ Patient will be free of infection with no complications from antimicrobial agents.
■ Patient will be free of seizure activity.
■ Patient will comply with isolation restrictions.

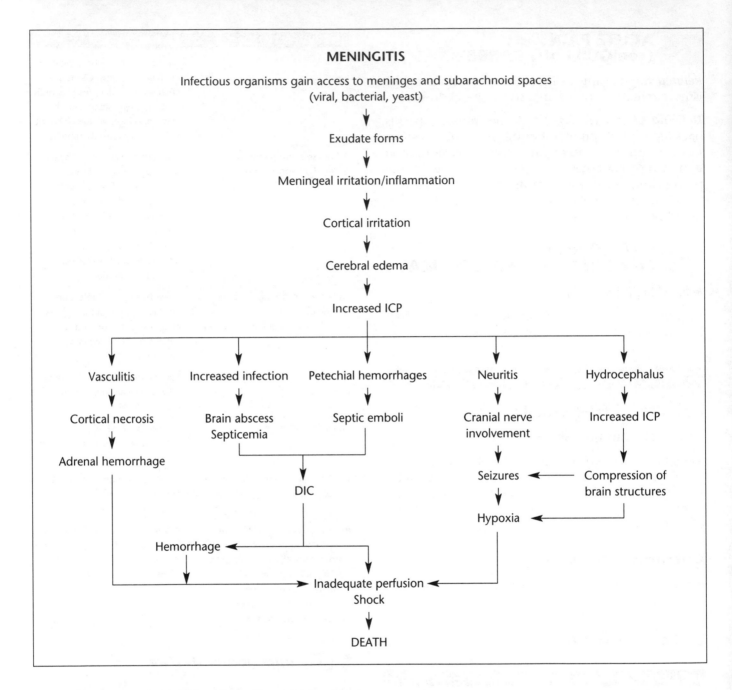

MENINGITIS

Infectious organisms gain access to meninges and subarachnoid spaces
(viral, bacterial, yeast)

↓

Exudate forms

↓

Meningeal irritation/inflammation

↓

Cortical irritation

↓

Cerebral edema

↓

Increased ICP

Vasculitis	Increased infection	Petechial hemorrhages	Neuritis	Hydrocephalus
↓	↓	↓	↓	↓
Cortical necrosis	Brain abscess Septicemia	Septic emboli	Cranial nerve involvement	Increased ICP
↓			↓	↓
Adrenal hemorrhage	DIC		Seizures ← Compression of brain structures	
			↓	
			Hypoxia ←	

Hemorrhage ←

→ Inadequate perfusion ←
Shock

↓

DEATH

CHAPTER 3.7

SPINAL CORD INJURIES

Spinal cord injuries are traumatic injuries to the spinal cord caused by contusion, compression, or transection of the cord as a result of dislocation of bones, rupture of ligaments, vessels, or vertebral discs, stretching of neural tissue, or impairment in blood supply. These lesions are classified as being complete or incomplete. Complete lesions involve the total loss of sensation as well as voluntary motor function, and incomplete lesions involve mixed losses of sensation and voluntary motor function.

The flexion, hyperextension and/or rotational types of injury that result in spinal cord injury are usually caused by trauma, motor vehicle accidents, falls, gunshot wounds, stab wounds, and diving injuries. The severity of the injury can vary depending on the amount of pathologic changes that are produced. Injury without intervention results in ischemia, edema, hemorrhage, and progressive destruction. After the initial cord compression, small hemorrhages occur in the central gray matter. The expansion and increase in number of hemorrhagic areas cause even more compression, edema, and finally, necrosis of the cord. The cervical area is the most vulnerable part of the spine because of the mobility of the head and poor support by the muscles, but cervical fractures do not necessarily cause neurologic problems.

The level of the injury relates to how much functional ability is retained. At the C1 to C8 levels, the patient is a quadriplegic with variances in muscle function from complete paralysis of respiratory function to limited use of the fingers. At T1 to L1 levels, paraplegia is noted with intact arm movement. At L2 level and below, there may be mixed dysfunction with bowel and bladder dysfunction.

In central cord syndrome, the central gray matter of the cord is contused, compressed, or hemorrhaged. This results in varying degrees of sensory loss and bowel/bladder dysfunction, and there is more motor loss in the arms than in the legs. In anterior cord syndrome, the injury has occurred to the anterior horn and spinothalamic areas resulting in a loss of motor function and pain/temperature sensation below the lesion. Sensations of touch, position, pressure and vibration may be maintained. In Brown-Sequard syndrome, as a result of a transverse hemi-transection of the cord, motor loss, touch, vibration, pressure, and position are involved ipsilaterally, with a contralateral loss of pain/temperature sensation. Posterior cord syndrome is exceedingly rare and results in the loss of light touch below the level of injury, with motor function and sensation of pain and temperature maintained intact.

When spinal lesions at or above the T6 level block sensory impulses from reaching the brain, an excessive and critical autonomic response to a stimulus occurs, and this is known as autonomic dysreflexia. It may be precipitated by bowel or bladder distention or by stimulation of the skin or pain receptors. Symptoms may include severe blood pressure increases, pounding headache, profuse sweating above the lesion, blurred vision, goosebumps, and bradycardia. Treatment is aimed at removing the stimulus that causes the problem, and treating the hypertensive episode.

Spinal shock occurs when there is an abrupt loss of continuity between the spinal cord and the higher nerve centers, with a complete loss of all reflexes and a flaccid paralysis below the level of injury. Normally, this spinal shock lasts 7–10 days and when it begins resolution, the flaccidity changes to a spastic type of paralysis.

MEDICAL CARE

Laboratory: CSF results may help to differentiate other pathology besides trauma

Arterial blood gases: used to identify hypoxemia and acid–base imbalances

Radiography: chest X-rays used to identify diaphragmatic changes or respiratory complications; spinal X-rays used to identify fracture or dislocation and identifies level of injury

CT scans: used to identify structural aberrancies and localize injury site; myelography, in conjunction, shows any impingement on the spinal canal by bony fragments or disks

Magnetic resonance imaging: used to identify cord lesions, compression, edema, or soft tissue injury

Surgery: may be required to align or stabilize fracture, or repair other traumatic injuries that may be concurrent

Traction: may be required to align and stabilize fracture or dislocation of the vertebral column

COMMON NURSING DIAGNOSES

ACUTE PAIN (see GUILLAIN-BARRÉ)

Related to: trauma, surgery, cervical traction

Defining Characteristics: burning pain below lesion, muscle spasms, phantom pain, hyperesthesia above lesion level, headaches, communication of pain, facial grimacing, irritability, restlessness

RISK FOR IMPAIRED SKIN INTEGRITY (see FRACTURES)

Related to: immobility, surgery, traction apparatus, changes in metabolism, decreased circulation, impaired sensation

Defining Characteristics: wounds, drainage, redness, pressure sores, abrasions, lacerations

DISTURBED SENSORY PERCEPTION (see CVA)

Related to: traumatic injury, sensory receptor and tract impairment, damaged sensory transmission

Defining Characteristics: decreased sensory acuity, impairment of position relation, proprioception, motor incoordination, mood swings, disorientation, agitation, anxiety, abnormal emotional responses, changes in stimulation response

ADDITIONAL NURSING DIAGNOSES

DECREASED CARDIAC OUTPUT

Related to: neurogenic shock, sympathetic blockade, spinal shock

Defining Characteristics: hypotension, bradycardia, vasovagal reflex, hypoxia, decreased venous return, decreased hemodynamic pressures, dysrhythmias

Outcome Criteria

✔ Patient will be able to maintain systolic blood pressure above 90 mm Hg and have stable vital signs and heart rhythm.

NOC: *Vital Sign Status*

INTERVENTIONS	RATIONALES
Monitor vital signs, especially blood pressure and heart rate.	Transection of the spinal cord above the T5 levels may result in vasodilation, decreased venous return, and hypotension. Sympathetic blockade may cause bradycardia.
Monitor ECG for changes in rhythm and conduction, and treat according to hospital protocol.	Sympathetic blockade may cause conduction problems such as escape rhythms, and vasovagal reflexes may provoke cardiac arrest.
Monitor hemodynamic parameters if feasible.	Fluid shifts, hypotension, and hemorrhage may be reflected in lowered pressures and lower cardiac output/index.
Administer oxygen as warranted, ensuring preoxygenation prior to suctioning or prolonged coughing exercises.	Assists in preventing hypoxia that can result in vasovagal reflex and cardiac arrest.
Administer vasopressors as warranted.	May be indicated if fluid resuscitation is not successful in maintaining systolic blood pressure above 90 mm Hg.
Administer IV fluids as ordered.	May require fluid replacement to maintain circulating volume and blood pressure.
Instruct patient in avoidance of Valsalva-type maneuvers.	May lower blood pressure and facilitate vasovagal response.

NIC: *Hemodynamic Regulation*

Discharge or Maintenance Evaluation

- Patient will exhibit no episodes of cardiac rhythm disturbances.
- Patient will have normotensive blood pressure with stable hemodynamic pressures.

- Patient will have optimal cardiac output and index.
- Patient will exhibit no hypoxic episodes and avoid desaturation with procedures.

INEFFECTIVE BREATHING PATTERN

Related to: trauma, spinal cord lesions at high levels, paralysis of respiratory musculature, ineffective coughing, pneumonia, pulmonary edema, pulmonary embolism

Defining Characteristics: dyspnea, use of accessory muscles, diaphragmatic breathing, decreased tidal volumes, sputum, abdominal distention, abnormal arterial blood gases, apnea, oxygen desaturation

Outcome Criteria

✔ Patient will maintain adequate oxygenation and ventilation without evidence of respiratory complications.

NOC: *Respiratory Status: Ventilation*

INTERVENTIONS	RATIONALES
Assess respiratory status for adequacy of airway and ventilation, rate, character, depth, increased work of breathing, or use of accessory muscles.	Spinal cord lesions below C4 level induce diaphragmatic breathing and hypoventilation. Patients with cervical cord lesions have paralysis of the abdominal and intercostal muscles, so as the patient inspires, the accessory muscles are used, and the diaphragm moves up, with inversion of the abdomen. The opposite occurs with expiration.
Auscultate lung fields for presence of adventitious sounds and other changes.	May reflect the presence of infiltrates, pneumonia, atelectasis, or fluid overload.
Assist with/measure pulmonary parameters, such as spontaneous tidal volume, vital capacity, and negative inspiratory force. Obtain arterial blood gases as warranted.	Measurement of pulmonary parameters may facilitate prompt identification of deterioration in respiratory status. ABGs are drawn to identify acid–base disturbances and hypoxemia that may result from restriction of lung expansion and ineffective cough mechanisms. Injuries below C4 level result in diaphragmatic breathing with

INTERVENTIONS	RATIONALES
	decreased tidal volumes and vital capacity.
Evaluate patient's ability to cough and assist with abdominal thrusting technique, or quad coughing, as warranted.	Paralysis of respiratory musculature may prevent sufficient pleural pressure to be produced to maintain effective cough. External technique can assist patient to cough effectively.
Monitor oxygen saturation continually and notify physician if levels stay below 90%.	Oximetry assists in identification of deterioration in ventilatory status, allowing for prompt intervention.
Suction patient only when required. Provide humidification of oxygen and utilize pulmonary toilette as required.	Suctioning may precipitate vasovagal reflexes, bradycardia, and cardiac arrest. Liquification of environmental air and secretions may prevent mucous plugs and thick mucoid secretions.
Prepare patient/family for placement on mechanical ventilation as warranted.	Hypoxemia that cannot be corrected with addition of supplemental oxygen may require intubation and ventilation to maintain airway and oxygenation.
Prepare patient for bronchoscopy as warranted.	May be required to remove obstructive secretions.
Monitor for signs/symptoms of pulmonary embolism, pneumonia, or pulmonary edema.	Edema may result from fluid resuscitation efforts, and pneumonia may develop from immobility and ineffective cough ability. Pulmonary emboli may result from venous thrombosis as a complication of immobility or hemorrhagic causes.
Instruct family member in techniques to assist patient with coughing, repositioning frequently, and suctioning techniques as warranted.	Provides information that will be used when patient is discharged and facilitates feelings of control over situation and self-esteem.

NIC: *Airway Management*

Discharge or Maintenance Evaluation

- Patient will maintain adequate airway and ventilation.
- Patient will exhibit no signs/symptoms of respiratory complications.
- Patient/family will be able to verbalize understanding of instructions and give adequate return demonstration.

INEFFECTIVE THERMOREGULATION

Related to: poikilothermism, injury to hypothalamic center or sensory pathways

Defining Characteristics: elevated body temperature, decreased body temperature, change of temperature based on environmental temperature

Outcome Criteria

✔ Patient will achieve and maintain core body temperature above 95 degrees.

NOC: *Thermoregulation*

INTERVENTIONS	RATIONALES
Monitor temperature every 2 hours until stabilized, then every 4 hours and prn.	Interruption of the sympathetic nervous system pathways to the temperature control center in the hypothalamus causes body temperature swings in an effort to match environmental temperatures.
Maintain a slightly cool environmental temperature. If patient is hypothermic, apply warm blanket.	Hyperthermia may occur during periods of spinal shock because the sympathetic activity is blocked and the patient does not perspire on paralyzed areas of body.
Instruct patient/family regarding variable body temperatures and methods to maintain comfort.	Provides knowledge and facilitates compliance.

NIC: *Temperature Regulation*

Discharge or Maintenance Evaluation

■ Patient will exhibit normal temperature and be able to maintain core body temperature using methods discussed.

IMPAIRED PHYSICAL MOBILITY

Related to: spinal cord lesion, trauma, paralysis, spasticity, physical restraint, traction

Defining Characteristics: contractures, inability to move as desired, spastic movements, muscle atrophy, muscle wasting, skin breakdown, redness, pressure areas

Outcome Criteria

✔ Patient will be able to achieve maximum mobility within limitations of paralysis and will avoid skin breakdown and contractures.

NOC: *Mobility Level*

INTERVENTIONS	RATIONALES
Assess motor strength and function at least every 4–8 hours, and prn. Identify level of tactile sensation, ability to move parts of body, spasticity, and so forth.	Identifies level of sensory–motor impairment and evaluates resolution of spinal shock. Specific injury level may have partially mixed or occult sensorimotor impairment.
Observe for muscle atrophy and wasting.	May be noted during flaccid paralysis stage of spinal shock.
Encourage independent activity as able.	C1–4 lesions result in quadriplegia with complete loss of respiratory function; C4–5 lesions result in quadriplegia with potential for phrenic nerve involvement that may result in loss of respiratory function; C5–6 lesions result in quadriplegia with some gross arm movement ability and some sparing of diaphragmatic muscle involvement; C6–7 lesions result in quadriplegia with intact biceps; C7–8 lesions result in quadriplegia with intact biceps and triceps but no intrinsic hand musculature intact; T1–L2 lesions result in paraplegia with variable amounts of involvement to intercostal and abdominal muscle groups; below L2 lesions result in mixed motor-sensory loss with bowel and bladder impairment.
Assist with/provide range of motion exercises to all joints.	Improves muscle tone and joint mobility, decreases risk for contractures, and prevents muscle atrophy.
Reposition every 2 hours and prn. Utilize kinetic bed therapy as warranted.	Decreases pressure on bony prominences and improves peripheral circulation. Kinetic beds can immobilize the unstable vertebral column and decrease potential for complications from immobility.

INTERVENTIONS	RATIONALES
Ensure proper alignment with each position.	Correct anatomic alignment prevents contractures and deformities.
Utilize footboards or high-top tennis shoes.	Prevents footdrop.
Observe for changes in skin status and provide frequent skin care.	Loss of sensation, paralysis, and decreased venous return predispose the patient for pressure wounds.
Assist with/consult physical therapists or occupational therapists to develop plan of care for patient.	Exercises help stimulate circulation and preserves joint mobility.
Maintain cervical traction apparatus as warranted.	Cervical traction provides for stabilization of vertebral column, reduction, and immobilization to maintain proper alignment. Halo brace/devices provide immobilization but can help facilitate patient with active participation with rehabilitation process.
Administer muscle relaxants as warranted.	May be required to reduce pain and spasticity.
Observe for redness and swelling to calf muscles. Measure circumference daily if problem is noted.	Thrombus formation may occur as a result of immobilization and flaccid paralysis.
Instruct family in rehabilitative therapy, exercises, and repositioning, and involve them with patient's care.	Facilitates adaptation to patient's health status and allows for family members to contribute to patient's welfare.
Avoid improper placement of footrests, headrests, or padding when repositioning patient.	May create pressure resulting in pressure sores or necrotic injury.
Instruct patient in methods for shifting weight.	Improves circulation by reducing pressure to body surfaces.

NIC: *Traction/Immobilization Care*

Discharge or Maintenance Evaluation

- Patient will maintain appropriate body alignment and maximal function within limit of injury.
- Patient will avoid complications of immobility.
- Patient will be able to verbalize understanding and demonstrate effective therapeutic modalities.
- Patient will exhibit suppleness of joints and muscles.

BOWEL INCONTINENCE

Related to: trauma, impairment of bowel innervation, impairment of perception, modifications of dietary intake, immobility

Defining Characteristics: inability to evacuate bowel voluntarily, inability to delay defecation, inability to feel rectal fullness, lack of urge to defecate, continual dribbling of soft or liquid stool, red perianal tissue, ileus, gastric distention, hypoactive bowel sounds, absent bowel sounds, nausea, vomiting, abdominal pain, constipation

Outcome Criteria

✔ Patient will be able to establish and maintain bowel elimination patterns.
✔ Patient/family will be able to perform bowel care routine with assistance as needed.

NOC: *Bowel Elimination*

INTERVENTIONS	RATIONALES
Observe for presence of abdominal distention.	Innervation may be impaired as a result of the injury with resultant decrease or loss of peristalsis, and potential for development of ileus. Bowel distention may precipitate autonomic dysreflexia after spinal shock recedes.
Auscultate for presence of bowel sounds, noting changes in character.	High-pitched tinkling bowel sounds may be heard when patient has an ileus, and bowel sounds may be absent during spinal shock phase.
Evaluate bowel habits, such as frequency, character, and amount of stools.	Establishes pattern and facilitates treatment options.
Establish bowel pattern by use of stool softeners, suppositories, or digital stimulation.	Effectively evacuates bowel. If anal reflex is intact, suppository insertion and response may be required. If patient has a flaccid rectal sphincter, enemas and/or digital removal of stool may be required. Regular patterns of evacuation encourage adaptation and routine physiologic bowel function, stimulates peristalsis, and promotes effective bowel elimination.

(continues)

(continued)

INTERVENTIONS	RATIONALES
Increase dietary bulk and fiber.	Promotes peristaltic movement through bowel and improves consistency of stool.
Provide frequent skin care.	Incontinence of stool increases potential for skin breakdown.
Instruct patient/family regarding method for daily bowel program.	Promotes independence and self-esteem.
Demonstrate and observe return demonstration from family regarding bowel care regime.	Decreases fear and anxiety, promotes knowledge of bowel routines, and involves family in giving care. Return demonstration allows for ensuring that family members understand regime and can adequately perform the care required.
Instruct patient/family in modifying diet to include foods and fluids that will promote elimination, and to avoid those that may result in diarrhea or constipation.	Identification of foods that irritate patient's system and cause painful flatulence and diarrhea allows for the elimination or minimization of use of these types of foods.
Instruct patient/family regarding use of protective padding and/or garments under clothing, and to change them frequently.	Helps to prevent leakage, patient embarrassment, odor, and skin breakdown.

NIC: *Bowel Incontinence Care*

Discharge or Maintenance Evaluation

- Patient/family will establish and maintain daily bowel pattern.
- Patient will be able to verbalize understanding and demonstrate appropriate methods to accomplish bowel care.
- Patient will be able to avoid complications that may be caused by gastric distention or ileus.

URINARY RETENTION

Related to: traumatic loss of bladder innervation, bladder atony

Defining Characteristics: urinary retention, incontinence, bladder distention, urinary tract infections, kidney dysfunction, stone formation, overflow syndrome, high urinary residual volume, continual urinary dribbling, bladder fullness, dysuria

Outcome Criteria

- ✔ Patient will be able to achieve and maintain balanced intake and output with no signs/symptoms of complications.
- ✔ Patient will not have bladder distention.
- ✔ Patient/family will be able to identify community and other resources for assistance post-discharge.

NOC: *Urinary Elimination*

INTERVENTIONS	RATIONALES
Monitor intake and output every shift, noting significant differences in amounts.	May identify urinary retention from an areflexic bladder.
Observe for ability to void and palpate for bladder distention. Insert Foley catheter as warranted.	Spinal shock is exhibited in the bladder when there is a loss of sensory perception and the bladder is unable to contract and empty itself. Bladder distention may precipitate autonomic dysreflexia.
Observe patient's voiding pattern.	Helps to identify pattern of incontinence.
Assist with bladder elimination procedures as ordered, such as Valsalva's maneuver every 3–4 hours, intermittent catheterization, or use of indwelling catheter.	Valsalva's maneuver helps to increase bladder pressure to pass urine. Intermittent catheterization every 2–4 hours helps to promote normal voiding, prevent infection from residual urine remaining in bladder, and helps to ensure integrity of ureterovesicular function. Indwelling catheter or suprapubic catheterization may be required to drain urine and decrease risk for development of bladder infection.
Encourage fluid intake, when appropriate, to at least 2–3 L/day, and attempt to limit fluid intake after 6 p.m.	Fluids help to maintain hydration and dilute toxic chemicals within the body. Avoidance of fluids in the evening, unless required, will help prevent nocturnia.
Monitor urinary output for changes in color or character.	Cloudiness, blood, concentration, or foul smell may indicate urinary tract infection.
Administer urinary antiseptic agents/acidifiers as ordered.	Vitamin C and mandelamine may be given to acidify the urine to hinder bacterial growth and prevent stone formation.

INTERVENTIONS	RATIONALES
Instruct patient/family in methods for intermittent catheterization when warranted.	Catheterization may be required for long-term due to injury and dysfunction to bladder. Intermittent catheterization is preferred and is performed at specific intervals to approximate physiological function and may decrease complications from indwelling catheter.
Increase fluid uptake, when warranted, up to 3–4 L/day, including acidic juices, such as cranberry juice.	Decreases formation of kidney and bladder stones, helps prevent infection, and ensures hydration.
Ensure sterile technique for catheter insertions.	Decreases potential for urinary tract infection.
Instruct patient/family in changing catheters, changing dressing to suprapubic catheter, avoidance of kinks in tubing, keeping drainage bag below the bladder level, methods of draining bag, use of leg bag, and taping of catheter tubing.	Promotes knowledge, reduces fear and anxiety, promotes comfort, and allows family to be a part of patient's care.
Instruct patient/family in sharing feelings and concerns about situation and provide opportunity for them to ask questions.	Verbalization allows patient and family to identify and address any fears they may have, and establishes trust. Allows for correction of misinformation or misperceptions.
Assist patient/family with consultation with community resources, such as counselors, enterostomal therapist, support groups, or home health care as needed.	Allows for assistance for patient to gain knowledge and independence with situation, and promotes personal growth. Community resources may provide services that the patient will require postdischarge, and support groups can be of benefit to both the patient and family to assist them in dealing with situational problems.

NIC: *Urinary Retention Care*

Discharge or Maintenance Evaluation

- Patient will have balanced intake and output without signs of urinary tract infection.
- Patient/family will be able to verbalize understanding of need for catheterization, and will be able to give return demonstration of procedure.

AUTONOMIC DYSREFLEXIA

Related to: spinal cord injury at T7 level and above, excessive autonomic reaction to stimulation

Defining Characteristics: hypertension, blurred vision, throbbing headache, diaphoresis above the level of the lesion, piloerection, nausea, bradycardia or tachycardia, red splotches on skin above injury level, pallor below injury, diffuse headache, chills, contracted pupils, partial ptosis, enophthalmos, paresthesias, blurred vision, chest pain, metallic taste, nasal congestion

Outcome Criteria

✔ Patient/nurse will be able to recognize signs/symptoms and take appropriate action to prevent complications.

✔ Cause of dysreflexia will be identified and eliminated/corrected.

✔ Patient will have few, if any, dysreflexia episodes.

✔ Patient will have vital signs within normal ranges.

NOC: *Neurologic Status*

INTERVENTIONS	RATIONALES
Observe for hypertension, tachycardia, bradycardia, sweating above level of lesion, pallor below level of injury, headache, piloerection, nasal congestion, metallic taste, blurred vision, chest pain, or nausea.	Identification of potential life-threatening complication facilitates prompt and timely intervention.
Assess for bowel or bladder distention, bladder spasms, or changes in temperature.	May be indicative of precipitating factor for autonomic dysreflexia.
Monitor vital signs frequently, especially blood pressure every 5 minutes during acute phase.	Hypotensive crisis may occur once stimulus is removed, but dysreflexia may recur and should be monitored.
Palpate abdomen *very* gently for bladder distention, and irrigate catheter *very* slowly with tepid solution.	Palpation should be done gently, if at all, so as to not increase stimulating factor and worsen condition. Irrigation may identify and correct catheter obstruction which may have been predisposing factor.
Check for rectal impaction *very* gently, and only after anesthetic-type rectal ointment has been applied.	May increase rectal stimulation and worsen dysreflexia.

(continues)

(continued)

INTERVENTIONS	RATIONALES
Position in high Fowler's position in bed.	Promotes decrease in blood pressure to avert intracranial hemorrhage or seizure activity. Position helps with venous drainage from brain, and lowers intracranial pressure, temporarily reducing blood pressure.
Administer medications as ordered.	Atropine may be required to increase heart rate if bradycardia is present; apresoline, hyperstat, or procardia may be required to decrease blood pressure.
Assess patient for any objects applying pressure to skin, or for cold drafts on patient.	May result in providing stimuli for dysreflexia.
If no other cause of dysreflexia is observed, obtain urine for analysis and culture.	Lack of other signs of dysreflexia may mean that patient has a urinary tract infection that has been undiagnosed.
Instruct patient/family on signs/ symptoms of syndrome, and methods for preventing occurrence.	Problem may be lifelong but can be prevented by avoiding pressure-causing sensation.
Administer antihypertensive drugs as ordered.	May be required for long-term use to alleviate chronic autonomic dysreflexia by relaxation of the bladder neck.

INTERVENTIONS	RATIONALES
Instruct patient/family about maintaining bowel and bladder regimes.	Lack of follow through with bowel/bladder elimination can result in stimuli that could cause a dysreflexic emergency.
Prepare patient for nerve block as warranted.	May be required if dysreflexia is unresponsive to other treatment modalities.

NIC: *Dysreflexia Management*

Discharge or Maintenance Evaluation

- Patient/family will be able to verbalize understanding of condition and methods to reduce occurrence.
- Patient will exhibit no signs/symptoms of autonomic dysreflexia, and have no complications.
- The cause of the autonomic dysreflexia will be identified and corrected in a timely manner.
- Patient will maintain bowel and bladder elimination programs.
- Patient's environment will have no noxious stimuli or pressure-causing objects.

SPINAL CORD INJURIES

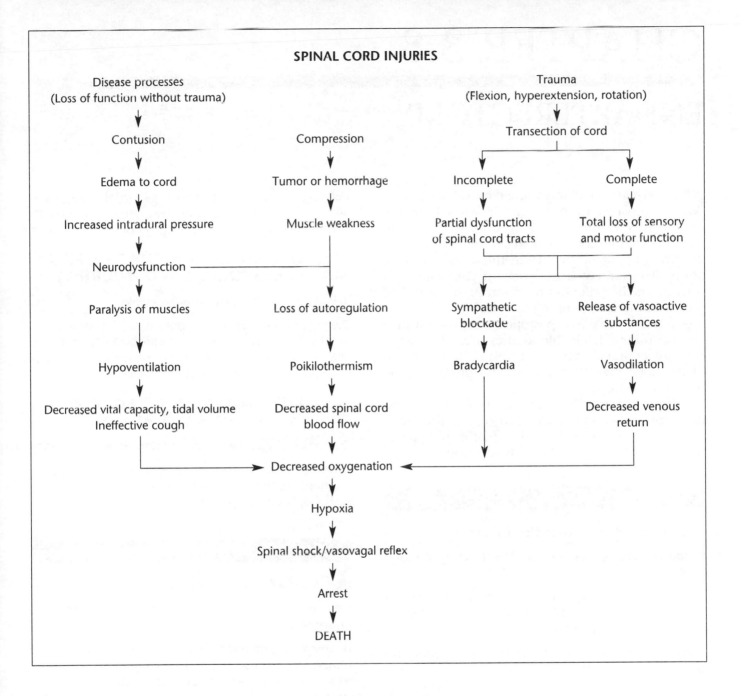

Disease processes
(Loss of function without trauma)

↓

Contution

↓

Edema to cord

↓

Increased intradural pressure

↓

Neurodysfunction ——————

↓

Paralysis of muscles

↓

Hypoventilation

↓

Decreased vital capacity, tidal volume
Ineffective cough

Compression

↓

Tumor or hemorrhage

↓

Muscle weakness

↓

Loss of autoregulation

↓

Poikilothermism

↓

Decreased spinal cord
blood flow

Trauma
(Flexion, hyperextension, rotation)

↓

Transection of cord

Incomplete   Complete

↓   ↓

Partial dysfunction   Total loss of sensory
of spinal cord tracts   and motor function

Sympathetic   Release of vasoactive
blockade   substances

↓   ↓

Bradycardia   Vasodilation

↓

Decreased venous
return

→ Decreased oxygenation ←

↓

Hypoxia

↓

Spinal shock/vasovagal reflex

↓

Arrest

↓

DEATH

CHAPTER 3.8

ENDARTERECTOMY

Carotid endarterectomy is the removal of a thrombus or plaque from the carotid artery to reduce the risk of stroke in patients who have had a transient ischemic attack (TIA). Circulation is augmented by increasing blood flow from the internal carotid artery. The surgery is not without risk of its own because of the potential for shearing off pieces of plaque or material resulting in a stroke.

Initially, the major postoperative problem may be controlling labile blood pressures that occur because of impairment in carotid sinus reflexes. These blood pressure variances also predispose the patient to a stroke.

Respiratory insufficiency may occur if the trachea is compressed or shifted by a growing hematoma at the wound site, or by lack of responses to hypoxia with impairment of carotid body function.

MEDICAL CARE

Surgery: performed as described above

Vasoactive drugs: may be required to control blood pressures

Laboratory: CBC used to identify potential bleeding problems, occult bleeding into neck; electrolytes used to identify imbalances

Arterial blood gases: used to identify hypoxemia and acid–base imbalances

COMMON NURSING DIAGNOSES

 ALTERATION IN TISSUE PERFUSION: CEREBRAL (see CVA)

Related to: occlusion, hemorrhage, vasospasms, cerebral edema, interruption of blood flow, surgery

Defining Characteristics: changes in vital signs, mental status changes, restlessness, anxiety, sensory deficits, confusion, decreased level of consciousness

DECREASED CARDIAC OUTPUT (see SPINAL CORD INJURIES)

Related to: vasospasm, surgery, stroke

Defining Characteristics: hypotension, hypertension, heart rate changes, decreased cardiac output/index, changes in systemic and peripheral vascular resistance, mental status changes, hypoxia

IMPAIRED SKIN INTEGRITY (see CARDIAC SURGERY)

Related to: surgical wounds, invasive lines, immobility

Defining Characteristics: presence of wounds, drainage, redness, swelling, abrasions, pressure, lacerations, bruises, open skin

ADDITIONAL NURSING DIAGNOSES

RISK FOR INJURY

Related to: surgery, predisposing health factors, injury to cranial nerves

Defining Characteristics: muscle weakness, nerve injury, airway obstruction, hypoxia, dysphagia, facial weakness, asymmetry of face, facial drooping, vocal cord paralysis

Outcome Criteria

✔ Patient will exhibit no complications from surgery and will have all cranial nerve function maintained.

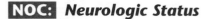 **NOC:** *Neurologic Status*

INTERVENTIONS	RATIONALES
Observe for deviation of tongue toward side of operation, or weakness of tongue muscles.	May indicate hypoglossal nerve damage.
Observe for dysphagia, dysphasia, or impairment of upper airway.	May indicate bilateral hypoglossal palsy.
Observe for facial asymmetry, drooping at corner of mouth, and inability to manage salivary secretions.	May indicate facial nerve damage.
Monitor for changes in voice quality and sound.	May indicate vocal cord paralysis, injury to the vagus nerve, or recurrent laryngeal nerve.

NIC: *Neurologic Monitoring*

Discharge or Maintenance Evaluation

- Patient will have facial symmetry and normal voice modulation.
- Patient will exhibit no signs/symptoms of cranial nerve injury.
- Patient will be free of any airway compromise and have stable vital signs.

UNIT 4

GASTROINTESTINAL/ HEPATIC SYSTEM

CHAPTER 4.1

GASTROINTESTINAL BLEEDING

Gastrointestinal bleeding may be massive and acute or occult and chronic in nature. GI bleeding results when irritation of the mucosal lining causes erosion through to the submucosal layer. Upper GI hemorrhage is considered to be a bleed from any site proximal to the cecum, and all ulcerative bleeding is arterial, with the exception of a tear that cuts across all vessels, malignant tumors, and in patients with esophagitis.

When erosion into an artery occurs, it usually produces two bleeding sites because of arterio-arterial anastomoses. When the bleeding occurs at the ulcer base artery, it may be a life-threatening emergency.

Bleeding may occur from the lower gastrointestinal tract as well. Causes of lower GI bleeding include hemorrhoids, diverticulosis, inflammatory bowel disease, rectal perforation, or intussusception.

Acute upper GI bleeding may result from many causes, such as gastritis, peptic ulcer, stress, drugs, hormones, trauma, head injuries, burns, and esophageal varices.

Differential diagnosis between gastric and duodenal ulcers must be obtained. Duodenal ulcers usually account for approximately 80% of all ulcers noted and rarely become cancerous. They are linked to increased hydrochloric acid levels as well, as with people with type A personalities, and the pylorus and first segment of the duodenum are the most common sites. Gastric ulcers, on the other hand, are related to a decrease in tissue resistance, and may become cancerous and are more likely to bleed.

Initial presenting symptoms of a GI bleed are either hematemesis, melena, or hematochezia. An acute bleed will have more than 60 cc/day of black tarry stool and usually greater than 500 cc, whereas occult bleeding is normally 15–30 cc/day. Stools can be positive for occult blood up to 12 days after an acute bleed. Of all GI hemorrhages, 80% usually stop spontaneously.

The goal of treatment is initially prevention and treatment of shock, with fluid volume replacement. Maintenance of circulating blood volume is imperative to prevent myocardial infarction, sepsis, and death. Endoscopic examination is the primary diagnostic procedure utilized. Once the lesion has been identified, treatment is used to control bleeding.

MEDICAL CARE

Laboratory: CBC to identify changes in blood volume and concentration, but may be normal during rapid loss because of the lapsed time required for equilibration of intravascular with extravascular spaces; MCV is useful to identify prolonged chronic loss with iron deficiency; B_{12} and folic acid levels used to identify anemia type; reticulocyte count may identify new RBC formation which occurs with an old bleed; platelet count, PT, PTT, and bleeding times to evaluate clotting status and platelet dysfunction; BUN and creatinine to evaluate effect on renal status; electrolytes to evaluate imbalances and treatment; ammonia levels may be used to identify liver dysfunction; gastric analysis to determine presence of blood and assess secretory activity of gastric mucosa; amylase elevated if duodenal ulcer has posterior penetration; pepsinogen level to help identify type of bleeding, with elevation seen in duodenal ulcer, and decreased levels seen in gastritis; guaiac testing used on nasogastric and stool specimens to identify blood; *Helicobacter pylori* testing for bacterial cause of ulceration

Arterial blood gases: may be used to show acid–base imbalances, compensation for decreased blood flow; initially respiratory alkalosis changing to metabolic acidosis as metabolic wastes accumulate

Esophagogastroduodenoscopy (EGD): primary diagnostic tool utilized for upper GI bleeding to visually identify lesion; can be performed as soon as lavage controls bleeding

Colonoscopy: used to evaluate lower gastrointestinal bleeding, perform biopsies, or remove polyps

Angiography: used when bleeding cannot be cleared for endoscopy; can identify bleeding site and allow for injection of vasopressin for active mucosal bleeding

Radiography: chest X-rays may be done to evaluate for free air/perforation; upper GI series may be done after endoscopy, but is never done before since the contrast media will adhere to mucosa and prevent further examination; may be done to identify other diagnosis; barium enema may be done once lower GI bleeding is stopped; radionuclide scanning, such as red cell tags, identify source of bleeding, but may take an extended time for results to show

Electrocardiogram: used to identify changes in heart rate and rhythm and identify conduction problems or dysrhythmias that may occur with fluid shifting or electrolyte imbalances

Blood products: blood, plasma, and platelets may be required for replacement based on severity of bleed

Nasogastric tubes: large bore NG tube or Ewald tube is usually inserted to allow for iced/saline lavage, confirmation of bleeding, and for decompression of stomach

Levophed: may be used in solution with saline for lavage when plain saline is not effective in stopping bleeding because of its vasoconstrictor effects

Vasopressin: may be used for direct infusion into the gastric artery to control bleeding, or via intravenous route for specified length of time

Antacids: used to alter pH so that platelets can aggregate and stop bleeding, and to prevent digestion of raw mucosal surfaces

Histamine antagonists: drugs such as cimetidine (Tagamet), famotidine (Pepcid), lansoprazole (Prevacid), misoprostol (Cytotec), nizatidine (Axid), omeprazole (Prilosec), pantoprazole sodium (Prontonix), rabeprazole sodium (Aciphex), or ranitidine (Tritec, Zantac) used to decrease acid secretion or inhibit ATP-ase pump

Sucralfate: used to help heal ulcer by forming protective barrier at site

Surgery: required in fewer than 10% of patients; may be necessary for control of hemorrhage

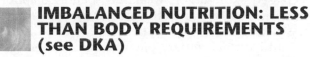

COMMON NURSING DIAGNOSES

IMBALANCED NUTRITION: LESS THAN BODY REQUIREMENTS (see DKA)

Related to: nausea, vomiting, nasogastric tube, inadequate intake, decreased absorption of nutrients, increased metabolic needs, gastric distress, trauma, surgery

Defining Characteristics: inability to ingest adequate amounts of food, weakness, fatigue, weight loss, decreased muscle mass, loss of subcutaneous fat, lethargy, ascites, poor wound healing, swelling of mouth and/or lips, poor dentition, bleeding gums, third spacing of fluids, fever, increased BUN, increased lactate levels

ACUTE PAIN (see MI)

Related to: muscle spasms, ulceration, gastric mucosal irritation, presence of invasive lines, surgery, or trauma

Defining Characteristics: verbalization of pain, facial grimacing, changes in vital signs, abdominal guarding

ANXIETY (see MI)

Related to: change in environment, change in health status, fear of the unknown, life-threatening crisis

Defining Characteristics: tension, irritability, restlessness, anxiousness, fearfulness, tremors, tachycardia, tachypnea, diaphoresis

DEFICIENT KNOWLEDGE (see MI)

Related to: hypoxia, lack of blood volume, lack of information, lack of understanding of medical condition, lack of recall

Defining Characteristics: verbalized questions regarding disease, care or instructions, inadequate follow-up on instructions given, misconceptions, development of preventable complications

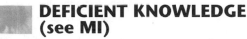

ADDITIONAL NURSING DIAGNOSES

DEFICIENT FLUID VOLUME

Related to: gastrointestinal bleeding, hemorrhage, sepsis, third spacing

Defining Characteristics: hypotension, tachycardia, decreased skin turgor, weakness, pallor, diaphoresis, decreased capillary refill, mental changes, restlessness, decreased filling pressures, decreased cardiac output and cardiac index, oliguria, anuria, increased specific gravity, increased BUN and creatinine, hypernatremia, hematemesis, melena, bloody drainage, decreased hemoglobin and hematocrit, decreased platelet count, increased clotting time, hypothermia, metabolic acidosis, fever, cyanosis, dyspnea, hypoxemia

Outcome Criteria

✔ Patient will have no further bleeding and vital signs will be stable.

✔ Patient will achieve and maintain adequate circulating fluid and blood volume.

NOC: *Fluid Balance*

NOC: *Coagulation Status*

INTERVENTIONS	RATIONALES
Monitor vital signs, including orthostatic changes when feasible.	Patients with major GI blood losses will present with supine hypotension and resting tachycardia greater than 110/min, orthostatic DBP decreases of at least 10 mm Hg, and orthostatic pulse increases of at least 15/min. Changes in vital signs may help approximate amount of blood loss and reflect decreasing circulating blood volume.
Monitor hemodynamic parameters when possible.	Facilitates early identification of fluid shifts. CVP values between 4–18 cm H_2O are considered adequate circulating volume.
Insert nasogastric tube for acute bleeding episodes, and monitor drainage for changes in bleeding character.	Facilitates removal of gastric contents, blood, and clots, relieves gastric distention, decreases nausea and vomiting, and provides for lavaging of stomach. Blood that is left in stomach can be metabolized into ammonia and can result in neurologic encephalopathy.
Actively lavage stomach via NG tube per hospital protocol with cold or room temperature saline until return is light pink or clear.	Saline solution is utilized to reduce washout of electrolytes that may occur with use of water. Flushing facilitates removal of clots to assist with visualization of bleeding site, and may assist with control of

INTERVENTIONS	RATIONALES
	bleeding through vasoconstrictive effect. The current consensus of opinion is that differences between using cold versus room temperature solutions is negligible, and in fact, iced solution may actually inhibit platelet function by lowering core body temperature.
Notify physician if bleeding clears and then becomes bright red again.	May indicate further bleeding or renewed bleeding.
Monitor intake and output, including amounts of lavage solution, bloody aspirate, blood products, and vomitus.	Helps facilitate estimation of fluid replacement required. Lavage amounts facilitate estimation of the magnitude of bleeding based on the volume of solution needed to clear the gastric return, and how long lavage is required before the aspirate clears.
Administer IV fluids through large bore catheters as ordered. Many facilities recommend at least two lines for active bleeding.	Facilitates rapid replacement of circulating volume prior to availability of blood products. Solutions of choice are normal saline or Ringer's lactate, and should be run wide open until blood pressure is stabilized, and titrated to match volume requirements after that.
Administer blood transfusions, fresh frozen plasma, platelets, or whole blood as ordered.	Fresh whole blood may be ordered when bleeding is acute and patient is in shock so as to ensure that clotting factors are not deficient. Packed red blood cells are utilized most often for replacement, especially when fluid shifting may create overload. Frequently, fresh frozen plasma (FFP) will be concurrently administered to replace clotting factors and facilitate cessation of an acute bleed. For each unit of blood that is transfused, a 3 point increase in the hematocrit should be noted. If this elevation is not noted, continued bleeding should be suspected.
Administer albumin as ordered.	May be used for volume expansion until blood products are available.
Administer vasopressin as ordered.	Intra-arterial infusion may be required for severe active bleeding and patient must be monitored closely for development of complications from the infusion.

INTERVENTIONS	RATIONALES
	Rates are usually 0.1–0.5 units/min into the artery supplying blood or peripherally at 0.3–1.5 units/min.
Administer histamine blockers and/or gastric acid pump inhibitors as ordered.	Histamine blockers decrease acid production, increase pH, and decrease gastric mucosal irritation. Gastric acid pump inhibitors can completely inhibit acid secretion.
Administer sucralfate as ordered.	Decreases gastric acid secretion and provides a protective layer over the ulcer site. May decrease or inhibit absorption of other medications.
Administer antacids as ordered.	Facilitates maintenance of pH level to decrease chance of rebleeding
Monitor lab work for changes and/or trends.	Hemoglobin and hematocrit help to identify blood replacement needs, but may not initially change as a result of loss of plasma and RBCs. BUN levels greater than 40 in the presence of normal creatinine may signify major bleeding, and BUN should normalize within 12 hours after bleeding has ceased.
Administer antibiotics when ordered.	May be indicated when infection is thought to be the cause of the gastritis or ulcer.
Assist with and prepare patient for EGD/sclerotherapy.	EGD provides direct visualization of an upper GI bleeding site, and a sclerosing substance may be injected at site to stop bleeding or prevent a recurrence.
Prepare patient for surgery.	May be required to control gastric hemorrhage. Vagotomy, pyloroplasty, oversewing of the ulcer, and total or subtotal gastrectomy may be procedure of choice based on severity of bleeding.

NIC: *Bleeding Reduction: Gastrointestinal*

Discharge or Maintenance Evaluation

- Patient will have stable fluid balance with normal vital signs and hemodynamic parameters.
- Patient will have adequate urine output.

- Patient will have no complications from fluid or blood replacement therapy.
- Patient will have lab work within normal limits.
- Patient will have no active bleeding or occult blood in stools.

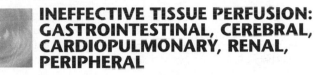

INEFFECTIVE TISSUE PERFUSION: GASTROINTESTINAL, CEREBRAL, CARDIOPULMONARY, RENAL, PERIPHERAL

Related to: hypovolemia, hypoxia, vasoconstrictive therapy

Defining Characteristics: decreased blood pressure, tachycardia, decreased peripheral pulses, decreased hemodynamic pressures, abnormal ABGs, abdominal pain, decreased urine output, confusion, mental status changes, dyspnea, headache

Outcome Criteria

✔ Patient will have adequate tissue perfusion to all body systems.

NOC: *Tissue Perfusion*

INTERVENTIONS	RATIONALES
Perform neurological checks every 4 hours and prn. Notify physician of changes in mentation or level of consciousness.	Decreases in blood pressure may result in decreased cerebral perfusion that may cause confusion. Increases in ammonia levels from residual blood may result in cerebral encephalopathy.
Monitor for complaints of increasing severity of abdominal pain, as well as pain radiating to shoulders.	May indicate ischemia and necrosis from vasoconstrictive medication which may result when intra-arterial catheter is displaced, or may indicate peritonitis or further bleeding.
Monitor ECG for changes and treat according to hospital protocols.	Decreased blood pressure, electrolyte imbalances, hypoxemia, or response to cold injectate solution may cause cardiac dysrhythmias or changes with perfusion loss.
Palpate peripheral pulses for presence and character of pulses. Monitor for changes in color and temperature of extremities.	Decreased circulating blood volume may result in peripheral vasoconstriction and shunting to core.
Monitor urine output for decreases or changes in color or	Renal perfusion may be affected by hypovolemia.

(continues)

(continued)

INTERVENTIONS	RATIONALES
specific gravity. Notify physician for abnormalities.	
Monitor for complaints of chest pain.	Myocardial ischemia and infarction may result if hypovolemic state decreases perfusion to crisis state.
Provide continuous pulse oximetry and notify physician for level below 90%.	Facilitates early identification of hypoxia and allows for timely intervention.

NIC: *Circulatory Care*

Discharge or Maintenance Evaluation

- Patient will have stable vital signs and hemodynamic parameters.
- Patient will have adequate and stable intake and output.
- Patient will have ABGs within normal limits, with no respiratory insufficiency or distress noted.
- Patient will have equally palpable pulses with equal color and temperature bilaterally to extremities.

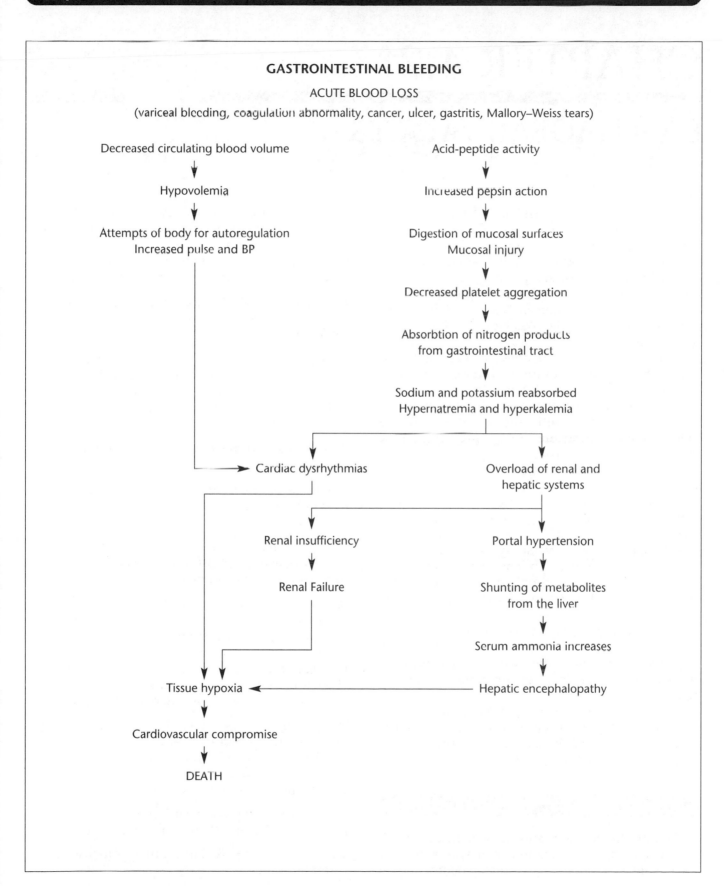

GASTROINTESTINAL BLEEDING

ACUTE BLOOD LOSS

(variceal bleeding, coagulation abnormality, cancer, ulcer, gastritis, Mallory–Weiss tears)

Decreased circulating blood volume

Hypovolemia

Attempts of body for autoregulation
Increased pulse and BP

Acid-peptide activity

Increased pepsin action

Digestion of mucosal surfaces
Mucosal injury

Decreased platelet aggregation

Absorbtion of nitrogen products
from gastrointestinal tract

Sodium and potassium reabsorbed
Hypernatremia and hyperkalemia

Cardiac dysrhythmias

Overload of renal and
hepatic systems

Renal insufficiency

Portal hypertension

Renal Failure

Shunting of metabolites
from the liver

Serum ammonia increases

Tissue hypoxia ◄─── Hepatic encephalopathy

Cardiovascular compromise

DEATH

CHAPTER 4.2

ESOPHAGEAL VARICES

Esophageal varices are twisting, dilated veins that are found in the gastrointestinal tract, but most frequently develop in the submucosal areas of the lower esophagus. Most esophageal varices occur as a result from liver disease and portal hypertension and the development of collateral esophageal veins. When these veins become eroded, the ensuing rupture causes extensive vigorous bleeding that is difficult to control.

Normally, the patient does not exhibit symptoms until coughing, vomiting, alcohol, or gastritis causes the varices to bleed. Mortality rates are high (above 60%) due to other complications of liver dysfunction, sepsis, or renal failure. Blood loss may be sudden, massive, and life-threatening, with shock and hypovolemia occurring.

Nearly all patients with esophageal varices have at least one of these precipitating factors: cirrhosis, Budd–Chiari syndrome (hepatic vein thrombosis), portal vein thrombosis, hepatic fibrosis, schistosomiasis, hepatic venous outflow obstruction, or splenic vein or superior vena caval abnormalities.

Variceal bleeding may be complex and other disease states must be ruled out, such as peptic ulcer disease, Mallory–Weiss tears of the esophagus, gastritis, or spontaneous esophageal rupture.

The initial goal of treatment is to replace blood loss and prevent shock from hypovolemia. Balloon tamponade, utilizing the Sengstaken–Blakemore or Minnesota tube, may be required to produce hemostasis.

Complications that occur in conjunction with bleeding may become irreversible and lethal, such as hepatic coma, renal failure, myocardial infarction, or congestive heart failure.

MEDICAL CARE

Laboratory: hemoglobin and hematocrit decreased; BUN increased; liver function tests may be abnormal due to liver involvement and disease; sodium may be elevated; clotting studies may be abnormal due to liver involvement; ammonia may be elevated; stools for guaiac; bilirubin may be elevated if cirrhosis is a factor; ALT and AST may be elevated; alkaline phosphatase may be elevated; platelets may be decreased

Esophagogastroduodenoscopy (EGD): used to identify and sometimes treat variceal bleeding with sclerotherapy

Radiography: arteriogram used to identify tortuous portal or hepatic veins, assess patency of blood flow, and measure the pressure gradients; chest X-ray used to identify other complicating problems with respiratory system

CT scan: used to rule out hepatomas and to identify cirrhosis

Arterial blood gases: may be used to identify acid–base imbalances; may show metabolic acidosis with bleeding

Nasogastric tube: used to keep stomach clear of blood and for lavage, but must be inserted cautiously so as to refrain from increasing bleeding

Balloon tamponade: Sengstaken–Blakemore (SB) or Minnesota tube is a multilumen tube that exerts pressure on part of the stomach and against bleeding varices to help control bleeding, and allows for removal of stomach contents; caution must be exercised as placement of this tube can create complications such as airway occlusion or esophageal rupture

Vasopressin: may be used as infusion through superior mesenteric artery or a peripheral vein to decrease splanchnic blood flow and promote hemostasis; may induce water intoxication or accentuate cardiac disease by increasing systemic vascular resistance

Nitroglycerin: may be used in conjunction with vasopressin to balance systemic vasoconstriction

Vitamin K: may be used to counteract increased prothrombin time

Cathartics: magnesium citrate or sobitol may be used to decrease risk of ammonia-induced neuroencephalopathy

Surgery: may require distal splenorenal shunt, mesocaval and portocaval anastomoses, or devascularization of the varices all in the effort to lower pressure in the portal system

 ## COMMON NURSING DIAGNOSES

(Care plans in GI bleeding section also apply to this diagnosis)

 ## INEFFECTIVE TISSUE PERFUSION: GASTROINTESTINAL, CARDIOPULMONARY, PERIPHERAL, RENAL (see GI BLEEDING)

Related to: variceal bleeding

Defining Characteristics: decreased peripheral pulses, hypotension, tachycardia initially, bradycardia, cold and clammy skin, diaphoresis, mental status changes, lethargy, pallor, abnormal ABGs, decreased oxygen saturation, decreased urine output

 ## DECREASED CARDIAC OUTPUT (see CARDIOGENIC SHOCK)

Related to: variceal bleeding, hemorrhage, exsanguination

Defining Characteristics: decreased peripheral pulses, hypotension, tachycardia, cold and clammy skin, decreased urinary output, mental status changes, pallor

INEFFECTIVE COPING (see MECHANICAL VENTILATION)

Related to: bleeding disorder, alcohol abuse, hepatic disease

Defining Characteristics: history of excessive alcohol usage, anxiety, fear, hostility, manipulative behavior, guilt, rationalization, blaming behavior

ADDITIONAL NURSING DIAGNOSES

RISK FOR INJURY

Related to: utilization of balloon tamponade to control esophageal bleeding

Defining Characteristics: increased bleeding, exsanguination, tube migration, air leakage, esophageal necrosis, encephalopathy, airway occlusion, asphyxia

Outcome Criteria

✔ Patient will be free of complications and injury to self.

NOC: *Risk Detection*

INTERVENTIONS	RATIONALES
Examine Sengstaken–Blakemore (or other type tube) balloons by testing inflation of balloons with air while tube is underwater.	Facilitates easier detection of leaks by escaping air bubbling, and ensures balloons are patent prior to insertion of tube into patient.
Refrigerate tube prior to insertion, and assist physician with insertion of tube into patient's nose/mouth by encouraging swallowing small sips of water.	Chilling firms the tube to facilitate easier placement.
Ensure that tube is patent in stomach by auscultating stomach for injected air bolus.	Proper positioning is crucial to ensure that the gastric tube is not inflated in the esophagus.
Obtain KUB X-ray after placement and securing of tube.	Verifies correct anatomical placement.
When placement is verified, inflate the gastric balloon with air and gently pull the tube back against the gastroesophageal junction. Secure tube, marking location at the nares, and clamp the gastric balloon.	Applies pressure against the cardia to attempt to control bleeding. Marking the tube facilitates prompt detection of accidental migration.
Balloon tubes should be adequately secured with some device (frequently used is a football helmet with face guard) with slight traction to the balloon tube.	Facilitates stable position of tube and prevents migration due to peristalsis or coughing, while exerting appropriate pull/pressure on anatomical sites.
Attach a Y-connector to the esophageal balloon opening, with a syringe on one side, and a manometer to the other. Fill balloon with air until manometer reading is between 25–35 mm Hg and clamp balloon.	Maintains sufficient pressure to tamponade bleeding with pressure lower than level that may result in esophageal ischemia and necrosis.
Connect gastric port to intermittent suction and irrigate every hour.	Facilitates removal of old blood from stomach, allows observation of changes in bleeding, and relieves gastric distention.
Insert nasogastric tube above the level of the esophageal balloon and connect to intermittent suction. If tamponade tube has an esophageal suction port, attach it to intermittent suction.	Facilitates removal of salivary secretions and monitors for bleeding above the esophageal balloon, and reduces aspiration risk.

(continues)

(continued)

INTERVENTIONS	RATIONALES
Clearly identify and label each port, checking connections frequently, and have scissors and resuscitative equipment at bedside.	Proper identification may prevent accidental deflation or improper irrigation. If the esophageal balloon migrates to the hypopharynx, the esophageal balloon must be cut immediately and removed to prevent airway obstruction.
Monitor for complaints of chest pain.	May indicate complication or esophageal rupture.
Monitor respiratory status for any changes, decrease in oxygen saturations, or changes in mental status.	May result from tube migration and asphyxia.
Keep head of bed elevated at least 30 degrees at all times.	Prevents regurgitation and decreases nausea.
Compare character and amounts of drainage coming from each lumen.	Facilitates identification of cessation of bleeding, as well as potentially identifying level of bleeding site.
Deflate esophageal balloon for 30 minutes every 12 hours, or as indicated per hospital protocol.	Decreases risk for esophageal mucosal ischemia and damage.
Instruct patient/family regarding need for balloon tamponade, procedure of insertion, what to expect, etc.	Promotes knowledge and facilitates compliance. Decreases fear of the unknown.
Observation of patient should be constant.	Deterioration in patient's status can occur rapidly and continuous observation facilitates prompt intervention to prevent injury.

NIC: *Hemorrhage Control*

Discharge or Maintenance Evaluation

- Patient will have bleeding from varices controlled with no injury or complication from treatment modalities.
- Patient will be able to comply with treatment.
- Patient will have stable vital signs and oxygenation.

RISK FOR DEFICIENT FLUID VOLUME

Related to: hemorrhage, gastrointestinal fluid loss, third space shifting

Defining Characteristics: hematemesis, melena, bloody drainage, changes in mental status, anxiety, decreased urinary output, concentrated urine, dry mucous membranes, dry skin, poor skin turgor, dry mouth, weight loss, thirst, weakness, decreased hemoglobin and hematocrit, increased blood pressure initially, with hypotension as a late sign, decreased pulse pressure and volume, decreased venous filling, abnormal electrolytes, increased BUN, decreased platelets and fibrinogen, tachycardia, dyspnea, metabolic acidosis

Outcome Criteria

✔ Patient will be free of esophageal variceal bleeding, with stable vital signs and hemodynamics.

NOC: *Fluid Balance*

INTERVENTIONS	RATIONALES
Monitor vital signs and hemodynamic readings q 1 hour and prn. Notify physician for significant abnormalities.	Changes in VS, such as tachycardia, hypotension, or dyspnea may indicate hypovolemic state from loss of blood.
Monitor I&O q 1 hour, including all irrigation solutions, aspirate, and blood loss.	Decreased urinary output may indicate hypovolemia. All amounts of fluids, including drainage and irrigation fluids should be carefully measured/estimated to provide a complete and accurate idea of fluid status.
If patient has wounds with copious amounts of drainage, use ostomy bags for collection, or if that is not feasible, weigh dressings at least q 8 hours and record output.	Excess drainage from wounds can also result in substantial fluid imbalances (1 kg dressing equals approximately 1 L of fluid.)
Administer IV fluids as ordered. Two separate IV sites should be used, with large gauge needles.	Allows for fluid hydration, maintenance of circulating fluid volume, and provides access for administration of emergency drugs and blood products.
Administer packed red blood cells, platelets, fresh frozen plasma, and clotting factors as ordered.	Replaces volume and blood that may be life-sustaining. Fresh frozen plasma helps to correct coagulopathies.
Maintain patent airway. Auscultate lung fields at least q 4 hours, and prn, and monitor saturation by oximetry. Notify physician if <90%.	Massive bleeding may result in aspiration, hypoxia, hypoxemia, and respiratory failure. Rapid transfusions may result in fluid shifting and fluid imbalances that will present as dyspnea with crackles (rales). Intubation and mechanical ventilation may be required if case is severe.

INTERVENTIONS	RATIONALES
Administer vasopressin as ordered.	May be required to halt bleeding. Angiographic therapy with intra-arterial infusions of vasopressin may be used, but should be observed for complications, such as necrosis.
Assist with, and provide balloon tamponade to varices using Sengstaken–Blakemore or Minnesota tube.	Attempts to control variceal bleeding by application of pressure using balloons on the tube against the areas of bleeding.
Instruct patient/family in use of blood products and IV fluids.	Promotion of hydration and maintenance of circulation of blood and fluid volume is essential for life. Preparation helps promote knowledge and compliance.
Instruct patient/family regarding use of Sengstaken–Blakemore or Minnesota tube.	Reduces fear, promotes knowledge, and assists in alleviating fear.
Prepare patient/family for surgical procedures.	If bleeding cannot be controlled via a pharmacologic method, surgery may be necessary to limit volume depletion. Surgical shunts procedures, such as a splenorenal shunt usually controls bleeding in about 90% of cases. Sometimes surgical devascularization is required if a shunt procedure is not appropriate and if bleeding is not controllable.

NIC: *Hypovolemia Management*

Discharge or Maintenance Evaluation

- Patient will have patent airway with clear lung fields to auscultation.

- Patient will have stable vital signs and hemodynamics and perfusion to all organs will be maintained.

- Patient will have normalized hemoglobin and hematocrit, and circulation fluid and blood volume will be adequate to meet his needs.

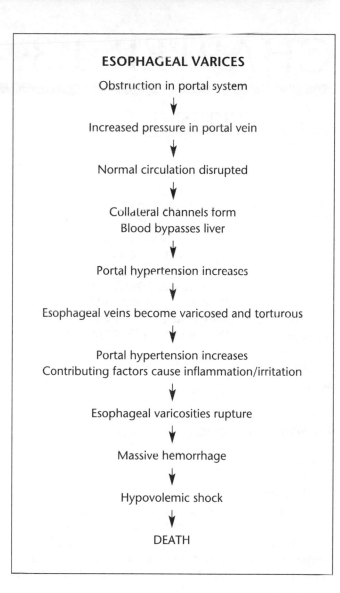

ESOPHAGEAL VARICES

Obstruction in portal system
↓
Increased pressure in portal vein
↓
Normal circulation disrupted
↓
Collateral channels form
Blood bypasses liver
↓
Portal hypertension increases
↓
Esophageal veins become varicosed and torturous
↓
Portal hypertension increases
Contributing factors cause inflammation/irritation
↓
Esophageal varicosities rupture
↓
Massive hemorrhage
↓
Hypovolemic shock
↓
DEATH

CHAPTER 4.3

HEPATITIS

Acute hepatitis is an infection of the liver that usually is viral in origin but may be induced by drugs or toxins, or may be related to an autoimmune process. There are currently five types of hepatitis, denoted HAV, HBV, NANB or hepatitis C, HDV, and HEV, with HAV being the most common type. Hepatitis B, or HBV, is more severe and because it can be acquired from exposure to individuals who are asymptomatic, the potential for transmission is increased many-fold.

Hepatitis A, or HAV, is transmitted via the fecal–oral route, with poor sanitation practices, with contamination of food, water, milk, and shellfish, or oral–anal sexual practices. HAV patients may exhibit no acute symptoms or have symptoms that are related to other causes. Formerly called infectious hepatitis, it is frequently misdiagnosed as an acute gastroenteritis because it is usually self-limiting.

Hepatitis B, or HBV, is transmitted via blood and blood products, breaks in the skin or mucous membranes, or from an asymptomatic carrier with Hepatitis B surface antigen (HBsAg). Formerly called serum hepatitis, it is actually a DNA virus that is transmitted by contaminated equipment, blood and blood products, promiscuous homosexual or heterosexual liaisons, IV drug abuse, and in mother-to-neonate transmission. Hepatitis B is associated with hepatitis D, which is an RNA virus that requires replication when activated by hepatitis B.

Hepatitis C, formerly non-A, non-B hepatitis, is transmitted via intravenous drug use, sexual contact, blood or blood products, and from asymptomatic carriers. It is an RNA virus and half of these cases have no known cause. This type also accounts for 90% or more of all posttransfusion hepatitis types, and is more chronic if related to a transfusion.

Hepatitis D, or HDV, is transmitted through the same routes as HBV but must have hepatitis B surface antigen to replicate. It is essential to Hepatitis D that it coexist with Hepatitis B because the delta virus is unable to replicate on its own and can only be activated with Hepatitis B infection.

Hepatitis E, or HEV, is seen in developing countries and not encountered in the United States. It is transmitted through food or water contamination. Formerly called epidemic non-A, non-B hepatitis, it is an RNA virus and thus similar in transmission to hepatitis A, but is more prevalent in younger adults.

Other types of hepatitis include non-A, non-B, non-C, hepatitis F, and hepatitis G. All of these deal with some type of virus in the herpesvirus group.

Once the disease has been contracted, treatment is symptomatic. Prophylactic therapy may assist in prevention of hepatitis from developing after being exposed to the virus. Immune globulin (IG) is generally given to provide temporary passive immunity. Hepatitis B vaccine provides active immunity and offers protection to people who are at high risk.

MEDICAL CARE

Laboratory: CBC shows decreased RBCs as a result of decreased life span from enzyme alterations or from hemorrhage; white blood cell count usually shows leukocytosis, atypical lymphocytes, and plasma cells; liver function studies are abnormal, up to 10 times normal values in some cases; decreased albumin, blood glucose may be decreased or elevated transiently because of liver dysfunction; Anti-HAV IgM presence shows either current infection or after 6 weeks, may indicate immunity; hepatitis B surface antigen and hepatitis Be antigen show presence of HBV; Anti-HBc in serum indicates carrier status; Anti-HBsAg indicates HBV immunity; antidelta antibodies present without HBsAg indicates HDV; urine bilirubin elevated; prothrombin time may be elevated with liver dysfunction; serology testing used to determine type of hepatitis

Liver biopsy: may be used to delineate type of hepatitis and degree of liver necrosis

Liver scans: may be performed to identify level of parenchymal damage

COMMON NURSING DIAGNOSES

SOCIAL ISOLATION (see TRANSPLANTS)

Related to: changes in health status, changes in physical status, imposed physical isolation, inadequate support system

Defining Characteristics: feelings of loneliness, feelings of rejection, absence of family members/friends, sad, dull affect, inappropriate behaviors

IMBALANCED NUTRITION: LESS THAN BODY REQUIREMENTS (see LIVER FAILURE)

Related to: metabolism changes, anorexia, tissue destruction

Defining Characteristics: nausea, vomiting, anorexia, abdominal pressure, malabsorption of fats, altered metabolism of protein, carbohydrates, and fat, weight loss, fatigue, edema

RISK FOR INFECTION (see TRANSPLANTS)

Related to: leukopenia, immunosuppression, malnutrition, exposure to causative organisms

Defining Characteristics: increased white blood cells, differential with a shift to the left, fever, chills, hypotension, tachycardia, positive cultures

RISK FOR IMPAIRED SKIN INTEGRITY (see LIVER FAILURE)

Related to: bile salt accumulations on skin

Defining Characteristics: jaundice, pruritus, itching, scratching

ADDITIONAL NURSING DIAGNOSES

ACTIVITY INTOLERANCE

Related to: infective process, decreased endurance

Defining Characteristics: easy fatiguability, lethargy, malaise, decreased muscle strength, reluctance to perform activity

Outcome Criteria

✔ Patient will achieve and maintain ability to perform normal activities without intolerance and fatigue.

NOC: *Endurance*

INTERVENTIONS	RATIONALES
Maintain bed rest and quiet environment, allowing rest periods between activities.	Decreases energy expenditure that is needed for healing. Activity can decrease hepatic blood flow and prevent circulation and healing to liver cells.
Reposition every 2 hours and provide good skin care.	Decreases potential for skin breakdown.
Increase activities as patient is able to tolerate.	Assists with return to optimal activity levels while enabling patient to have some measure of control over the situation.
Monitor lab work for liver function studies.	May assist with identification of appropriate levels of activity.
Administer medications as warranted.	Sedatives and antianxiety drugs may be required to effect needed rest. Caution should be taken to ensure drugs used are not hepatotoxic.
Administer antidotes/therapeutic treatment modalities to remove causative agent with toxic hepatitis.	Removal of substance may restrict amounts of tissue damage.
Instruct patient/family on disease process and need for extended rest.	Promotes knowledge and facilitates compliance with treatment.

NIC: *Exercise Promotion*

Discharge or Maintenance Evaluation

■ Patient will be able to verbalize understanding of disease process and treatment program.

■ Patient will be able to perform usual activities without fatigue.

■ Patient will be able to gradually increase level of activities performed.

DEFICIENT KNOWLEDGE

Related to: lack of information about hepatitis, lack of recall, unfamiliarity of resources, misinterpretation of information received

Defining Characteristics: questions, requests for information, statements of misperceptions, development of preventable complications

Outcome Criteria

✔ Patient will be able to verbalize understanding of disease, treatment, and causative behaviors.

NOC: *Knowledge: Disease Process*

INTERVENTIONS	RATIONALES
Discuss patient's perceptions of disease process.	Identifies knowledge base and misconceptions to facilitate appropriate teaching plan.
Instruct patient/family on disease process, prevention and transmission of disease, and isolation requirements.	Types of isolation will vary according to type of hepatitis and personal situation. Family members may require treatment depending on type of hepatitis.
Instruct patient/family in appropriate home sanitation.	Dirty environment and poor sanitation methods may be responsible for transmission of the disease.
Instruct patient/family on activity limitations.	Complete resumption of normal activity may not take place until liver returns to its normal size and patient begins to feel better and this may take up to several months.

INTERVENTIONS	RATIONALES
Instruct patient/family on all medications, side effects, effects, contraindications, and dangers of administration of over-the-counter drugs without physician approval.	Promotes knowledge and facilitates compliance. Some medications are hepatotoxic or are metabolized by the liver, increasing its workload.
Instruct patient/family to refrain from blood donation.	Most states do not allow anyone who has a history of any type of hepatitis to donate blood or blood products to prevent possible spread of the infection.
Instruct patient on avoidance of recreational drugs or alcohol.	May jeopardize recovery from infection and increases liver dysfunction.
Consult with counselors, ministers, drug or alcohol treatment facilities as warranted.	May be required for assistance with substance withdrawal and for long-term support once discharged.

NIC: *Teaching: Individual*

Discharge or Maintenance Evaluation

- Patient will be able to accurately verbalize understanding of all instructions given.
- Patient/family will be able to modify environment to control spread of disease.
- Patient will be able to effectively access community resources for treatment programs and discharge follow-up care.
- Patient will be able to effectively manage medical regimen with follow-up from physician.

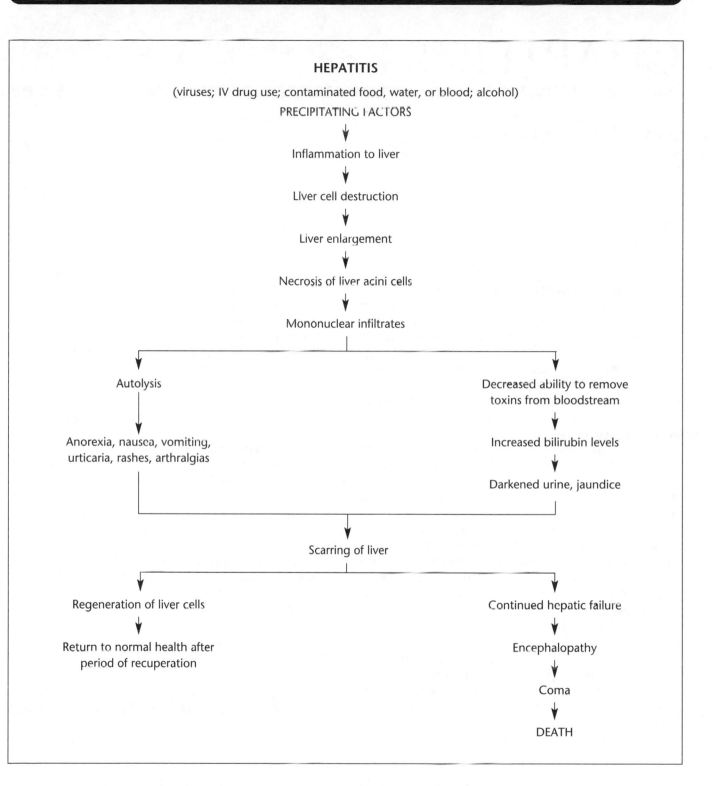

HEPATITIS

(viruses; IV drug use; contaminated food, water, or blood; alcohol)

PRECIPITATING FACTORS

↓

Inflammation to liver

↓

Liver cell destruction

↓

Liver enlargement

↓

Necrosis of liver acini cells

↓

Mononuclear infiltrates

Autolysis

↓

Anorexia, nausea, vomiting,
urticaria, rashes, arthralgias

Decreased ability to remove
toxins from bloodstream

↓

Increased bilirubin levels

↓

Darkened urine, jaundice

Scarring of liver

Regeneration of liver cells

↓

Return to normal health after
period of recuperation

Continued hepatic failure

↓

Encephalopathy

↓

Coma

↓

DEATH

CHAPTER 4.4

PANCREATITIS

Acute pancreatitis is a life-threatening inflammatory response to an injury, in which pancreatic enzymes are abnormally activated and these enzymes destroy tissues and fat in and surrounding the pancreas by autodigestion. Precipitating factors for the abnormal activation may be caused by effects of ethanol and its metabolite, acetaldehyde, diseases of the biliary tract, obstruction of the common bile duct, bile reflux into the pancreatic duct, ischemia, trauma, infections, surgical or invasive procedures, neoplasms, metabolic aberrations, use of oral contraceptives, corticosteroids, thiazide diuretics, antihypertensives, cyclosporines, sulfonamides, or tetracycline, or stimulation of vasoactive substances. Obstruction may result in widespread edema to the pancreas, which increases pressure in the pancreatic system. This increase in pressure results in the rupture of the ducts which allows the enzymes to spill into the cells, and begin the autodigestion process.

Trypsin activates the pancreatic enzymes, phospholipase A, elastase, and kallikrein. Trypsin may cause edema, necrosis, and hemorrhage in the pancreas. Elastase may attack the walls of smaller blood vessels and facilitate hemorrhage. Phospholipase A allows damage to the acinar cell membrane to occur, and may alter coagulation. Vasomotor changes and increases in vascular permeability may be caused by kallikrein, and this may also be the cause of the pain experienced with pancreatitis. If the disease is allowed to progress, the inflammation leads to massive hemorrhage, destruction of the pancreas, diabetes mellitus, acidosis, shock, coma, and death.

Pancreatitis can be further classified as being acute, recurrent acute, chronic and recurrent chronic pancreatitis. In acute pancreatitis a single episode is noted with resolution of pancreatic dysfunction in mild interstitial forms. A more severe variety, such as necrotizing pancreatitis, has a 50% mortality rate, caused in part by concurrent and resultant complications, such as MODS, DIC, and sepsis. Recurrent acute pancreatitis occurs if more than one incident happens, but pancreatic function may return to normal in between these events. Chronic pancreatitis patients usually have persistent pain because of the progressive damage and fibrosis to the acinar cells, and recurrent chronic pancreatitis patients may have occasional pain-free phases even with the destruction and inflammation to the acinar cells. Even mild forms of pancreatitis may be fatal in compromised or elderly individuals because of pancreatic edema and shifts of up to 6 liters of fluid into the interstitial spaces.

One of the predominant symptoms of this disease is the unrelenting abdominal pain located in the epigastric and/or periumbilical areas that may radiate to the chest and back. Nausea, continuous vomiting, low-grade fever, anorexia, diarrhea, weight loss, jaundice, diaphoresis, dehydration, and poorly defined abdominal mass may also be encountered.

Pseudocysts and abscesses in and around the pancreas may occur as a result of localized necrosis, and may exert pressure on the stomach or colon. They may develop slowly and may result in fistula formation.

The goal of therapy is to maintain adequate circulatory fluid volume with electrolyte replacement, pain relief, treatment of infection and treatment of hyperglycemia.

MEDICAL CARE

Laboratory: serum amylase is elevated up to 40 times the normal limit in the early stages and then decreases over 2–3 days; urine amylase elevated and lasts longer than serum amylase; elevated glucose, which reflects beta-cell connection; elevated levels of bilirubin, alkaline phosphatase, lactic dehydrogenase, aspartate transferase, potassium, triglycerides, cholesterol, and lipase; decreased albumin, calcium, sodium, and magnesium; white blood cell counts from 8,000–20,000 with increased polymorphonuclear cells; hematocrit may exceed 50%; prothrombin time may be increased; fat content in the stool increased; amylase–creatinine clearance ratio may indicate pancreatic disease; renal profiles used to evaluate renal function and hypovolemia

Radiography: abdominal X-rays may be used to identify dilation of duodenum or transverse colon; chest X-ray used to assess for complications, lung involvement, and heart size

CT scans: used to identify size, shape, density, masses, necrosis, or infiltrates in the pancreas

Ultrasonography: used to identify neoplasms, edema, inflammation, cysts, abscesses, or infiltrates in the pancreas, but cannot confirm the diagnosis of pancreatitis

Angiography: helps to visualize early pancreatic tumors or problems with vasculature

Endoscopic retrograde cholangiopancreatography (ERCP): used to directly visualize the pancreatic duct system by use of endoscopy and radiography; used to identify cysts, calculi, stenosis, pancreatic and biliary duct disease when other diagnostic tools are not conclusive; if stone extraction via sphincterotomy is done early, the course of biliary pancreatitis may be improved

Surgery: may be necessary to drain abscesses or pseudocysts, or to anastomose the pseudocysts to an adjacent structure to provide internal drainage; chronic pancreatitis may require a pancreaticojejunostomy to relieve obstruction of the duct to relieve pain; experimental surgery for transplantation of the pancreas or islet cells may be performed

COMMON NURSING DIAGNOSES

IMBALANCED NUTRITION: LESS THAN BODY REQUIREMENTS (see DKA)

Related to: nausea, vomiting, anorexia, digestive enzyme leakage, increased metabolic needs, sepsis

Defining Characteristics: increases in nausea and vomiting, retching, absent bowel sounds, decreased bowel sounds, anorexia, increased metabolism, lack of adequate food ingested

DEFICIENT FLUID VOLUME (see DKA)

Related to: nausea, vomiting, fever, diaphoresis, nasogastric drainage, fluid shifting, diarrhea

Defining Characteristics: nausea, vomiting, ascites, nasogastric suctioning, hypotension, tachycardia, decreased urinary output

IMPAIRED GAS EXCHANGE (see MECHANICAL VENTILATION)

Related to: complications from disease, pulmonary endothelial capillary damage, acute respiratory distress, SIRS, MODS, sepsis

Defining Characteristics: altered arterial blood gases, dyspnea, use of accessory muscles, tachypnea, bradypnea, cough, sputum

ADDITIONAL NURSING DIAGNOSES

ACUTE PAIN

Related to: pancreatic obstruction, autodigestion of pancreas, leakage of pancreatic enzymes, inflammation

Defining Characteristics: unrelenting epigastric pain, patient curled up with both arms over abdomen, nausea, vomiting, tenderness, facial grimacing, groaning

Outcome Criteria

✔ Patient will exhibit periods without pain.

✔ Patient will be able to obtain relief of pain from medications administered.

NOC: *Pain Control*

INTERVENTIONS	RATIONALES
Obtain pain history from patient/ family and patient's ability to handle pain.	Pain is specific to each individual and each person has their own coping strategies to deal with their discomfort. Use of pre-existing strategies may assist in pain relief.
Assess patient for pain level.	Helps to establish plan of care and shows concern for the patient.

(continues)

(continued)

INTERVENTIONS	RATIONALES
Administer medications (usually meperidine [Demerol]) IV as ordered.	Demerol is the drug of choice for pancreatitis. Morphine should not be given because most opiate-type narcotics cause spasms of the sphincter of Oddi, increasing the patient's pain. Large dosages may be required for patient's relief of pain, and may even be ineffective at relieving discomfort.
Utilize other medications, such as histamine blockers, enzymes, and so forth as ordered.	These medications may be able to decrease secretion of enzymes and acids so as to decrease pain.
Use relaxation techniques, biofeedback, guided imagery, and other alternatives to ease pain.	Alternative nonmedicinal therapeutics may be significantly helpful in reducing anxiety and discomfort.
Consistently assess patient for nonverbal cues as to discomfort and pain.	Some patients are reluctant to verbalize pain and will let pain escalate to the point where significantly more analgesia is required to achieve pain relief.
Administer pain medications on a routine basis, as ordered.	May help to keep analgesic levels maintained and requires less pain medication to keep patient comfortable.
Instruct patient to notify nurse of pain when it first begins.	Allows for timely intervention to preclude pain from becoming exquisite and requiring extensive analgesic administration.
Instruct patient/family regarding medication administration, and be available to answer all questions.	Patient and/or family may believe that patient will become addicted to medication and try to refuse pain relief. False misconceptions should be illuminated. Knowledge will foster compliance.
Instruct family in the use of touch, and other soothing measures to help with patient's pain.	Allows family the ability to participate in patient's care, and the patient may be more willing to allow familiar people to provide care and express concerns.

NIC: *Pain Management*

Discharge or Maintenance Evaluation

- Patient will be free of pain for longer periods of time.
- Patient will be able to utilize alternative methods to ease pain and discomfort.

- Patient will be compliant with notifying nurse when pain begins and accepting medications on a routine basis to prevent exacerbation of pain.

RISK FOR INJURY

Related to: sepsis, pseudocysts, fistula formation, abscess formation, complications from disease

Defining Characteristics: fever, abdominal pain, drainage, increased white blood cell count, shift to the left, systemic infection symptoms, DIC, electrolyte imbalances

Outcome Criteria

✔ Patient will be afebrile and have no complications from disease.

NOC: *Risk Detection*

INTERVENTIONS	RATIONALES
Monitor vital signs at least every 2 hours, and note changes.	Allows for prompt identification of early signs of infection to facilitate timely treatment. Third spacing, bleeding, and secretion of vasodilating substances may result in hypotension.
Monitor hemodynamic pressures if possible.	Allows for actual measurement of cardiac output and other parameters to identify fluid shifts and hemodynamic alterations which may precede systemic complications.
Monitor ECG for cardiac rhythm, rate, and changes, and treat dysrhythmias per protocol.	Hypovolemia and electrolyte imbalances may precipitate cardiac dysrhythmias.
Auscultate heart sounds for changes, gallops, or murmurs.	JVD in conjunction with a new S_3 gallop may indicate heart failure or pulmonary edema.
Observe for changes in respiratory status, especially when occurring concurrently with fever and jaundice.	Gram negative sepsis may be seen symptomatically with cholestatic jaundice and decreases in pulmonary function.
Observe for increasing complaints of abdominal pain or tenderness, chills, fever, or hypotension.	May indicate formation of abscess, especially if symptoms occur while patient is receiving vigorous medical treatment. Abdominal rigidity or rebound tenderness may indicate peritonitis.

INTERVENTIONS	RATIONALES
Observe for presence of petechiae, continued bleeding, or hematoma formation.	May indicate impending DIC as a result of circulating pancreatic enzymes.
Measure and monitor abdominal girth changes.	Identifies increases in fluid retention and ascites.
Monitor intake and output every 2 hours, noting hematuria, or significant imbalance.	Oliguria may occur as a result of renal involvement caused by increases in vascular resistance or decreased renal blood flow. Hematuria may occur as a result from circulating pancreatic enzymes.
Strict aseptic technique should be maintained when dealing with invasive lines or dressings.	Failure to maintain technique may result in sepsis, which is responsible for over 80% of deaths associated with pancreatitis.

INTERVENTIONS	RATIONALES
Prepare patient/family members for surgical procedures as warranted.	Surgical drainage of abscesses or pseudocysts may be required.
Instruct patient in usage of pancreatic enzyme supplements/ bile salts.	Long-term replacement may be required for exocrine deficiencies from permanent pancreatic damage.

NIC: *Surveillance*

Discharge or Maintenance Evaluation

- Patient will be free of complications from pancreatitis, and will exhibit timely healing of all wounds.
- Patient will be able to accurately verbalize all instructed information.

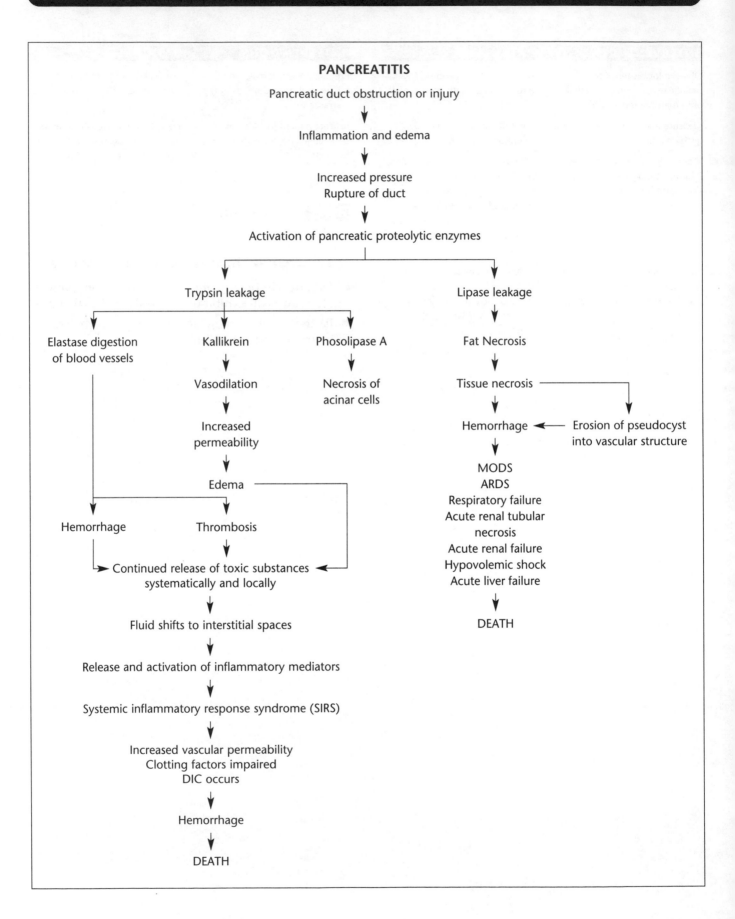

PANCREATITIS

Pancreatic duct obstruction or injury

↓

Inflammation and edema

↓

Increased pressure
Rupture of duct

↓

Activation of pancreatic proteolytic enzymes

Trypsin leakage   Lipase leakage

Elastase digestion   Kallikrein   Phosolipase A   Fat Necrosis
of blood vessels   ↓   ↓   ↓
                            Vasodilation   Necrosis of   Tissue necrosis ──────────┐
                                ↓   acinar cells   ↓   │
                            Increased   Hemorrhage ◄──── Erosion of pseudocyst
                            permeability   ↓   into vascular structure
                                ↓   MODS
                              Edema ───────────┐   ARDS
                                ↓   │   Respiratory failure
Hemorrhage   Thrombosis   │   Acute renal tubular
      │   ↓   │   necrosis
      └──► Continued release of toxic substances ◄──┘   Acute renal failure
              systematically and locally   Hypovolemic shock
                                ↓   Acute liver failure
                   Fluid shifts to interstitial spaces   ↓
                                ↓   DEATH
            Release and activation of inflammatory mediators

                                ↓

          Systemic inflammatory response syndrome (SIRS)

                                ↓

                   Increased vascular permeability
                      Clotting factors impaired
                            DIC occurs

                                ↓

                            Hemorrhage

                                ↓

                              DEATH

CHAPTER 4.5

ACUTE ABDOMEN/ABDOMINAL TRAUMA

When someone is said to have an acute abdomen, it generally indicates that they have a sudden onset of severe abdominal pain that typically requires surgery to prevent peritonitis from contaminated materials spilling into the peritoneal cavity. There are numerous situations that could be responsible for this diagnosis, such as perforation of the appendix, peptic ulcer, bowel, gallbladder, diverticuli, or abdominal aortic aneurysm, ruptured ectopic pregnancy, or an abdominal injury.

Abdominal injuries may be caused from either blunt trauma or penetrating damage. Blunt trauma, with compression of abdominal structures against the vertebral column, can result from sports injuries, accidents, or falls, and can be caused as a result of a direct impact, rotary or shearing forces, or rapid deceleration. Any of these mechanisms can cause tearing of body structures that may involve substantial bleeding into the peritoneal cavity.

Penetrating injuries can cause perforation of the bowel or hemorrhage from lacerations to major vessels. These types of trauma can either be low-velocity, which damages tissues at the injury site, or high-velocity, in which tissues and organs surrounding the penetration path are damaged.

All of the types of injuries discussed have significant potential for critical emergencies, based on the severity of the wound, and how much damage it has caused. Mortality is approximately 10% from abdominal trauma caused in part by the presence of structures involving many body systems being located in the abdomen. The goals of immediate treatment involve maintaining the hemodynamic status, control of hemorrhage, and preparation for surgical procedures.

MEDICAL CARE

Surgery: usually the treatment of choice because of potential or presence of peritonitis from injury; procedure is dependent on source of bleeding or contamination

Laboratory: urinalysis to identify bleeding or urinary tract injuries; CBC to identify sepsis and changes in hematologic status; WBC is normally elevated in trauma; differential used to identify shifts to the left; amylase elevated with pancreatic injury or gastrointestinal perforations; renal and liver profiles used to discern damage to the particular system; clotting profiles to monitor for coagulation status; myoglobin levels elevated with crush injuries; peritoneal fluid analysis for bleeding or infection; cultures done to identify source of pathogenic cause as well as to ascertain which antimicrobial agent is required to eradicate the specific organism

Radiography: chest and abdominal X-rays used to identify pneumothorax, free air below the diaphragm, foreign body that may have caused injury, or other complications; loss of psoas muscle outline indicates retroperitoneal bleeding

Arteriography: used to identify areas of bleeding and infection

Magnetic resonance imaging (MRI): used to identify vascular problems, masses, pseudocysts, and infection

Endoscopic retrograde cholangiopancreatography (ERCP): used to identify biliary or pancreatic stones or any obstruction of ducts

CT scans: may be used to identify abdominal and retroperitoneal injuries that may not be overt with regular X-rays; can identify cysts or abscesses that may require surgical intervention

Intravenous pyelogram: used to detect hematuria and trauma to renal structures

Retrograde urethrography/cystography: used to identify urethral or bladder injury

Ultrasound: use is limited; may be useful to distinguish between splenic hematoma from peritoneal blood or ascites

Paracentesis: may be used to identify presence of pus, blood, or other substance, and may be used for peritoneal lavage to identify effects of abdominal trauma and prevent unnecessary surgical intervention

EGD/Colonoscopy: used to identify bleeding sites, presence of esophageal tears, varices, ulcers, lower gastrointestinal ulcers, perforation, abscesses, ischemia, or bleeding

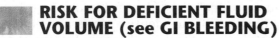

COMMON NURSING DIAGNOSES

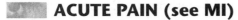

RISK FOR DEFICIENT FLUID VOLUME (see GI BLEEDING)

Related to: fluid shifts, hemorrhage, nasogastric suctioning, bowel obstruction

Defining Characteristics: hypotension, tachycardia, decreased urinary output, decreased hemoglobin and hematocrit, decreased filling pressures, electrolyte imbalances, presence of peritonitis

ACUTE PAIN (see MI)

Related to: trauma, surgery, edema

Defining Characteristics: grimacing, complaints of pain, restlessness, splinting, shallow respirations, abdominal rigidity

IMBALANCED NUTRITION: LESS THAN BODY REQUIREMENTS (see DKA)

Related to: trauma, surgery, nasogastric suctioning, hypermetabolic state

Defining Characteristics: abdominal pain, ordered nutritional status of NPO, increased metabolism, weight loss, nitrogen and electrolyte imbalance, decreased albumin and protein levels, vitamin deficiencies

ADDITIONAL NURSING DIAGNOSES

INEFFECTIVE TISSUE PERFUSION: GASTROINTESTINAL

Related to: intestinal infarction, peritonitis, hemorrhage, hypovolemia

Defining Characteristics: severe abdominal pain, especially in periumbilical region, constant generalized abdominal pain, rebound tenderness, abdominal dis-

tention, ileus, hyperactive bowel sounds (early sign), nausea, vomiting, bloody diarrhea, increased gastric secretion, free air in intestine on X-ray, fever, chills, increased WBC, hypoactive bowel sounds (late sign), weight loss, hypoxia, hypoxemia, decreased breath sounds

Outcome Criteria

✔ Patient will have intestinal bleeding, perforation, or trauma repaired.

✔ Patient will have no further complications from abdominal wound/injury.

NOC: *Tissue Perfusion: Gastrointestinal*

INTERVENTIONS	RATIONALES
Monitor VS and hemodynamics q 1–2 hours and prn. Notify physician of significant changes.	Decreased blood pressure, increased heart rate and respirations, and fever may all be symptoms of infection related to acute abdomen.
Auscultate and palpate abdomen. Notify physician for significant findings.	Increased abdominal tenderness to palpation may signal increased gastrointestinal ischemia. Changes in bowel sounds may indicate an impending or present obstruction or perforation.
Maintain NPO status as ordered.	Restriction of fluids and food may be required if patient has a perforation or ileus, requiring nasogastric suctioning to allow the stomach and intestine to rest.
Monitor I&O q 2–4 hours and notify physician if urinary output <30 cc/hr for 2 hours.	Decreased urinary output may be a symptom of decreased perfusion and ischemia caused by hypovolemia.
Insert and maintain nasogastric suctioning as ordered.	Decompresses stomach, alleviates nausea and vomiting, and may decrease risk of inflammation to gastric lining from accumulated acidic secretions.
Administer IV fluids as ordered.	Maintains hydration and provides access for administration of medications.
Administer antimicrobials as ordered.	May be required to eradicate gram-negative anaerobic infections.

INTERVENTIONS	RATIONALES
Administer vasoactive drugs as ordered.	Low-dose dopamine may be required to help increase splanchnic blood flow and nitroglycerin may be required to decrease abdominal pain by means of vasodilation.
Administer enteral or parenteral feeding as ordered.	May be required to maintain nutritional status while allowing bowel to rest and adjust to the increased metabolic demands for perfusion.
Administer pain medication as ordered.	Narcotic analgesics decrease gastric motility. Care should be utilized to avoid overmedicating patient; instead other pain relief techniques should be utilized to provide relief without pharmacologic help when possible.
Monitor lab work, especially CBC, electrolytes, and liver function studies.	Decreased hemoglobin and hematocrit may indicate hemorrhage and ischemia, and increased WBC with shift to the left on the differential diagnoses infection. Increased liver function tests may be seen when hepatic system is involved. Electrolytes may be depleted because of nasogastric suctioning, lack of nutrition, and metabolic demands.
Instruct patient/family in medications to avoid that decrease peristalsis.	Decreased peristalsis contributes to decreases in perfusion and can lead to ischemia.
Instruct patient/family regarding checking all stools for blood.	Assists to monitor for blood loss that could lead to anemia.
Prepare and instruct patient in all procedures/surgery.	Promotes knowledge, decreases fear, and facilitates compliance.

NIC: *Emergency Care*

Discharge or Maintenance Evaluation

- Patient will be free of abdominal pain and distention.
- Patient will have normal vital signs and intake and output will be equivalent.
- Patient will have no further abdominal perfusion complications.
- Patient/family will verbalize understanding of all instructions and comply.

RISK FOR INFECTION

Related to: perforation of abdominal structures, laceration of vasculature, open wounds, peritoneal cavity contamination

Defining Characteristics: fever, trauma, elevated white blood cell count, sepsis

Outcome Criteria

✔ Patient will be free of infection, with stable vital signs and lab work within normal parameters.

NOC: *Risk Control*

INTERVENTIONS	RATIONALES
Monitor vital signs, especially temperature q 2–4 hours.	May indicate presence of or impending infection and sepsis. Decreasing pulse pressure, hypotension and tachycardia may signify impending septic shock from endotoxic vasodilation.
Observe skin color, temperature, and monitor for changes.	Patient may have warm, flushed, dry skin in shock's warm phase, changing to cold and clammy pale skin as shock progresses.
Obtain blood, urine, sputum, drainage, or other cultures as ordered.	Identifies causative organism and facilitates appropriate selection of antimicrobial agents.
Monitor intake and output every 1–2 hours.	Sepsis may impair renal perfusion and result in oliguria or anuria.
Administer antimicrobials as ordered.	Cephalosporins and aminoglycosides are frequently used to fight these types of infections.
Ensure that universal precautions are utilized, and that sterile or aseptic technique is used when caring for wounds or inserting invasive lines or catheters.	Assists in preventing spread of infection by cross-contamination, as well as preventing other bacterial growth from invasion of skin/body.
Administer tetanus toxoid as ordered.	Decreases risk of development of tetanus.
Prepare for surgery as warranted.	Surgical intervention may be the treatment of choice to drain abscesses or remove or repair perforated structures.
Assist with peritoneal aspiration as warranted.	May be performed to remove fluid and identify causative organism.
Change wound dressings as ordered.	Dressings protect wound and prevent spread of infection.

(continues)

(continued)

INTERVENTIONS	RATIONALES
Monitor CBC, especially WBC count.	Facilitates assessment of effectiveness of antimicrobial therapy, as well as identifies blood loss or changes in infection.
Limit visitors as indicated, utilizing appropriate isolation precautions as warranted.	Decreases potential for cross-contamination.

NIC: *Infection Control*

Discharge or Maintenance Evaluation

- Patient will have stable vital signs and hemodynamic status.
- Patient will have white blood cell count within normal limits.
- Patient will have negative cultures.
- Patient will not exhibit further signs/symptoms of infection.
- Patient will not develop secondary infection.
- Family members will adhere to isolation regulations.

RISK FOR INJURY

Related to: trauma

Defining Characteristics: hemorrhage, peritonitis, altered arterial blood gases, mental status changes, hypotension, tachycardia, bradycardia, arterial injuries, fractures, electrolyte imbalances

Outcome Criteria

✔ Patient will be free of injury to self, and free of complications that may ensue from trauma.

NOC: *Symptom Control*

INTERVENTIONS	RATIONALES
Monitor vital signs every 1–2 hours, and prn. Check blood pressure readings in both arms and legs.	Decreases in blood pressure or changes with orthostatic readings may indicate impending hypovolemia. Pulse pressures may increase during the latent effects of shock or with head injuries, and may decrease in early stages of shock. Differences between right and left sides greater than 20 mm Hg may indicate aortic injury.

INTERVENTIONS	RATIONALES
Monitor respiratory status, noting changes in breath sounds.	Injury to lungs or diaphragm may result in tachypnea and dyspnea. Breath sounds that are distant or absent may indicate pneumothorax or hemothorax.
Observe chest for symmetry, paradoxical movement, anatomic deformity, swelling, bruising, or crepitus.	Splinting by patient or obvious deformity or swelling may be seen if ribs are fractured. Paradoxical movement may indicate flail chest. Palpable crepitus may be present if lung or mediastinum has been punctured.
Auscultate heart sounds for changes or abnormalities.	Extra heart sounds or murmurs may indicate injury to valves or heart, and distant, muffled heart tones may signal cardiac tamponade.
Observe abdomen for wounds, masses, swelling, pulsations, hematomas, protrusion of organs or viscera, lacerations, and abrasions; auscultate for bowel sounds.	Bluish discolorations around the umbilicus may indicate retroperitoneal bleeding accumulating in abdomen. An odd number of bullet holes may indicate the remaining presence of a foreign object/bullet in the body. Decreased or absent bowel sounds may indicate ileus or peritonitis. Abdominal bruits may result when a vessel is partially occluded, venous hums auscultated over the upper abdomen or liver may indicate hepatic or splenic vein thrombosis, and friction rubs heard over the spleen may indicate infarction or inflammation of spleen.
Percuss abdomen for changes, dullness or tympany.	Dullness that is decreased over liver may indicate presence of free air below the diaphragm. Upper abdominal distention and increased tympany over the stomach may indicate gastric dilation. Flank area dullness may indicate retroperitoneal hemorrhage.
Cover protruding abdominal viscera with saline-soaked sterile gauze or sterile towels, and position patient with knees flexed.	Protects viscera from drying, and positioning prevents additional protrusion/evisceration.
Palpate peripheral pulses for presence, quality, and character. Notify physician for significant changes.	Changes in pulse characteristics may indicate arterial or venous impairment which may require immediate treatment.

INTERVENTIONS	RATIONALES
Observe for Grey Turner's and Coopernail's signs.	Grey Turner's sign is a bluish discoloration on flank that indicates retroperitoneal bleeding accumulation in abdomen. Coopernail's sign is ecchymoses on scrotum or labia and may indicate pelvic fracture.
Monitor for complaints of pain at the tip of the left shoulder or right shoulder.	May indicate rupture of spleen or irritation of the diaphragm from blood or other substance with left shoulder pain, and possible liver laceration with right shoulder pain.
Assist with peritoneal tap and lavage.	Done to identify intraperitoneal bleeding which is diagnosed when fluid is analyzed.
Instruct patient on all procedures and testing; prepare for surgery as warranted.	Promotes knowledge and decreases anxiety which facilitates compliance with medical regimen.

INTERVENTIONS	RATIONALES
Instruct patient/family to notify physician for fever or abdominal pain.	Abdominal injury signs and symptoms may not appear for several hours to days.

NIC: *Shock Prevention*

Discharge or Maintenance Evaluation

- Patient will have no evidence of abdominal injury complication.
- Patient will have no intraperitoneal bleeding or structural damage to organs.
- Patient will be compliant with regimen.
- Patient will have successful surgical intervention with no postoperative complications.

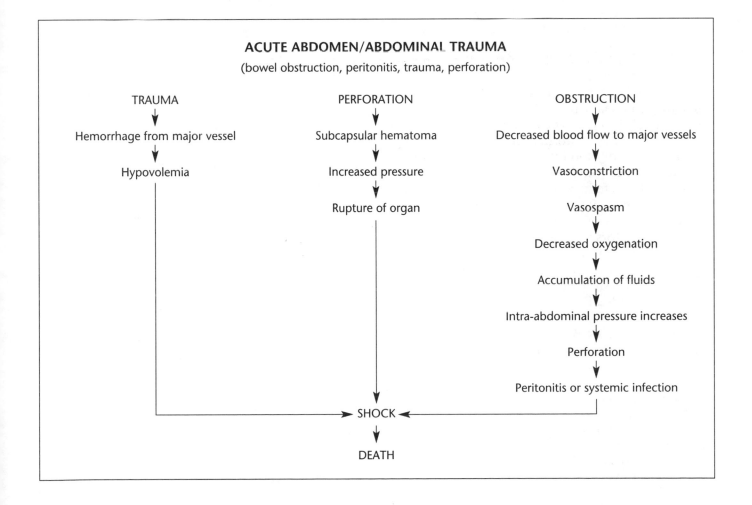

ACUTE ABDOMEN/ABDOMINAL TRAUMA
(bowel obstruction, peritonitis, trauma, perforation)

TRAUMA
↓
Hemorrhage from major vessel
↓
Hypovolemia

PERFORATION
↓
Subcapsular hematoma
↓
Increased pressure
↓
Rupture of organ

OBSTRUCTION
↓
Decreased blood flow to major vessels
↓
Vasoconstriction
↓
Vasospasm
↓
Decreased oxygenation
↓
Accumulation of fluids
↓
Intra-abdominal pressure increases
↓
Perforation
↓
Peritonitis or systemic infection

→ SHOCK ←
↓
DEATH

CHAPTER 4.6

LIVER FAILURE

The liver plays a vital role by providing multiple functions, such as, metabolism of carbohydrates, proteins, and fats, storing fat-soluble vitamins, vitamin B_{12}, copper, and iron, synthesis of blood clotting factors, amino acids, albumin, and globulins, detoxification of toxic substances, and phagocytosis of microorganisms, and plays a role in glycolysis and gluconeogenesis. Liver functioning can be preserved until up to 75% of the hepatocytes become damaged or necrotic, at which time the liver can no longer perform its normal operation.

Early hepatic failure presents as a type of cirrhosis of the liver. Liver cells become inflamed and obstructed, which results in damage to the cells around the central portal vein. When the inflammation decreases, the lobule regenerates, and this cycle is repeated until the lobule is irreversibly damaged and fibrotic tissue replaces liver tissue.

Advanced hepatic failure develops when all compensatory mechanisms fail, causing the serum ammonia level to rise. The already-damaged liver is unable to synthesize normal products, so acidosis, hypoglycemia, or blood dyscrasias develop, and the patient becomes comatose.

Acute liver failure, also known as fulminant hepatic failure, may be precipitated by a stress factor that aggravates a pre-existing chronic liver disease. Some stress factors include alcohol intake, ingestion of Amanita mushrooms, large amounts of dietary protein, gastrointestinal bleeding, and portacaval shunt surgery. An acute type of liver failure may occur as a result of viral or toxic hepatitis, biliary obstruction, cancer, acute infective processes, acute Wilson's disease or Budd–Chiari syndrome, graft-versus-host disease following bone marrow transplantation, veno-occlusive disease, drugs, such as acetaminophen, isoniazid, and rifampin, severe dehydration, Reye's syndrome, or shock states.

Fulminant hepatic failure may begin in stage I as hepatic encephalopathy, progressing to drowsiness and asterixis, stupor and incoherent communication, finally to stage IV with deep coma. The stages may progress over as little as two months.

The goal of treatment is to halt progression of the encephalopathy that occurs with increasing ammonia levels, and is accomplished with use of cathartics, decreasing dietary protein, and electrolyte replacement. Even with treatment, mortality rates are as high as 90%, depending on the age of the patient and severity of disease.

In chronic liver failure, or cirrhosis, changes in the liver become irreversible after the progressive formation of connective tissue and nodular liver regeneration after necrosis and inflammation occur. This type of liver failure may lack any serious signs or symptoms for several years until the functioning portion of the liver no longer can maintain homeostasis, portal hypertension ensues, and the disease becomes life-threatening.

MEDICAL CARE

Laboratory: ALT, AST, GGT, and alkaline phosphatase not usually elevated in advanced cirrhosis, but increased in acute liver failure; bilirubin not usually elevated in advanced cirrhosis with the exception of biliary stasis diseases, but increased with acute liver failure; Protime is the most sensitive indication of liver failure and is usually increased in both acute and chronic failure; serum ammonia level increased; hemoglobin and hematocrit decreased; BUN and creatinine decreased in chronic failure and increased in acute failure; platelet count may be decreased; glucose decreased; lactate increased; serology for hepatitis positive; cultures of body fluids and urine toxicology screening positive; ascitic fluid usually shows WBC >250 polymorphonuclear neutrophil leukocytes/mm^3, and *Escherichia coli* and *Klebsiella* species common; magnesium level may be decreased with alcoholic cirrhosis and toxic, if magnesium replacement has been used; albumin decreases and globulin increases with liver failure

Radiography: chest X-ray used to identify infiltrates or pneumonia that may occur

CT scan: used to identify increased liver size and volume, or increase in spleen size; used to identify masses or cysts; can be used to detect degenerative cirrhotic changes or focal liver disease

Ultrasonography: abdominal ultrasound used to identify presence and amount of ascites

Medication: Neomycin or Kanamycin frequently used to prevent intestinal bacteria from converting protein/amino acids to ammonia; lactulose or sorbitol used to induce catharsis to empty intestines to decrease conversion to ammonia; thiazide diuretics may be given to decrease fluid retention

Hyperalimentation: may be used as diet of choice because of ability to control concentration of nutrients, electrolytes, and vitamins

Paracentesis: abdominal paracentesis done to detect presence of ascites, and obtain fluid for laboratory analysis

Electroencephalography: used to show slowing of brain wave activity with hepatic encephalopathy

Hemodialysis: may be used as a temporary measure for severe hepatic encephalopathy

Liver biopsy: may be done to establish diagnosis by study of biopsied tissue

COMMON NURSING DIAGNOSES

DEFICIENT FLUID VOLUME (see GI BLEEDING)

Related to: osmotic changes, hydrostatic pressure changes

Defining Characteristics: presence of ascites, oliguria, anuria, dry skin, decreased skin turgor, hypotension

ADDITIONAL NURSING DIAGNOSES

DISTURBED THOUGHT PROCESSES

Related to: serum ammonia levels, hepatic encephalopathy

Defining Characteristics: increased ammonia, increased BUN, mental status changes, decreasing level of consciousness, changes in personality, handwriting changes, tremors, coma

Outcome Criteria

✔ Patient will be conscious and stable, with ammonia levels within normal ranges.

NOC: *Neurologic Status: Consciousness*

INTERVENTIONS	RATIONALES
Monitor neurologic status every 1–2 hours, and prn. Notify physician for abnormalities.	Identifies onset of problem and potential trend.
If possible, have patient write name each day and do simple mathematic calculation.	As hepatic failure progresses, the ability to write becomes more difficult, and writing becomes illegible at precoma stage. Inability to perform mental calculations may indicate worsening failure.
Assess patient and identify grade of encephalopathy present. Monitor for changes and notify physician.	With encephalopathy, grade I signs include total consciousness, orientation with progression to confusion and disorientation to time and place, slowness to answer questions, impaired handwriting, subtle intellectual function changes, forgetfulness, irritability, mood swings from euphoria to depression, muscular tremors, incoordination, and yawning. Grade II signs include decreased consciousness but patient will be able to open eyes spontaneously, disorientation to time and place with severe confusion, amnesia of past events, lethargy, decreased inhibitions, paranoia, apathy, hypoactive reflexes, asterixis, ataxia, and slurred speech. Grade III signs include reusability with verbal and pain stimuli, but patient does not open eyes spontaneously, total disorientation, inability to formulate computations, bizarre behavior, increased apathy, inability to cooperate with neuromuscular testing, nystagmus, clonus, decorticate and decerebrate posturing, rigidity, and seizures. Grade IV, which is the worst classification, has signs including complete coma with no response to pain, seizures, rigidity decreasing to flaccidity, and pupillary dilatation.

(continues)

(continued)

INTERVENTIONS	RATIONALES
Monitor lab work, especially ammonia levels. Ensure lab test is done properly, with placement of vial on ice and immediate processing.	Increasing serum ammonia may indicate increasing encephalopathy, but patients may have developed a tolerance to high ammonia levels and, thus, levels may not correlate to their specific level of encephalopathy. Incorrect processing of lab test may result in inaccurate data.
Maintain patent airway.	As encephalopathy progresses, patient may not be able to maintain airway, and artificial airway may be required.
Administer cathartic agents as ordered. Administer Kanamycin or Neomycin as ordered.	Lactulose minimizes formation of ammonia and other nitrogenous byproducts by altering intestinal pH. Neomycin or Kanamycin help prevent conversion of amino acids into ammonia. Sorbitol-type cathartics cause an osmotic diarrhea to empty the intestines to decrease ammonia production.
Observe for asterixis or other tremors.	Rapid wrist flapping when arms are raised in front of body with hands dorsiflexed may indicate presence of encephalopathy.
Provide safe environment for patient.	Decreases risk of injury caused by altered consciousness levels.
Provide low protein diet.	Decreased dietary protein may lessen serum ammonia levels.
Avoid sedatives and narcotics if at all possible.	May worsen decreasing level of consciousness and make identification of cause of decreased sensorium more difficult.
Instruct patient/family in potential for altered sensorium and encephalopathy signs. Reorient patient as needed.	Provides knowledge and facilitates family involvement with maintaining optimal orientation level. Provides support with realistic expectations of disease process since outcome is poor.
Instruct patient in side effects of drugs used to facilitate decrease in ammonia levels.	Diarrhea will occur, and lactulose should be titrated to where patient has 3 stools per day.

NIC: *Cerebral Perfusion Promotion*

Discharge or Maintenance Evaluation

- Patient will be awake, alert, and oriented.
- Patient will have serum ammonia levels within acceptable ranges.

- Patient and/or family will be able to verbalize understanding of instructions and be able to communicate concerns.

IMBALANCED NUTRITION: LESS THAN BODY REQUIREMENTS

Related to: metabolism changes, increased ammonia level, major tissue destruction, hypermetabolic state

Defining Characteristics: anorexia, nausea, vomiting, malabsorption of fats, malabsorption of vitamins, altered carbohydrate, fat, and protein metabolism, malnutrition, weight loss, fatigue, edema, ascites, actual inadequate food intake, weight loss, anorexia, absent bowel sounds, decreased peristalsis, muscle mass loss, changes in bowel habits, abdominal distention

Outcome Criteria

✔ Patient will be able to achieve positive nitrogen balance and have stable weight.

NOC: *Nutritional Status: Nutrient Intake*

INTERVENTIONS	RATIONALES
Provide diet that has protein in ordered amounts, with supplementation of vitamins and other nutrients.	Protein metabolism is altered with liver disease and results in increased ammonia levels. Vitamin/nutrient supplementation may be required because of malabsorption of element.
Ensure that patient is positioned in sitting position for meals.	Decreases abdominal tenderness and fullness, and prevents potential for aspiration.
Avoid sodium intake of amounts greater than ordered.	Sodium should be restricted to less than 500 mg per day to decrease edema and ascites.
If patient is unable to ingest adequate dietary intake, administer tube feedings or TPN as ordered.	Provides needed nutrients when patient is unable to eat.
Instruct patient/family if patient requires long-term feeding tubes.	Patient may require enteral feeding for several months if GI tract is dysfunctional. If patients have upper gastrointestinal tract obstruction or is in danger of aspiration complications, a percutaneously placed PEG tube may be required.

INTERVENTIONS	RATIONALES
Instruct patient/family in care of skin at placement site of tube for enteral feedings.	Patient is already compromised, and lack of adequate care to sites may result in necrosis of tissue, infection, or other complications.
Instruct patient/family in weighing patient on a weekly basis, with set parameters in which to notify physician.	Assists in monitoring nutritional status and sets boundaries for which to notify physician if weight is not being maintained to allow for changes in enteral solutions or feeding techniques.

NIC: *Nutrition Therapy*

Discharge or Maintenance Evaluation

- Patient will be able to ingest adequate amounts of prescribed diet to maintain weight and ammonia levels at acceptable levels.
- Patient will comply with dietary regimen and limitations.
- Patient will have no complications from enteral or parenteral therapies.

IMPAIRED SKIN INTEGRITY

Related to: poor nutrition, renal involvement, bile deposits on skin

Defining Characteristics: edema, ascites, jaundice, pruritus

Outcome Criteria

✔ Patient will maintain skin integrity.

NOC: *Tissue Integrity: Skin and Mucous Membranes*

INTERVENTIONS	RATIONALES
Observe skin for changes, abrasions, rashes, scaling, wounds, bleeding, redness, and so forth.	Facilitates identification of potential complications.
Turn at least every two hours and prn.	Prevents pressure area compromise of skin.
Apply lotions frequently when providing skin care; do not use soap when bathing; apply cornstarch or baking soda prn.	Soap may dry skin further and result in breach of integrity. Lotions and other agents may decrease itching.

INTERVENTIONS	RATIONALES
Administer medications for pruritus as ordered.	Decreases itching which may cause wounds. Bile salts that are deposited on the skin of patients with hepatic or renal involvement cause chronic and severe pruritus.
Instruct patient in methods to decrease itching: soothing massages, avoidance of extra covers, and use of clean white gloves at night.	Helps prevent patient from scratching during the night and reduces tendency to scratch.
Provide attention-diverting activity.	May refocus concentration to decrease scratching.

NIC: *Skin Surveillance*

Discharge or Maintenance Evaluation

- Patient will exhibit no evidence of skin breakdown.
- Patient will be able to use discussed methods to avoid scratching.
- Patient will have no complications from lack of skin integrity.

INEFFECTIVE BREATHING PATTERN

Related to: increased pressure from ascites, elevated ammonia levels, decreased lung expansion, fatigue

Defining Characteristics: presence of ascites, weakness, tachypnea, dyspnea, decreased lung expansion, altered arterial blood gases

Outcome Criteria

✔ Patient will maintain effective respiration with normal ABGs and hemodynamics.

NOC: *Respiratory Status: Ventilation*

INTERVENTIONS	RATIONALES
Monitor respiratory status for changes in rate and depth, use of accessory muscles, increased work of breathing, nasal flaring, and symmetric chest expansion.	Ascites may cause pressure and increase the effort of breathing. Depending on the severity and amount of ascitic fluid, the depth of the respirations may vary, and chest expansion may be decreased.

(continues)

(continued)

INTERVENTIONS	RATIONALES
Provide supplemental oxygen via nasal cannula or mask as ordered. Monitor saturation by oximetry and notify physician if <90%.	Provides needed supplementation of oxygen and may decrease work of breathing. If oximetry is <90%, further measures may be required, including changing oxygen sources and potential mechanical ventilation.
Monitor for presence of cough and character of any sputum.	Liver failure may result in abnormal coagulation, which in turn, can result in bloody secretions. Atelectasis from decreased chest excursion may occur and result in infection.
Auscultate lung fields for adventitious breath sounds or rubs.	Breath sounds may be decreased because of decreased chest expansion from increasing ascites.
Encourage deep breathing and coughing exercises.	Improves lung expansion and helps to remove secretions.
Assist with paracentesis.	May be required to remove ascitic fluid if respiratory insufficiency cannot be corrected by other methods.
Prepare patient for placement of peritoneovenous shunt.	Surgical intervention may be required to provide method to return accumulations of fluid in abdominal cavity to the systemic circulation and provides long-term ascites relief.

NIC: *Respiratory Monitoring*

Discharge or Maintenance Evaluation

■ Patient will be free of shortness of breath and will have normal lung expansion with optimal arterial blood gases and oxygenation.

INEFFECTIVE TISSUE PERFUSION: CEREBRAL

Related to: hepatic necrosis

Defining Characteristics: changes in mental status, confusion, disorientation, amnesia of past events, apathy, paranoia, forgetfulness, irritability, disobedient, depressed, euphoric, muscle tremors, muscle incoordination, insomnia, hypoactive reflexes, asterixis, ataxia, slurred speech, changes in level of consciousness, coma, bizarre behavior, nystagmus, Babinski sign, clonus, decorticate or decerebrate posturing, muscle rigidity, muscle flaccidity, seizures, pupillary dilation, abnormal electroencephalogram

Outcome Criteria

✔ Patient will maintain adequate cerebral perfusion until transplantation can be accomplished.

✔ Patient will suffer no complications from decreased cerebral perfusion.

NOC: *Tissue Perfusion: Cerebral*

INTERVENTIONS	RATIONALES
Assess patient completely, especially for grade of encephalopathic involvement.	Provides initial baseline from which to gauge deterioration in status. As encephalopathy worsens, patient's level of consciousness and ability to cooperate diminish to the point of coma.
Monitor airway and oxygenation via pulse oximetry.	As encephalopathy increases, metabolic changes take place and may result in inability of patient to maintain adequate airway requiring artificial intubation and placement on mechanical ventilation to maintain oxygenation.
Administer IV fluids as ordered.	Maintains hydration status and allows access for emergency and other medication administration.
Administer antimicrobials as ordered.	May be required if liver failure is caused by bacterial or viral pathogenic source.
Assist with insertion of ICP monitoring as needed.	Distinguishing attributes between acute and chronic liver failure are the presence of cerebral edema and increased intracranial pressure. ICP monitoring allows for continuous observance and identification of significant changes in ICP that can result in timely intervention to preserve cerebral perfusion.
Administer barbiturates or sedatives to place patient in coma if ordered.	May be required to decrease cerebral metabolism in order to preserve perfusion.
Administer mannitol as ordered.	Mannitol helps to decrease ICP and increase cerebral perfusion pressure.
Instruct patient/family regarding need for mechanical ventilation, ICP monitoring, or other procedures.	Promotes knowledge, decreases fear, and helps to ensure family that everything is being done for the patient.
Prepare patient/family for potential liver transplant.	Liver transplantation is the only essential treatment for acute fulminant liver failure, unless the

INTERVENTIONS	RATIONALES
	failure is caused by acetaminophen toxicity. Otherwise, the mortality rate is 100% without transplantation.

NIC: *Cerebral Perfusion Promotion*

Discharge or Maintenance Evaluation

- Patient will have cerebral perfusion maintained until transplantation.

- Patient will maintain airway, or be able to be kept oxygenated by artificial means.

- Patient will have perfusion to all vital organs and cerebral perfusion pressure will be maintained at greater than 50 mm Hg.

INEFFECTIVE TISSUE PERFUSION: CEREBRAL, CARDIOPULMONARY, RENAL, GASTROINTESTINAL, PERIPHERAL

Related to: complications from liver transplantation, transplant rejection, allergic reactions, infection

Defining Characteristics: absence of bile production, abnormal coagulation, increased lactate levels, hypothermia, hypoglycemia, hyperglycemia hypovolemia, elevated blood pressure, atelectasis, ileus, ulcers, elevated AST, ALT, GGT, alkaline phosphatase and bilirubin, abnormal arterial blood gases, dysrhythmias, dyspnea, use of accessory muscles, changes in mental status, changes in behavior, speech difficulties, weakness, paralysis in extremity, abdominal pain, tenderness, abdominal distention, nausea, vomiting, hypoactive bowel sounds, edema, weak or absent pulses, skin discolorations, increased BUN and creatinine, hematuria, oliguria, anuria, increased white blood cell count, differential shift to the left, blood dyscrasias, decreased platelet count, abnormal heart tones

Outcome Criteria

✔ Patient will have stable vital signs without complications of liver transplantation.

✔ Patient will have no signs or symptoms of altered tissue perfusion.

✔ If patient does have changes in perfusion, the symptoms will be recognized and treated promptly.

NOC: *Vital Sign Status*

INTERVENTIONS	RATIONALES
Monitor VS and hemodynamics q 1 hour and prn. Notify physician of significant changes.	Hypothermia may result from prolonged surgical procedure, which decreases perfusion, and vasodilation that occurs during the warming phase of hypothermia may cause cardiovascular instability. Hypertension and fluid volume increases may increase cardiac workload, myocardial oxygen demand, and myocardial oxygen consumption, which can lead to cardiac failure. Blood pressures below 70 mm Hg systolic interferes with autoregulatory mechanisms.
Monitor ECG for dysrhythmias or changes in cardiac rhythm, and treat per protocol.	Kidney failure, electrolyte imbalances, and liver failure may predispose patient to dysrhythmias and conduction problems. Hyperkalemia may be reflected with peaked T waves, widened QRS complex, increased PR interval, and flattened P wave. Hypokalemia may be reflected with flat T wave, peaked P wave, and sometimes the presence of a U wave. Treatment of potentially-lethal cardiac dysrhythmias may prevent death from complications of transplant failure.
Monitor neurologic status for changes in mentation or level of consciousness.	Decreasing neurologic status may be first indicator of electrolyte imbalances, worsening liver or renal failure, or other complication associated with transplant.
Monitor peripheral pulses for presence and character, skin color, turgor, and capillary refill time.	Vasoconstriction or anemia may cause pallor of extremities, and skin may be cyanotic or mottled with pulmonary edema or cardiac failure. Coagulopathy may contribute to bruising and potential symptoms of DIC.
Auscultate lung fields for adventitious breath sounds, and heart tones for abnormalities or changes, and notify physician.	Fluid overload and decreased perfusion may result in development of gallops and a pericardial friction rub may indicate the presence of uremic pericarditis. Posttransplantation complications include unresolved intrapulmonary shunting and hepatopulmonary syndrome. Paresis of the right hemidiaphragm may result in decreased breath sounds and lead to atelectasis and infiltrate formation.

(continues)

(continued)

INTERVENTIONS	RATIONALES
Monitor for complaints of paresthesias, muscle cramps, muscle weakness, or paralysis.	May indicate impairment of neuromuscular activity, hypocalcemia, and potential for decreased cardiac perfusion and function.
Monitor I&O q 1–2 hours and prn. Notify physician of output <30 cc/hr.	Oliguria and anuria may be seen with fluid volume excess or decreased perfusion states. Decreases in urinary output that do not respond to fluid challenges cause renal vasoconstriction and decreased perfusion from increased renin secretion. Immunosuppressant drug toxicity may result in acute tubular necrosis, and renal system compromise because of unresolved hepatorenal syndrome.
Provide oxygen via nasal cannula or mask as ordered. Monitor oxygen saturation by oximetry and notify physician if <90%.	Facilitates oxygenation of tissues in the presence of decreased perfusion and increased workload.
Monitor lab work, especially electrolytes, clotting profiles, renal function, liver function, and glucose levels.	Hypoglycemia and the absence of bile production may indicate that the transplanted liver is nonfunctional because of ischemia, preservation injury, procurement injury, or hepatic artery thrombosis. Coagulation abnormalities may result because of massive blood replacement or nonfunctioning liver transplant. Hyperglycemia may be seen if gastrointestinal or endocrine system is dysfunctional. Renal and liver abnormalities may indicate decreased perfusion and ischemia, and potential rejection of liver. Increased white blood cell count, with shift to the left on differential may indicate bacterial infection that is a complication of surgery or surgical error, or is the result of immunocompromise. Increases in AST, ALT, GGT, alkaline phosphatase and bilirubin all signal acute cellular rejection of liver.
Administer IV fluids as ordered.	Maintains hydration and provides access for administration of medications and blood products.
Administer antimicrobials as ordered.	May be required if patient develops infection.

INTERVENTIONS	RATIONALES
Administer immunosuppressant drugs as ordered.	These drugs are required in order to facilitate patient's body's acceptance of donor liver.
Instruct patient/family in symptoms of organ rejection.	Provides knowledge, and ensures that patient and family will be alert for rejection and can seek timely intervention when it occurs.
Instruct patient/family on isolation techniques.	Patient may require isolation because of immunocompromise resulting from immunosuppressant drug use.

NIC: *Surveillance*

Discharge or Maintenance Evaluation

- Patient will have stable liver function from donor transplant.
- Patient will be able to acknowledge signs and symptoms to be aware of in regards to transplant rejection.

RISK FOR INJURY

Related to: hemorrhage, altered clotting factors, portal hypertension

Defining Characteristics: bleeding, exsanguination, decreased hemoglobin and hematocrit, decreased prothrombin, decreased fibrinogen, decreased clotting factors VIII, IX, and X, vitamin K malabsorption, thromboplastin release

Outcome Criteria

✔ Patient will exhibit no evidence of bleeding.

NOC: *Symptom Control*

INTERVENTIONS	RATIONALES
Monitor all bodily secretions for presence of blood; test stools and nasogastric drainage for guaiac.	GI bleeding may occur because of altered clotting factors and changes that occur with cirrhosis and liver disease.
Observe for bleeding from puncture sites, presence of hematomas or petechiae, or bruising.	May indicate a form of disseminated intravascular coagulation as a result of altered clotting factors.

INTERVENTIONS	RATIONALES
Monitor vital signs and hemo-dynamic parameters. Avoid rectal temperatures.	Changes in vital signs may indicate loss of circulating blood volume. Vasculature in rectum may be susceptible to rupture.
Insert nasogastric tube gently and lavage as ordered.	Esophageal vasculature may be susceptible to rupture. Removal of blood from the stomach decreases synthesis to ammonia.
Administer vitamins as ordered.	Vitamin K facilitates synthesis of prothrombin and coagulation if liver is functional. Vitamin C may reduce potential for GI bleeding and facilitates healing process.
Administer stool softeners as needed.	Prevents straining to pass stool which may result in rupture of vasculature or increase in intra-abdominal pressures.
Monitor lab work for CBC and clotting factors.	Helps to identify blood loss or impending DIC.

NIC: *Bleeding Reduction*

Discharge or Maintenance Evaluation

- Patient will have no active bleeding and lab work will be within normal limits.
- Patient will not exhibit any hemorrhagic compli-cations from invasive line/tube placement.

DISTURBED BODY IMAGE

Related to: changes in physical appearance, ascites

Defining Characteristics: presence of ascites, biophys-ical changes, negative feelings about body, fear of rejection, fear of reaction from others, fear of death, fear of the unknown

Outcome Criteria

✔ Patient will be able to verbalize concerns and accept body/self perception within situational limits.

NOC: *Acceptance: Health Status*

INTERVENTIONS	RATIONALES
Encourage patient to discuss concerns, fears, and questions regarding diagnosis being careful to recognize and accept his fears without minimizing them.	Validates patient's feelings and concerns regarding changes in body.

INTERVENTIONS	RATIONALES
Discuss causes of alteration of appearance with patient and family members.	Validates realistic changes and allows for reinstruction on areas that may not have been under-stood. Jaundice, bruising, and ascites may be considered unattractive by patient and/or family, and may precipitate feelings of low self-esteem and body worth.
Encourage family to support patient without rejection or fear of his appearance.	Patient and family may experience guilt, especially if the cause is alcohol or drug-related. Emo-tional support from loved ones may enhance patient's ability to accept changes.
Consult with social services, counseling, psychiatric services, minister, or other community resources.	Additional professional and community resources may be required to deal with alcohol or drug rehabilitation, or with perceptions of body image.
Instruct patient/family regarding all procedures.	Promotes knowledge and facilitates compliance.
Instruct patient and family about importance of discussing feelings and concerns about changes in body appearance.	Discussion helps to provide emotional support and correct inaccurate information and misperceptions.
Instruct patient/family regarding loose-fitting clothes and other items for comfort.	Abdominal swelling may pre-clude patient from wearing previous clothing, and patient may feel isolated. Loose-fitting clothing provides patient with as much comfort for changes in body shape and size.

NIC: *Body Image Enhancement*

Discharge or Maintenance Evaluation

- Patient will be able to verbalize concerns over his appearance.
- Patient will be able to verbalize understanding of disease process and changes that may occur.
- Patient will be able to effectively utilize methods for coping with changes.
- Family will be supportive of patient's altered appearance and self-esteem.
- Patient will be able to effectively access commu-nity resources for continuing needs.

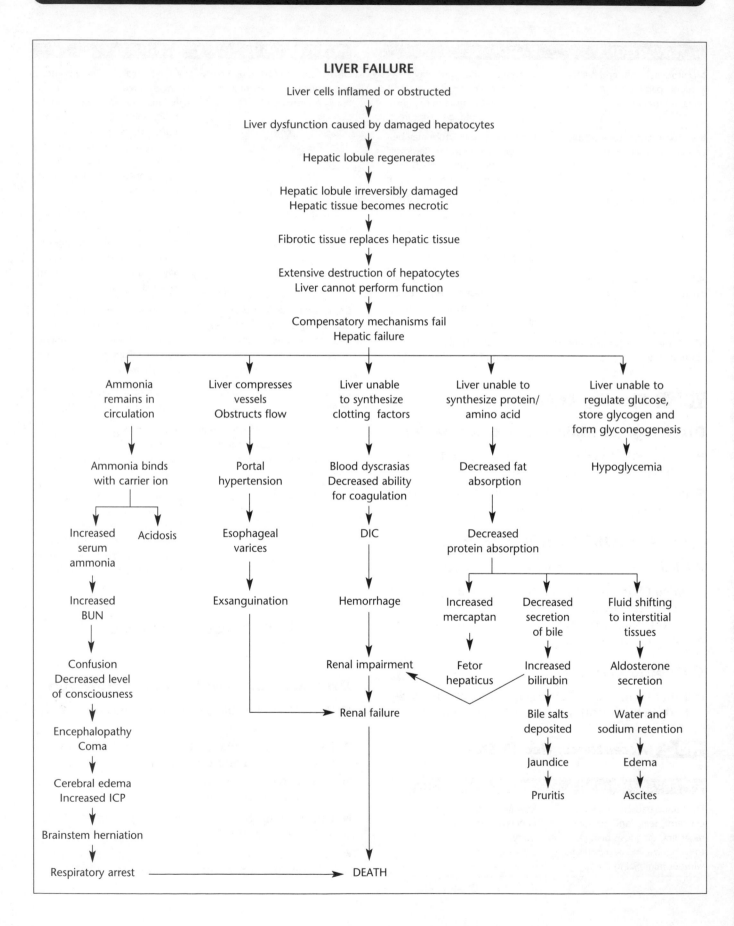

UNIT 5

HEMATOLOGIC SYSTEM

CHAPTER 5.1

DISSEMINATED INTRAVASCULAR COAGULATION

Disseminated intravascular coagulation, also known as consumptive coagulopathy, defibrinogenation syndrome, or DIC, is an acute disorder that accelerates the activation of the intrinsic and/or extrinsic cascade clotting mechanism and depletes both clotting factors and platelets. DIC is usually a complication of another disease process in which excessive thrombin is produced, converting fibrinogen to fibrin, and the fibrin creates damaging thrombi in the microcirculation. Fibrin blocks the capillary flow to the organs and results in ischemic tissue damage, and as the clotting factors, platelets, and fibrin split products (FSP) are consumed, hemorrhage and shock result. As the fibrin and FSP repolymerize, a secondary fibrin mesh forms in the microcirculation and when blood travels through this, the red blood cells become damaged and a hemolytic anemia can occur.

Some of the precipitating factors include sepsis, neoplasm necrosis, eclampsia, abruptio placentae, saline-induced abortions, retained dead fetus, amniotic fluid embolus, hemolysis, giant hemangiomas, systemic lupus erythematosus, transfusions, trauma, crush injuries, shock, burns, head injuries, transplant rejection, snake bite, fractures, anoxia, heat stroke, surgery utilizing cardiopulmonary bypass, and necrotizing enterocolitis.

Bleeding in a patient with no other previous history of bleeding or coagulopathy problems should raise questions as to the possibility of the presence of DIC. DIC may be acute or chronic (usually seen with neoplasms) and can vary in severity from mild oozing to exsanguination from all orifices. Treatment is aimed at correction of the underlying problem, correction of shock, acidosis, and sepsis, supportive care to restore circulatory volume and adequate oxygenation of tissues, and to replace blood loss resulting from hemorrhage.

MEDICAL CARE

Laboratory: prothrombin time (PT) to measure activity level and patency of the extrinsic and final pathways, increased in DIC; partial thromboplastin time (PTT) to measure activity level and patency of the intrinsic and final pathways, increased in DIC; thromboplastin time increased, platelet count decreased; fibrinogen usually decreased showing increased hypercoagability and decreased bleeding tendency; FSP elevated, usually >10; clotting factor analysis used to identify factors being depleted; increased D-dimers; prolonged TT; CBC used to evaluate anemia and RBC fragmentation; BUN and creatinine used to assess renal involvement from thrombosis; guaiacs on all body fluids to identify occult bleeding; cultures of sputum, blood, urine, CSF, and other drainage used to identify causative organism of infection and to ascertain appropriate antimicrobial therapy

Blood components: used as replacement therapy for significant blood loss; RBCs given to increase the oxygen-carrying capability; whole blood, plasma, plasmanate and albumin used to expand volume; fresh frozen plasma (FFP) and albumin used to replace proteins; FFP, cryoprecipitate, and fresh whole blood used to replace coagulation factors; platelet concentrate used to replace platelets

IV fluids: used to treat hypovolemia and shock

Antimicrobials: used to treat infection that may cause DIC

Heparin: use is controversial; heparin inhibits microthrombi formation by neutralizing free circulating thrombin; should not be used unless bleeding is unmanageable by replacement therapy of FFP and platelets

COMMON NURSING DIAGNOSES

IMPAIRED GAS EXCHANGE (see GI BLEEDING)

Related to: bleeding, disease

Defining Characteristics: decreased PaO$_2$ below 80 mm Hg, dyspnea, tachypnea, increased work of breathing, restlessness, irritability, mental status changes, changes in blood pressure and pulse, decreased hemoglobin and hematocrit

RISK FOR DEFICIENT FLUID VOLUME (see GI BLEEDING)

Related to: blood loss, altered coagulability

Defining Characteristics: weight loss, oliguria, abnormal electrolytes, hypotension, tachycardia, decreased central venous pressures, decreased filling pressures, altered coagulation studies, lethargy, mental status changes

ADDITIONAL NURSING DIAGNOSES

RISK FOR INJURY

Related to: hemorrhage, blood loss, altered coagulability

Defining Characteristics: bleeding, exsanguination, decreased hemoglobin and hematocrit levels, increased fibrin split products, increased prothrombin time, decreased platelet count, increased partial thromboplastin time, decreased fibrinogen, bruising, prolonged bleeding, petechiae, ecchymoses, hematomas, purpura, hematemesis, hemoptysis, hematochezia, melena, menorrhagia, hematuria

Outcome Criteria

✔ Patient will be free of unexplained bleeding and will have stable vital signs and hemodynamic pressures.

✔ Patient will have coagulation lab values within set parameters.

✔ The patient and family will be able to accurately verbalize pathologic causes and bleeding precautions that are required.

NOC: *Symptom Control*

INTERVENTIONS	RATIONALES
Identify and treat underlying disorder.	Treatment of cause and correction of coagulation problem is major goal of treatment. DIC is most often seen as the complication of an underlying infection, malignant disease, trauma, or shock state.
Administer IV fluids as ordered.	Large volumes may be required to maintain circulating volume because of bleeding, and to maintain hemodynamic status.
Administer blood and blood by-products, such as cryoprecipitate, fresh frozen plasma, and so forth as ordered.	May be required to replace circulating blood volume and to help correct thrombocytopenia or hypofibrinogenemia. If platelet transfusion is planned prior to performance of procedures, the transfusion should be given just prior to the procedure to ensure that the maximum number of platelets will be available to stop the bleeding caused by the procedure.
Administer supplemental oxygen as warranted.	Decreased blood volume impairs oxygen carrying capability and supplemental oxygen may be required to maintain oxygenation.
Observe patient for petechiae, bruising, overt and occult bleeding.	May be present with impending DIC.
Avoid prolonged tourniquet use. When possible take manual blood pressure readings and inflate cuff only until the pulse is obliterated.	Helps to prevent petechiae formation along arm.
Avoid taking rectal temperatures when possible. Avoid administering suppositories and enemas; instead utilize increased fiber in diet or use of stool softeners.	Helps to avoid injury to rectal mucosa that may instigate bleeding. Use of fiber and stool softeners may help prevent constipation and straining at stool, which may result in rectal bleeding.
Monitor for dyspnea, hemoptysis, and decreased saturation; auscultate lung fields for adventitious breath sounds.	Crackles may be present and patient may exhibit these signs if microemboli in the pulmonary circulation are present.
Monitor intake and output.	Microemboli or deposits of fibrin within the renal system may present as renal insufficiency or failure.

(continues)

(continued)

INTERVENTIONS	RATIONALES
Administer heparin therapy as ordered.	Controversial treatment may be given to disperse clumped clotting factors, but is rarely used today. Heparin reduces the conversion of prothrombin to thrombin and slows the coagulation cycle, which is thought by some physicians to allow the body to replenish platelets and clotting factors. Other clinicians believe that heparin exacerbates the patient's bleeding.
Monitor lab work for coagulation studies and CBC.	Provided identification of effectiveness of therapy or worsening of condition.
Instruct patient in use of soft toothbrush, toothette, or mouth rinses.	Maintains oral hygiene while decreases incidence of oral bleeding.
Instruct patient to use electric razor and avoid other types of razors.	Decreases chance for patient to nick skin and cause bleeding.
Instruct patient/family regarding disease process, precautions against bleeding, and symptoms of which to notify nurse or physician.	Provides knowledge of disease, helps to lessen risk of bleeding and hemorrhage, and assists with prompt identification of complications to allow for timely intervention.

INTERVENTIONS	RATIONALES
Instruct patient/family regarding medications to avoid, such as aspirin, Pepto-Bismol, oxycodone, and NSAIDs.	These drugs interfere with platelet function and can cause bleeding and hemorrhage.

NIC: *Hemorrhage Control*

Discharge or Maintenance Evaluation

- Patient will have stable vital signs and hemodynamic pressures.
- Patient will exhibit no bleeding tendencies or active hemorrhage.
- Patient will exhibit no complications from other disease processes.
- Patient will achieve and maintain adequate blood volume.
- Patient will have underlying disease process corrected.
- Patient/family will be able to accurately verbalize risks of bleeding, methods of avoiding risks, avoidance of medications that may cause bleeding, and understanding of disease process.

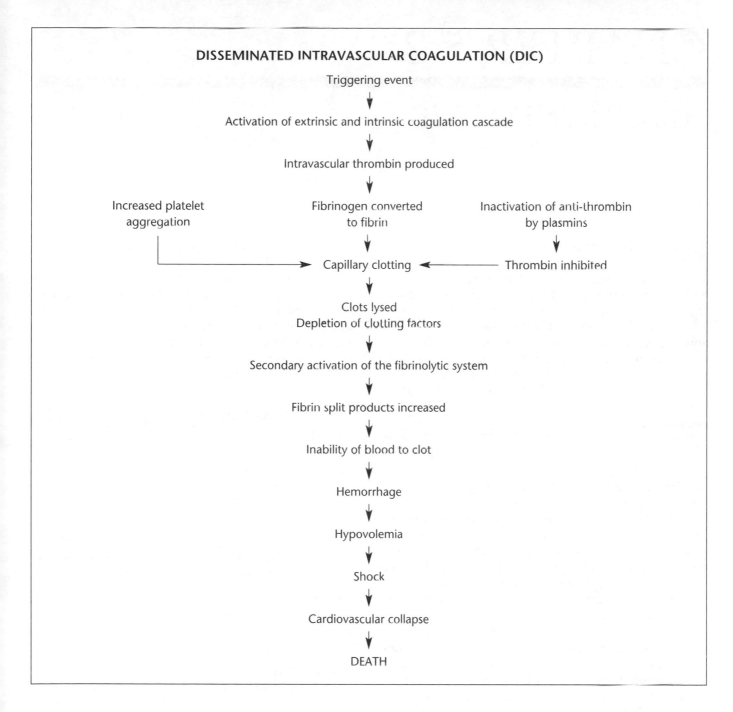

DISSEMINATED INTRAVASCULAR COAGULATION (DIC)

Triggering event

↓

Activation of extrinsic and intrinsic coagulation cascade

↓

Intravascular thrombin produced

↓

Increased platelet aggregation	Fibrinogen converted to fibrin	Inactivation of anti-thrombin by plasmins

Capillary clotting

↓

Clots lysed
Depletion of clotting factors

↓

Secondary activation of the fibrinolytic system

↓

Fibrin split products increased

↓

Inability of blood to clot

↓

Hemorrhage

↓

Hypovolemia

↓

Shock

↓

Cardiovascular collapse

↓

DEATH

CHAPTER 5.2

HELLP SYNDROME

HELLP syndrome is an acute and severe complication that presents as a multiorganic disease process occurring concurrently with pregnancy-induced hypertension (PIH). The initials are compiled from the symptoms that comprise the syndrome: hemolysis, elevated liver enzymes and low platelets. These same findings may also be associated with DIC and frequently are diagnosed as such.

PIH usually occurs after the twentieth week of gestation in approximately 5% of all pregnancies, and most often in the primigravida patient. PIH results in increased edema, proteinuria, and hypertension. Although the cause is unknown, theories often involve immunologic, endocrine, and chorionic villi exposure.

HELLP may represent an acute autoimmune state in which the red blood cells lyse, liver enzymes are elevated as a result of fibrin thrombi blocking blood flow to the liver, and platelets decrease because of vasospasm and platelet aggregation. Vasospasm results in increases in systemic and peripheral vascular resistance, which increase blood pressure further. Sensitivity to angiotensin II is increased, and vasoconstriction may result in increases in vascular permeability and hemoconcentration.

The pathologic changes in the liver may develop because of generalized activation of the intravascular coagulation process. Fibrin deposits and hemorrhagic necrosis develops in periportal areas and may lead to subcapsular hematomas or liver rupture. A decrease in antithrombin III and an increase in thrombin–antithrombin III complex (TAT) and the appearance of fibrin monomers and D-dimers is found in almost all cases of HELLP, but decompensated intravascular coagulation with increased PT and PTT and decreased fibrinogen levels is found only in severe forms. Decompensated coagulation occurs with other complications such as liver hematoma, abruptio placentae, renal failure, and pulmonary edema.

There is usually a low recurrence rate (5% or less), and the HELLP syndrome usually resolves with delivery of the baby. Treatment involves prophylaxis against postpartum worsening, curettage of the uterus, and treatment with calcium antagonists and decadron, as well as intense monitoring for a decline in liver function and for potential for bleeding.

MEDICAL CARE

Laboratory: hematocrit used to assess intravascular fluid status; protime and partial thromboplastin time used to evaluate clotting; magnesium levels used to evaluate therapeutic levels for treatment; urine collection for protein used to diagnose complications

Magnesium: used to prevent and treat convulsions by decreasing the neuromuscular irritability and depressing the central nervous system

Antihypertensives: apresoline is the drug of choice; used to relax arterioles and stimulate cardiac output and is utilized with diastolic blood pressures greater than 110 mm Hg

Beta-blockers: drugs such as acebutolol (Sectral), atenolol (Tenormin), betaxolol hydrochloride (Kerlone), bisoprolol fumarate (Zebeta), carteolol hydrochloride (Cartrol), carvedilol (Coreg), esmolol (Brevibloc), metoprolol (Toprol XL, Betaloc, Lopressor), labetalol hydrochloride (Normodyne, Trandate), nadolol (Corgard), pindolol (Visken), propranolol (Inderal), sotalol hydrochloride (Betapace), and timolol (Blocadren) occasionally used to control acute hypertensive crises

Valium: used to control seizure activity

COMMON NURSING DIAGNOSES

IMPAIRED GAS EXCHANGE (see GI BLEEDING)

Related to: bleeding, disease

Defining Characteristics: decreased PaO_2 below 80 mm Hg, dyspnea, tachypnea, increased work of breathing, restlessness, irritability, mental status changes, changes in blood pressure and pulse, decreased hemoglobin and hematocrit

RISK FOR DEFICIENT FLUID VOLUME (see GI BLEEDING)

Related to: blood loss, altered coagulability

Defining Characteristics: weight loss, oliguria, abnormal electrolytes, hypotension, tachycardia, decreased central venous pressures, altered coagulation studies, lethargy, mental status changes

ADDITIONAL NURSING DIAGNOSES

RISK FOR INJURY

Related to: administration of magnesium

Defining Characteristics: CNS depression, venous irritation, dyspnea, shallow respirations, decreased oxygen saturation, oliguria, absence of deep tendon reflexes, changes in vital signs

Outcome Criteria

✔ Patient will receive medication without experiencing side effects.

NOC: *Risk Detection*

INTERVENTIONS	RATIONALES
Montor for convulsions or tremors.	Identifies precipitation of problem.
Administer magnesium sulfate as ordered.	Magnesium is used to prevent and treat convulsions by decreasing the neuromuscular irritability and depression of the central nervous system. Normally, $MgSO_4$ is given IV, with a loading dose of 3–4 gm, followed by an infusion of 1–4 gm/hr. It may be given IM with dosage of 5 gm

INTERVENTIONS	RATIONALES
	gm in each hip every 4 hours using the Z-tract method. Some facilities add xylocaine to the medication to decrease the pain of IM injections.
Monitor vital signs every 1–2 hours, and prn, especially respiratory status.	Depression of central nervous system can result in respiratory insufficiency or paralysis. Hypothermia may occur with toxicity of drug. $MgSO_4$ should be held for respirations less than 16 per minute.
Monitor ECG for changes and dysrhythmias, and treat per protocol.	Dysrhythmias may occur with administration of magnesium or with its antidote, calcium.
Monitor I&O every 2 hours.	Magnesium sulfate may cause toxicity with large doses and result in renal insufficiency and oliguria.
Monitor fetal heart tones every hour.	Fetal heart rate may decrease with use of magnesium sulfate.
Assess deep tendon reflexes (DTRs).	Absence of DTRs may indicate hypermagnesemia and toxicity. Decreased DTRs may occur with therapeutic ranges.
Have calcium gluconate at bedside and give as warranted/ordered.	Calcium gluconate is the antidote for magnesium sulfate.
Monitor lab work for magnesium sulfate.	Normal levels are 4–7.5 mEq/L, with toxic levels above that.
Instruct patient on signs and symptoms to report to nurse/physician.	Facilitates prompt identification of problem to allow for timely intervention.
Observe IM injection sites for redness, firm areas, warmth, and pain.	May indicate presence of sterile abscess from injections which have a variable rate of absorption given in this manner.

NIC: *High-Risk Pregnancy Care*

Discharge or Maintenance Evaluation

- Patient will have stable vital signs.
- Patient will be free of convulsions.
- Fetal heart rates will remain unaffected and activity will be within normal range.
- Patient will exhibit no signs of magnesium toxicity or complications from therapy.

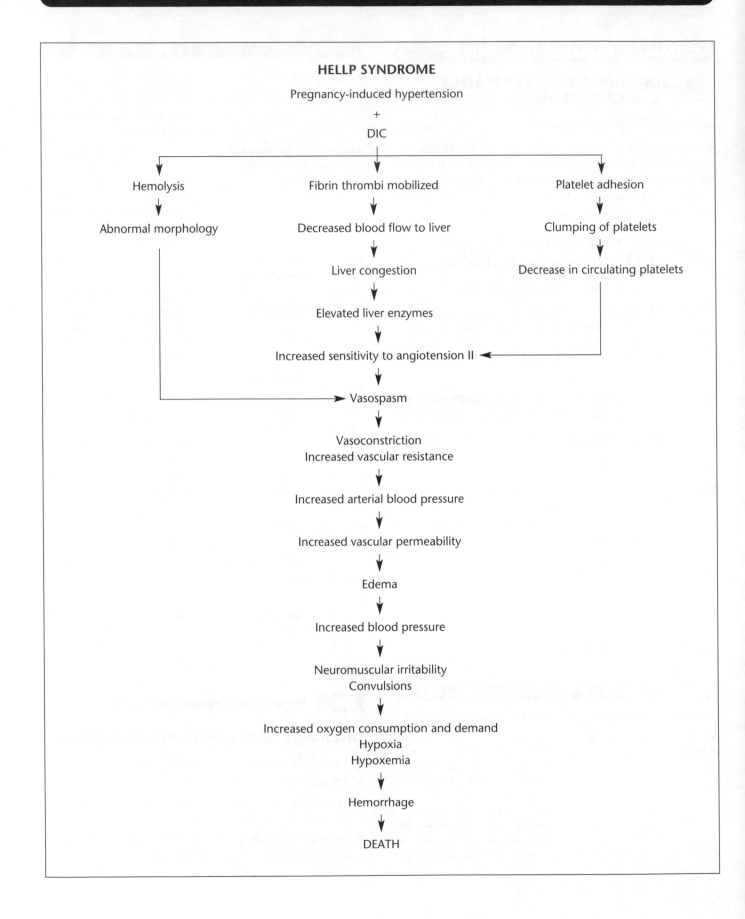

HELLP SYNDROME

Pregnancy-induced hypertension

+

DIC

Hemolysis	Fibrin thrombi mobilized	Platelet adhesion
Abnormal morphology	Decreased blood flow to liver	Clumping of platelets
	Liver congestion	Decrease in circulating platelets
	Elevated liver enzymes	

Increased sensitivity to angiotension II

Vasospasm

Vasoconstriction
Increased vascular resistance

Increased arterial blood pressure

Increased vascular permeability

Edema

Increased blood pressure

Neuromuscular irritability
Convulsions

Increased oxygen consumption and demand
Hypoxia
Hypoxemia

Hemorrhage

DEATH

CHAPTER 5.3

ANEMIA

Anemia is a condition in which the red blood cell count, hemoglobin, and hematocrit are decreased. This decrease results in a decrease in the oxygen-carrying capability and causes tissue hypoxia. As the body tries to compensate, blood is shifted from areas that have a plentiful amount in tissues that have low oxygen requirements to those areas that require higher oxygen concentrations, such as the heart and brain.

There are several types of anemias; those that are caused by decreased red blood cell production, those that are caused by blood loss, and the hemolytic anemias caused from G6PD deficiency, autoimmunity, or physical causes. Microcytic, or iron deficiency anemia, develops when the transportation of iron by transferrin is insufficient to meet requirements of the erythropoietic cells. Macrocytic, or megaloblastic anemia, occurs because of a deficiency in vitamin B_{12} or folic acid. Pernicious anemia is a type of megaloblastic anemia in which the absence of vitamin B_{12} as well as a lack of the intrinsic factor is noted. Normocytic, or aplastic anemia, is caused from the failure of the bone marrow or destruction of bone marrow by either chemical or physical means. Autoimmune anemia is an acquired condition that involves premature erythrocyte destruction from the person's own immune system. Hemolytic anemia results when erythrocyte destruction is increased and cells have a shortened life span. Sickle cell anemia is an inherited condition in which hemoglobin S is present in the blood resulting in sickling and abnormal hemolyzation that obstructs capillary flow. Thalassemia is a group of inherited anemias that results from faulty production of alpha or beta-hemoglobin polypeptides.

Anemia can occur as the direct result of prosthetic heart valves or extracorporeal circulation and the destruction of red blood cells. Anemias can also be precipitated by toxic substance exposure or chronic disease processes, such as uremia or chronic liver disease.

MEDICAL CARE

Laboratory: CBC to help differentiate type of anemia—RBCs reduced; hemoglobin decreased with mild considered 10–14 m/dl, moderate 6–10 m/dl, and severe below 6 m/dl; hematocrit decreased; MCH, MCHC variable dependent on type of anemia; MCV 80–100 fl with normocytic, greater than 100 fl with macrocytic, and less than 80 fl with microcytic; platelet count usually decreased, but may be elevated after hemorrhage; RDW increased in iron depletion anemia; B_{12} level decreased, folate decreased; serum iron and TIBC may be decreased; stool guaiac may be positive if blood loss is from GI tract; increased reticulocyte count, decreased ferritin level, positive Coombs' testing, increased indirect bilirubin; urinalysis may show hematuria

Radiography: chest X-ray used to discern pulmonary or cardiac complications; upper and lower gastrointestinal series may be done to identify active or current bleeding

Bone marrow aspiration: may be performed to determine type of anemia; evaluates bone marrow production of red blood cells and can identify malignant cells infiltrated throughout bone marrow

Bone marrow transplants: may be required for severe aplastic anemia

Blood transfusions: may be required to replace blood volume in hemorrhage

COMMON NURSING DIAGNOSES

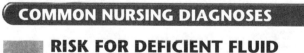

RISK FOR DEFICIENT FLUID VOLUME (see GI BLEEDING)

Related to: bleeding

Defining Characteristics: hypotension, tachycardia, decreased skin turgor, weakness, decreased urinary output, pallor, diaphoresis, decreased capillary refill, mental changes, restlessness, decreased filling pressures

ACTIVITY INTOLERANCE (see COPD)

Related to: decreased oxygen-carrying capability

Defining Characteristics: weakness, lethargy, fatigue, dyspnea, activity intolerance, chest pain, palpitations, tachycardia, decreased oxygen saturation, increased respiratory rate with exertion, hypertension

IMBALANCED NUTRITION: LESS THAN BODY REQUIREMENTS (see DKA)

Related to: inability to absorb required nutrients for red blood cell production

Defining Characteristics: weight loss, activity intolerance, dyspnea, fatigue, weakness, loss of muscle tone, anorexia

ADDITIONAL NURSING DIAGNOSES

INEFFECTIVE TISSUE PERFUSION: CARDIOPULMONARY, RENAL, CEREBRAL, GASTROINTESTINAL, PERIPHERAL

Related to: altered oxygen-carrying capability, blood loss

Defining Characteristics: decreased hematocrit and hemoglobin, chest pain, palpitations, pallor, dry mucous membranes, cold intolerance, oliguria, nausea, vomiting, abdominal pain, abdominal distention, increased capillary refill time, confusion, lethargy, changes in pulse rate and blood pressure

Outcome Criteria

✔ Patient will have adequate perfusion to all body systems with stable vital signs and hemodynamics

NOC: *Tissue Perfusion*

INTERVENTIONS	RATIONALES
Monitor vital signs every 1–2 hours and prn	Facilitates identification of changes that may require intervention.

INTERVENTIONS	RATIONALES
Monitor neurologic status for mental confusion or level of consciousness changes.	May be indicative of impaired cerebral perfusion.
Auscultate lung fields for adventitious breath sounds. Auscultate for abnormal heart tones.	Crackles and/or new presence of cardiac gallops may indicate impending or present congestive failure that may have resulted from the body's compensatory mechanism of increasing cardiac output. Mild anemia can cause exertional dyspnea and palpitations; moderate anemia can cause increased palpitations and dyspnea at rest; severe anemia causes tachycardia, increased pulse pressure, systolic murmurs, intermittent claudication, angina, congestive heart failure, orthopnea, and tachypnea.
Administer supplemental oxygen as warranted.	Decreases in red blood cells decreases oxygen-carrying capability as oxygen is bound to the hemoglobin for transport, and may require supplementation to maintain oxygenation.
Monitor ECG for changes in cardiac rhythm or conduction. Treat per protocol.	Changes may occur with imbalances of electrolytes, with fluid shifts, or with hypoxia.
Monitor for complaints of chest pain, pressure, palpitations, or dyspnea.	May indicate decreased cardiac perfusion from hypoxia or ischemia.
Administer blood and/or blood products as warranted.	Blood replacement may facilitate improved oxygen-carrying ability because of increased number of red blood cells and correct volume deficiency.
Monitor lab work for changes.	May facilitate identification of deficiencies and allow for assessment of effectiveness of treatment.
Maintain environment temperature within normal ranges.	Reduction of peripheral perfusion may result in cold intolerance to vasoconstriction. Excessive heat may cause vasodilation and further reduce organ perfusion.
Prepare patient/family for surgical procedures as warranted.	May require transplantation of bone marrow, or surgical repair for site of bleeding.

NIC: *Bleeding Precautions*

Discharge or Maintenance Evaluation

- Patient will achieve and maintain adequate perfusion to all body systems.
- Patient will have stable vital signs and hemodynamic pressures.
- Patient will exhibit no evidence of GI bleeding.
- Patient will exhibit no signs of complications of disease or therapy.

DEFICIENT KNOWLEDGE

Related to: lack of information, unfamiliarity with information, lack of recall, misinterpretation of information, hypoxia

Defining Characteristics: questions, communication of misconceptions, development of preventable complications, incorrect follow-up with instructions

Outcome Criteria

✔ Patient will be able to verbalize understanding of disease process, treatment regimen, and procedures, and comply with therapy.

NOC: *Knowledge: Disease Process*

INTERVENTIONS	RATIONALES
Instruct patient/family on particular type of anemia that patient has developed.	Provided knowledge and facilitates compliance.
Instruct patient/family on lab work and other procedures.	Decreases anxiety and fear of the unknown.

INTERVENTIONS	RATIONALES
Instruct patient/family on dietary requirements.	Increasing iron sources from red meat, egg yolks, dried fruits and green leafy vegetables may facilitate correction of anemia. Folic acid and vitamin C which augments iron absorption may be found in green vegetables, whole grains, citrus fruits, and liver.
Instruct patient/family on signs and symptoms of which to notify physician.	Decreased leukocyte count may potentiate the risk of infection and patient should seek medical assistance for timely intervention.
Instruct patient/family on medications, effects, side effects, contraindications, and avoidance of over-the-counter medications without physician approval.	Iron or vitamin B_{12} replacement may be necessary for life, and knowledge regarding therapeutic management will increase compliance with treatment and allow for prompt identification of complications that may require changes in dosages, types of medication, or schedule of administration.

NIC: *Teaching: Disease Process*

Discharge or Maintenance Evaluation

- Patient will be able to verbalize and demonstrate understanding of all instructed information.
- Patient will be knowledgeable about his particular type of anemia.
- Patient will be able to recognize signs and symptoms of infection or hemorrhage and notify physician.

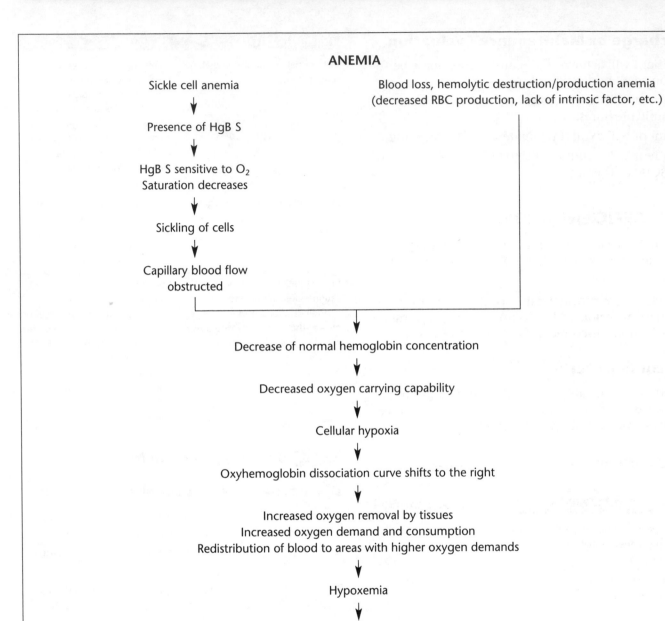

ANEMIA

Sickle cell anemia

↓

Presence of HgB S

↓

HgB S sensitive to O₂
Saturation decreases

↓

Sickling of cells

↓

Capillary blood flow
obstructed

Blood loss, hemolytic destruction/production anemia
(decreased RBC production, lack of intrinsic factor, etc.)

Decrease of normal hemoglobin concentration

↓

Decreased oxygen carrying capability

↓

Cellular hypoxia

↓

Oxyhemoglobin dissociation curve shifts to the right

↓

Increased oxygen removal by tissues
Increased oxygen demand and consumption
Redistribution of blood to areas with higher oxygen demands

↓

Hypoxemia

↓

Organ dysfunction

↓

Organ failure

↓

DEATH

UNIT 6

RENAL/ENDOCRINE SYSTEMS

CHAPTER 6.1

ACUTE RENAL FAILURE

Acute renal failure (ARF) is noted when there is a sudden deterioration in function of the renal system that may be caused by renal circulation failure or glomerular or tubular dysfunction. The buildup of waste materials that accumulates affects multiple organ systems.

ARF can be subclassified according to the etiology of condition, such as prerenal, intrarenal, and postrenal. Prerenal conditions occur when blood perfusion is inadequate, such as with hypotension, hemorrhage, myocardial infarction, congestive heart failure, pulmonary embolism, burns, third spacing, septic shock, diuretic abuse, or volume depletion. This dysfunction causes glomerular filtration rates to decrease, and decreased reabsorption of sodium in the tubules.

Intrarenal renal failure occurs either from damage to the tubular epithelium, known as acute tubular necrosis (ATN), or from damage to glomeruli and the small vessels. This condition causes renal capillary swelling that decreases the glomerular filtration rate (GFR), or decreased GFR is secondary to the obstruction of the glomeruli by edema and cellular debris. ATN is the most common type of ARF and is the result of nephrotoxins or ischemia. Intrarenal failure may take many weeks to repair damage and is usually seen with trauma, sepsis, DIC, transfusion reactions, renal vasculature blockages, heavy metal poisoning, and with use of aminoglycosides, penicillins, tetracylines, dilantin, and amphotericin. Glomeruli damage is seen with acute glomerulonephritis, polyarteritis nodosa, lupus erythematosus, Goodpasture's syndrome, endocarditis, abruptio placentae, abortion, serum sickness, malignant hypertension, or hemolytic uremic syndromes.

Postrenal failure may occur as a result of an obstruction anywhere in the system from the kidney to the urethra. Some clinical conditions in which this type of failure is seen includes urethral obstruction, prostatic hypertrophy, bladder carcinoma, bladder infection, neurogenic bladder, renal calculi, and abdominal tumors.

There are four phases in ARF—an onset phase, an oliguric phase, a diuretic phase, and a recovery phase. The initial, or onset, phase occurs prior to the actual necrotic injury and is associated with alterations in renal function and hemodynamics. Sympathetic activity or an increase in renal vascular resistance help to contribute to decreased renal perfusion. The renal blood flow and glomerular filtration rate (GFR) are decreased, as is cardiac output.

The oliguric phase occurs when the tubule obstruction caused by cellular debris, casts, or tubular swelling, creates damage to the renal system and makes absorption unstable. BUN, creatinine, and potassium levels increase. The damage causes development of necrotic areas that result in fluid leakage from the cells of ATP and potassium, and calcium is able to leak into the cells. Vasoconstriction occurs and continues contributing to decreased GFR.

The nonoliguric phase, which is usually synonymous with the diuretic phase, suggests that some tubular function is restored. The patient must be monitored for excessive diuresis with loss of electrolytes, and it is not uncommon for urine output to exceed 1–3 liters/hour. This phase usually lasts between 5–8 days. Obstruction is relieved, but cellular edema continues to be a problem as scar tissue forms over necrotic areas.

When diuresis is no longer excessive, the recovery phase begins with gradual improvement in kidney function over the period of up to one year. GFR may remain impaired, and there may be a permanent decrease in renal function that, depending on the severity, may require dialysis.

MEDICAL CARE

Laboratory: CBC—hemoglobin decreased with anemia, RBCs decreased because of fragility, white blood cell count elevated if sepsis or trauma is precipitating event; BUN and creatinine elevated with ratio of 10:1; prerenal failure usually has urine sodium <10 mEq/L, specific gravity >1.020, BUN/creatinine ratio >25:1, little or no proteinuria, and normal urinary sedimentation; intrarenal (cortical) failure usually has urine sodium <10 mEq/L, variable specific gravity, moderate to heavy proteinuria, BUN/creatinine ratio elevated but remains in 10:1 ratio, hematuria, urine with erythrocyte casts and leukocytes; intrarenal (medullary) failure usually has urine sodium >20 mEq/L, specific gravity 1.010, minimal to moderate proteinuria, BUN and creatinine elevated, urine sediment with numerous epithelial cells, tubular casts, and rare erythrocytes; postrenal failures usually has BUN and creatinine elevate if obstruction is complete, and bacterial cultures positive; serum osmolality increased above 285 mOsm/kg; electrolytes used to show imbalances, with elevated potassium caused by retention, hemolysis, or acidosis; sodium usually increased, but may be normal; bicarbonate, pH, and calcium decreased; magnesium, phosphorus, and chloride increased; complement studies may be used to identify lupus nephritis; serum electrophoresis may be used to identify abnormal proteins that may damage kidneys permanently; ASO titer may be used to diagnose recent streptococcal infection that could cause poststreptococcal glomerulonephritis; UA: Urine color is dirty, tea-colored brown, volume is less than 400 cc/day, specific gravity less than 1.020 indicates renal disease and fixed at 1.010 indicates severe renal damage; pH greater than 7.0 seen with UTI, ATN, and chronic renal failure; osmolality less than 350 mOsm/kg indicates tubular damage; creatinine clearance decreased; sodium decreased but may be greater than 40 mEq/L if kidney does not reabsorb sodium; RBCs may be present if infection, renal stones, trauma, or tumor is cause; protein of 3+ or 4+ indicates glomerular damage, 1+ or 2+ may indicate infection or interstitial nephritis; casts indicate renal disease or infection, brownish casts and numerous epithelial cells indicate ATN, and red casts indicate acute glomerular nephritis; complement studies may be done with decreases seen in active complement-mediated glomerulonephritis and lupus nephritis; serum electrophoresis for immunoglobulin levels are used to show abnormal protein formation that are seen in multiple myeloma and can do irreversible kidney damage; antiglomerular basement membrane titers used to diagnose diseases of pulmonary hemorrhage and renal failure

Electrocardiogram: used to identify dysrhythmias and cardiac changes that may occur with acid–base imbalances or electrolyte imbalance

Radiography: KUB to identify size of structures, cysts, tumors, stones, or abnormal kidney location; chest X-ray to identify fluid overload that may occur with fluid shifts

Radionuclide imaging: may be used to identify hydronephrosis, calicectasis, or delayed filling or emptying, or other causes of ARF

Retrograde pyelogram: may be used to identify abnormalities of ureters or renal pelvis

Renal arteriogram: may be used to identify extravascular irregularities or masses, and provides visualization of renal circulation

Magnetic resonance imaging: may be used to evaluate soft tissue

CT scans: may be used to detect presence of renal disease or masses

Dialysis: emergency and chronic dialysis may be required for ARF; ultrafiltration and CAVH may also be utilized

Surgery: may be required for renal calculi removal, resection of the prostate, or placement of fistula for long-term dialysis

Diuretics: furosemide (Lasix, Furosemide, Luramide), bumetanine (Bumex), chlorothiazide (Diuril), hydrochlorothiazide (Esidrex, Hydrochlorthiazide, HydroDiuril, Thiuretic), chlorthalidone (Chlorthalidone, Hygroton, Hylidone, Thalitone), indapamide (Lozol), metolazone (Diulo, Zaroxolyn), ethacrynic acid (Edecrin), torsemide (Demadex), acetazolamide (Acetazolamide, Diamox), methazolamide (Neptazane), amiloride (Amiloride, Midamor), spironolactone (Aldactone), triamterene (Dyrenium), mannitol (Mannitol, Osmitrol), and urea (Ureaphil) may be used to increase urinary output

COMMON NURSING DIAGNOSES

FATIGUE (see DKA)

Related to: anemia, restriction on diet, increased metabolic needs

Defining Characteristics: lack of energy, inability to maintain normal activities, lethargy, disinterest

ANXIETY (see MI)

Related to: change in health status, fear of death, threat to role functioning, threat to body image

Defining Characteristics: restlessness, insomnia, anorexia, increased respirations, heart rate, and/or blood pressure, dry mouth, poor eye contact, decreased energy, irritability, crying, feelings of helplessness

INEFFECTIVE COPING (see ARDS)

Related to: sudden onset of acute renal failure, ineffective or insufficient comfort by support system

Defining Characteristics: inability to meet expectations, inability to solve problems, failure to comply with treatment, decreased socialization, destructive behavior, verbalizing inability to cope, inability to ask for help

ADDITIONAL NURSING DIAGNOSES

EXCESS FLUID VOLUME

Related to: impairment of renal system regulation, retention of water, oliguric phase

Defining Characteristics: oliguria, anuria, intake greater than output, weight gain, elevated blood pressure, edema, ascites, increased central venous pressure, neck vein distention, dyspnea, orthopnea, crackles, muffled heart tones, decreased hemoglobin and hematocrit, altered electrolytes, increased filling pressures, restlessness, anxiety, water intoxication; specific gravity 1.015 or less, dilute urine, pulmonary congestion

Outcome Criteria

✔ Patient will have balanced intake and output, stable weight, stable vital signs and hemodynamic parameters, and have effective dialysis when required.

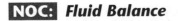 **NOC:** *Fluid Balance*

INTERVENTIONS	RATIONALES
Monitor vital signs and hemodynamic parameters every 1–2 hours.	Hypertension with increases in heart rate may occur when kidneys fail to excrete urine, changes occur within the renin-angiotensin cascade, or with fluid resuscitation. Hemodynamic pressures can facilitate identification of changes with intravascular volume.

INTERVENTIONS	RATIONALES
Monitor intake and output every 2 hours and prn, noting balance or imbalance per 24 hour period. Estimate insensible losses through lungs, skin, and bowel.	Facilitates identification of fluid requirements based on renal function. Insensible losses can add up to 800–1000 cc/day and metabolism of carbohydrates can liberate up to 350 cc/day of fluid from ingested foods.
Weigh daily.	Changes in body weight help to identify fluid status. Gains over 1–2 pound/day indicate fluid retention. Fluid amounts of 500 cc are equivalent to 1 pound.
Auscultate lungs for adventitious breath sounds.	Adventitious breath sounds, such as crackles, will be heard with development of pulmonary edema or congestive heart failure.
Measure urine specific gravity, and note changes in character of urine output.	Specific gravity is less than 1.010 in intrarenal failure and signifies inability to appropriately concentrate the urine.
Administer fluids as warranted with restrictions per physician orders.	Prerenal failure is treated with fluid replacement, occasionally with use of vasopressors. Management of fluids is based on replacement of output from all sources.
Administer diuretics as ordered.	May be given to convert oliguric phase to nonoliguric phase, to flush debris from tubules, decreased hyperkalemia, or foster improved urine output.
Insert Foley catheter as warranted.	Catheterization eliminates potential lower GU tract obstruction and provides for accuracy of measurement of urine output, but may not be treatment of choice due to potential for infection.
Observe for presence and character of edema.	Dependent edema may be present, but pitting edema may not be discernable until the patient has more than 10 pounds of fluid in body. Periorbital edema may be the first clinical evidence of edema and indication of fluid shifting.
Monitor for mental status changes.	May indicate impending hypoxic state, electrolyte imbalances, acidosis, or sepsis.
Prepare for and assist with dialysis procedures as warranted.	Fluid imbalance may require rapid removal of fluid and/or

INTERVENTIONS	RATIONALES
	toxic substances by the use of hemodialysis or hemofiltration when the patient has recurring episodes of symptomatic hypervolemia.
Monitor arterial blood gases.	May indicate presence of acidosis and facilitate intervention for hypoxemia.
Monitor lab work for alterations.	Electrolyte imbalances may occur from impaired sodium reabsorption, fluid overload, or lack of excretion of potassium. Hyperkalemia may occur as body attempts to correct acidosis, hypernatremia may indicate total body water deficit, and hyponatremia may result from fluid overloading or inability to conserve sodium. BUN/creatinine ratio, which is normally 10:1 is greater than 20:1 with prerenal failure.
Monitor urine specimen lab work for changes.	Urine sodium less than 20 mEq/L, osmolality above 450 mOsm/kg, and urine creatinine above 40 indicates prerenal failure. Urine sodium above 40 mEq/L, osmolality below 350 mOsm/kg, and urine creatinine below 20 indicates ATN.
Identify and correct any reversible reason for ARF.	Improvement of perfusion, enhancing cardiac output and hemodynamics, or removal of obstruction may facilitate recovery from ARF and limit residual effects.
Obtain chest X-rays and compare with previous films.	May be used to identify increasing cardiac silhouette, effusions, infiltrates, pulmonary edema, or other complications that may occur with fluid overload.
Administer antihypertensives as warranted/ordered.	May be required to treat hypertension that occurs from decreased renal perfusion or fluid overload.
Instruct patient/family on necessity for fluid restriction.	Promotes understanding and facilitates compliance.
Prepare patient/family for dialysis treatment as warranted.	Dialysis may be required to remove toxic wastes and to correct electrolyte, acid–base, and fluid imbalances.

NIC: *Hypervolemia Management*

Discharge or Maintenance Evaluation

- Patient will achieve and maintain urinary output within normal limits for character and amount.
- Patient will have stable weight, vital signs, and hemodynamic parameters.
- Patient will exhibit no respiratory dysfunction and have normal arterial blood gases.
- Patient/family will be able to verbalize understanding of instructions and comply with treatment.
- Patient will have no signs of edema.
- Patient will tolerate dialysis procedure without complications.

RISK FOR DEFICIENT FLUID VOLUME

Related to: fluid loss, diuretic phase

Defining Characteristics: weight loss, output greater than intake, hypotension, tachycardia, decreased central venous pressure, decreased hemodynamic pressures, increased temperature, dilute urine with low specific gravity, oliguria with high specific gravity, weakness, stupor, lethargy, decreased skin turgor, large volume of dilute urine with low specific gravity during polyuric phase, oliguria, concentrated urine, and elevated specific gravity with dehydration and normal renal function

Outcome Criteria

✔ Patient will exhibit equivalent intake and output, have stable vital signs and weight, and will have urine output within acceptable levels.

NOC: *Fluid Balance*

INTERVENTIONS	RATIONALES
Monitor vital signs and hemodynamic pressures.	Hypovolemia may result in hypotension and tachycardia.
Observe for complaints of thirst, dry mucous membranes, poor skin turgor, or lethargy.	May indicate presence of dehydration. When extracellular fluid or sodium is depleted, the thirst center is activated. Continued losses without adequate replacement may lead to hypovolemia and shock.
Measure intake and output every 1–2 hours, or prn, including insensible fluid losses. Compare for balance at least every 24 hours.	Facilitates identification of fluid loss and replacement requirements.

(continues)

(continued)

INTERVENTIONS	RATIONALES
Supply allowed amounts of fluid throughout the day ensuring that all fluids are counted.	Lack of fluid intake maintenance may predispose nocturnal dehydration.
Administer IV fluids as ordered.	May require intermittent fluid boluses to challenge fluid shifting.
Instruct patient/family regarding fluid intake and any dietary restrictions.	Promotes knowledge of disease process and facilitates compliance with medical regimen.
Instruct/prepare family for potential complications from renal failure, such as lethargy and stupor.	Symptoms may occur with water intoxication or severe hypovolemia.

NIC: *Fluid Management*

Discharge or Maintenance Evaluation

- Patient will have stable weight.
- Patient will have equivalent intake and output.
- Patient will have stable vital signs and hemodynamic parameters.
- Patient will have urine output within normal limits.
- Patient will have normal neurological status.

INEFFECTIVE TISSUE PERFUSION: RENAL, CARDIOPULMONARY, CEREBRAL, GASTROINTESTINAL, PERIPHERAL

Related to: fluid shifts, renal obstruction, impairment of renal function, septic shock, trauma, burns, uremia, hypertension, hypotension

Defining Characteristics: oliguria, anuria, dehydration, hypotension, abnormal vital signs, abnormal blood gases, abnormal electrolytes, mental status changes, lethargy, nausea, vomiting, skin changes, elevated blood pressure, headache, dizziness, blurry vision, decreased peripheral pulses, skin color changes, abdominal distention, absent or minimal bowel sounds, ileus, peritonitis, elevated white blood count

Outcome Criteria

✔ Patient will have adequate perfusion to all body systems.

NOC: *Tissue Perfusion*

NOC: *Systemic Toxin Clearance: Dialysis*

INTERVENTIONS	RATIONALES
Monitor vital signs and hemodynamic parameters.	Hypertension and fluid volume increases may increase cardiac workload, increase myocardial oxygen demand, and possibly lead to cardiac failure. Blood pressure below 70 mm Hg interferes with autoregulatory mechanisms.
Monitor ECG for dysrhythmias or changes in cardiac rhythm, and treat appropriately.	Renal failure and electrolyte imbalances may predispose patient to dysrhythmias and conduction problems. Hypokalemia may be reflected with flat T wave, peaked P wave, and sometimes the presence of a U wave. Hyperkalemia may be reflected with peaked T wave, widened QRS complex, increased PR interval, and flattened P wave. Hypocalcemia may be manifested with QT prolongation. Treatment may prevent death from potentially-lethal cardiac dysrhythmias caused by complications of renal failure.
Monitor neurologic status for changes in mentation or level of consciousness.	Decreased perfusion may result in cerebral perfusion decreases resulting in lethargy, weakness, and stupor, or from uremic syndrome.
Monitor for peripheral pulse presence and character, skin color, appearance of mucous membranes, turgor, capillary refill time.	Pallor may be present with vasoconstriction or anemia, and skin may be cyanotic or mottled with pulmonary edema or cardiac failure.
Auscultate for breath sounds and heart tones, and notify physician of abnormalities.	Fluid overload and decreased perfusion may result in development of S_3 or S_4 gallops, and pericardial friction rub may indicate the presence of uremic pericarditis.
Monitor for complaints of numbness, paresthesias, muscle cramps, tremors, twitching, or hyperreflexia.	May indicate impairment of neuromuscular activity, hypocalcemia, and potential for decreased cardiac perfusion and function.
Monitor intake and output every 1–2 hours and prn. Measure specific gravity and note changes in character of urine.	Oliguria, with output less than 400 cc/day, and anuria, or no output, may be seen with fluid volume excess or decreased perfusion states. Decreases in urinary output that do not respond to fluid challenges cause

INTERVENTIONS	RATIONALES
	renal vasoconstriction and decreased perfusion from increased renin secretion.
Monitor lab work for electrolyte changes.	May have hyperkalemia in oliguric phase changing to hypokalemia with diuretic phase. Potassium levels above 6.5 mEq/L should be treated as a medical emergency. Hypocalcemia produces adverse cardiac effects and potentiates potassium. Hypermagnesemia may occur with use of antacids and cause neuromuscular dysfunction, or cardiac or respiratory arrest.
Maintain oximetry of at least 90% by using supplemental oxygen.	Facilitates oxygenation of tissues in the presence of decreased perfusion and increased workload.
Monitor arterial blood gases.	Facilitates measurement of actual oxygen levels and identifies acid–base disturbances that may require further intervention.
Administer inotropic agents as ordered.	May be required to improve cardiac output, increase myocardial contractility, and improve perfusion.
Administer glucose/insulin combination as ordered.	May be used as temporary emergent treatment to decrease serum potassium by shifting potassium into the cells.
Administer polystyrene sulfonate as ordered.	May be used to lower serum potassium by exchanging sodium for potassium in the GI tract. Solutions that also contain sorbitol may also decrease potassium levels by osmotic diarrhea.
Administer mannitol as ordered.	May be used with muscle trauma for osmotic diuresis, but should not be given repeatedly if response is not achieved because accumulations of hyperosmolar compounds may result in further renal damage and decreased perfusion.
Prepare patient/family for dialysis as warranted.	Dialysis may be required to remove toxins and excess fluids from body and maintain life until kidney function is restored.
Instruct patient/family on specifics of peritoneal dialysis.	Peritoneal dialysis, or PD, may be intermittent, continuous ambulatory peritoneal dialysis (CAPD), or continuous cycling peritoneal

INTERVENTIONS	RATIONALES
	dialysis for use overnight. With PD, the peritoneum becomes the dialyzing membrane with dialysate solution infused into the peritoneal cavity, allowed to remain there for 30 minutes and then siphoned out through a closed system. The duration of this dialysis depends on the severity of the renal condition and proportions of the patient. Peritonitis may occur and antibiotics may be added to the dialysate prophylactically.
Instruct patient/family on specifics of hemodialysis.	Hemodialysis, or HD, may be used for chronic renal failure patients as well as acute renal failure patients who require short-term dialysis. Blood passes through a semipermeable membrane or kidney, to the dialysate fluid where toxic substances move from the blood to the dialysate solution and are then discarded. Requires circulatory access, and takes 3–4 hours 3 times per week. Complications may include infection, bleeding, or obstruction of vascular access.

NIC: *Shock Management*

Discharge or Maintenance Evaluation

- Patient will achieve normalized perfusion of all body systems.
- Patient will have no long-term effects from perfusion impairment.
- Patient will have normal urine output with no symptoms or signs of ARF.
- Patient will have stable vital signs and hemodynamic pressures.
- Patient will have balanced intake and output with stable weight.
- Patient will have precipitating illness stabilized/resolved.

RISK FOR INJURY

Related to: early uremia, progressive uremia, pulmonary edema, bleeding

Defining Characteristics: changes in mental status, lethargy, nausea, vomiting, weight loss, stomatitis, uremic frost, uremic odor, edema, weight gain, heart murmur, skin changes, electrolyte imbalances, especially hyperkalemia and hyponatremia, carbohydrate intolerance, increased peripheral neuropathy, diuresis, oliguria, anuria, acidosis, increased BUN over 100 mg/dl, increased creatinine, toxic levels of drugs, pericardial friction rubs, pericarditis, ascites, decreased immunity, peritonitis, increased WBC count, infection, hypoglycemia

Outcome Criteria

✔ Patient will achieve and maintain BUN and creatinine at levels to diminish uremic symptoms.

✔ Patient will be able to tolerate dialysis procedures, with no long-term adverse complications.

NOC: *Symptom Control*

INTERVENTIONS	RATIONALES
Assess patient's dietary and fluid consumption, and restrict protein, potassium, and sodium intake.	Protein is metabolized through the kidneys and increases the workload on an already-impaired organ function. Potassium and sodium may need to be decreased to reduce the amount of fluid retention that exacerbates the renal impairment.
Monitor vital signs and hemodynamics, if available, and notify physician of significant abnormalities.	Poor renal function can result in toxic levels of normal dosages of drugs, which can result in lethal dysrhythmias, hemodynamic instability, and fluid overload. CVP and PCWP should be monitored to identify the presence of fluid status changes, especially overload.
Auscultate for pericardial friction rubs, cardiac murmurs and gallops, and adventitious breath sounds.	Crackles (rales) will be heard as fluid accumulates within the interstitial tissues in the lungs. Increasing fluid can result in pleuritis and pericarditis, resulting in pericardial friction rubs, murmurs, and/or gallops.
Assess neurologic status and report significant changes.	As renal function decreases, toxins build up and decrease perfusion to all organs and tissues, including the brain, causing lethargy and memory impairment. Sometimes, these symptoms may be the first

INTERVENTIONS	RATIONALES
	indicator of identification of the renal failure. Stupor may occur in severe cases of hypovolemia.
Monitor I&O q 1 hr, and notify physician for abnormal increases (>200 cc/hr) or decreases (<30 cc/hr).	Urinary output may represent how well the kidneys are compensating for increasing toxins, BUN, and creatinine that they are no longer able to clear. In the polyuric phase of renal failure, a large amount of very dilute urine with a low specific gravity may be produced leading to dehydration.
Assess for uremic signs and symptoms, such as edema, increasing BUN and creatinine levels, uremic odor, severe pruritis, pale yellow tinged skin, ecchymoses, and azotemia.	Itching occurs from the uremic deposits on the skin. If case is severe, uremic frost may be noted on the skin, especially on the facial areas. Uremia occurs when the kidneys can no longer excrete toxins and waste products, and usually symptoms occur when BUN >100 mg/dl or GFR <10–15 ml/min. Increasing BUN and creatinine levels indicate failing kidneys and will require dialysis to maintain life.
Assess for nausea, vomiting, or any bleeding from the GI tract.	Bleeding may be caused by platelet dysfunction that occurs frequently with renal failure. Blood in the gastrointestinal tract is a protein source that is metabolized to ammonia and urea, which cannot be managed by impaired kidney function, and eventually will lead to coma and death. Nausea and vomiting may be caused by the toxins that are circulating throughout the body, by drug toxicity, or by electrolyte imbalances, all of which are a result of poor renal function.
Assess patient for signs that hemodialysis is indicated.	Increased BUN and creatinine levels despite usual conservative treatment measures, such as reducing fluids, sodium, potassium, and protein, or when medication in chronic renal failure patients no longer is able to maintain renal status are indications for the use of hemodialysis. Sometimes, with acute poisoning hemodialysis is used for rapid removal of drugs such as alcohol, aspirin, poisons, or barbiturates.

INTERVENTIONS	RATIONALES
Assess patient for contraindications for types of dialysis.	Hemodialysis may be contraindicated if patient is hemodynamically unstable with rapid changes in fluid volume status, if their cardiovascular condition is unstable, or if the patient is unable to tolerate heparinization. Peritoneal dialysis, which is usually the second option for acute renal failure, may be contraindicated if the patient has peritonitis, bleeding disorders, recent abdominal surgery, or abdominal adhesions.
Assess patient for other continuous renal replacement therapies (CRRT), including slow continuous ultrafiltration (SCUF), continuous arteriovenous hemodialysis or hemodiafiltration (CAVHD), continuous arteriovenous hemofiltration (CAVH), or continuous venovenous hemodialysis or hemodiafiltration (CVVHD).	CRRTs have been shown to be beneficial for dialysis and blood decontamination when hemodialysis or peritoneal dialysis are not options. CAVH is used for fluid overload, cardiovascular instability, azotemia, acute renal failure, pulmonary edema, postoperative cardiac surgery, ascites, or recent MIs. CAVH should not be utilized if the patient's hematocrit is >45%. SCUF and CAVH use ultrafiltration and exchange plasma water with particulate by convection. CAVHD uses peritoneal dialysis fluid with ultrafiltration principles. CVVHD uses a filter that is capable of removing fluid rapidly during hypotensive and low blood flow states, and uses the principles of diffusion, osmosis, and ultrafiltration.
Prepare patient for and assist with hemodialysis procedure as warranted.	Some facilities have nurses who specialize in dialysis care. Dialysis removes the toxins from the systemic circulation by osmosis, diffusion, and convection or ultrafiltration.
Administer heparin as ordered prior to and during the procedure as ordered.	Anticoagulation is performed to keep the blood anticoagulated within the machine to prevent clotting of the semipermeable membrane that filters out the toxic wastes.
If AV fistula is utilized to administer hemodialysis, auscultate and palpate area for bruit and thrill at least q 4 hr.	Identifies patency of the shunt. Loss of bruit or thrill must be reported immediately and may require surgical intervention, including declotting or revision

INTERVENTIONS	RATIONALES
	of the shunt, or possible replacement. Blood pressure readings, lab draws, and IV insertion should never be done on the same arm as the AV graft so as to minimize potential for clotting and impairment of circulation.
Prepare for and assist with beginning peritoneal dialysis, as warranted.	Peritoneal dialysis may be the preferred method for patients who are too hemodynamically unstable to tolerate rapid removal of fluid and toxins. It utilizes diffusion and osmosis by instilling a dialysate solution (its contents based upon the patient's condition and lab values) into the peritoneal cavity, allowing it to remain for a determined length of time, and then allowed to drain out. The solution is usually made up of a glucose solution, heparin, potassium chloride, insulin, lidocaine and/or antibiotics.
Weigh patient before and after procedure.	Helps to identify amount of fluid removed from patient; 500 cc fluid approximates 1 pound of weight loss.
Observe the fluid that is drained out from patient and notify physician for significant abnormalities.	Typically, a normal drainage should be clear and pale yellow in color. If solution is cloudy, it indicates an infective process or the potential for peritonitis. If the solution is brown, it may indicate a bowel perforation, and an amber color may indicate a bladder perforation. Some blood noted in the solution may be normal, but if the bleeding continues after the fourth exchange, it may indicate that the patient has a uremic coagulopathy, and the physician should be notified.
Monitor vital signs and hemodynamics, if available, during procedure, especially during the draining phase.	Changes in vital signs or cardiac rhythm may indicate impending shock, hypoglycemic reaction, or fluid excess.
Observe peritoneal catheter site for signs or symptoms of infection, and perform wound care with dressing changes after each treatment and prn.	Catheter provides direct access to peritoneal cavity for bacterial invasion and aseptic wound care helps to decrease the potential for wound infection.

(continues)

(continued)

INTERVENTIONS	RATIONALES
Monitor lab work for abnormalities.	Renal failure patients normally have abnormal electrolytes caused by decreased glomerular filtration and impaired function, especially with potassium and sodium. Drug toxicity may occur even if the patient is taking an appropriate dosage of medication because of the lack of renal clearance.
Instruct patient/family regarding the specific type of dialysis procedure.	Promotes knowledge of disease process, need for therapy, and facilitates compliance.
Instruct patient in care of AV fistula or peritoneal catheter.	Provides for reduction of infection and for prompt recognition of potential problems that may require emergent medical attention.

NIC: *Hemodialysis Therapy*

NIC: *Peritoneal Dialysis Therapy*

Discharge or Maintenance Evaluation

- Patient will tolerate dialysis procedure without hemodynamic compromise.
- Patient will have BUN level decreased and maintained at an acceptable level determined by physician that will minimize complications.
- Patient/family will be able to accurately verbalize understanding of wound care of dialysis access.

IMBALANCED NUTRITION: LESS THAN BODY REQUIREMENTS

Related to: dietary restrictions, hypercatabolic state, negative nitrogen balance, uremia

Defining Characteristics: elevated BUN and creatinine levels, anorexia, nausea, vomiting, distorted taste perception, fatigue, weakness, loss of weight (dietary restriction), weight gain (noncompliance with fluid restriction), pain, depression, lethargy, oral mucosal lesions, glucose intolerance, lipid clearance reduction, fatty acid metabolic disturbances

Outcome Criteria

✔ Patient will achieve and maintain nutritional requirements and stable weight.

NOC: *Nutritional Status*

INTERVENTIONS	RATIONALES
Determine patient's dietary habits and intake. Perform calorie count.	Identifies nutritional deficiencies, noncompliance with restrictions, and metabolic requirements.
Provide several small meals rather than 3 large ones.	Decreases nausea that may occur because of diminished peristalsis. Smaller meals may not be as overwhelming and may facilitate compliance with restrictions.
Give patient high caloric, low protein, low potassium, low sodium diet as ordered.	Protein requirements for renal failure patients are much less than normal to compensate for their impaired renal function. Increased carbohydrates satisfy energy requirements while restricting catabolism and preventing acid formation from protein and fat metabolism. Restriction of potassium, sodium, and phosphorus may be required to prevent further renal damage.
Administer hyperalimentation as ordered.	If patient is unable to take in enough oral nutrients, hyperalimentation may be utilized to maintain a positive nitrogen balance and nutritional status. In acute renal failure, acceleration of protein catabolism combines with other factors to produce a negative nitrogen balance and hypercatabolic state. Amino acids are usually administered at 2 gm/kg/day to prevent catabolism. Hyperalimentation and daily dialysis have been shown to increase survival in ARF and also assist with renal tubular cell restoration.
Avoid excess usage of vitamin supplementation, especially vitamin C.	Increased amounts of vitamin C may result in exacerbation of ARF. Vitamin A toxicity can occur in the absence of renal excretion of this fat soluble vitamin.
Monitor lab work, such as albumin, prealbumin, protein, hemoglobin and hematocrit, and BUN levels.	Assesses efficacy of nutritional supplementation.
Assist with/encourage frequent oral care.	Reduces distaste and freshens oral mucosa that may be inflamed.
Weigh daily.	Patient may lose up to 1 pound per day during NPO status.

INTERVENTIONS	RATIONALES
Administer vitamins/minerals as ordered.	Patient may have iron deficiency secondary to protein restriction, anemia, or impaired GI function and need supplemental iron. Calcium may be given to replace levels and facilitate coagulation and metabolism of bone. Vitamin B complexes are required to maintain cell growth.
Instruct patient/family member on renal diet.	Protein and electrolytes are adjusted to prevent uremia and electrolyte imbalances. Instruction provides knowledge and may facilitate compliance.
Consult dietician and/or other dietary resources.	May be helpful to discuss choices for meals, replacements for foods previously enjoyed but now restricted, and to allow patient some measure of control over his situation.

NIC: *Total Parenteral Nutrition (TPN) Administration*

Discharge or Maintenance Evaluation

- Patient will achieve and maintain desired weight.
- Patient will be able to tolerate diet without nausea/vomiting.
- Patient will exhibit no evidence of mucosal lesions in mouth.
- Patient will adhere to dietary restrictions.
- Patient will comply with medical regimen and supplementation.

RISK FOR INFECTION

Related to: renal failure, uremia, debilitation, septic shock, invasive procedures and lines, malnutrition, impaired immune system

Defining Characteristics: increased white blood cell count, shift to the left, BUN greater than 100 mg/dl, history of repeated infections, fever, chills, cough with or without sputum production, wound drainage, hypotension, tachycardia, impaired skin integrity, wounds, positive blood, urine, or sputum cultures, cloudy concentrated urine

Outcome Criteria

✔ Patient will exhibit no signs or symptoms of infection.

NOC: *Risk Detection*

INTERVENTIONS	RATIONALES
Monitor vital signs and hemodynamic pressures.	Systemic vascular resistance decreases, cardiac output initially increases, blood pressure decreases, and patient has tachycardia, tachypnea, and hyperthermia with warm flushed skin in early stages of septic shock.
Obtain urine culture as ordered.	Urinary tract infections may be asymptomatic initially.
Avoid insertion of invasive lines, catheters, and procedures whenever possible. Use aseptic/sterile technique for changing IV sites, dressing changes, or caring for catheters.	Decreases potential of bacteria gaining entrance to body and prevents risk of cross-contamination.
Observe wounds for drainage, noting changes in amount, color, and character. Change IV sites per hospital protocol.	Allows for identification of detrimental changes in wound status and facilitates timely intervention. Early detection of infection may preclude the development of septicemia.
Observe PD return fluid for cloudiness.	May indicate presence of peritonitis from perforation or loss of albumin.
Maintain adequate nutrition.	Facilitates healing and body metabolism.
Utilize appropriate isolation techniques when warranted.	Prevents cross-contamination and minimizes patient's risk of secondary infection.
Reposition patient every 2 hours, and encourage coughing and deep breathing.	Decreases potential for atelectasis and facilitates mobilizing secretions to avoid respiratory infection.
Obtain cultures as ordered.	Facilitates identification of causative organism and allows for appropriate antimicrobial treatment.
Administer antimicrobials as ordered.	May be required to combat infection.
Instruct patient to avoid scratching and to maintain skin integrity.	May precipitate infection and worsen renal dysfunction.
Monitor lab work, especially BUN and creatinine, CBC, and differential.	BUN should be maintained lower than 100 mg/dl to decrease potential for infection. CBC will identify presence of infection, and will be helpful to monitor therapeutic response to antimicrobials.

NIC: *Infection Protection*

Discharge or Maintenance Evaluation

- Patient will be free of infection.
- Patient will be able to verbalize understanding of instructions to prevent infection complications.
- Patient will not develop septic shock.

 RISK FOR IMPAIRED SKIN INTEGRITY

Related to: uremia, malnutrition, immobility

Defining Characteristics: dry skin, edema, presence of wounds, presence of invasive lines/grafts/fistulas, uremic frost, bruising, erythema, pruritus, changes in skin texture and thickness

Outcome Criteria

✔ Patient will maintain skin integrity or will have wound healing in a timely manner.

NOC: *Tissue Integrity: Skin and Mucous Membranes*

INTERVENTIONS	RATIONALES
Observe skin for wounds, pressure areas, abrasions, drainage, redness, rashes.	Prompt identification allows for timely intervention.
Bathe patient daily using oil in bath, and scant soap. Provide skin care with lotion or creams.	Removes waste products from skin while keeping skin supple and moist.
Administer antipruritic drugs as ordered.	Persistent itching may cause patient to scratch body to the point of bleeding and medication will help allay strong urge to scratch. Open areas of skin are more susceptible to infection.
Reposition every 2 hours. Avoid constricting garments.	Decreases potential for skin breakdown.
Instruct patient in avoidance of scratching.	Scratching may result in worsened skin integrity problems.
Instruct patient to avoid confining clothing or shoes.	May produce pressure to areas that are vulnerable to breakdown.
Instruct patient/family regarding signs and symptoms of infection.	Promotes knowledge and assists with early identification of symptoms to allow for prompt intervention.

NIC: *Skin Surveillance*

Discharge or Maintenance Evaluation

- Patient will have clean, dry, intact skin.
- Patient will be free of itching.
- Patient will have no signs/symptoms of infection.
- Patient will have timely wound healing with no complications.

RISK FOR INJURY

Related to: altered metabolism and excretion of medications, kidney failure, electrolyte imbalances

Defining Characteristics: decreased cardiac output states, acidosis, decreased protein binding, presence of uremia, competition for binding sites, decreased body stores of fat, decreased GI motility, changes in gastric pH, decreased protein binding, present renal failure, hyperkalemia, hypokalemia, hypocalcemia, hypercalcemia, hyperphosphatemia, hypophosphatemia, hyponatremia

Outcome Criteria

✔ Patient will be able to tolerate all pharmacological agents without adverse effects on renal or other body systems.
✔ Patient will have normal electrolyte levels within patient's parameters.

NOC: *Symptom Control*

INTERVENTIONS	RATIONALES
Determine methods of action and excretion of all drugs being taken, as well as interactions among them.	Facilitates understanding of how uremia may affect drug effects. Conditions that reduce renal perfusion limit the amount of drug that the kidney is exposed to and decrease the amount of metabolism or excretion of the drug.
Monitor for presence of acidosis.	Acidosis may interfere with absorption of some drugs.
Ensure that nephrotoxic drugs are utilized only when absolutely necessary.	Nephrotoxics will further impair renal failure.
Monitor patient for signs and symptoms of drug toxicity, and obtain serum drug levels for specific drugs in use.	Excretion of drugs may be hindered by renal failure and result in toxic levels with normally safe dosages.
Assess patient for irritability, hyporeflexia, hyperreflexia,	Usually most electrolyte imbalances appear as symptoms of

INTERVENTIONS	RATIONALES
seizures, weakness, confusion, changes in respiratory rate and depth, abdominal cramping, cardiac dysrhythmias, paralysis, numbness in extremities.	neuromuscular dysfunction and/or cardiac or respiratory aberrancies. Hyperkalemia causes deep and rapid respirations when it occurs in conjunction with acidosis, but may be exhibited by shallow respirations as a result of neuromuscular paralysis. Hyperkalemia causes elevation of T waves, widening of the QRS complex, prolongation of the PR interval, and can progress to flattened or absent P waves and asystole, depending on the level of potassium excess. Hypokalemia causes intracellular shifting of potassium, with symptoms of polyuria, dizziness, nausea, vomiting, weakness, and fatigue. This causes depression of the ST segment, flattened or inverted T waves, and a present U wave, leading to ventricular dysrhythmias. Hypernatremia causes increased sodium and water retention, and has symptoms of weight gain, dyspnea, decreased urinary output, dry mucous membranes, and dry, flushed skin. Cardiac manifestations include tachycardia changing to bradycardia as dehydration worsens. Hyponatremia involves sodium loss that exceeds fluid loss, and patients will have thirst, muscle weakness, and decreased urinary output. Cardiac manifestations include rapid heart rate with fluid overload, increased or decreased CVP, and BP may run the gamut from hypotension to hypertension. Hypercalcemia alters the tubular reabsorption of calcium, with symptomatic fatigue, constipation, and nausea with vomiting. Renal calculi can occur, and patients who have concurrent diagnoses of carcinoma will have hypercalcemia caused by the release of calcium into the plasma by the lesions. ECG changes may include shortening of the ST segment and advanced AV blocks that can result in cardiac arrest, depending on the level of calcium excess. Hypo-

INTERVENTIONS	RATIONALES
	calcemia may occur because of the binding of phosphate and precipitation into the tissues. Symptoms include bone pain and lethargy, tetany, stridor, and labored, shallow respirations, and cardiac manifestations include prolongation of the ST segment and QT interval, impairment of contractility that can result in heart failure and, ultimately, cardiac arrest. Hyperphosphatemia occurs if the glomerular filtration rate is reduced to such a point that phosphate is unable to be excreted, and result in symptoms of neurologic complaints, seizures, hypocalcemia, and metastatic calcifications. Cardiac changes are similar to those in hypocalcemia. Hypophosphatemia occurs because of renal phosphate wasting, loss of proximal tubular function, increased cell uptake, or decreased phosphate absorption from the gut. Dyspnea occurs from hypoxia that is seen with the erythrocyte deficit for 2,3-DPG. Tachycardia occurs as a result of decreased cardiac output and potential cardiac failure.
Assess for complaints of blurred vision, thirst, urinary retention, rhinitis, and fluid and electrolyte imbalances.	May indicate side effects from osmotic diuretics.
Assess for complaints of intermittent hearing loss, abdominal pain or discomfort, and monitor lab for agranulocytosis, thrombocytopenia, hypokalemia, hypochloremic alkalosis, and hyperglycemia.	May indicate side effects from loop diuretics that act on the medullary ascending loop of Henle. Prolonged use of these drugs without appropriate electrolyte replacement may result in other electrolyte imbalances and dysrhythmias.
Assess for rash and monitor lab for leukopenia, thrombocytopenia, and hypercalcemia.	May indicate side effects of thiazide diuretics that act on sodium reabsorption inhibition in the ascending loop of Henle and beginning portion of distal tubule.
Assess for complaints of headache, nausea, vomiting, diarrhea, urticaria, menstrual dysfunction, or gynecomastia, and monitor lab for hyperkalemia and hyponatremia.	May indicate side effects of potassium-sparing diuretics that promote secretion of sodium and reabsorption of potassium in the distal tubule.

(continues)

(continued)

INTERVENTIONS	RATIONALES
Assess for complaints of rash, nausea, vomiting, anorexia, and monitor lab for hyperchloremic acidosis and deterioration in renal function.	May indicate side effects from carbonic anhydrase inhibitor diuretics that increase excretion of sodium by impeding reabsorption of sodium bicarbonate.
Monitor lab work for BUN, creatinine, and specific drug levels. Notify physician of significant changes.	Some antibiotics are nephrotoxic and antibiotic peak and trough levels may rise to toxic levels even when given in recommended dosages.
Instruct patient on all medications being taken, with symptoms to be reported.	Facilitates knowledge and increases compliance.
Give reduced drug dosages with longer time intervals between doses.	Decreases potential for toxic reaction to dosage with impaired excretion and metabolism.

NIC: *Electrolyte Management*

Discharge or Maintenance Evaluation

- Patient will comply and tolerate therapeutic regimen with no adverse drug effects noted.
- Patient will have serum drug levels within therapeutic ranges.
- Patient will exhibit no signs of toxicity to drugs.
- Patient will have stable renal function.
- Patient will be able to verbalize understanding of all instructions and be able to identify medications being taken.

IMPAIRED GAS EXCHANGE

Related to: inability of excretion of hydrogen ions by kidneys because of acute renal failure, renal dysfunction

Defining Characteristics: pH <7.35, bicarbonate level <22 mEq/L, hypotension, headache, dysrhythmias, conduction defects, fatigue, Kussmaul's respirations, lethargy, stupor, coma, seizures, abnormal arterial blood gases, concurrent physiologic processes, such as burns, trauma, septic shock, or MODS, skeletal system disorders, such as fibrosis and osteomalacia

Outcome Criteria

✔ Patient will have normal pH and arterial blood gas values will be within normal limits, with no signs or symptoms of metabolic acidosis exhibited.

NOC: *Respiratory Status: Gas Exchange*

INTERVENTIONS	RATIONALES
Assess patient for risk of ARF, and treat appropriately.	Patients who are in high risk of development for ARF include those who have unstable hemodynamic parameters, significant multiple trauma, rhabdomyolysis, IV hemolysis, MODS, surgical patients who have had significant blood loss or prolonged hypotension, and those receiving nephrotoxic drugs.
Monitor VS q 1 hour and prn. Notify physician for significant changes.	If patient is hypotensive, and mean arterial blood pressure is <70 mm Hg, GFR decreases because of decreased renal perfusion. Renal vasoconstriction occurs when cardiac output is decreased.
Monitor I&O q 1 hour and notify physician of urine output <30 cc/hr.	Oliguria may be first symptom of impending prerenal failure.
Administer IV fluids as ordered.	Assists to maintain hydration status and helps to increase cardiac output which promotes renal perfusion. Correction of fluid imbalance, hypotension, and renal hypoperfusion may not salvage the renal tubules from damage, but may limit the amount of damage done.
Administer oxygen as ordered.	Supplemental oxygen may be required to compensate for patient's decreasing respiratory status.
Identify and correct, when possible, causes for metabolic acidosis.	Metabolic acidosis is caused by acids that accumulate in renal failure, uremia, and anaerobic metabolism states, such as shock and sepsis. Treatment is aimed at compensating for the metabolic acidosis by hyperventilation in order to reduce the $PaCO_2$.
Administer sodium bicarbonate IV slowly and only as ordered by physician.	The overuse of sodium bicarbonate may cause a considerable overload of sodium and can predispose the patient to pulmonary edema. This treatment should only be utilized in emergent situations, with repeated episodes of acidosis being treated with dialysis.
Administer vasoactive drugs and diuretics as ordered.	May be required to reduce tubular obstruction, preserve urine output, maintain renal blood flow, increase glomerular

INTERVENTIONS	RATIONALES
	filtration rates, and increase cardiac output.
Instruct patient/family regarding disease process.	Acute renal failure may result in chronic failure and knowledge of the disease process will assist in dealing with changes that will be required. Promotion of knowledge decreases fear and increases compliance with medical regimen.
Instruct patient/family regarding respiratory testing, such as ABGs.	Provides information and rationale for assessment of respiratory acid–base balance.
Instruct patient/family regarding all medications and procedures.	Knowledge of effects, side effects, and adverse reactions may assist with timely intervention of unfavorable conditions.

NIC: *Acid–Base Management: Metabolic Acidosis*

Discharge or Maintenance Evaluation

- Patient will have arterial blood gases within normal limits for patient parameters.
- Patient will have no complications from dialysis treatment used to correct acidotic state.
- Patient will have stable vital signs and enhanced renal perfusion.

▨ INEFFECTIVE PROTECTION

Related to: anemia, lack of erythropoietin secretion by the kidneys, bleeding

Defining Characteristics: hemorrhage, decreased RBC count, decreased platelet count, prolonged coagulation profile times, petechiae, purpura, ecchymoses, hematomas, conjunctival bleeding, gingival bleeding, hematuria, melena, hematochezia, menorrhagia, hematemesis, hemoptysis

Outcome Criteria

- ✔ Patient will exhibit no evidence of spontaneous hemorrhage and can achieve and maintain adequate platelet and RBC counts.
- ✔ Patient will achieve and maintain an asymptomatic level of anemia.

NOC: *Coagulation Status*

INTERVENTIONS	RATIONALES
Assess patient and identify type of anemia or bleeding dyscrasia.	Patient may have a chronic anemia associated with his renal failure, or may have a suppression of erythropoietin or tangible blood loss. Identification of the cause allows for appropriate treatment modalities.
Administer blood or blood products as ordered.	Packed RBCs are usually given and the nurse can expect the hemoglobin count to increase approximately 1 gm/dl/unit and the hematocrit to rise approximately 3% per unit. If more than 8–10 units of RBCs are given, fresh frozen plasma (FFP) may be required to correct dilutional coagulopathies by providing clotting factors that are missing in RBCs, or for rapid reversal of warfarin effects. Platelets may be given if the patient has thrombocytopenia and will increase the platelet count by approximately 12,000/mm^3 per unit. Cryoprecipitate is given to provide coagulation factors I and VIII for patients with hemophilia and DIC. Albumin may be given for shock. Intravenous immunoglobulin (IVIG) is given to treat ITP, AIDS, following bone marrow transplants, and for severely immunodeficient individuals.
Monitor vital signs but use manual cuffs when possible and only inflate the cuff until the pulse is obliterated.	Reduces potential for damage to fragile vessels and prevents petechiae formation.
Monitor patient's medications, noting any drugs that have potential for increasing bleeding.	NSAIDs, oxycodone, aspirin-containing drugs, and aspirin interfere with platelet function and cause increased bleeding.
Avoid invasive procedures that are performed on the patient as much as is possible.	Venipunctures may result in prolonged bleeding. Rectal temperatures, suppository and enema insertion, and constipation may damage rectal mucosa and may create bleeding complications.
Administer iron orally or intramuscularly as ordered.	Provides for replacement of necessary element.
Administer folic acid and vitamin B$_6$ as ordered.	If patient is receiving dialysis, these vitamins are removed during the dialysis procedure, and may increase bleeding with their absence.

(continues)

(continued)

INTERVENTIONS	RATIONALES
Administer anabolic steroids, such as nandrolone decanoate as ordered.	Helps to encourage erythrocyte formation.
Administer erythropoietin (EPO) as ordered.	Helps to stimulate the production of erythrocytes and prevents chronic renal failure anemia, but does not start working acutely. Helps to decrease the number of transfusions the patient must receive to combat his anemia.
Instruct patient regarding the need to notify nurse or physician of any bleeding source.	Provides for prompt detection to allow for timely intervention.
Instruct patient to use soft-bristled toothbrush for oral care, or to use mouth rinses or toothettes as needed.	Reduces the trauma to fragile tissues and the potential for bleeding to occur.
Instruct patient/family regarding anemia and the disease that has put him at risk for bleeding problems. Discuss bleeding precautions.	Provides information and allows family to maintain some control in patient's care.
Instruct patient/family in dietary measures to increase fiber and/or the use of stool softeners.	Constipation may result in patient straining at stool, which in turn can result in bleeding complications.

NIC: *Bleeding Precautions*

Discharge or Maintenance Evaluation

- Patient will exhibit no overt signs of bleeding.
- Patient will be able to maintain hemoglobin and hematocrit at a prescribed level.
- Patient will be able to accurately verbalize understanding of need of notification of medical personnel for bleeding.
- Patient/family will be able to accurately verbalize understanding of disease entity, bleeding precautions, and ways of reducing risk for the patient.

IMPAIRED ORAL MUCOUS MEMBRANE

Related to: uremia, restriction on fluids, lesions, thrush

Defining Characteristics: dry mouth, dry mucous membranes, taste distortion, presence of lesions, inflammation, white patches on mucosa, coated tongue, stomatitis, gingivitis

Outcome Criteria

✔ Patient will have moist mucous membranes and be free of oral lesions and inflammation.

NOC: *Oral Health*

INTERVENTIONS	RATIONALES
Observe mouth and oral cavity at least every shift, noting lesions, redness, drainage, vesicles, lacerations, or ulcers.	Facilitates identification of problem to permit prompt treatment and resolution.
Differentiate inflammation of the mucosa from thrush, and administer nystatin suspension as ordered.	Thrush is initially identified as white patches on the tongue and mucosa, and occurs frequently in the presence of multiple antimicrobial agents as a fungal growth. Nystatin is the drug of choice for thrush.
Provide oral care at least every 2 hours, with peroxide rinses or normal saline as ordered.	Removes buildup of debris, moistens mouth, and decreases bad taste.
Use topical anesthetics as ordered.	Viscous xylocaine or Chloraseptic may be used to anesthetize mucosal pain receptors.
Instruct patient in signs/symptoms to report to nurse or physician: pain in mouth, sores on tongue or mouth, foul taste, drainage, and so forth.	Provides prompt identification of complications to oral mucosa and allows for prompt intervention.
Instruct patient/family in medications utilized.	Nystatin is the drug of choice for thrush.

NIC: *Oral Health Restoration*

Discharge or Maintenance Evaluation

- Patient will be free of oral mucosal lesions and pain.
- Patient will exhibit no evidence of inflammation or infection to mouth.
- Patient will be able to swallow without discomfort.
- Patient will have no taste distortion and will be able to ingest adequate nutrition.

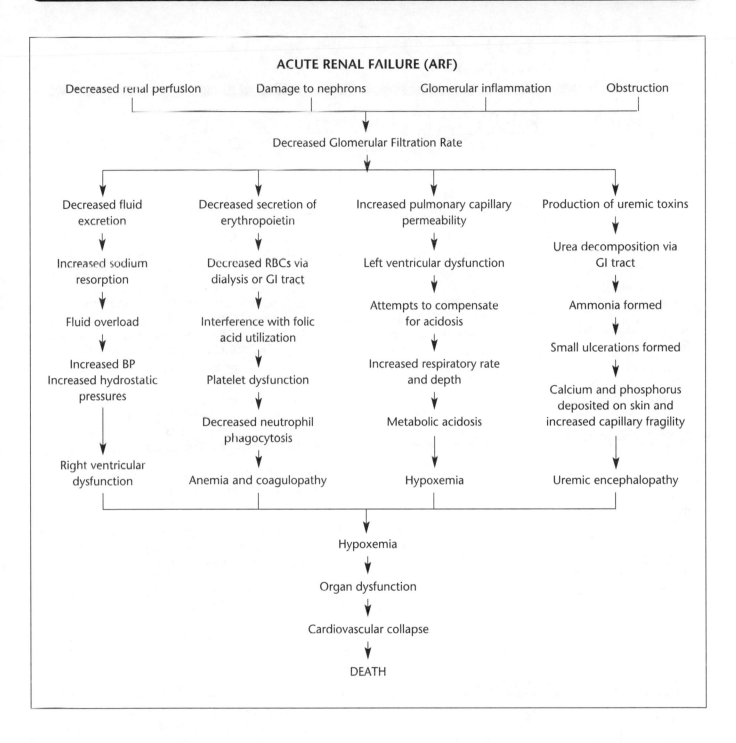

CHAPTER 6.2

DIABETIC KETOACIDOSIS

Diabetic ketoacidosis, or DKA, is a critical emergency state that is caused by a deficiency of insulin in patients with either type I or type II diabetes mellitus with a concurrent increase in glucagon, catecholamines, cortisol, and growth hormone to counterbalance the lack of insulin. The hormonal changes lead to increases in liver and renal glucose production and glucose utilization dysfunction in the peripheral tissues that results in hyperglycemia and changing osmolality of the extracellular spaces. Free fatty acids also are released into the circulation from the fat tissues, which ultimately results in ketonemia and a metabolic acidotic state. This deficiency can be caused by physiologic causes, or by failure to take an adequate amount of insulin. Precipitating causes include failure to take an adequate amount of insulin on a daily basis or failure to increase and compensate for infection processes, surgery, trauma, pregnancy, or other acute stress events. Early symptoms include polyuria, polydipsia, fatigue, drowsiness, headache, muscle cramps and nausea/vomiting. Later symptoms, such as Kussmaul breathing, sweet, fruity breath odor, hypotension, and weak and thready pulses will precede stupor and coma.

Treatment is aimed at correction of the acidotic state, hyperglycemia, hyperosmolality, hypovolemia, and potassium deficits, in conjunction with treatment of the underlying cause of the problem.

MEDICAL CARE

Laboratory: serum glucose level is increased above 300 mg/dl and may be greater than 1000 mg/dl; serum acetone positive; lipids and cholesterol levels elevated; osmolality increased but normally less than 330 mOsm/L; potassium initially normal or elevated because of cellular shifting, then later decreased; sodium may be decreased, normal, or elevated; calcium levels decreased in approximately one-third of patients; phosphorus is often decreased; amylase can be elevated if pancreatitis is precipitating cause;

serum insulin may be decreased in type I DM or normal to high in type II, suggesting that there is improper utilization of insulin or that insulin resistance may have developed secondary to antibody formation; BUN may be elevated if dehydration is severe and renal perfusion is decreased; urinalysis will show positive for glucose and acetone, specific gravity and osmolality may be elevated; hemoglobin A_{1C} helps to differentiate whether episode is caused by poor control of DM over previous few months or whether episode is incident-related; hematocrit may be elevated with dehydration; elevation of WBCs may occur in response to hemoconcentration or to stress; cultures may be helpful to discern potential cause of infection which may be precipitating factor

Arterial blood gases: pH will be less than 7.3, bicarbonate levels will be decreased, usually less than 15 mEq/L; usually metabolic acidosis

Electrocardiogram: may show changes associated with electrolyte imbalances, especially hyperkalemia, with peaked T waves

IV fluids: required to combat dehydration, to provide fluids, and to provide method of administration of electrolyte replacement; fluids are usually begun with 0.9% NaCl solution and when patient's blood sugar lowers to a specific range, 5% dextrose is added to prevent hypoglycemia

Insulin: required to lower severely elevated blood glucose levels; normally given as a bolus of regular insulin, followed by an infusion that is titrated for patient's specific glucose levels; subcutaneous insulin is begun once the blood sugar levels are low enough, but prior to the discontinuation of the IV infusion to prevent a recurrent rebound hyperglycemia and ketosis

Antimicrobials: may be given if precipitating event was infectious in nature, with specific antimicrobial being given to eradicate infectious agent

COMMON NURSING DIAGNOSES

DEFICIENT FLUID VOLUME

Related to: hyperglycemic-induced osmotic diuresis, vomiting, inadequate oral intake

Defining Characteristics: dry mucous membranes, decreased skin turgor, thirst, hypotension, orthostatic changes, tachycardia, weak and thready pulse, weight loss, intake less than output, increased urinary output, dilute urine

Outcome Criteria

✔ Patient will have stable vital signs, adequate skin turgor, intake and output equivalent, and electrolyte levels within acceptable ranges.

NOC: *Hydration*

INTERVENTIONS	RATIONALES
Monitor vital signs, especially noting respiratory status changes or alterations in blood pressure.	Tachycardia and hypotension are classic symptoms of hypovolemia. When systolic BP drops more than 10 mm Hg when position is changed, it may indicate severity of hypovolemic state. Kussmaul's respirations may be present depending on degree of hyperglycemia, and respiratory changes may occur as the lungs attempt to remove acids by creating a compensatory respiratory alkalosis. Fever, in conjunction with flushed, dry skin, may indicate dehydration.
Monitor I&O q 2–4 hours.	Facilitates measurement and effectiveness of volume replacement and maintenance of adequate circulating fluid volume.
Administer IV fluids per protocol, usually at least 2–3 L/day, and usually initially, 3+ L.	Amounts and solution types may vary based upon the degree of dehydration and patient status. Usual solutions of normal or half-normal saline, with or without dextrose, are used, as well as occasional use of plasma expanders depending on unsuccessful fluid rehydration. The initial fluid therapy is aimed at the expansion of the intravascular and extravascular volume in

INTERVENTIONS	RATIONALES
	order to restore perfusion to renal tissues. If the patient is not compromised by cardiac status, isotonic saline is usually infused at a rate of 15–20 cc/kg/hr or more for the first hour (approximately 1 L), and is followed by either 0.45% NaCl if serum sodium is normal or increased, or 0.9% NaCl if sodium is decreased, at a rate of 4–15 cc/kg/hr. When renal perfusion and function has been guaranteed, the IV fluids should include 20–30 mEq/L of potassium until the patient becomes stable and can tolerate oral fluids and supplementation. Successful fluid resuscitation should occur within the first 24 hours. If the patient is compromised either with renal or cardiac status, serial monitoring of osmolality and frequent assessments are required to avoid fluid overload.
Administer insulin infusion as ordered.	For DKA, continuous IV infusion of regular insulin is the normal treatment, after a bolus of regular insulin of 0.15 units/kg body weight is given. The infusion of insulin should normally be given at 0.1 unit/kg/hr (5–7 units/hr in an adult), and can be expected to lower blood glucose levels by 50–75 mg/dl/hr. Once serum glucose levels have reached 250 mg/dl, the insulin infusion may be decreased, and dextrose added to the IV fluid solution, and carefully maintained until the desired effect is achieved.
Weigh every day.	Assesses fluid status.
Observe for complaints of nausea/vomiting, abdominal bloating, or distention.	Gastric motility may be affected by fluid deficits, and vomiting or other gastric losses may potentiate fluid and electrolyte imbalances.
Auscultate lungs for crackles, and assess patient for presence of edema, or bounding pulses.	Congestive heart failure or circulatory overload may occur with rapid rehydration.
Insert catheter as ordered.	Provides for more accurate assessment of output, especially if urinary retention or incontinence is present.

(continues)

(continued)

INTERVENTIONS	RATIONALES
Monitor lab work for BUN, creatinine, osmolality, hematocrit, and electrolytes. During the acute phase of DKA, monitor blood glucose levels, venous pH, and ketone levels every 1–2 hours. Monitoring of ß-OHB is preferred, if the facility is capable of performing this test.	Hematocrit may be increased because of hemoconcentration following osmotic diuresis. Dehydration may result in cellular destruction and may result in renal insufficiency. Dehydration will result in elevated osmolality. Potassium is usually elevated initially in response to the acidosis, but with diuresis, a hypokalemic state will ensue. Sodium may be decreased with shifting of fluids, and high sodium levels may indicate either a severe fluid loss or sodium reabsorption in response to aldosterone secretion. Blood glucose levels must be used to ensure that the patient is not becoming hypoglycemic or dropping his glucose level too quickly. Venous pH is usually approximately 0.03 units lower than arterial pH and is used to identify and monitor metabolic acidosis. ß-OHB is the test of choice for monitoring ketonemia, which requires a longer time to clear than does the hyperglycemia, because it is the strongest and most common acid formed in DKA.
Administer electrolyte replacements per doctor's orders.	Phosphate replacement may help with plasma buffering capacity, but excessive replacement can cause hypocalcemia. Potassium supplementation is usually done as soon as urinary output is adequate to prevent hypokalemic states. As insulin replacement occurs and acidosis is corrected, hypokalemia usually occurs. If urine output is sufficient, potassium replacement is begun when serum levels go below 5–5.5 mEq/l. Potassium levels must be kept normalized to preclude dysrhythmias, cardiac arrest, or respiratory muscle debility.
Assess patient's mental status and observe for significant changes in status.	Mental status changes can occur with exceedingly high or low glucose levels, electrolyte imbalances, acidotic states, hypoxia, or with decreases in cerebral perfusion pressure.

INTERVENTIONS	RATIONALES
Instruct patient/family members regarding signs/symptoms of hyperglycemia.	Provides information and promotes more timely identification of complications.
Instruct patient in seeking medical attention for infective processes or illness that may deplete circulating volume.	Infection may predispose the patient to fever and a hypermetabolic state which may increase volume depletion.

NIC: *Fluid/Electrolyte Management*

Discharge or Maintenance Evaluation

- Patient will have vital signs and hemodynamic parameters within acceptable ranges.
- Patient will have normal skin turgor with adequate output.
- Patient will have electrolytes and glucose levels within normal ranges.
- Patient will exhibit no signs or symptoms of dehydration

IMBALANCED NUTRITION: LESS THAN BODY REQUIREMENTS

Related to: insulin deficiency, excessive amounts of epinephrine, growth hormone, and cortisol, increased protein-fat metabolism, decreased oral intake, nausea, vomiting, altered mental status, infection

Defining Characteristics: weakness, fatigue, increased levels of glucose and ketones, weight loss in spite of polyphagia, lack of adequate food intake, glycosuria

Outcome Criteria

✔ Patient will be able to have intake of appropriate amounts and types of calories and nutrients, and have glucose levels within acceptable range for patient.

NOC: *Nutrutional Status: Nutrient Intake*

INTERVENTIONS	RATIONALES
Obtain weight every day.	Facilitates assessment of nutritional utilization and fluid shifts.
Provide high-nutrient liquids as soon as patient is able to tolerate oral intake, with progression to solid food as tolerated.	Provides nutrition and helps restore bowel function.

INTERVENTIONS	RATIONALES
Auscultate bowel sounds every 4–8 hours, and observe for abdominal distention or pain.	Elevated glucose levels can cause altered electrolyte levels and both may decrease gastric function. DKA may also mimic an acute surgical abdomen.
Monitor for changes in level of consciousness, cool or clammy skin, tachycardia, extreme hunger, anxiety, headache, light-headedness, tremors, or irritability.	When carbohydrate metabolism begins and blood glucose level decreases, hypoglycemia can occur. Comatose patients may not exhibit any noticeable change in mentation status and should be monitored closely. Long-standing diabetic patients may not show normal signs of hypoglycemia caused in part by their diminished response to low glucose levels.
Administer regular insulin, either by continuous infusion after an IV bolus dose has been given, or by subcutaneous injection.	Subcutaneous route may be an option if the patient's peripheral perfusion is adequate but the response will not be as rapid as with IV administration. Regular insulin is rapid acting and will assist in movement of glucose into cells. The continuous IV method is normally preferred because it optimizes transition to carbohydrate metabolism, and helps to reduce hypoglycemia. Normally, the infusion rate is 5–10 Units/hr until glucose levels decrease within a stated parameter. Another goal of IV administration of insulin is to decrease the acidosis.
Monitor serum glucose every hour while on insulin IV infusion, and notify physician per parameters or when blood glucose has dropped to 250 mg/dl.	Blood glucose levels will decrease with insulin therapy usually in increments of 75 to 100 mg/dl/hr. Once the blood sugar has dropped to 250 mg/dl, and depending upon the degree of acidosis that is present, dextrose is added to the IV infusion, and the insulin infusion should be stopped to prevent hypoglycemic episodes.
Administer subcutaneous insulin 1–2 hours before stopping the continuous insulin infusion.	Prevents recurrence of ketosis and rebound hyperglycemia.
Administer IV solutions containing dextrose as ordered.	Dextrose solutions are usually added after the blood glucose levels have decreased to 250 mg/dl in order to avoid hypoglycemia.

INTERVENTIONS	RATIONALES
Administer metoclopramide (Reglan) IV or PO as ordered by physician.	May be used to treat symptoms related to neuropathies that affect the GI tract, and facilitate oral intake and nutrient absorption.
Assess patient for presence of any eating disorders.	Fear of weight gain and psychological problems that are complicated by eating disorders may contribute to the recurrence of DKA in some patients, especially younger patients.
Evaluate patient's current drug regimen for any contributing causes for precipitating factors.	Corticosteroids, thiazides, and sympathomimetic drugs, such as terbutaline and dobutamine, affect the metabolism of carbohydrates and can precipitate DKA.
Instruct patient/family member in dietary management, with ideal amounts of 60% carbohydrates, 20% fats, and 20% proteins to be divided in designated number of meals and snacks.	Complex carbohydrates decrease the amounts of insulin needs, reduce serum cholesterol, and help to satiate patient. Food should be scheduled for peak effects with insulin as well as patient preference. Snacks are important to prevent Somogyi responses and hypoglycemia during sleep.
Obtain consult with dietician.	Assists in facilitating adjustments to diet for patient's special needs, and can facilitate development of workable meal plans.
Instruct patient in correct procedure for fingerstick glucose testing, with return demonstration as needed.	Monitoring blood glucose levels is more accurate than urine glucose testing, and can facilitate identification of alterations in levels of glucose to promote tighter control of varying glucose levels/insulin usage.
Ensure that at least 50 cc of solution is flushed through the tubing prior to connection to patient when intravenous insulin drips are utilized.	Promotes saturation of binding sites on plastic tubing to decrease incidence of insulin adhering to tubing rather than staying in solution.

NIC: *Diet Staging*

Discharge or Maintenance Evaluation

- Patient will have normalized blood glucose levels within their own special parameters.
- Patient will be able to ingest oral food of sufficient amounts and nutrients to maintain and stabilize weight.
- Patient will be free of ketosis.

- Patient/family member will be able to verbalize understanding of instructions and able to provide acceptable return demonstration of procedure.

IMPAIRED GAS EXCHANGE

Related to: accumulation of ketones and acids secondary to insulin deficiencies and excessive production of stress hormones

Defining Characteristics: acid–base imbalances, acetone breath, tachypnea, Kussmaul respirations, serum and urine ketones present, decreased pH, decreased bicarbonate levels, hyperkalemia, decreased level of consciousness, confusion, increased anion gap

Outcome Criteria

✔ Patient will have normalized acid–base balance with stable vital signs and mentation level.

NOC: *Electrolyte and Acid–Base Balance*

INTERVENTIONS	RATIONALES
Monitor respiratory status for changes in rate, rhythm and depth, and for presence of acetone smell on breath.	Acetone breath is due to breakdown of acetoacetic acids. The lungs remove carbonic acid through respiration process, and may produce a compensatory respiratory alkalosis for ketoacidosis. Increased work of breathing may indicate that the patient is losing the ability to compensate for the severe acidosis or respiratory fatigue.
Monitor for changes in neurologic status.	Acidosis, hypoxia, or decreased cerebral perfusion may cause changes in mentation. Impairment in consciousness may predispose the patient to aspiration and its complications.
Administer IV fluids and insulin as ordered.	Promotes correction of acidosis with DKA.
Administer sodium bicarbonate, if ordered, for severe acidosis only.	Current recommendations are for use only where pH is below 7.0 because excessive use of sodium bicarbonate may induce hypokalemia as well as alter the oxygen dissociation curve causing prolongation of the comatose state. When the pH is above 7.0, the replacement of insulin helps to block the lipolysis and assists in resolving ketoacidosis without

INTERVENTIONS	RATIONALES
	the addition of bicarbonate administration.
Monitor lab work for hypokalemia.	May occur as acidosis and volume deficits are corrected.
Administer supplemental oxygen as necessary.	Provides needed oxygen, especially in patients that may not be able to obtain adequate oxygenation with room air, and helps to improve acidosis.
Monitor arterial blood gases as ordered and prn.	Hypoxemia can result in complications in the treatment of DKA. Hypoxia and hypoxemia reduces colloid osmotic pressure and increases lung fluid content and decreases the lung's compliance. DKA patients having a widened A-a gradient may be at greater risk for pulmonary edema.
Instruct patient in relaxation techniques.	Helps to reduce oxygen demand and consumption.
Instruct patient/family regarding energy conservation techniques.	Activity increases tissue oxygen demands and rest periods help to improve tissue perfusion.

NIC: *Acid–Base Monitoring*

Discharge or Maintenance Evaluation

- Patient will have pH, bicarbonate, potassium, serum and urine ketones within normal limits.
- Patient will have stable vital signs with respiratory rate within normal limits.
- Patient will be free of acetone on breath.

RISK FOR INFECTION

Related to: elevated glucose levels, alterations in circulation, pre-existing infection, especially URI or UTI, decreased leukocyte function

Defining Characteristics: increased serum and urine glucose levels, temperature elevation, chills, fever, elevated white blood cell count, differential with shift to the left

Outcome Criteria

✔ Patient will be free of infection and able to verbalize methods to prevent or reduce risk of infection.

NOC: *Knowledge: Infection Control*

INTERVENTIONS	RATIONALES
Monitor for fever, facial flushing, drainage from wounds, urine cloudiness, changes in sputum, and tachycardia.	Patient may have been admitted with undiagnosed infection or have developed a nosocomial infection.
Auscultate for changes in breath sounds.	Accumulation of bronchial secretions may be heard as rhonchi and may indicate the presence of bronchitis or pneumonia, either of which may be the precipitating cause of the DKA. Crackles may indicate fluid overload or congestive failure as a result from rapid fluid replacement.
Provide perineal or catheter care frequently.	Elderly female diabetics are prone to the development of urinary tract and vaginal infections.
Reposition patient and provide skin care every 2 hours.	Facilitates lung expansion, decreases risk of skin irritation and breakdown, and improves peripheral circulation.
Obtain culture specimens as ordered or per hospital policy.	Assists with identification of causative organism and appropriate antimicrobial therapy.
Administer antimicrobials as ordered.	Early intervention may reduce the risk of sepsis or multisystem involvement.
Ensure proper handwashing techniques are used by staff and patient.	Prevents cross-contamination and decreases risk of spread of infection.
Maintain aseptic technique with administration of IV medications, insertion of catheters and invasive lines, and maintenance care. Restart IVs per hospital protocol.	Elevated glucose levels provide an excellent culture medium for bacterial growth.
Instruct patient in perineal care and disposal of secretions and infected materials.	Promotes compliance, minimizes risk of spread of infection, and cross-contamination.
Instruct patient in importance of oral care.	Reduces risk of oral or gum disease.

NIC: *Infection Protection*

Discharge or Maintenance Evaluation

- Patient will be able to identify actions to reduce or prevent infection and cross-contamination.
- Patient will be free of infective process.

- Patient will be able to adequately demonstrate techniques to prevent or reduce infection risk.

RISK FOR INJURY

Related to: hypoglycemia, insulin therapy, decreased insulin-antagonist hormones circulating in body, rebound action

Defining Characteristics: blood glucose levels below 60 mg/dl, altered mental state, decreased level of consciousness, cool and clammy skin, pallor, tremors, tachycardia, irritability, visual disturbances, paresthesias, dizziness, hunger, nausea, fatigue, diaphoresis

Outcome Criteria

✔ Patient will have stable blood glucose levels and be able to identify methods of treatment and identification of hypoglycemic episodes.

NOC: *Risk Detection*

INTERVENTIONS	RATIONALES
Monitor for signs/symptoms of hypoglycemia.	Prompt identification of problem will facilitate prompt treatment and help prevent further complications.
Change IV fluid to solution containing glucose when blood glucose level reaches 250 mg/dl, as well as change infusion rate on insulin drip.	Prevents excessive drop in blood glucose level and allows time for blood chemistry to normalize.
If hypoglycemia occurs, give the patient oral (if awake and able to tolerate fluids) or parenteral glucose solutions, as ordered.	Glucagon, 10–50% solutions, may be given IV, or 15 grams of a rapid-acting carbohydrate will be effective in elevating the blood sugar level. Milk and crackers will assist in protecting patient from recurrences of hypoglycemic episode.
Instruct patient/family in signs of hypoglycemia and treatment for this condition.	Promotes knowledge and facilitates compliance. Assists patient and family to feel in control.

NIC: *Hypoglycemia Management*

Discharge or Maintenance Evaluation

- Patient will have stable blood glucose level above 80 mg/dl.

- Patient/family member will be able to identify signs and symptoms of hypoglycemia and interventions for treatment.
- Patient will have no hypoglycemic symptoms.

FATIGUE

Related to: insufficient insulin, increased metabolic demands, decreased metabolic energy production, infection

Defining Characteristics: lack of energy, inability to perform normal routine, decreased performance, accident prone, lethargy, tiredness, alterations in consciousness

Outcome Criteria

✔ Patient will have increased energy and be able to participate adequately in normal activities.

NOC: *Activity Tolerance*

INTERVENTIONS	RATIONALES
Observe patient for activity tolerance.	Provides baseline information so that identification of problem and interventions may be planned. Elevations in pulse, blood pressure and respiratory rate may indicate physiologic intolerance of activity.
Provide period of rest or sleep alternated with periods of activity as patient can tolerate.	Prevents excessive fatigue.
Increase activity and patient participation gradually.	Provides time to build up tolerance, and increases self-esteem.
Discuss with patient/family member the importance of activity, planning schedules with alternating rest and activity, and methods of conserving energy.	Information may facilitate motivation to increase activity level knowing that decreased energy will be expended and he will be able to accomplish more activity.

NIC: *Exercise Promotion*

Discharge or Maintenance Evaluation

- Patient will be able to tolerate increased activity with stable vital signs.
- Patient/family will be able to verbalize and/or demonstrate techniques to conserve energy while performing activities.

DEFICIENT KNOWLEDGE

Related to: management of hyperglycemia, new diagnosis of diabetes mellitus, lack of information, lack of recall, misinterpreted information, unfamiliarity with resources

Defining Characteristics: requests for information, questions, misrepresentation of facts, inaccurate follow-through of instructions, development of preventable complications, inability to verbalize management of sick days, delays in notifying doctor about worsening condition, inability to verbalize troubleshooting information

Outcome Criteria

✔ Patient will be able to verbalize understanding of diabetes disease process, identify signs and symptoms of complications, correctly demonstrate all procedures, and access community resources adequately.

NOC: *Knowledge: Diabetes Management*

INTERVENTIONS	RATIONALES
Instruct patient/family member about disease process, normal ranges for blood glucose, glucometer use, relationship between insulin and glucose levels, type of diabetes the patient has, and so forth.	Provides knowledge base on which further instruction can be performed.
Instruct patient/family member in glucometer use and urine testing, with return demonstration by patient.	Promotes tighter control of diabetes with self-monitoring at least four times per day, and may help prevent or delay long-term complications.
Instruct patient/family in dietary plan, allowances, caloric intake, meals outside the home, and so forth.	Dietary control will assist with maintenance of decreased blood glucose levels. Fiber may slow glucose absorption and decrease fluctuations in serum levels.
Instruct patient/family in medication regime, with actions, side effects, and contraindications noted.	Promotes understanding of drug use and facilitates compliance with regimen. Proper techniques with administration of insulin assist with understanding and identification of potential problems so that interventions may be found.

INTERVENTIONS	RATIONALES
Instruct patient/family in activity and other factors that determine diabetic control.	Promotes control of diabetes and may help reduce incidence of ketoacidosis. Aerobic exercises promote effective utilization of insulin and strengthen the cardiovascular system. Illness management and management of other stress-type factors facilitate equilibrium with disease process during these episodes.
Instruct patient/family in avoidance of smoking.	Nicotine causes constriction of blood vessels which restricts insulin absorption up to 30%.
Instruct patient/family in examination and care of feet.	Identifies potential complications that may occur because of peripheral neuropathy or circulatory impairment, and allows for early intervention.
Instruct patient/family in protocols for sick days—to take medications, to notify physician, to monitor blood sugar every 2–4 hours, to check urine ketones if blood sugar is >240 mg/dl, and to replace carbohydrates with liquids.	Provides plan for complications that occur, and gives the patient the knowledge to enable patient to adequately care for self during times of illness.
Instruct patient in maintaining medical maintenance, including vision checks, and follow-up care.	Vision changes may be gradual and may be more pronounced in poorly-controlled diabetics. Visual acuity may deteriorate to retinopathy and eventual blindness. Follow-up care can assist in

INTERVENTIONS	RATIONALES
	preventing exacerbations of diabetic complications and delay development of systemic problems.
Discuss sexual function and questions patient/family member may ask.	Impotence may occur as an initial symptom of diabetes mellitus. Penile prosthesis and/or counseling may be of help.
Instruct patient in avoidance of use of over-the-counter medications without physician approval.	May contain increased sugar content and may interact with other medications being taken.
Instruct patient/family in available community resources, support groups like the American Diabetic Association, smoking and weight loss clinics, and so forth.	Provides continued support post discharge, and assists to support lifestyle changes.

NIC: *Teaching: Disease Process*

Discharge or Maintenance Evaluation

- Patient/family member will be able to accurately verbalize knowledge base regarding diabetic disease process.
- Patient/family member will be able to accurately verbalize all information given.
- Patient/family member will be able to accurately return demonstration for all necessary procedures.

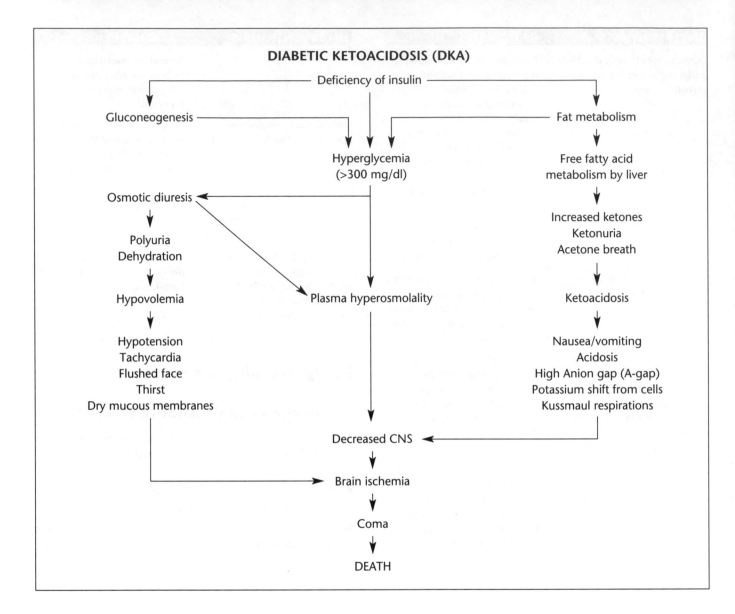

DIABETIC KETOACIDOSIS (DKA)

CHAPTER 6.3

HYPEROSMOLAR HYPERGLYCEMIC STATE

Hyperosmolar hyperglycemic state (HHS), once known as HHNK, or hyperglycemic, hyperosmolar nonketotic coma, or hyperglycemic nonacidotic diabetic coma, presents a life-threatening emergency. It can occur in both types I and II diabetes and the morbidity rate is high at approximately 15%. Glucose transportation across the cell membrane is impaired by enough of an insulin deficiency that causes hyperglycemia without inhibiting lipolysis or ketogenesis in the liver. The hyperosmolality occurs from the hypernatremia and hyperglycemia, and may further impair the secretion of insulin and prevent fatty acid release from adipose tissues. Extracellular fluid volume deficits occur as a result of osmotic diuresis in the body's attempt to offset increasing plasma osmolality. As fluid volume deficits increase, glomerular filtration rates decrease and reduce the ability of the kidneys to excrete the glucose.

HHS occurs when insulin action or secretion is inadequate, and may occur in patients who have no previous history of diabetes mellitus. The elderly are especially prone to this because of lower body water content and dehydration, which may alter their buffering ability to respond to changes in osmolality. Illnesses, and other stress-provoking episodes, may either cause or hasten the development of HHS by increasing glucose production in response to excessive stress hormone production.

HHS has almost the same pathophysiologic pattern as DKA, but the difference is that with HHS, a sufficient amount of insulin is being released to prevent the development of ketosis.

HHS has also been associated with usage of thiazide diuretics, glucocorticoids, phenytoin, sympathomimetics, diazoxide, chlorpromazine, sedatives, cimetidine, calcium channel blockers, and immunosuppressive agents because of their effects with glucogenesis and/or insulin.

Mortality is caused in part by common complications that occur, such as shock, coma, acute tubular necrosis, and vascular thrombosis. Correction of the problem is the main goal of treatment, with fluid balance the initial concern. The lack of insulin may be corrected by supplemental insulin administration and usually requires 100 units or less in the first 24 hour period. Electrolyte imbalances are corrected and may require large amounts of potassium supplementation.

MEDICAL CARE

Laboratory: blood sugar level elevated, frequently over 1000 mg/dl; plasma osmolality elevated, frequently as high as 450 mOsm/kg; hematocrit elevated because of hemoconcentration; urine and serum acetone levels negative; BUN and creatinine elevated; marked leukocytosis; electrolytes to evaluate deficiency; hypernatremia usually present

Arterial blood gases: used to identify acidosis; pH is usually greater than 7.30, bicarbonate is usually greater than 15 mEq/L; acidosis is mainly caused by lactic acid or renal dysfunction

Electrocardiogram: used to identify dysrhythmias that may result as a consequence of electrolyte and fluid disturbances

IV fluids: required to combat dehydration, to provide fluids, and to provide method of administration of electrolyte replacement; fluids are usually begun with 0.9% NaCl solution and when patient's blood sugar lowers to a specific range, 5% dextrose is added to prevent hypoglycemia; unlike DKA, the patient's fluid needs are usually increased

Insulin: required to lower severely elevated blood glucose levels; normally given as a bolus of regular insulin, followed by an infusion that is titrated for patient's specific glucose levels; subcutaneous insulin is begun once the blood sugar levels are low enough, but prior to the discontinuation of the IV infusion to prevent a recurrent rebound hyperglycemia

COMMON NURSING DIAGNOSES

DEFICIENT FLUID VOLUME (see DKA)

Related to: osmotic diuresis, hyperosmolality, lack of insulin, increased gluconeogenesis, decreased glucogenolysis

Defining Characteristics: increased temperature, tachycardia, hypotension, dry mucous membranes, decreased skin turgor, thirst, intake less than output, increased urinary output, polydipsia, increased BUN and sodium, decreased potassium, lethargy, cardiac dysrhythmias, gastrointestinal stasis, renal dysfunction

IMBALANCED NUTRITION: LESS THAN BODY REQUIREMENTS (see DKA)

Related to: insulin deficiency, excessive amounts of epinephrine, growth hormone, and cortisol, increased protein–fat metabolism, decreased oral intake, nausea, vomiting, altered mental status, infection

Defining Characteristics: weakness, fatigue, increased levels of glucose, weight loss in spite of polyphagia, lack of adequate food intake, glycosuria

RISK FOR INJURY: HYPOGLYCEMIA (see DKA)

Related to: hypoglycemia, insulin therapy, decreased insulin-antagonist hormones circulating in body, rebound action

Defining Characteristics: blood glucose levels below 60 mg/dl, altered mental state, decreased level of consciousness, cool and clammy skin, pallor, tremors, tachycardia, irritability, visual disturbances, paresthesias, dizziness, hunger, nausea, fatigue, diaphoresis

ADDITIONAL NURSING DIAGNOSES

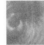

INEFFECTIVE TISSUE PERFUSION: PERIPHERAL

Related to: dehydration, increased platelet aggregation, increased viscosity of blood

Defining Characteristics: cool extremities, decreased peripheral pulses, extremity pallor or cyanosis, unequal extremity temperatures, hypotension

Outcome Criteria

✔ Patient will have bilaterally equal pulses, color, and temperature to extremities, with no complications.

NOC: *Tissue Perfusion: Peripheral*

INTERVENTIONS	RATIONALES
Monitor and assess lower extremities for color, temperature, presence of pulses, and equality.	Identifies the status of circulation in the extremities and assists with prompt identification of complications.
Test for positive Homan's sign, redness, warmth, tenderness, or swelling to legs.	May indicate thrombus formation, but is not always present with thrombus formation.
Remove TED hose at least every 8 hours for 30 minutes to 1 hour.	Provides opportunity for thorough assessment and identification of changes, as well as for comfort of patient.
Assist with passive range of motion/encourage active range of motion exercises.	Prevents venous stasis.
Instruct patient/family member to avoid constricting apparel, crossing legs or ankles, or any other activity that impedes circulation.	Prevents circulatory impairment and risk of complications.
Notify physician for any evidence of thrombus formation.	Prompt identification can lead to timely intervention.

NIC: *Embolus Care: Peripheral*

Discharge or Maintenance Evaluation

- Patient will have equal pulses, color, and temperature to lower extremities bilaterally.
- Patient will have no evidence of thrombus formation.
- Patient/family will be compliant with methods to reduce risk of thrombus formation.

HYPERGLYCEMIC HYPEROSMOLAR NONKETOTIC COMA (HHNK)

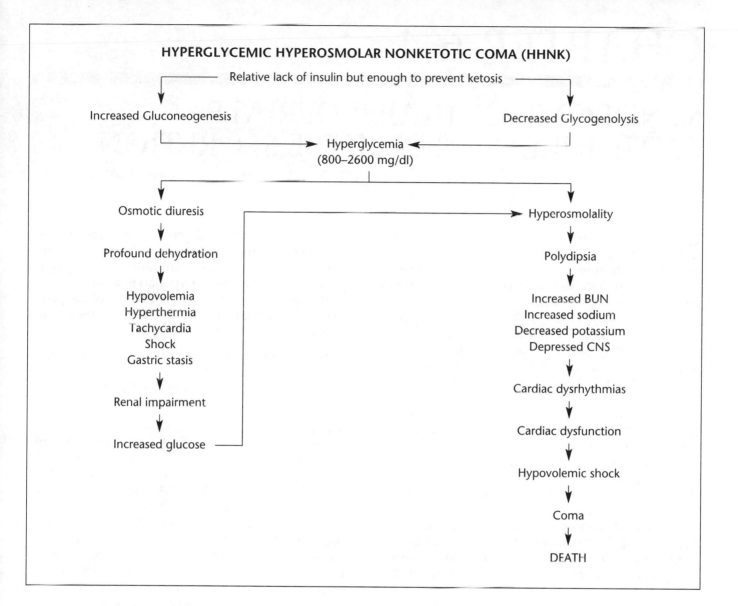

CHAPTER 6.4

SYNDROME OF INAPPROPRIATE ANTIDIURETIC HORMONE SECRETION

Syndrome of inappropriate antidiuretic hormone secretion (SIADH) is another dysfunction of the antidiuretic hormone in which there is increased secretion or production of ADH. The increase is not related to osmolality, and therefore causes a slight increase in body water. Sodium concentration is decreased in the extracellular fluid and plasma. SIADH is usually caused by bronchogenic or pancreatic cancer, but can occasionally result from pituitary tumors. Other etiologies include skull fractures, subdural hematoma, subarachnoid hemorrhage, cerebral contusion, meningitis, encephalitis, Guillain–Barré syndrome, stroke, aneurysm, infections, tumors, pulmonary diseases, Addison's disease, hypopituitarism, AIDS, and use of tricyclic drugs, oral hypoglycemics, acetaminophen, chlorpropamide, thiazide diuretics, cytotoxic agents, and excessive vasopressin therapy.

Unlike diabetes insipidus, SIADH has a failure of the negative feedback system in which continued ADH secretion creates water intoxication because of low plasma osmolality and expanded volume. The primary initial goal is to restrict fluid intake and correct electrolyte imbalances. With severe cases, 3% hypertonic saline and IV lasix are used.

MEDICAL CARE

Laboratory: serum sodium decreased, plasma osmolality decreased, urine sodium and osmolality increased, elevated ADH levels; renal profiles used to assess renal status changes from imbalances and from nephrotoxic medications; thyroid profiles to assess thyroid function; electrolytes to evaluate concurrent imbalances

Electrocardiogram: used to identify cardiac dysrhythmias that may occur as a result of electrolyte or fluid imbalances

IV fluids: fluids will be given or restricted based on the patient's urinary output and insensible fluid losses; hypertonic sodium chloride may be given if patient develops severe hyponatemia but its use is controversial in many facilities because of the prevalence of potential fluid overload, heart failure and cerebral osmotic demyelination syndrome

Electrolyte replacement: should be given based upon patient's specific lab values; replacement may be required because of the use of diuretics to treat water intoxication

Diuretics: furosemide (Lasix, Furosemide, Luramide), bumetanine (Bumex), chlorothiazide (Diuril), hydrochlorothiazide (Esidrex, Hydrochlorthiazide, HydroDiuril, Thiuretic), chlorthalidone (Chlorthalidone, Hygroton, Hylidone, Thalitone), indapamide (Lozol), metolazone (Diulo, Zaroxolyn), ethacrynic acid (Edecrin), torsemide (Demadex), acetazolamide (Acetazolamide, Diamox), methazolamide (Neptazane), amiloride (Amiloride, Midamor), spironolactone (Aldactone), triamterene (Dyrenium), mannitol (Mannitol, Osmitrol), and urea (Ureaphil) may be used to treat water intoxication and fluid overload

Antimicrobials: may be required to treat the precipitating cause of this syndrome and should be specific to the causative organism

COMMON NURSING DIAGNOSES

RISK FOR INJURY (see STATUS EPILEPTICUS)

Related to: impairment of cognitive ability, physical inactivity, seizure activity

Defining Characteristics: confusion, lethargy, memory impairment, irritability, personality changes, level of consciousness changes, restlessness, fatigue, weakness, seizures, imposed physical inactivity

ADDITIONAL NURSING DIAGNOSES

EXCESS FLUID VOLUME

Related to: inability to excrete water, inappropriate antidiuretic hormone secretion, failure of negative feedback system

Defining Characteristics: hyponatremia, decreased plasma osmolality, increased urine osmolality, weight gain, neurologic disturbances, seizures

Outcome Criteria

✔ Patient will exhibit no signs or symptoms of excessive fluid overload and will have equivalent intake and output with normalized electrolytes

NOC: *Fluid Balance*

INTERVENTIONS	RATIONALES
Monitor for changes in level of consciousness, fatigue, weakness, headache or generalized pain.	May be early indication of impending water intoxication.
Monitor heart rhythm and hemodynamics as ordered.	Fluid shifts and electrolyte disturbances can precipitate cardiac dysrhythmias and changes in hemodynamic status.
Weigh patient every day, and maintain accurate I&O.	Assists with identification of fluid status/balance.
Administer IV and PO fluids as ordered, maintaining fluid restriction.	Restriction of fluid may be based partially on urine, nasogastric, or other fluid losses.
Administer hypertonic saline IV when ordered.	These types of infusions are generally reserved for severe hyponatremia or when accompanied by seizure activity. Fluid overload may worsen and deteriorate into heart failure. There are controversial theories that sudden increases in serum sodium can result in osmotic demyelination syndrome which may have adapted to the lower level of sodium.
Administer diuretics as ordered.	Assists with decreasing the action of ADH, but can also cause electrolyte losses.

INTERVENTIONS	RATIONALES
Administer other drugs that help inhibit ADH action, as ordered.	Lithium and demeclocycline interfere with ADH at the renal tubular level, but can be nephrotoxic. Phenytoin inhibits ADH release.
Administer supplemental electrolytes as ordered.	Facilitates replacement of required electrolytes to maintain function.
Monitor lab studies, especially renal profiles for changes in renal perfusion.	Some medications are nephrotoxic and can worsen renal function.
Instruct patient/family regarding fluid balance, seizure precautions, drug therapy, procedures, lab studies, etc.	Promotes knowledge, and encourages compliance with medical regimen. Facilitates patient taking active part in his care.

NIC: *Hypervolemia Management*

Discharge or Maintenance Evaluation

- Patient will be neurologically stable with approximately equivalent intake and output, and vital signs will be stable.
- Patient will have normalized weight and be able to maintain weight.
- Patient will have laboratory values within normal parameters.
- Patient/family will be able to accurately verbalize understanding of all instructions.

CONSTIPATION

Related to: decreased gastric motility secondary to hyponatremia, fluid restriction, decreased activity

Defining Characteristics: inability to pass stool, hard stools, painful, small stools

Outcome Criteria

✔ Patient will be free of constipation.

NOC: *Bowel Elimination*

INTERVENTIONS	RATIONALES
Assess bowel habits of patient; normal routines, frequency of stools, use of cathartics, etc.	Provides baseline from which to plan interventions.

(continues)

(continued)

INTERVENTIONS	RATIONALES
Administer laxatives or stool softeners as ordered. Tap water enemas should be avoided.	Caution must be used in selection of pharmacological agent so as to not further add to fluid volume overload. Water in the enemas can be absorbed and increase overload.
Instruct patient in importance of responding to urge to defecate.	Responsiveness of patient to urge is essential to normal bowel functioning and to avoid discomfort.
Instruct patient in massaging abdomen along transverse and descending colon each day.	Massage may assist to stimulate peristalsis.
Instruct patient/family in appropriate use of laxatives, stool softeners, and enemas.	Overuse of purgative may increase fluid and electrolyte loss, create laxative dependence, and damage intestinal mucosa.

 NIC: *Constipation/Impaction Management*

Discharge or Maintenance Evaluation

- Patient will have normal bowel function with no complications to fluid status.
- Patient will not exacerbate fluid imbalances.
- Patient will be able to use laxatives and stool softeners appropriately.

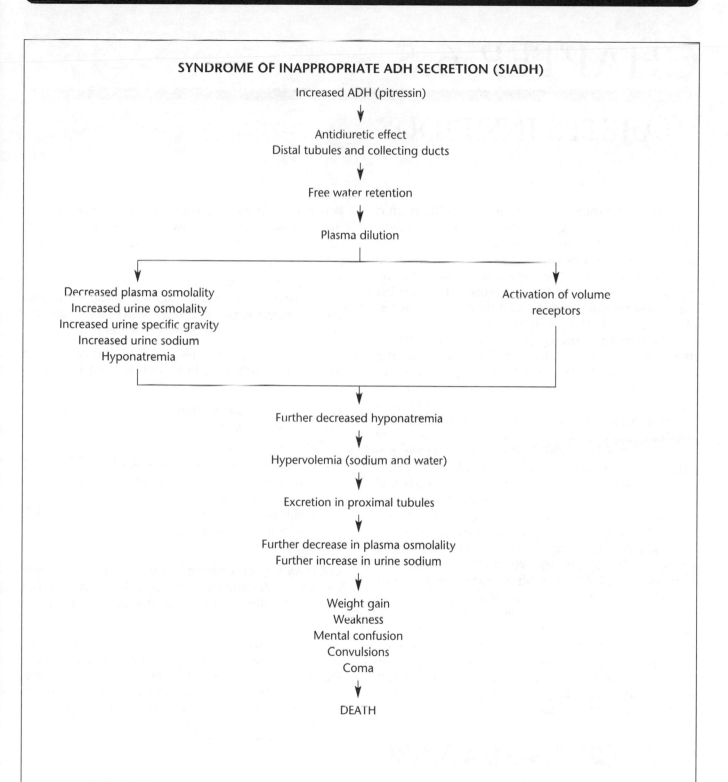

SYNDROME OF INAPPROPRIATE ADH SECRETION (SIADH)

Increased ADH (pitressin)

↓

Antidiuretic effect
Distal tubules and collecting ducts

↓

Free water retention

↓

Plasma dilution

Decreased plasma osmolality
Increased urine osmolality
Increased urine specific gravity
Increased urine sodium
Hyponatremia

Activation of volume
receptors

Further decreased hyponatremia

↓

Hypervolemia (sodium and water)

↓

Excretion in proximal tubules

↓

Further decrease in plasma osmolality
Further increase in urine sodium

↓

Weight gain
Weakness
Mental confusion
Convulsions
Coma

↓

DEATH

CHAPTER 6.5

DIABETES INSIPIDUS

Diabetes insipidus, or DI, is a condition that results when damage or destruction of the neurons of the hypothalamus causes decreased levels of antidiuretic hormone (ADH) and severe diuresis and dehydration occur. The deficiency results in the inability to conserve water, and if the patient's thirst mechanism is not adequate, or if fluids are not accessible, the fluid balance will be altered.

The two main etiologies of DI are tumors of the hypothalamus or pituitary and closed head injuries that may have damage to the supraoptic nuclei or hypothalamus. Head injuries, neurosurgery, or hypophysectomy may lead to a loss of osmoreceptor function and/or damage to the areas that produce antidiuretic hormone. Sometimes, a transient type of DI occurs after surgical procedures, histiocytosis, sarcoidosis, aneurysms, meningitis, encephalitis, or neoplastic conditions. All the above respond to vasopressin.

DI that is nephrogenic is usually vasopressin-insensitive, and is seen in polycystic kidney disease, pyelonephritis, multiple myeloma, sarcoidosis, sickle cell disease, or any disorder that affects the kidneys. Usage of ethanol and phenytoin inhibit ADH secretion, and drugs such as lithium and demeclocycline inhibit ADH action in the kidney.

The main goal for treatment is to prevent dehydration and electrolyte imbalances, while determination and treatment of the underlying cause occurs. Vasopressin administration will control diabetes insipidus; D-amino-D-arginine vasopressin (DDAVP) is a nasal spray that has prolonged antidiuretic effects with minimal side effects.

MEDICAL CARE

Laboratory: serum osmolality elevated, usually greater than 295 mOsm/kg; urine osmolality decreased, generally less than 500 mOsm/kg and can be as low as 30 mOsm/kg; urine specific gravity low, generally 1.001 to 1.005; plasma ADH levels decreased in central diabetes insipidus; serum sodium elevated

Water deprivation test: used to demonstrate that in the presence of simple dehydration, kidneys cannot concentrate urine; used to differentiate psychogenic polydipsia from diabetes insipidus

Vasopressin test: used in conjunction with water deprivation test to identify that the kidneys can concentrate urine with exogenous ADH and differentiates nephrogenic from central diabetes insipidus

IV fluids: required because of potential or present fluid deficits resulting from the body's inability to conserve water

Electrolyte replacement: required based upon patient's lab levels; hypernatremia is frequently seen, so potassium levels may be low

Hormonal replacement: vasopressin (Pitressin) or desmopressin acetate (DDAVP, Stimate) are used to replace endogenous hormone; drugs increase the permeability of the renal tubular epithelium which increase reabsorption of water and allowed for concentration of urine

Chlorpropamide: diabenese used for its antidiuretic effect with DI patients; stimulates the release of ADH and helps the response of the renal tubules to ADH effects

Thiazide diuretics: chlorothiazide (Diuril), hydrochlorothiazide (Esidrex, Hydrochlorthiazide, Hydro-Diuril, Thiuretic), chlorthalidone (Chlorthalidone, Hygroton, Hylidone, Thalitone), indapamide (Lozol), and metolazone (Diulo, Zaroxolyn) used to reduce the solute load and deplete sodium in order to increase water reabsorption

NURSING DIAGNOSES

DEFICIENT FLUID VOLUME

Related to: inability to conserve water, dehydration, decreased levels of ADH

Defining Characteristics: extreme thirst, decreased skin turgor, dry mucous membranes, hypotension, tachycardia, weight loss, dilute urine output, increased urine output, hemoconcentration, hyperosmolality, increased serum sodium

Outcome Criteria

✔ Patient will have fluid volume balance restored and be able to maintain adequate fluid volume.

NOC: *Hydration*

INTERVENTIONS	RATIONALES
Assess and monitor vital signs.	Tachycardia and hypotension may result from hypovolemia.
Measure intake and output every 1–2 hours, and notify physician for changes. Record specific gravity measurements per protocol.	Provides information to identify fluid imbalances and volume depletion. I&O should be continued in postoperative patients, especially neurosurgical patients, to ensure that DI has not transiently resolved and then reappear only to become permanent. Urinary output may be as much as 15 L/day, and specific gravity is usually between 1.001 and 1.005.
Administer IV fluids as ordered. If able to take oral fluids, encourage patient PO intake.	Helps to restore circulating fluid volume.
Weigh patient daily.	Provides identification of fluid balances and water losses.
Administer replacement therapy for central diabetes insipidus.	Aqueous pitressin (IV or SQ) is a short-acting ADH useful in transient DI. Nasal spray vasopressin is also short-acting and may be erratic in patients with respiratory infections or nasal problems. DDAVP (nasal or SQ) is a synthetic ADH that has a longer duration and can be given q 12–24 hours. Vasopressin tannate in oil can last 24–72 hours and is not utilized as initial treatment due to inability to titrate dose.
Administer medication therapy for nephrogenic diabetes insipidus.	Chlorpropamide is used to stimulate ADH release and can

INTERVENTIONS	RATIONALES
	augment the renal tubular response to ADH. Thiazide diuretics in conjunction with sodium restriction will reduce solute load and enhance water reabsorption.
Ensure that vasopressin tannate in oil is warmed and vigorously agitated prior to injection.	Reduces pain from injection and ensures complete mixture.
Observe for water intoxication with pharmacologic replacement therapies.	May occur with shifting fluid balances.
Assist with diagnostic procedures such as water deprivation and vasopressin tests by obtaining accurate weights, vital signs, I&O, lab specimens at proper intervals, and maintaining deprivation for required amount of time.	Ensures that correct sequence will be maintained for specimens and that procedure data will be accurate. The water deprivation test is usually terminated if the patient has a 3% weight loss.
Instruct patient/family member in methods to prevent dehydration when on long-term ADH therapy, as well as when hospitalized.	Promotes knowledge and facilitates compliance with medical regimen.

NIC: *Hypovolemia Management*

Discharge or Maintenance Evaluation

- Patient will have stable vital signs and balanced intake and output.
- Patient will be able to maintain normal hemodynamic parameters.
- Patient will have weight restored and be able to maintain weight.
- Patient/family will be able to verbalize accurately any information related to them.

DEFICIENT KNOWLEDGE

Related to: potential self-care management for permanent diabetes insipidus

Defining Characteristics: newly diagnosed DI, requests for information, questions, inaccurate follow-through with instructions or medications, development of preventable complications, inability to recall information vital to disease process

Outcome Criteria

✔ Patient/family member will be able to accurately verbalize medical regimen to manage diabetes insipidus.

NOC: *Knowledge: Treatment Regimen*

INTERVENTIONS	RATIONALES
Assess for patient/family member comprehension of disease and medications.	Provides baseline of knowledge and facilitates plan for interventions.
Instruct patient in all medications, action, side effects, adverse reactions, schedule to be taken, method of administration, and importance of adherence to medical regime.	Promotes knowledge and facilitates compliance.
Instruct patient to notify physician for excessive water retention or urinary frequency and increased amount.	Prompt identification may facilitate timely intervention and treatment.

INTERVENTIONS	RATIONALES
Discuss reasons for nonadherence to medication, if patient has previously been diagnosed with DI.	Explores patient's rationale and identifies any misconceptions he might have regarding his medical regimen.
Discuss obtaining medical alert bracelet identifying patient as having DI.	Promotes fast recognition of medical condition in cases where patient is not able to identify problems.

NIC: *Teaching: Disease Process*

Discharge or Maintenance Evaluation

■ Patient will be able to accurately verbalize purpose, side effects, and schedule of medications.

■ Patient will adhere to medical therapeutics and take medication as prescribed.

■ Patient/family will be able to accurately recall all information related to them.

■ Patient/family will be able to identify fluid balance alterations that should be reported to physician.

■ Patient will be compliant in obtaining medical identification bracelet.

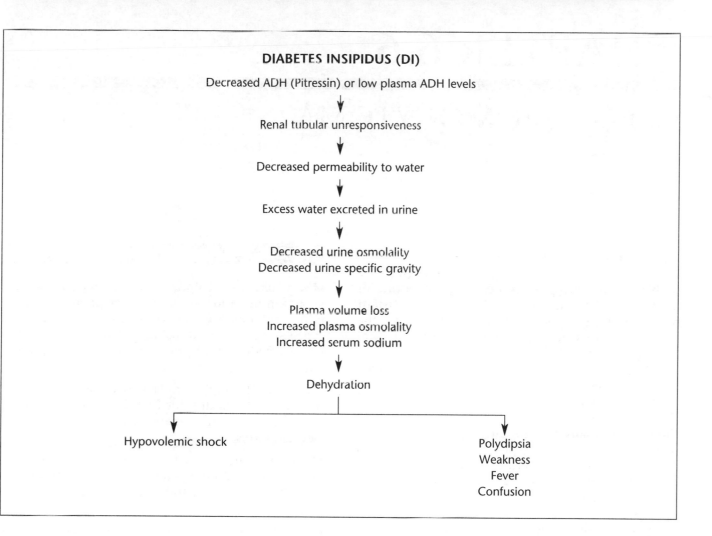

DIABETES INSIPIDUS (DI)

Decreased ADH (Pitressin) or low plasma ADH levels

↓

Renal tubular unresponsiveness

↓

Decreased permeability to water

↓

Excess water excreted in urine

↓

Decreased urine osmolality
Decreased urine specific gravity

↓

Plasma volume loss
Increased plasma osmolality
Increased serum sodium

↓

Dehydration

Hypovolemic shock

Polydipsia
Weakness
Fever
Confusion

CHAPTER 6.6

PHEOCHROMOCYTOMA

Pheochromocytoma is a vascular tumor, composed of chromaffin cells that secrete catecholamines or their precursors (epinephrine, norephinephrine, or dopamine). This, in turn, causes severe persistent or intermittent hypertension resulting from the severe vasoconstriction in response to the catecholamine excess.

Usually the tumor is encapsulated and located within the medulla of the adrenal glands, but can occur in the sympathetic paraganglionic areas of the abdomen, chest, brain, or cervical areas. These tumors are usually benign, but can be malignant in up to 10% of patients. Frequently occurring between the ages of 30 and 50, attacks may occur paroxysmally if the tumor releases catecholamines on an intermittent basis. These episodes may range from once per year to several times per day. Attacks may be spontaneous, or be caused by palpation of the tumor, emotional stress or trauma, exposure to cold, beta-blockers, postural changes, abdominal compression, anesthesia induction, urination, defecation, or heavy lifting.

The tumor's hallmark symptom is high blood pressure with fluctuations up to 220/150 or higher. The catecholamine secretion causes symptoms of "flight or fight" reactions, typically beginning with palpitations, headache, pallor, cool, moist hands and feet, flushing, profuse sweating, and extreme anxiety. Pheochromocytoma is also a part of the multiple endocrine neoplasia (MEN) syndromes and may be found in conjunction with neurofibromatoses, hemangiomas, and medullary thyroid cancers. Other diagnoses, such as angina, essential hypertension, hyperthyroidism, acute anxiety reactions, transient ischemic attacks, and menopause, must be ruled out. Pheochromocytoma always leads to death, if untreated.

MEDICAL CARE

Medications: use of alpha- and beta-blockers (phenoxybenzamine and propranolol, or phenoxylbenzamine and metyrosine) to control catecholamine excess symptoms; IV infusions of trimethaphan camsylate or sodium nitroprusside to control vasopressor effects

Laboratory: fasting serum glucose elevated, increased hematocrit; 24-hour urine for catecholamines, vanillymandelic acid and metanephrines used to identify elevated levels

Electrocardiogram: used to identify tachycardia, bradycardia, LV enlargement and strain from elevated blood pressure, and cardiac dysrhythmias

Radiography: chest and abdominal X-rays used to localize and identify tumor; CT scans, IVP, radionuclide imaging and selective venographic angiography also used to localize tumors; caution must be used because of potential for test to exacerbate hypertensive crisis

Surgery: surgical removal of the pheochromocytoma may be required

COMMON NURSING DIAGNOSES

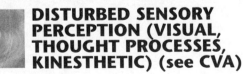

DISTURBED SENSORY PERCEPTION (VISUAL, THOUGHT PROCESSES, KINESTHETIC) (see CVA)

Related to: altered sensory reception, chemical alterations caused by hypoxia, chemical alterations due to glucose/insulin and electrolyte imbalances, restricted environment, psychologic stress, vasoconstriction

Defining Characteristics: confusion, anxiety, fear, disorientation, change in behavior patterns, hyperesthesia, restlessness, irritability, impaired decision-making

IMBALANCED NUTRITION: LESS THAN BODY REQUIREMENTS (see MECHANICAL VENTILATION)

Related to: hypermetabolic state, nausea, vomiting, anorexia, malabsorption

Defining Characteristics: inadequate food intake, weight loss, muscle weakness, fatigue

IMPAIRED GAS EXCHANGE (see MECHANICAL VENTILATION)

Related to: increased respiratory workload, impaired oxygen to heart, hypoventilation, altered oxygen supply, altered blood flow, change in vascular resistance, altered oxygen-carrying capacity of blood, shift of the oxyhemoglobin dissociation curve, hypermetabolic state

Defining Characteristics: confusion, restlessness, hypercapnia, hypoxia, cyanosis, dyspnea, tachypnea, changes in ABG values, changes in A-a gradient, changes in vital signs, activity intolerance, changes in mental status

ADDITIONAL NURSING DIAGNOSES

INEFFECTIVE TISSUE PERFUSION: CARDIOPULMONARY, CEREBRAL, GASTROINTESTINAL, PERIPHERAL, AND RENAL

Related to: excessive catecholamine secretion

Defining Characteristics: pulse and blood pressure changes, changes in cardiac output, changes in peripheral resistance, impaired myocardial oxygenation, chest pain, cardiac dysrhythmias, ECG changes, dyspnea, tachypnea, palpitations, nausea, vomiting, epigastric pain, constipation, slow digestion, weight loss, headaches, visual disturbances, paresthesias, oliguria, anuria, electrolyte imbalances, cold and clammy skin, decreased peripheral pulses, flushing, diaphoresis

Outcome Criteria

✔ Patient will maintain adequate perfusion to all vital organs and will have adequate peripheral and systemic circulation.

NOC: *Tissue Perfusion*

INTERVENTIONS	RATIONALES
Monitor vital signs, including lying, sitting, and standing BP.	Provides information about heart rate and perfusion pressure that will affect blood flow and tissue perfusion. Chronic excessive secretion of catecholamines will affect the reflexes that are responsible for maintaining upright blood pressure and may result in orthostatic hypotension.
Monitor functional abilities in relation to the affected system.	Interrelationships of the body systems can cause overlapping signs and symptoms associated with tissue perfusion and can cause changes in oxygenation, cardiac output, metabolic demands, neurologic function, renal function, and nutrition.
Assess for presence and character of pulses, capillary refill time, skin color and temperature, urine output, mentation, gastric distention, presence of bowel sounds, and appetite.	May indicate decreased perfusion related to the particular body system.
Position patient in Fowler's position.	Helps to decrease the blood volume returning to the heart by pooling blood in dependent parts of the body. Decreases BP by use of orthostatic changes associated with the chronic catecholamine secretion.
Avoid any non-essential activities, especially pressure-causing movement. Avoid straining with bowel movements or urination.	Ambulation, exercise, and Valsalva-type efforts may provoke an attack, increasing blood pressure and decreasing tissue perfusion.
Administer medications as ordered.	Alpha- and beta-blockers may stabilize the condition prior to surgical intervention. Metyrosine interrupts the catecholamine synthesis, decreases levels of norepinephrine production, decreases levels of VMA, and decreases BP.

(continues)

(continued)

INTERVENTIONS	RATIONALES
Titrate IV meds as needed to keep systolic blood pressure less than 170 mm Hg, and diastolic pressure less than 100 mm Hg.	Reduces risk of complications from severely elevated pressure.
Weigh every day.	Weight loss may occur from increased metabolism, decreased appetite, nausea, or vomiting.
Monitor I&O q 1 hour, and notify physician for urine output <30 cc/hr.	Decreased renal perfusion may lead to decreased urinary output, renal impairment, and failure.
Avoid palpation of abdomen; post sign near bed to refrain from palpation during assessments.	Prevents possible palpation of tumor and triggering of acute crisis.
Monitor lab work, especially FBS, hematocrit and renal function levels.	Catecholamine release can increase glycolysis and inhibit insulin release. Excess catecholamines can also increase erythropoietin stimulation and can elevate hematocrit, as well as decrease blood flow to the kidney resulting in renal impairment.
Assist with obtaining 24-hour urine specimen for diagnosis.	Elevated levels may be diagnostic for pheochromocytoma, but coma and increased stress states must be ruled out. Normal values for VMA are <10 mg/24 hrs, metanephrines <1.3 mg/24 hrs, free epinephrine and norepinephrine <100 mcg/24 hrs.
Avoid use of rauwolfia alkaloids, tetracycline, quinine, methyldopa, catecholamines, large quantities of vanilla, coffee, chocolate, nuts, bananas, guaifenesin, and salicylates for at least 2 days prior to 24-hour test, if possible.	These substances may interfere with the results and hamper determination of diagnosis.
Instruct patient/family in causes of exacerbations or attacks, and methods to reduce frequency of occurrence.	Promotes understanding of the condition and risk of decreased perfusion to vital organs.
Instruct patient/family to avoid exposure to cold temperatures.	Cold may cause vasoconstriction, decreased circulation, and perfusion, as well as precipitate an attack.
Instruct patient/family in medications, effects, side effects, adverse reactions, complications, and symptoms to report to physician.	Promotes knowledge and facilitates compliance with medical regimen.
Instruct patient/family in methods to decrease emotional stress, such as relaxation techniques.	Reduces stress and lessens precipitating factors with intermittent attacks by facilitating vasodilation.

INTERVENTIONS	RATIONALES
Instruct patient/family in having frequent blood pressure checks, keeping log of trends, ranges to report to physician, etc.	Primary indicator of the tumor activity is blood pressure increase, which cause decreased perfusion to tissues and organs. Increased knowledge will decrease fear and increase compliance with treatment, and provide opportunity for prompt treatment to prevent serious complications.
Instruct patient/family in avoiding rapid changes in position.	Facilitates body's attempt to cope with orthostatic hypotension by allowing time for body and circulatory system to adjust to changes.
Instruct patient/family to avoid wearing any clothing that may be tight or constrictive.	May result in an attack by compression of abdomen or tumor region.

NIC: *Shock Management: Vasogenic*

Discharge or Maintenance Evaluation

- Patient will have normalized vital signs.
- Organ function will be within patient's normal parameters.
- Extremities will be warm, with normal color and sensation, and have equally palpable pulses.
- Patient will have adequate urinary output with equivalent intake and output.
- Patient will be free of abdominal or epigastric pain, and able to ingest adequate nutritional intake to maintain weight.

ANXIETY

Related to: excessive catecholamine release, threat to health status, changes in health status, life-threatening crisis, possibility of surgical intervention

Defining Characteristics: apprehension, sense of impending doom, fear of death, restlessness, fear, fear of surgery, fear of the unknown, feelings of helplessness, anxiousness, worry, communication of uncertainty, voiced concern over changes in life events

Outcome Criteria

✔ Patient will have less anxiety or anxiety will be within an acceptable and manageable level.

NOC: *Anxiety Control*

INTERVENTIONS	RATIONALES
Assess anxiety level, noting verbalizations of fear or sense of doom.	Catecholamine increases can produce marked anxiety which then increases oxygen demand on tissues.
Provide calm environment for patient to express fears, concerns, and feelings. Allow time for patient to ask questions.	Provides an opportunity to vent feelings and to obtain information. Decreases anxiety and promotes a caring and trusting atmosphere.
Encourage visits from family and friends who do not increase or provide patient with emotional stress.	Provides emotional support and relieves anxiety when familiar people are available.
Decrease stimuli in environment.	Prevents further stressors.
Administer medications as ordered.	Assists to allay fear and anxiety.
Instruct patient/family members about disease process, what to expect with procedures, pre- and postoperative care.	Decreases anxiety caused by fear of the unknown, and promotes knowledge and understanding.
Instruct patient on emotional stress and other precipitating triggers for attacks, and methods to reduce stress and anxiety.	Reduces anxiety and provides patient with some measure of control over the situation.
Instruct patient on medications, effects, side effects, contraindications, and symptoms to report to physician.	Promotes knowledge and understanding which facilitates compliance with medical regimen.

NIC: *Anxiety Reduction*

Discharge or Maintenance Evaluation

- Patient will have reduced anxiety and be able to vent feelings and concerns.
- Patient/family will be able to verbalize understanding of disease process, medications, and treatments, and will be compliant with regimen.
- Patient will be able to avoid stressful visitors, situations, or other provoking events, and will be able to perform relaxation exercises when stressed.

HYPERTHERMIA

Related to: increased metabolic rate in response to catecholamines, decreased heat loss caused by vasoconstriction

Defining Characteristics: increase in body temperature greater than normal range, flushed warm skin, increased heart rate, increased respiratory rate, diaphoresis, delirium

Outcome Criteria

✔ Patient will have temperature within normal range.

NOC: *Thermoregulation*

INTERVENTIONS	RATIONALES
Monitor temperature every 1–2 hours or use continuous monitoring.	Fluctuations in temperature can occur rapidly and temperature elevations can increase metabolism needs.
Adjust room temperature for patient comfort and maintain at or below 72 degrees.	Assists patient with comfort and decreases temperature.
Administer antipyretics as ordered.	Decreases fever.
Provide frequent tepid sponge baths and change linens if patient is diaphoretic.	Promotes patient comfort and reduces temperature by evaporation.
Avoid chilling or shivering of patient.	Shivering may increase metabolic requirements and actually increase temperature.
Place covered ice packs to groin, axillae, and/or behind neck, if warranted.	Decreases temperature by means of conduction.
Use cooling blanket for temperatures greater than 103 degrees if warranted. Cool body slowly—no faster than 1 degree/15 minutes. Blanket should be covered and continuous monitoring of temperature should be performed.	Assists in lowering temperatures by conduction. Blankets should be covered to prevent burns and tissue injury. Cooling that is done too rapidly can produce ventricular ectopy.
Administer thorazine IM/IV as ordered.	Thorazine is an alpha-adrenergic blocking agent that causes peripheral vasodilation which helps heat to dissipate and also can assist in decreasing shivering.
Instruct patient/family in procedures, what to expect with cooling blanket application, and so forth.	Promotes knowledge and reduces anxiety.

NIC: *Temperature Regulation*

Discharge or Maintenance Evaluation

- Patient will achieve and maintain normal body temperature.
- Patient will be compliant with medical regimen.

CONSTIPATION

Related to: inadequate dietary/fluid intake, GI distress, changes in level of activity, decreased blood flow slowing digestion, malabsorption

Defining Characteristics: nausea, vomiting, decreased appetite, epigastric pain, hard-formed stool, absence of stool, abdominal pain

Outcome Criteria

✔ Patient will have normal elimination pattern reestablished and maintained.

NOC: *Bowel Elimination*

INTERVENTIONS	RATIONALES
Determine patient's bowel habits, lifestyle, ability to sense urge to defecate, painful hemorrhoids, and history of constipation.	Assists with identification of an effective bowel regime and/or impairment and need for assistance. GI function may be decreased as a result of decreased digestion.
Auscultate bowel sounds for presence and quality.	Presence of abnormal sounds, such as high-pitched tinkles, suggest complications like ileus.
Monitor diet and fluid intake.	Adequate amounts of fiber and roughage provide bulk and adequate fluid intake (greater than 2 L/day) is important in determining stool consistency.
Monitor for abdominal pain and distention.	Gas, abdominal distention, or ileus could be a factor. Lack of peristalsis from impaired digestion can create bowel distention and worsen to the point of ileus.
Provide bulk, stool softeners, laxatives, or suppositories as warranted.	May be required to stimulate evacuation of stool.
Provide high-fiber, whole grain cereals, breads and fresh fruits.	Improves stool consistency and promotes elimination.
Determine pre-existing habits of laxative/enema usage.	Laxative dependence can predispose patient to constipation.
Instruct patient to avoid frequent use of enemas.	Promotes enema dependence and causes fluid loss which results in more difficult elimination.
Provide activity or exercise within limits of disease process.	Promotes peristalsis.

NIC: *Constipation/Impaction Management*

Discharge or Maintenance Evaluation

■ Patient will have improved dietary and fluid intake.

■ Patient will achieve bowel elimination pattern establishment and be able to maintain elimination of soft-formed stool without cramping or straining.

■ Daily exercise will be maintained within level of confinement in ICU.

DECREASED CARDIAC OUTPUT

Related to: altered preload, altered afterload, inotropic changes in the heart from increased blood pressure and TPR, left ventricular enlargement and strain, and from accumulation of extra fluid in the lungs or systemic venous system, myocardial compromise caused by vasoconstriction, decreased coronary blood flow, increased myocardial oxygen demands, hyperthermia, increased catecholamine receptor sensitivity

Defining Characteristics: increased blood pressure and pulse, cold and clammy skin, jugular vein distention, dyspnea, crackles, edema, cough, frothy blood-tinged sputum, confusion, restlessness, nocturia, decreased urinary output, increased mean arterial pressure, increased systemic vascular resistance, decreased cardiac output and cardiac index

Outcome Criteria

✔ Patient will have adequate cardiac output to maintain hemodynamic stability and perfusion to all organs.

NOC: *Circulation Status*

INTERVENTIONS	RATIONALES
Identify other pre-existing conditions and assess cardiac function.	Other factors and disease states may further stress an already compromised heart and place an extra burden of myocardial oxygen supply.
Monitor blood pressure, heart rate and rhythm, apical and peripheral pulses, pulse deficits, respiratory status, presence of cough or adventitious breath sounds, presence and character of any sputum, and oxygenation.	Cardiac output and blood volume is decreased with elevated blood pressure. Afterload increases, pulse increases, and changes in contractility and conduction occur. Respiratory changes may result in decreased oxygen intake and hypoxia.

INTERVENTIONS	RATIONALES
Measure cardiac output/cardiac index and other hemodynamic parameters as indicated.	Cardiac output <4 L/min or cardiac index <2.5 L/min/m² indicates severe vasoconstriction and decrease in myocardial oxygenation, leading to myocardial ischemia, cardiac failure, and death.
Monitor ECG for presence of dysrhythmias, and treat according to protocol.	Dysrhythmias decrease the heart's pumping efficiency which affects the cardiac output. Dysrhythmias may indicate inadequate myocardial perfusion. Tachydysrhythmias decrease ventricular filling time and coronary blood flow; bradydysrhythmias decrease cardiac output and result in left ventricular failure.
Auscultate heart sounds for presence of gallops and/or murmurs.	Accumulations of extra fluid can be heard as these abnormal heart sounds.
Monitor for edema to extremities, sacral region, or other dependent areas; assess for jugular vein distention, cold peripheral extremities, decreased urinary output, and sluggish capillary refill.	May indicate decreased venous return to the heart and a decrease in cardiac output. Fluid retention may result in a decrease in urinary output as a result of decreased venous return and perfusion.
Weigh every day.	Weight gain may indicate fluid retention.
Monitor intake and output every 2 hrs and prn.	Intake and output should approximate each other. A fluid deficit between output and intake indicates fluid retention and a weight gain (500 cc approximately = 1 lb).
Position in semi-Fowler's or high Fowler's position.	Semi-Fowler's positioning prevents blood pooling and facilitates breathing and improved air exchange. High Fowler's positioning reduces preload quickly by pooling blood but does not decrease stroke volume significantly. Afterload decreases by dilating peripheral arteries and decreasing LVEDP.
Balance rest with short, planned periods of activity; provide atmosphere that is conducive to rest.	Prevents increased demand on heart and myocardial oxygen supply.
Monitor for mental status changes, decreases in orientation, restlessness, agitation, or dizziness.	Central nervous system disturbances can occur with decreased cardiac output due to decreases in perfusion to these areas.
Administer vasoactive drugs as ordered, with titration based on ordered parameters.	These agents promote optimum cardiac output by changing blood pressure, and can reduce afterload and preload.
Administer antidysrhythmic drugs as ordered.	These agents decrease pacemaker activity, modify areas of impaired conduction, and block sympathetic effects of the heart; myocardial contractility is decreased, heart rate is slowed, and oxygen consumption is preserved. Blood pressure decreases and coronary perfusion and myocardial oxygen supply are increased due to the decrease in the heart rate.
Instruct patient to elevate legs when sitting or lying down.	Promotes venous return.
Instruct patient in signs to report: edema, weight gain, chest pain, headache, blood pressure or pulse rate changes.	May indicate complications as a result of decreased cardiac output and facilitate prompt intervention.

NIC: *Cardiac Care*

Discharge or Maintenance Evaluation

- Patient will have stable vital signs and hemodynamics will be within patient's acceptable parameters.
- Patient will have stable cardiac rhythm with no dysrhythmias, and perfusion to organs will be maintained.
- Patient will have clear lung fields with no adventitious breath sounds.
- Patient will have palpable peripheral pulses with warm, dry extremities.
- Patient will have adequate urinary output, with no edema or extra weight gain.

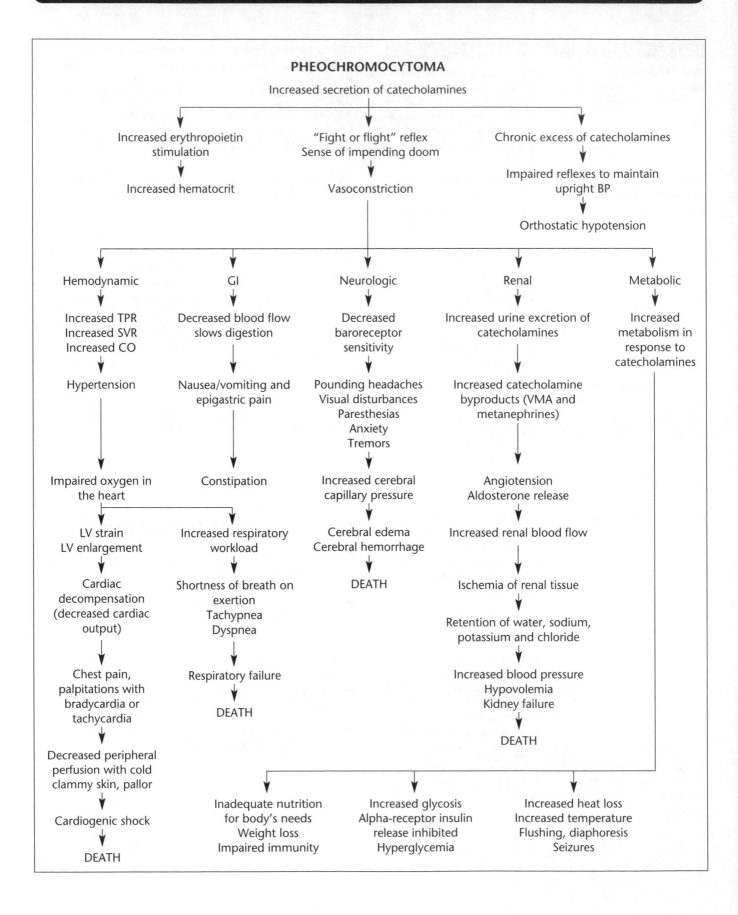

PHEOCHROMOCYTOMA

Increased secretion of catecholamines

Increased erythropoietin stimulation → Increased hematocrit

"Fight or flight" reflex / Sense of impending doom → Vasoconstriction

Chronic excess of catecholamines → Impaired reflexes to maintain upright BP → Orthostatic hypotension

Hemodynamic
Increased TPR
Increased SVR
Increased CO → Hypertension → Impaired oxygen in the heart → LV strain / LV enlargement → Cardiac decompensation (decreased cardiac output) → Chest pain, palpitations with bradycardia or tachycardia → Decreased peripheral perfusion with cold clammy skin, pallor → Cardiogenic shock → DEATH

GI
Decreased blood flow slows digestion → Nausea/vomiting and epigastric pain → Constipation → Increased respiratory workload → Shortness of breath on exertion / Tachypnea / Dyspnea → Respiratory failure → DEATH

Neurologic
Decreased baroreceptor sensitivity → Pounding headaches / Visual disturbances / Paresthesias / Anxiety / Tremors → Increased cerebral capillary pressure → Cerebral edema / Cerebral hemorrhage → DEATH

Renal
Increased urine excretion of catecholamines → Increased catecholamine byproducts (VMA and metanephrines) → Angiotension / Aldosterone release → Increased renal blood flow → Ischemia of renal tissue → Retention of water, sodium, potassium and chloride → Increased blood pressure / Hypovolemia / Kidney failure → DEATH

Metabolic
Increased metabolism in response to catecholamines

Inadequate nutrition for body's needs / Weight loss / Impaired immunity

Increased glycosis / Alpha-receptor insulin release inhibited / Hyperglycemia

Increased heat loss / Increased temperature / Flushing, diaphoresis / Seizures

CHAPTER 6.7

THYROTOXICOSIS

Hyperthyroid crisis, also known as thyroid storm and thyrotoxicosis, is a life-threatening emergency characterized by greatly exaggerated signs of hyperthyroidism. Mortality is high, and symptoms appear rapidly when triggered by infection, trauma, surgery, diabetes, or abrupt withdrawal of thyroid medication. Thyroid storm may be difficult to diagnose because the precipitating illness may mask its detection.

Hyperthyroid patients are more susceptible to catecholamines because of the increased number of catecholamine receptors they possess. A triggering illness creates an outpouring of catecholamines, and so the elevated levels of thyroid and increased number of receptors create the crisis. A hypermetabolic state then ensues causing increased oxygen and nutrient consumption, fluid and electrolyte imbalances, and a catabolic state.

Patients in crisis typically have hyperthermia, tachydysrhythmias, dehydration, nausea, vomiting, weight loss, and neurologic changes. Treatment is usually begun without waiting for confirmation of lab tests and is aimed at supporting vital functions. Reversal of excessive thyroid hormone decreases the hypermetabolic state, and reduction of the circulating thyroid hormones further decreases the crisis. Once vital functions are preserved, treatment of the precipitating cause is begun. If the crisis is untreated, heart failure, exhaustion, and death will ensue.

MEDICAL CARE

Laboratory: serum total, and serum free T_4 and T_3 are increased; TSH levels are decreased; thyroglobulin is increased; electrolytes are used to identify imbalances; thyroid antibodies positive in Graves' disease; glucose levels elevated from insulin resistance, increased glycogenolysis, or impaired insulin secretion; serum cortisol decreased by lower adrenal reserve; alkaline phosphatase increased; serum calcium increased; liver function abnormal, decreased serum catecholamines; urine creatinine increased

TRH test: used in some cases to identify TSH suppression with administration of TRH hormones

Electrocardiogram: used to identify cardiac rhythm changes due to elevated thyroid levels or electrolyte imbalances; atrial fibrillation may be present; cardiomegaly in elderly with masked hyperthyroidism

Oxygen: used to provide supplemental oxygen because of increased oxygen consumption and increased metabolic demands

Radiography: chest X-rays used to identify cardiac enlargement that may occur in response to increased circulatory demands, to identify presence of cardiac overload and congestion, respiratory infiltrates or other precipitating causes

Radioactive iodine uptake test: used to differentiate types of thyroid problems; usually high in Graves' disease and toxic goiter, but low in thyroiditis

Thyroid scan: may be used to aid diagnosis when thyrotoxicosis is caused from cancer or a multinodular goiter

Iodine solutions: used to slow the release of thyroid hormones; common solutions are Lugol's solution and sodium iodide

Beta-adrenergic blockers: used to reverse peripheral effects of excessive thyroid hormones and to decrease the hypermetabolic state; commonly used is propranolol; reserpine IM also helps to reduce peripheral effects and may help decrease tachycardias

Corticosteriods: high doses of hydrocortisone help support body functions during hypermetabolic state

Digoxin: may be required for congestive heart failure patients prior to initiating beta-blockade

Diuretics: may be required if congestive heart failure occurs, and may also help decrease calcium level if neuromuscular function is compromised

Nutrients: high doses of vitamin B complex are used to provide necessary nutrient support for the catabolism state, as well as to facilitate increased glucose, protein, and carbohydrate absorption

Thyroid hormone antagonists: used to block the thyroid hormone production and effects; usually propylthiouracil (PTU) or methimazole (Tapazole) are used; lithium carbonate can also inhibit thyroid hormone synthesis and may be used in patients who cannot tolerate other drugs

Sedatives: may be required to help patient rest and reduce myocardial oxygen consumption and cardiac workload, as well as control of shivering that may increase metabolic rate

Surgery: thyroidectomy or subthyroidectomy may be required

COMMON NURSING DIAGNOSES

IMBALANCED NUTRITION: LESS THAN BODY REQUIREMENTS (see DKA)

Related to: hypermetabolic state, excessive thyroid hormone secretion, nausea, vomiting, elevated glucose levels

Defining Characteristics: weakness, fatigue, weight loss, lack of inadequate food intake, increased glucose level

ANXIETY (see PHEOCHROMOCYTOMA)

Related to: hypermetabolic state, increased catecholamine stimulation

Defining Characteristics: apprehension, loss of control, panic, shakiness, distorted perception, restlessness, tremors, mental changes, lack of attention

FATIGUE (see DKA)

Related to: hypermetabolic state, increased thyroid hormone secretion, increased energy requirements, changes in body chemistry, central nervous system irritability, increased oxygen consumption and demand

Defining Characteristics: lack of energy, inability to perform normal activities, inability to concentrate, lethargy, irritability, nervousness, tension, apathy, depression

ADDITIONAL NURSING DIAGNOSES

HYPERTHERMIA

Related to: accelerated metabolic rate secondary to excessive thyroid hormone secretion, increased beta-adrenergic responses, increased sodium-potassium exchange in cells

Defining Characteristics: increase in body temperature over 100 degrees, flushed warm skin, diaphoresis, tachypnea, tachycardia, delirium, lethargy

Outcome Criteria

✔ Patient will have normal body temperature restored and be able to maintain temperature within acceptable range.

NOC: *Thermoregulation*

INTERVENTIONS	RATIONALES
Monitor temperature for elevation and/or pattern of elevation, chilling, shaking, or diaphoresis.	Hyperthermia up to 106 degrees may result from the acceleration of the metabolic rate caused from excessive thyroid hormone secretion. Chills may precede temperature elevation.
Monitor other vital signs and heart rhythm for alterations. Treat dysrhythmias appropriately.	Elevated temperatures may result in elevations of blood pressure, respiration, and pulse. Cardiac dysrhythmias as a result of heart failure, electrolyte imbalance, or fluid overload may be noted promptly to allow timely intervention.
If required, use cooling methods such as cooling blankets, ice packs, and so forth, being careful to not cause shivering.	Assists in reducing temperature, but may cause shivering, which increases metabolic rate and may worsen condition.
Administer antipyretic medications as ordered by physician, but avoid the use of aspirin.	Assists with reduction of temperature. Aspirin should be avoided because it increases free thyroid hormone levels and may worsen condition.
Administer antithyroid medications as ordered.	PTU or methimazole inhibits thyroid hormone synthesis, and PTU inhibits conversion of T_4 to T_3 in peripheral tissues. Iodine-containing agents inhibit the release of stored thyroid hormones and help to inhibit synthesis. Glucocorticosteroids block conversion of T_4 to T_3.

INTERVENTIONS	RATIONALES
Administer beta-adrenergic blockers as ordered.	Propranolol and nadolol block the peripheral effects from excessive thyroid hormone and may block conversion of T_4 to T_3.
Administer IV fluids and electrolytes as ordered.	Replaces fluid losses from fever and diaphoresis.
Administer antimicrobials as ordered.	Assist in fighting infection when that is believed to be a precipitating factor in the crisis.
Ensure comfort of patient by frequent repositioning, changing of linens and clothing, cool cloths, lowering room temperature, and so forth.	Assists in reducing and maintaining temperature.
Instruct patient/family in all medications being utilized.	Promotes knowledge and facilitates compliance with regimen.
Observe for depression, tremors, nausea, vomiting, or increased urine output.	Symptoms may indicate adverse effects from lithium carbonate.
Instruct in watching for fever, sore throat, or rashes, and to notify physician if he develops these symptoms.	May be indicative of an agranulocytosis caused from medication.

NIC: *Temperature Regulation*

Discharge or Maintenance Evaluation

- Patient will have stable vital signs and be able to maintain values within normal ranges.
- Patient will have no adverse reactions to medications or treatment.
- Patient will be able to accurately recall all instructed information.

DECREASED CARDIAC OUTPUT

Related to: excessive demands on cardiovascular system caused by hypermetabolic state, increased cardiac workload, hyperthermia, increased sensitivity of catecholamine receptors, changes in venous return, changes in peripheral and systemic vascular resistance, changes in heart rhythm or conduction.

Defining Characteristics: elevated blood pressure, elevated mean arterial pressure, elevated systemic vascular resistance, elevated peripheral vascular resistance, decreased cardiac output or cardiac index, tachycardia, decreased or absent peripheral pulses, ECG changes, hypotension, gallops, decreased uri-

nary output, diaphoresis, deterioration in mental status, impending cardiovascular collapse.

Outcome Criteria

✔ Patient will be able to maintain cardiac output at an acceptable level for tissue perfusion.

NOC: *Tissue Perfusion: Peripheral*

INTERVENTIONS	RATIONALES
Monitor vital signs, especially blood pressure for widening pulse pressures.	Peripheral vasodilatation and decreased fluid volume may result from excessive catecholamine secretion. Widening of pulse pressure may indicate compensatory changes in stroke volume and decreasing systemic vascular resistance.
Observe heart rate and respiratory rate while patient is sleeping.	Provides accurate assessment of tachycardia without increase demand of activity.
Auscultate heart tones for extra sounds, gallops, and murmurs.	Hypermetabolic states create prominent S_1 sounds and murmurs due to the forcefulness of the cardiac output, and S_3 gallop development may indicate impending cardiac failure.
Monitor cardiac rhythm for changes, and treat accordingly per protocol.	Excessive thyroid hormone secretion creates excessive catecholamine stimulation to myocardium which can result in tachycardia and dysrhythmias, and may worsen condition by decreasing cardiac output.
Assess for weak or thready pulses, decreased capillary refill, decreased urinary output, and decreased blood pressure.	May indicate dehydration and reduction in circulating volume which compromises cardiac output.
Auscultate lung fields for changes in breath sounds.	Adventitious breath sounds may indicate early signs of pulmonary congestion or impending cardiac failure.
Administer IV fluids as ordered.	Fluid replacement may be indicated to increase circulating volume, but may result in cardiac failure or overload.
Administer atropine if indicated.	Beta-blockers that are given to control tachycardia and tremors during the crisis may decrease heart rate, and may result in symptomatic bradycardia requiring treatment.

(continues)

(continued)

INTERVENTIONS	RATIONALES
Administer digoxin if indicated.	CHF patients may require digitalization prior to initiating beta-blockers.
Administer sedatives and/or muscle relaxants as ordered.	Reduces metabolic demands by promoting rest, and may be helpful to reduce shivering that occurs with fever.
Administer supplemental oxygen as ordered.	Assists to support increased metabolic needs and increased oxygen consumption.
Assist patient by restricting activity or assisting with activity when required.	Reduces energy expenditure that increases oxygen consumption and contributes to increased metabolic needs.
Identify patients who may be at most risk from complications of disease, such as elderly, pre-existing coronary disease or cardiac risk, pregnancy, asthma, or bronchoconstrictive diseases.	Allows for closer assessment and monitoring of patients who may develop cardiovascular compromise from therapeutic measures designed to relieve thyroid crisis, and enable appropriate choices of beta-blockers or other agents.
Once PTU therapy has begun, avoid abrupt withdrawal of drug.	May result in further thyroid crisis. PTU may not have rapid effect on thyroid crisis.
If oral iodine solution is utilized, it should be started 1–3 hours after beginning anti-thyroid medication.	Minimizes hormone formation from the iodine. Iodine may interfere with radioactive iodine treatment and has been known to exacerbate the crisis in some individuals.
Monitor lab studies, for example, potassium, calcium, and so forth.	Hypokalemia may cause cardiac dysrhythmias and hypercalcemia may interfere with contractility, both of which decrease cardiac output and function.
Monitor cultures for infection.	Identifies causative organism that may be responsible for thyroid crisis. The most frequent factor of thyrotoxicosis is respiratory infection.
Assist with hemofiltration, hemodialysis, or plasmapheresis procedures.	May be used in severe crisis to rapidly decrease thyroid hormone.
Prepare patient/family for surgery as indicated.	Subtotal or total thyroidectomy may be required once euthyroid state is attained.

NIC: *Cardiac Precautions*

Discharge or Maintenance Evaluation

- Patient will have stable vital signs and hemodynamic parameters will be within normal limits.
- Patient will have stable cardiac rhythm with no dysrhythmias.
- Patient will exhibit no signs/symptoms of cardiac failure.
- Patient will be able to tolerate activity without circulatory compromise.
- Patient will be able to accurately verbalize instructed information.

RISK FOR INJURY

Related to: cognitive impairment, altered protective mechanisms of body, hypermetabolic state

Defining Characteristics: diminished attention span, agitation, restlessness, impaired judgment, weakness, impaired body functions, eye pain, photophobia, tearing, difficulty closing eyes, periorbital edema, blurred vision, decreased visual acuity, corneal abrasion

Outcome Criteria

✔ Patient will be free of personal injury with all body systems functioning normally.

NOC: *Risk Control*

INTERVENTIONS	RATIONALES
Monitor patient for complaints of eye pain, photophobia, eye irritation, tearing, difficulty closing eyelids, and presence of periorbital edema.	May result from excessive catecholamine stimulation, and may require care until crisis is resolved.
Assess for decreasing visual acuity or blurring of vision.	May be a result of Graves' disease in which increased tissue behind the orbit causes exophthalmos and infiltration of extraocular muscles and weakness. Vision may worsen or improve without basis on medical therapy or disease progression.
Administer medications as indicated, especially eye lubricant drops and ointment.	Prevents eyes from drying and protects cornea when patient is unable to close eyelids completely because of edema.

INTERVENTIONS	RATIONALES
Ensure interventions to prevent injury to patient are in place, such as bed in lowest position, side rails raised, restraints when necessary, and so forth.	Prevents injury due to physical risks in environment.
Assess for changes in mental status and ability; reorient patient as necessary.	Assists with identification of changes that may occur as a result of exhaustion, electrolyte or other chemical imbalance, or physiological problems and allows for prompt intervention.
Discuss patient's feelings regarding alterations in appearance, methods to enhance self-image, and exercises for eyes.	Assists patient in verbalizing concerns regarding perceptions of unattractiveness and allows for discussion of methods to enhance appearance with makeup, shaded glasses, and exercises for extra-ocular muscles that can help maintain mobility of eyelids.

NIC: *Eye Care*

Discharge or Maintenance Evaluation

- Patient will be free of personal injury to any body system.
- Patient's eyes will remain moist, with decreased edema, and will have the ability to completely close the eyelids.
- Patient will be able to freely discuss concerns and problems and be able to utilize problem-solving skills.

DEFICIENT KNOWLEDGE

Related to: hyperthyroidism, lack of information, unfamiliarity with resources, misinterpretation of information, lack of recall

Defining Characteristics: requests for information, questions, misrepresentation of facts, inaccurate follow-through of instructions, development of preventable complications

Outcome Criteria

✔ Patient will be able to accurately recall measures for managing hyperthyroidism and be able to decrease risk of complications.

NOC: *Knowledge: Treatment Regimen*

INTERVENTIONS	RATIONALES
Discuss patient's perceptions and knowledge of disease.	Establishes knowledge base of patient and helps identify interventions and appropriate plan of care.
Ensure that family members are included in discussions and allowed to verbalize their concerns and questions.	Patient's physical condition may interfere with his ability to concentrate which can hinder the learning process. Instruction to the family can assist with reinstruction when needed.
Instruct patient in all medications, effects, side effects, complications, and symptoms to report to physician.	Provides knowledge and facilitates compliance with regimen. Antithyroid therapy will require long-term use in order to inhibit hormone production. Alternative drugs may be chosen if the patient develops symptoms of agranulocytosis from his therapy.
Instruct patient to notify physician for fever, sore throat, or rashes.	May be indicative of adverse reactions to thiourea therapy and facilitates prompt treatment.
Instruct patient to avoid taking over-the-counter medications unless advised to do so by physician.	Antithyroid medicines can affect and/or be affected by several OTC drugs and may cause dangerous interactions.
Instruct patient in diet needs, avoidance of caffeine, artificial preservatives and dyes.	Hypermetabolic states require increased nutrients to maintain well-being and meet demand. Stimulants and additives may result in systemic problems.
Instruct patient in need/rationale for continued medical follow-up.	Compliance with monitoring medical regimen and identification of potential complications can be assessed for timely intervention.

NIC: *Teaching: Disease Process*

Discharge or Maintenance Evaluation

- Patient/family members will be able to accurately recall all instructional information provided to them.
- Patient will be free of preventable complications.
- Patient will be able to correctly recall all medications and effects.
- Patient will be able to manage hyperthyroidism without crisis.

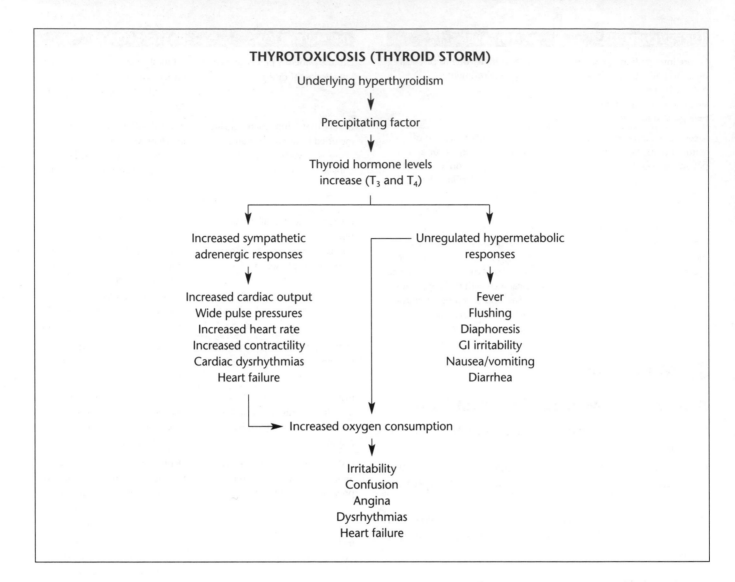

THYROTOXICOSIS (THYROID STORM)

Underlying hyperthyroidism

↓

Precipitating factor

↓

Thyroid hormone levels
increase (T$_3$ and T$_4$)

Increased sympathetic adrenergic responses	Unregulated hypermetabolic responses
Increased cardiac output Wide pulse pressures Increased heart rate Increased contractility Cardiac dysrhythmias Heart failure	Fever Flushing Diaphoresis GI irritability Nausea/vomiting Diarrhea

Increased oxygen consumption

↓

Irritability
Confusion
Angina
Dysrhythmias
Heart failure

UNIT 7

MUSCULOSKELETAL SYSTEM

CHAPTER 7.1

FRACTURES

A fracture is a break in a bone that occurs when direct or indirect pressure is placed on the bone in a force sufficient to exceed the bone's normal elasticity and causes deformation. There are many types of fractures, but the major classifications include open or compound, closed or simple, complete, incomplete, and pathologic fractures.

In closed fractures, there is no contact of the bone with the environment. In open fractures, the skin surrounding the area of the break is open and the bone is exposed to the environment. The major goal in these types of fractures involves the prevention of infection in conjunction with achieving proper alignment. Many patients have severe bleeding associated with this type of fracture. A complete fracture is one that involves the complete cross-section of the bone and it is visibly misaligned. In an incomplete fracture, the actual break may only involve a part of the cross-section of the bone in which one side of the bone is broken and the other part is merely bent. Pathologic fractures occur without or with minimal trauma and are usually seen in diseases such as osteoporosis and cancer.

Fractures not only cause damage to the bone involved, but to the soft tissues, nerves, tendons, and vascular system as well. These structures are in close proximity to the bones and help to support skeletal weight and to facilitate joint movement. When the fracture occurs, this stability is lost, and in turn, results in pain, swelling and splinting. The surrounding muscles are usually flaccid initially after the injury, but within an hour or less, may begin to spasm and this may impair venous circulation and displace the fracture further.

Another complication that frequently occurs is called compartmental syndrome. After a fracture occurs to the arm or leg, the fascia surrounding the muscles form compartments with small openings for major arteries, nerves, and tendons. Edema can compress these structures and cause ischemia to muscle tissues. The initial ischemic changes result in a histamine release that causes dilation of the capillary bed and edema to the area. The edema further compresses the larger arteries, which in turn creates further ischemia, further histamine release, and a vicious cycle is formed. The nerves, veins, arteries, and muscles may receive irreversible damage within 6 hours, and contractures, paralysis, and paresthesia may occur within 24–48 hours, without intervention.

Healing begins when the blood around the end of the bone forms a clot and is related to the revascularization process. An inflammatory response occurs with blood vessel dilatation, then the increased permeability of the capillaries allow protein and granulocytes to leak into the tissue. Fibrinogen converts to fibrin that collects proteins and other types of cells, and the granulation tissue allows for debris removal. When the pH of the fluid surrounding the bone fragments decreases, calcium goes into the solution and this begins the process that helps to form new bone. After a couple of weeks, the pH of the tissues rises, and calcium precipitates into the meshwork and a callus is formed as a bridge within the fragments of bone.

Frequently, if open fractures are present, fat particulate may embolize, and the patient must be monitored for this complication (see Fat Embolus).

MEDICAL CARE

X-rays: used to identify type, location, and severity of fractures or traumatic injuries and to evaluate healing process stage

Bone scans, CT scans, MRI scans: used to identify fractures and/or soft tissue damage

Arteriography: may be used to identify presence and severity of vascular damage associated with fracture

Laboratory: CBC may identify hemorrhage or hemoconcentration; WBC is usually increased from the stress response after an injury but may indicate infection; coagulation profiles may be used to identify problems related to blood loss, liver injuries, or after blood transfusions

Surgery: may be required to repair and realign bone structure, nerve injury, soft tissue injury, or vascular injuries; may be required to stabilize skeletal integrity; may be required to relieve compartmental syndrome compression

Traction: used to realign fractured bones and to facilitate healing in proper alignment

Analgesics: used to reduce pain

NURSING DIAGNOSES

ACUTE PAIN

Related to: pain, muscle spasm, fracture, trauma, soft tissue injury, nerve injury, vascular injury, tendon injury, traction apparatus

Defining Characteristics: communication of pain, moaning, facial grimacing, guarding of injured area, inability to be distracted, anxiety

Outcome Criteria

✔ Patient will be free of pain or pain will be controlled to patient's satisfaction.

NOC: *Pain Level*

INTERVENTIONS	RATIONALES
Immobilize injured body part.	Reduces pain and prevents further skeletal displacement. Splinting the fracture stabilizes the damaged bones and prevents unwanted movement, that could result in increased tissue damage.
Support injured extremity gently and elevate using pillows as warranted.	Decreases edema, promotes venous return, and may help to decrease pain.
Administer analgesics as warranted, and especially prior to painful activities.	Reduces pain, promotes muscle relaxation, and facilitates patient cooperation with medical treatment.
Provide backrubs, massage, position changes, and other comfort measures.	Helps to reduce pressure areas, enhances circulation, and may decrease pain.

INTERVENTIONS	RATIONALES
Administer muscle relaxants as warranted.	Reduces muscle spasms which can decrease pain.
Instruct patient on relaxation techniques, deep breathing exercises, visualization, guided imagery, therapeutic touch, and so forth.	Redirects attention from pain and provides patient with feelings of control; may assist patient in coping with discomfort.
Instruct patient in use of PCA as warranted.	Provides patient with control over his pain relief and has been shown to reduce the amount of narcotic analgesic the patient requires for pain control.
Instruct patient to notify nurse or physician of sudden different pain or pain that is unrelieved with analgesics.	May indicate infection, ischemia, or compartmental syndrome.

NIC: *Pain Management*

Discharge or Maintenance Evaluation

■ Patient will have no complaints of pain.

■ Patient will be able to control pain management by use of PCA with satisfaction.

■ Patient will be able to recall information accurately and will notify medical personnel for signs/symptoms of complications.

■ Patient will be able to demonstrate accurately and effectively the use of relaxation activity skills for use with controlling pain.

IMPAIRED PHYSICAL MOBILITY

Related to: fractures, pain, immobilization, traction, neurovascular impairment

Defining Characteristics: inability to move at will, limited range of motion, decreased muscle strength, decreased muscle control, reluctance to move injured body part

Outcome Criteria

✔ Patient will achieve and maintain optimal mobility and function of injured area.

NOC: *Mobility Level*

NOC: *Skeletal Function*

INTERVENTIONS	RATIONALES
Evaluate degree of immobility that has resulted from injury and patient's perception of his limitations.	After trauma, patient's perception of limitations may be out of proportion with their physical levels of activities and may require further information to dispel false concepts.
Maintain bedrest and move injured limbs gently, supporting areas above and below the fracture.	Decreases potential for further injury and impairment in alignment while stabilizing the injured area.
Reposition patient every 2 hours and prn.	Prevents formation of pressure areas and improves circulation.
Assist patient with range of motion exercises of all extremities as warranted.	Prevents muscle atrophy, increases blood flow, improves joint mobility, and helps prevent reabsorption of calcium resulting from disuse.
Encourage isometric exercises once bleeding and edema has resolved.	Helps to contract muscles without bending joints or moving extremities to facilitate maintenance of muscle strength. These exercises can exacerbate bleeding or edema if these problems are not resolved.
Ensure that adequate numbers of personnel are present for repositioning.	Casts and/or traction apparatus may be cumbersome and heavy and may require increased personnel to avoid injury to the patient or the nurses.
Evaluate integrity of traction apparatus and set-up.	Traction provides for a pulling force on the long axis of a fractured bone to facilitate proper alignment and healing.
Maintain free hanging weights and unobstructed ropes when traction is utilized.	Ensures that the prescribed amount of weight is maintained on traction and reduces muscle spasms and pain.
If patient requires traction, observe for wrinkles in the material covering the inner aspect of the traction apparatus.	May result in pressure to tissue and cause blisters on skin.
Observe patient for complaints of itching, burning, or pain while in traction.	May indicate a possible allergic reaction to components of traction apparatus.
Apply antiembolic hose and remove for 1 hour every 8 hours.	Prevents venous stasis and decreases potential for thrombophlebitis.
Observe for redness, tenderness, pain, or swelling to the calf; assess for positive Homan's or Pratt's signs.	May indicate thrombophlebitis.

INTERVENTIONS	RATIONALES
Instruct patient in use of spirometer and coughing and deep breathing exercises to be done every 2 hours.	Prevents atelectasis and facilitates lung expansion.
Do not routinely elevate the knees.	Elevation may place pressure on the lower extremities and decrease venous return and blood flow.

NIC: *Traction/Immobilization Care*

Discharge or Maintenance Evaluation

- Patient will achieve and maintain increased mobility and function of injured area.
- Patient will be free of complications that may occur as a result of immobility.
- Patient will be able to effectively demonstrate exercises to increase mobility.
- Patient will be able to recall accurately all information instructed.

RISK FOR PERIPHERAL NEUROVASCULAR DYSFUNCTION

Related to: vascular injury, soft tissue injury, interruption of blood flow, edema, thrombus, hypovolemia

Defining Characteristics: decreased or absent pulses, cyanosis, mottling, pallor, cold extremities, mental changes, abnormal vital signs, decreased urinary output

Outcome Criteria

✔ Patient will be able to maintain adequate tissue perfusion.
✔ Patient will not suffer any disability related to peripheral neurovascular dysfunction after treatment or injury.
✔ Patient will exhibit no signs or symptoms of neurovascular compromise.

NOC: *Tissue Perfusion: Peripheral*

INTERVENTIONS	RATIONALES
Monitor vital signs 1–2 hours.	Systemic perfusion will be impaired if circulating blood volume is inadequate.

INTERVENTIONS	RATIONALES
Provide immobilization to joints above and below fracture site, leaving enough room to assess pulses.	Facilitates monitoring of circulatory status of extremity.
Palpate peripheral pulses and identify changes in equality or character of pulses distal to injury.	Decreased or absent pulse may indicate vascular injury that requires immediate intervention.
Monitor extremity involved for rapid capillary refill, skin color, warmth, and sensation.	Circulatory impairment may result in delayed refill times greater than 5 seconds. Arterial compromise may occur when skin is cool to cold and white, and venous compromise may occur with cyanosis. Sudden ischemic signs may be caused with joint dislocation resulting from injury to adjacent arterial structures.
Monitor for changes in neurovascular integrity every 1–2 hours as warranted. Notify physician for significant changes.	Paresthesias, numbness, tingling, or diffused pain may occur when nerves have been damaged or when circulation is impaired, and may require intervention.
Evaluate complaints of pain that are abnormal for the type of injury sustained, pain with passive muscle stretching, or decreases in muscle movement distal to the injury, and notify physician as warranted.	Hemorrhage and/or edema within the muscle fascia can impair blood flow and cause compartmental syndrome that will require emergency intervention to restore circulation. Compartmental syndrome can result in permanent dysfunction and deformity within 24–48 hours and irreversible damage may occur after 6 hours without intervention.
Assist with monitoring of compartmental pressures as warranted.	Increases in pressure above 30 mm Hg requires immediate intervention to prevent permanent damage.
Assess skin around cast edges for redness or pressure points, or for complaints of burning under the cast. Cover rough edges of cast with tape.	Rough edges of the cast may produce pressure and result in ischemia or tissue breakdown. Burning pain may indicate pressure areas that are inside cast and not visible.
Monitor cast for presence of flattened or dented areas.	May indicate that the cast is placing pressure to areas and may result in tissue necrosis.
Cut/bivalve cast as needed per hospital/physician protocol for circulatory impairment.	Relieves circulatory impairment that may occur from edema and swelling to injured area.
Apply ice packs to fracture site as warranted.	Reduces edema and hematoma formation.

INTERVENTIONS	RATIONALES
Remove patient's jewelry from injured extremity.	May impair circulation when extremity swells.
Perform testing for tendon damage: Immobilize the two fingers on either side of the patient's middle finger and ask him to wiggle the middle finger; immobilize the proximal interphalangeal joint of a lacerated/injured finger and ask him to flex the finger.	May indicate superficial tendon damage if the patient cannot wiggle his finger, and deep tendon damage if the patient cannot flex the finger.
Position extremity in proper alignment.	Circulation may be compromised if correct alignment is not maintained.
Elevate extremity above heart level after surgery or injury, but keep extremity at heart level if compartmental syndrome and increasing pressure is evident.	Elevation may reduce hazard of edema, but if intracompartmental pressure is increased, elevation will only increase the pressure further.
Avoid flexion of fractured extremity.	May result in decreased venous circulation and increase potential for neurovascular compromise.
Administer vasodilators, as ordered.	May be required to control vasospasms and decrease impairment of perfusion to tissues.
Prepare patient for surgery as warranted.	Surgical intervention may be required to relieve compartmental pressure in order to avoid permanent dysfunction.
Instruct patient in signs/symptoms to notify nurse/physician: increased pain, decreased sensation or movement, or changes in temperature or color of injured part.	Provides knowledge and allows for patient involvement in care. Provides method for prompt detection of potential complications to facilitate prompt intervention.
Instruct patient/family in correct positioning techniques, and methods to use to obtain relief from pressure.	Provides knowledge and helps to avoid venous pooling and potential pressure ulcerations.

NIC: *Circulatory Precautions*

Discharge or Maintenance Evaluation

- Patient will have equally palpable pulses, warm and dry skin, and stable vital signs.
- Patient will have normal sensation to injured part.
- Patient will be able to recall information accurately and will be able to avoid potential complications.

IMPAIRED SKIN INTEGRITY

Related to: compound fracture, traumatic injury, surgery, use of traction pins or other devices, use of fixation devices, immobilization

Defining Characteristics: disruption of skin surface or other tissue layers, open wounds, pain, paresthesias

Outcome Criteria

✔ Patient will achieve optimal wound healing and have no skin breakdown.

NOC: *Wound Healing: Primary Intention*

INTERVENTIONS	RATIONALES
Observe skin for open wounds, redness, discoloration, duskiness, cyanosis, mottling, or pallor.	Changes may indicate problems with circulation that may be caused by traction, casts, or splints, or by edema.
Apply eggcrate mattress, flotation mattress, air mattress, sheepskins, or use kinetic-type bed.	Helps prevent formation of pressure areas caused by immobility.
Encourage patient to use trapeze bar and reposition frequently.	May minimize potential for abrasions to elbows from friction during movement. Positioning helps to decrease pressure to skin areas.
Monitor integrity of traction setup; pad areas that come in contact with patient's skin.	Improper setup or positioning of apparatus may result in tissue injury or skin breakdown. Padding prevents pressure areas from forming on skin and enhances moisture evaporation to prevent skin excoriation.
Cover the ends of any traction pins or wires with cork or other protectors.	Prevents injury to other skin tissues.
Apply skin traction as ordered. Apply traction tape lengthwise on both sides of the injured limb after applying tincture of benzoin and extend the tape beyond the limb.	Benzoin provides a protective layer to prevent skin abrasion with removal of tapes. Traction tape that encircles a limb may impair circulation.
Mark a line on the tapes at the point when the tape extends beyond the limb.	Provides identification marker to assess whether traction tape has slipped.
Using elastic bandage, wrap the limb and tape (and padding, if needed) being careful to avoid wrapping too tight.	Allows prescribed traction without impairing circulation.

INTERVENTIONS	RATIONALES
Remove skin traction at least daily and observe for any reddened or discolored areas. Provide skin care.	May provide evidence of any skin impairment and allows for cleansing of area to remove debris or drainage.
If cast is present, cleanse plaster off skin while still damp.	Dry plaster can flake and result in skin irritation.
Use padding, tape, and/or plastic to protect cast near perineal area.	Prevents skin breakdown and helps to prevent contaminants from adhering to cast.
Avoid use of lotions or oils around cast edges.	These agents can create a seal and prevent the cast from "breathing." Powder should be avoided because of the potential for accumulation inside the cast.
Instruct the patient to avoid putting objects inside cast, such as fly swatters, coat hangers, and so forth.	Objects used for scratching may damage tissue.
Instruct patient in cast care.	Provides knowledge for future patient care and involves the patient in his medical treatment.
Instruct patient/family to position patient every 2 hours and avoid pressure points to bony prominences.	Facilitates patient and family compliance and helps to reduce pressure and avoid skin breakdown.

NIC: *Skin Surveillance*

Discharge or Maintenance Evaluation

- Patient will have no further skin breakdown.
- Patient will have healed wounds without complications.
- Patient will be able to avoid complications of immobility.
- Patient will be able to accurately recall all instructive information.

RISK FOR INFECTION

Related to: broken skin, disrupted tissues, exposed bone structure, traction devices, surgery, invasive procedures

Defining Characteristics: temperature elevation, elevated white blood cell count, shift to the left, purulent drainage, redness, warmth, and tenderness

Outcome Criteria

✔ Patient will be free of signs/symptoms of infection and wounds will heal without complications.

NOC: *Risk Control*

INTERVENTIONS	RATIONALES
Monitor vital signs. Observe for fever, chills, and lethargy.	Increased temperature and heart rate may indicate impending or present sepsis. Gas gangrene may result in hypotension and mental changes.
Observe wounds for redness, drainage, dehiscence, failure to heal, and so forth.	May indicate presence of infection.
Perform wound care/pin care utilizing sterile technique.	Removes drainage and debris from wound which may prevent infection.
Obtain cultures as ordered.	Identifies causative organism and allows for specific antimicrobial therapy to eradicate the infection.
Observe prescribed isolation techniques.	Isolation may be required depending on type of infective organism. Precautions will prevent cross-contamination and spread of infection.
Observe wounds for presence of crepitus or fruity-smelling/frothy drainage.	May indicate the presence of gas gangrene infection.
Evaluate patient's complaints of sudden increase of pain or difficulty with movement in injured area.	May indicate development of compartmental syndrome or osteomyelitis.
Observe for hyperreflexia, muscle rigidity, spasticity in facial and jaw muscles, and decreases in ability to speak or swallow.	May indicate development of tetanus.
Utilize proper handwashing techniques and aseptic technique when changing dressings, suctioning, inserting lines and catheters, and so forth.	Hand washing is the single most effective method of preventing the spread of pathogens. Using gloves when handling dressings or providing care promotes protection against cross-contamination and avoidance of spreading pathogens.
Monitor lab work, especially WBC and differentials.	Elevation of total WBC count indicates presence of infection. Significant decreases in WBCs may reflect decreased cell production caused by extreme

INTERVENTIONS	RATIONALES
	debilitated state, severe lack of necessary nutrients, or bone marrow damage.
Instruct patient to avoid touching wounds or pin sites.	Decreases potential for spread of infection.
Instruct patient/family in isolation procedures.	Provides knowledge and ensures compliance with procedures and decreases chance of cross-contamination.
Prepare patient for surgical procedures as warranted.	Surgical intervention may be required to remove necrotic bone or tissue to facilitate healing process and to prevent further infection.
Encourage coughing and deep breathing exercises every 2–4 hours after surgery.	Assists in prevention of pulmonary complications, such as atelectasis and pneumonia.
Instruct patient/family as to increasing fluid intake up to 3–4 L/day, unless contraindicated.	Assists to thin viscous secretions and promote expectoration.
Instruct patient/family in dietary changes, such as increasing protein, unless contraindicated.	High-protein supplementation may enrich muscle tone and mass, and assists with wound healing.
Change IV site every 72 hours and IV fluids every 24 hours, or per protocol.	Reduces risk of infection.

NIC: *Wound Care*

Discharge or Maintenance Evaluation

■ Patient will have appropriate wound healing with no signs/symptoms of infection.

■ Patient will have stable vital signs with normal temperature.

■ Patient will have negative culture results.

■ Patient will have white blood cell count and differential within normal range.

■ Patient will have healing wounds that are free of purulent drainage, and are well approximated.

■ Patient will be able to accurately recall all instructions and avoid potential complications.

DEFICIENT KNOWLEDGE

Related to: fractures, lack of information, misunderstanding of information, inability to recall information

Defining Characteristics: verbal requests for information, questions, inaccurate statements, lack of compliance with instructions, lack of follow-through, development of preventable complications

Outcome Criteria

✔ Patient will be able to accurately verbalize understanding of disease process and treatment.

NOC: *Knowledge: Treatment Procedures*

INTERVENTIONS	RATIONALES
Evaluate patient's understanding of disease process, injury, and treatment.	Provides baseline of patient's knowledge and helps identify need for instruction.
Instruct patient/family regarding mobility concerns.	Fractures usually require casts or splints during healing, and improper use may delay wound/bone healing.
Instruct patient in exercises to perform.	Prevents joint stiffness and muscle wasting.
Instruct patient/family in wound care/fixator pin care.	Enables patient to understand need for sterile/aseptic wound

INTERVENTIONS	RATIONALES
	care to prevent further injury and infection.
Instruct patient to keep all follow-up appointments.	Provides for identification of complications and promotes patient compliance with medical regimen.
Instruct in signs/symptoms to notify physician: pain, elevated temperature, chills, paresthesias, paralysis, color changes, edema, dislodged fixator, cracks in casts, and so forth.	Provides for prompt identification of problem to ensure prompt intervention.

NIC: *Teaching: Procedure/Treatment*

Discharge or Maintenance Evaluation

■ Patient will be able to accurately recall all instructional information.

■ Patient will be free of preventable complications.

■ Patient/family will be able to accurately perform demonstration of wound/pin care.

FRACTURES

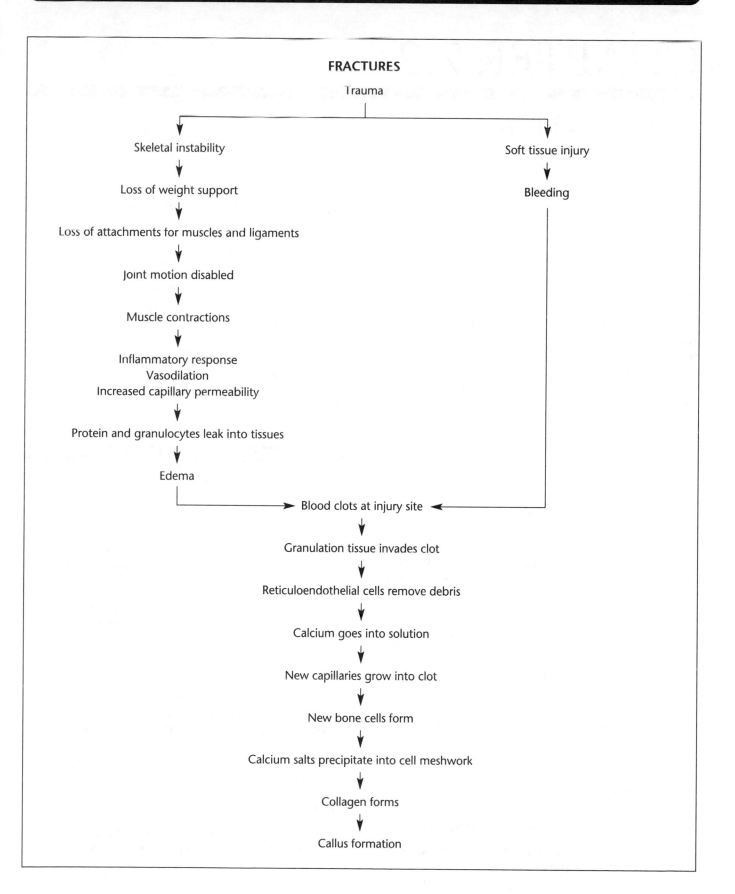

Trauma

Skeletal instability

Loss of weight support

Loss of attachments for muscles and ligaments

Joint motion disabled

Muscle contractions

Inflammatory response
Vasodilation
Increased capillary permeability

Protein and granulocytes leak into tissues

Edema

Soft tissue injury

Bleeding

Blood clots at injury site

Granulation tissue invades clot

Reticuloendothelial cells remove debris

Calcium goes into solution

New capillaries grow into clot

New bone cells form

Calcium salts precipitate into cell meshwork

Collagen forms

Callus formation

CHAPTER 7.2

AMPUTATION

Amputation may be caused by trauma, disease, or congenital problems. It may be required for uncontrolled infection, intractable pain, or gangrene resulting from inadequate tissue perfusion, and is usually performed as distally as possible to preserve viable tissue and bony structure for use with prosthetics.

A closed amputation utilizes a flap of skin for closure over the residual limb, and an open amputation requires future revisions and the wound heals by granulation. The open amputation is utilized in patients who are poor surgical candidates and with the presence of infection. Traumatic amputation is an accidental loss of a body part and is classified as complete when the part is totally severed, and partial when there is some connection with soft tissues.

Amputation may be considered as a last option when trying to salvage an extremity, and the surgeon may try revascularization, resection, or hyperbaric oxygenation in an attempt to save the limb. A lower extremity amputation is still considered a life-threatening procedure, especially when the patient is elderly or has peripheral vascular disease. With the advances in microsurgery, reimplantation of severed digits and limbs have become more successful.

MEDICAL CARE

Laboratory: culture and sensitivity of the wound may be done to identify the infection organism and the optimal antimicrobial agent required to eradicate the infection; sedimentation rate usually increased from inflammatory response; CBC with differential used to identify elevated white blood cell count and presence of a shift to the left representing an infection process

Angiography, arteriography: used to assess blood flow and to identify the optimal amputation level

CT scans: used to identify neoplasms, osteomyelitis, or hematoma formation

Doppler ultrasound or flowmetry: used to assess blood flow to tissue areas

Analgesics: meperidine (Demerol), morphine, or other narcotics are used to control pain

Surgery: may be required to remove a gangrenous limb, or may be required to replant or try to revascularize severed parts; revisional surgery may be required if stump deteriorates or if revascularization procedures do not succeed

Antimicrobials: may be required because of open wound, infection, or potential for infection, and should be specific to the causative organism

COMMON NURSING DIAGNOSES

ACUTE PAIN (see FRACTURES)

Related to: injury, trauma, surgical procedure, stump pain

Defining Characteristics: complaints of pain, guarding of area, facial grimacing, moaning, discomfort

ADDITIONAL NURSING DIAGNOSES

CHRONIC PAIN

Related to: amputation, phantom pain

Defining Characteristics: complaints of pain in amputated limb, discomfort, facial grimacing, irritability, restlessness, inability to focus on anything but oneself, inability to continue with previous activities, atrophy of muscle groups, depression, weight gain, weight loss

Outcome Criteria

✔ Patient will be able to recognize characteristics of pain and use techniques effectively to deal with phantom pain.

✔ Patient will be able to assist in the development of a pain management program that does not rely on analgesia.

NOC: *Pain Control*

INTERVENTIONS	RATIONALES
Assess patient for symptoms of pain, complaints of discomfort, and participation in daily activities.	Relationship of pain to activity may enable nurse to modify activity, or provide analgesia prior to painful procedures or activities.
Administer pain medication as ordered.	Relieves pain and discomfort, but may also be patient's way of removing self from facing changes in body image and other psychological issues.
Encourage patient to participate in self-care, and allow patient to assist with developing schedules of activities.	Assists patient to gain sense of control over situation and decreases dependency on others.
Provide adequate time for patient to discuss feelings and emotions regarding pain, loss of limb, and other issues.	Assists in establishing a trusting relationship and aids patient in dealing with concerns.
Instruct patient regarding phantom pain phenomenon.	Phantom pain is a sensation of a painless awareness of the amputated limb, sometimes occurring concurrently with tingling or nerve-type sensations. Amputees may sense only a part of the missing limb, and this is frequently related to the position of the limb at the time of amputation. Most amputees will develop this and the symptoms may last several months to several years. Usually these sensations decrease and disappear without any treatment.
Instruct patient in use of relaxation techniques, guided imagery, massage, music therapy, and so forth, during painful experiences.	Reduces pain without the use of analgesia, and also helps in conjunction with the use of medication to facilitate improvement with smaller dosages of narcotics.
Instruct patient/family in massage techniques, exercises, and use of ice or heat.	Relieves pain and encourages independence.
Provide time for family and staff to discuss patient's care, goals, and treatment plans.	Care conferences may facilitate pain management and achieve treatment plan goals while assisting family to aid patient to gain independence.

INTERVENTIONS	RATIONALES
Instruct patient/family in behavior modification techniques and behavior-oriented plan of care.	Behavioral and cognitive measures assist patient to modify previously learned pain behavior. Decreasing talk focused on patient's pain and pain behaviors assist patient to refocus on other important matters.

NIC: *Pain Management*

Discharge or Maintenance Evaluation

- Patient will be able to describe pain, rate pain on scale of severity, and will be able to identify activities that increase and decrease pain.
- Patient will be able to manage pain with the use of a pain management program including activity, exercise, and medication.
- Patient will be able to increase activity and have less dependence on caregivers.
- Patient will understand the concept behind phantom limb pain and will effectively utilize techniques to decrease discomfort.
- Patient and family will be able to verbalize understanding of alternative therapies to use in place of medications.

INEFFECTIVE TISSUE PERFUSION: PERIPHERAL

Related to: disease, surgical procedure, decreased blood flow, edema, hypovolemia

Defining Characteristics: absent or diminished pulses, color changes, mottling, blanching, cyanosis, necrosis, gangrene, temperature changes, swelling

Outcome Criteria

✔ Patient will have adequate peripheral perfusion with equal pulses, warm, pink skin, and optimal wound healing.

NOC: *Tissue Perfusion: Peripheral*

INTERVENTIONS	RATIONALES
Assess presence of peripheral pulses, strength, equality, and character. Notify physician for significant changes.	Changes in equality between limbs, diminished strength or absence indicates problems with perfusion.

(continues)

(continued)

INTERVENTIONS	RATIONALES
Perform neurovascular checks every 1–2 hours, noting changes in color, temperature, movement, or sensation.	Circulation may become impaired due to edema or tight dressings and may result in necrosis of tissues. Prompt detection of problems will allow for prompt intervention.
Evaluate nonoperative leg for edema, inflammation, erythema, or positive Homan's or Pratt's signs.	Peripheral vascular disease may increase the incidence of post-operative thrombus formation.
Instruct patient to report changes in sensation to operative site or any swelling.	Paresthesias may occur as a result of nerve damage or with impaired circulation. Swelling may result from fluid shifting or from continued bleeding which would require intervention.

NIC: *Amputation Care*

Discharge or Maintenance Evaluation

- Patient will have strong, equal peripheral pulses, with no changes in sensation or temperature.
- Patient will be able to accurately recall signs/symptoms to report to nurse/physician.
- Patient will experience optimal wound healing.

RISK FOR INFECTION

Related to: trauma, surgical incisions, open skin, invasive procedures, disease, decreased nutritional status

Defining Characteristics: temperature elevation, elevated white blood cell count, shift to the left, sepsis, purulent drainage, reddened wound site, swelling, wound dehiscence

Outcome Criteria

✔ Patient will be free of infection with no threat to wound healing.

NOC: *Risk Detection*

INTERVENTIONS	RATIONALES
Monitor vital signs and notify physician for significant changes.	Sepsis may result in temperature elevation, tachycardia, and tachypnea.
Observe wound for signs of infection: redness, warmth,	Prompt recognition of infection may result in prompt intervention

INTERVENTIONS	RATIONALES
drainage changes, swelling, or dehiscence.	and decrease the potential for further complications.
Culture wound drainage as warranted, and as per hospital protocol.	Identifies causative organism and allows for choice of optimal antimicrobial agent to eradicate infection.
Change dressing using aseptic or sterile technique as warranted.	Reduces spread of or introduction of bacteria to wound.
Ensure that drainage systems are functioning properly, and that measurement/emptying of drainage is being performed.	Drainage systems facilitate removal of drainage from wound which can decrease the chance of infection from stagnant body fluids. Measurement of drainage provides a trend to identify loss of fluid as well as potential heal-ing or deterioration of wounds.
Administer antimicrobials as ordered.	Drug therapy may be given prophylactically using a broad-spectrum antibiotic until specific sensitivity reports are available to identify organism-specific antimicrobials.
Instruct patient on signs/symptoms of infection to report.	Allows for prompt recognition of problems to facilitate prompt intervention.
Instruct patient/family on anti-microbial effects, side effects, and contraindications.	Provides knowledge and facilitates cooperation in the medical regimen.
Instruct patient/family on infec-tion control procedures, isolation requirements, and so forth.	Provides knowledge and facilitates compliance with treatment; involves the family in patient care and reduces the potential for spread of infection.

NIC: *Infection Precautions*

Discharge or Maintenance Evaluation

- Patient will remain free of signs and symptoms of infection process.
- Patient will be able to assist family or others with changing of dressings as required.
- Patient will exhibit no toxic reactions to antimi-crobials that may be required.
- Patient will be able to accurately identify and ver-balize signs and symptoms of infection to report to medical personnel.
- Patient/family will be able to understand the use of and perform isolation precautions as needed.

IMPAIRED SKIN INTEGRITY

Related to: amputation, surgical procedure, invasive procedures, broken skin

Defining Characteristics: surgical wounds, puncture sites, abraded skin, disrupted skin or tissues

Outcome Criteria

✔ Patient will have healed wounds with no skin or tissue disruption.

NOC: *Wound Healing: Primary Intention*

INTERVENTIONS	RATIONALES
Inspect wound daily to assess for healing, deterioration, color, character and amount of drainage, signs/symptoms of infection, and so forth.	Prompt detection of changes can facilitate prompt intervention for complications. Decreases in drainage amounts may indicate appropriate healing, whereas increasing amounts of drainage, or purulent/odiferous drainage may indicate the presence of fistulas, hemorrhage, or infective process.
If drainage amount is large, apply collection devices/bags over sites, recording amounts every 8 hours.	Helps reduce skin trauma by reducing surface area in contact with drainage, and facilitates more accurate measurement of drainage.
Cleanse wound per protocol at ordered frequency utilizing sterile or aseptic technique. (Many facilities use hydrogen peroxide followed by normal saline rinse.)	Helps reduce potential for infection; removes debris and caustic drainage from skin surface to preserve skin integrity and promote healing.
Utilize benzoin or other skin barrier products prior to the application of tape during dressing changes, or use Montgomery straps or stretch netting for dressings that may require more frequent changes.	Protects skin from abrasion with removal of tape. Use of netting or Montgomery straps prevent repeated removal of tape which can further disrupt skin integrity.
Leave wound open to air, or cover with a light gauze dressing as soon as feasible.	Helps to facilitate healing; a light dressing may be required to prevent sutures or wound from becoming irritated by linens, clothes, etc.
Instruct patient to avoid touching wound.	Prevents spread of infection or contamination of the wound.
Instruct patient in wound care as warranted.	Promotes knowledge and provides for patient involvement in his care.

INTERVENTIONS	RATIONALES
Instruct patient/family regarding stump care. Stump should be monitored each day and cleansed with soap and water and dried completely. Talcum powder may be placed on the stump once the wound is completely healed. If the skin on the stump is excessively dry, lanolin or petrolatum may be utilized. If the skin is damaged, the prosthesis should not be worn until the wound has completely healed.	Prosthesis should be removed prior to sleeping as it is intended only for ambulation. Application of powder or lotions may assist with maintenance of skin integrity, but may create infection if used on broken skin.
Instruct patient/family to observe stump and report any changes in appearance, or development of new and different pain.	May indicate the presence of an amputation neuroma or spur formation at the end of the amputated bone, requiring medical treatment.

NIC: *Amputation Care*

Discharge or Maintenance Evaluation

- Patient will have healed wounds with no impairment of skin integrity.
- Patient will be able to accurately perform wound care utilizing appropriate infection control techniques.
- Patient will be able to use supportive devices as needed to prevent wound dehiscence.
- Patient will be able to demonstrate appropriate behavior to prevent wound healing complications.

RISK FOR DEFICIENT FLUID VOLUME

Related to: nausea/vomiting, fever, excessive wound drainage, urine output, changes in vascular integrity, fluid shifts, oral fluid restriction

Defining Characteristics: imbalance between intake and output, dehydration, poor skin turgor, tenting of skin

Outcome Criteria

✔ Patient will achieve and maintain an adequate fluid balance, with stable vital signs and hemodynamic parameters, and palpable pulses.

NOC: *Fluid Balance*

INTERVENTIONS	RATIONALES
Monitor vital signs every 1–2 hours.	Fluid deficit symptoms may be manifested in low blood pressure, and increases in respiratory and heart rates. Changes in pulse quality or cool and clammy skin may indicate decreased perfusion and peripheral circulation and the need for replacement fluids.
Monitor I&O q 1–2 hours, and notify physician of significant fluid imbalances or urine output less than 30 cc/hr for 2 hours.	Prompt recognition of imbalance and fluid loss provides for prompt intervention and replenishment of necessary fluids.
Evaluate for presence of nausea/ vomiting; medicate as warranted.	Immediate postoperative nausea may result due to length of anesthesia and predisposition for nausea. Nausea/vomiting lasting longer than 3 days may result from adverse reactions to analgesics or other medications.
Observe wound sites for increases in drainage, swelling to area, or lack of drainage in drain tubes.	Sudden cessation of previously noted wound drainage may indicate an obstruction in the drainage system, with potential drainage then routed to tissues and other cavities. Edema to wound sites may indicate the formation of a hematoma or hemorrhage from the wound. Lack of swelling does not mean that hemorrhage is not occurring—retroperitoneal bleeding may not be visually noted until long after the patient has shown vital sign changes.
Administer IV fluids, blood and blood products as warranted.	Replaces necessary fluids and increases circulating volume.
Administer antiemetic drugs as warranted; may administer these in combination with analgesics.	Relieves nausea and vomiting which can result in the ability to ingest adequate fluid amounts. Concurrent administration with analgesics may potentiate the analgesic in addition to controlling nausea and vomiting related to the pain medication.
Monitor lab values for hemoglobin and hematocrit, and notify physician for significant changes.	Hematocrit provides an indicator of fluid volume status and hydration. Blood losses that are not replaced may result in further fluid deficits.
Instruct patient to report increases in wound drainage,	Pressure sensation may result from retroperitoneal hemorrhage

INTERVENTIONS	RATIONALES
leakage, or feelings of pressure sensation to wound areas.	and should be evaluated immediately. Including the patient in his care provides for cooperation with medical regimen and provides for prompt recognition of potential problems that may lead to circulatory collapse from hypovolemia.

NIC: *Fluid Monitoring*

Discharge or Maintenance Evaluation

- Patient will be adequately hydrated, normotensive, with equal palpable pulses.
- Patient will have a balanced fluid intake with adequate urinary output.
- Patient will have normal skin turgor and moist mucous membranes.
- Patient will be able to accurately recall signs/ symptoms to notify nurse/physician.

DISTURBED BODY IMAGE

Related to: loss of body part, disease process, disfigurement, loss of function

Defining Characteristics: negative feelings about body, preoccupation with missing part, avoidance of looking at missing part, perceptions of changes in lifestyle, preoccupation with previous function of missing part, feelings of helplessness

Outcome Criteria

✔ Patient will be able to adapt and cope with changes in body image and demonstrate ability to accept self.

NOC: *Body Image*

INTERVENTIONS	RATIONALES
Evaluate patient's ability to deal with amputation and his perception of need for amputation.	Provides input as to level of understanding of patient. Traumatic amputees most often have trouble in dealing with body image problems, as opposed to those who have reconciled that amputation may have been a life-saving procedure.

INTERVENTIONS	RATIONALES
Observe for withdrawal, denial, or negativity regarding self.	Patients may not be able to deal with the trauma initially and may require time to come to terms with their new self. Recognition of stages of grief provides opportunity for interventions.
Provide time to discuss patient's concerns over the change in body structure and his perceptions of needs for a new/different lifestyle.	Provides opportunity to dispel false concerns and allows time for problem solving with realistic goals.
Encourage patient to help participate in his care and provide opportunities for patient to observe stump.	Promotes feelings of independence and allows time for patient to accept his body image. Positive reinforcement regarding the progress toward healing may further help his self-worth.
Discuss the availability of visits by another amputee.	Another person who has gone through the same experience may facilitate recovery and help the patient to recognize how he may attain a normal lifestyle.
Encourage family members to assist with care and assess their ability to support patient.	Provides opportunity for family members to deal with the loss and to help in the rehabilitation phase.
Instruct patient/family as to pre- and postoperative care, rehabilitation, and use of prosthetics.	Promotes knowledge and provides opportunity for patient to verbalize concerns and questions. May enhance postoperative recovery and facilitate compliance with medical treatment.
Obtain consultations as warranted with counselors or therapists.	May enhance patient's rehabilitation and ability to adapt to new body image.
Discuss concerns regarding sexuality as warranted.	Provides knowledge and helps with adjustment to body image, as well as provides opportunity to dispel any misconceptions.

NIC: *Body Image Enhancement*

Discharge or Maintenance Evaluation

- Patient will adapt and accept new situation and body image changes.
- Patient will be able to identify methods to adapt to changes and will be able to have positive self-esteem.

- Patient will be able to identify realistic goals and plans for rehabilitation and adapting to modification in body image.

ANTICIPATORY GRIEVING

Related to: actual loss of physical well-being

Defining Characteristics: expressions of anger or distress at loss, crying, sadness, guilt, alterations in sleep patterns, activity, eating or libido

Outcome Criteria

✔ Patient will be able to express feelings appropriately and work through the stages of grief and grieving.

NOC: *Psychosocial Adjustment: Life Change*

INTERVENTIONS	RATIONALES
Evaluate emotional status.	Anxiety, depression, and anger are normal reactions to loss of body parts. The patient may progress through the various stages of grief at their own rate and changes may be related to their physical condition as well.
Identify patient's stage in the grieving process.	Shock may be the initial response associated with the amputation, especially if it was traumatic. The patient may be so acutely ill that he is unable to express his feelings and concerns. Denial may initially be useful for patient's ability to cope with the injury, but continued denial may impair the patient's ability to effectively deal with the problem. Anger may be expressed either verbally, non-verbally, or physically, and the patient may displace his anger by placing blame. Depression may last from weeks to years and acceptance and support for these feelings will facilitate recovery.
Provide factual information to patient/family in regard to the diagnosis/prognosis. Do not give false reassurance.	Family may be where the initial instruction is directed if the patient's awareness is diminished due to his injury. The final

(continues)

(continued)

INTERVENTIONS	RATIONALES
	outcome of a patient's injuries may not be initially known and so information should be kept simple.
Assist patient to focus on needs he has now before changing focus to long-term goals. Encourage patient to take control in decisions regarding his care whenever possible.	Reduces frustration of facing an uncertain future, and allows the patient some control in dealing with current problems.
Provide acceptance of anger, hopelessness, and depression, but set limits on unacceptable behavior when warranted.	Acceptance of the patient's feelings acknowledges him as being worthwhile and a non-judgmental attitude is important in establishing trust and care. Limits may be needed to protect the patient and others from violent behavior while allowing the patient to express his negative feelings.
Provide consultation with therapists, social workers, or minister as warranted.	Physical and spiritual distress will be faced by the patient and his family and they will require long-term assistance and counseling in order to cope with the changes required by this injury.

NIC: *Grief-work Facilitation*

Discharge or Maintenance Evaluation

- Patient will be able to progress through the various stages of grief and grieving effectively.
- Patient will be able to express his feelings and concerns appropriately without unacceptable violent behavior.
- Patient will be able to access community resources for long-term counseling and assistance to deal with his injury.
- Patient and family will be able to gain adequate support throughout the grieving process.

POST-TRAUMA SYNDROME

Related to: traumatic amputation, loss of limb, accidental injury

Defining Characteristics: exaggerated startle response, flashbacks, hypervigilance, nightmares, inability to concentrate, irritability, panic attacks, amnesia of events, repression, shame, guilt, headaches, compulsive behaviors, denial, grief, fear, anxiety, anger, aggression, mood swings, detachment from surroundings and others

Outcome Criteria

- ✔ Patient will be able to express feelings and concerns related to the traumatic event and loss of body part.
- ✔ Patient will be able to use coping skills effectively to reduce fear and be able to have feelings of well-being and safety.
- ✔ Patient will achieve or maintain social interaction with family and others.

NOC: *Coping*

INTERVENTIONS	RATIONALES
Maintain and address patient's physical needs during this period.	Patient needs are primary concern and must be dealt with first before effective intervention can take place regarding his traumatic situation.
Provide adequate time to spend with patient and provide emotional support.	Reduces patient's fear of being alone and facilitates establishment of a trusting relationship.
Allow patient to express feelings and be accepting of them.	Helps to support patient and assures him that his feelings are valid and appropriate.
Assess patient's orientation and reorient as needed.	Post-traumatic numbing may impair orientation, perceptions of reality, and memory.
Decrease competing stimuli in room. Speak softly and announce your entrance to his room.	Environmental stimuli may become excessive and result in intensifying symptoms associated with trauma.
Instruct patient in methods to reduce fear.	The ability to cope with trauma will increase as the patient learns to decrease fear.
Instruct family in methods to lower patient's anxiety.	Involves family in care and assists with patient improvement and coping skills.
Be sympathetic to family members and allow them time to express feelings and concerns.	Helps to reduce family members' anxiety level and allow them to work through their own feelings, which in turn, will assist patient to deal with his problem.
Consult support groups, minister, mental health providers, and/or trauma support groups as needed.	Other sources may be required to assist patient to share and deal constructively with feelings, and provides for resources post-discharge.

NIC: *Milieu Therapy*

Discharge or Maintenance Evaluation

- Patient will be able to express feelings associated with traumatic event and will be able to feel safe.
- Patient will be able to reduce fear by using coping skills.
- Patient will be able to interact with family and others to lessen distress and fear.
- Patient will be able to resume usual activities as much as possible.
- Patient and family will be able to access support services and groups to help intervene with problems.

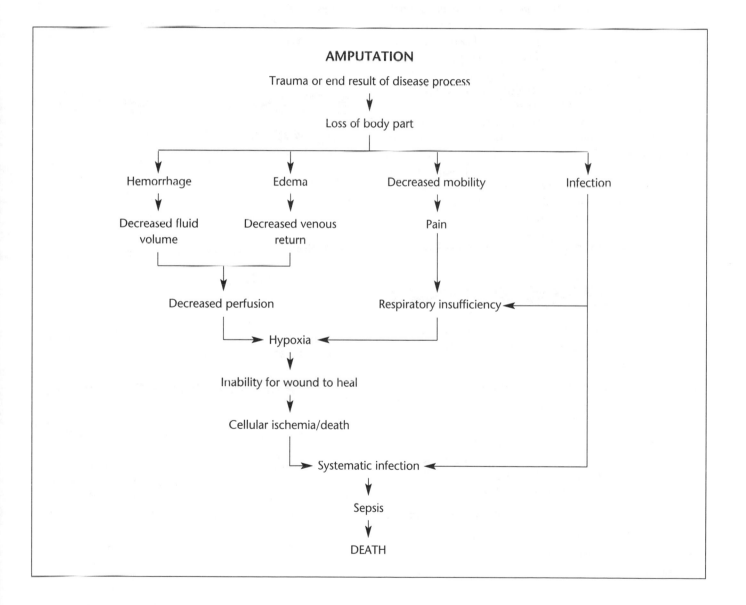

AMPUTATION

CHAPTER 7.3

FAT EMBOLISM

A fat embolism usually occurs in patients with multiple fractures or fractures that involve the long bones or pelvis, when particles of bone marrow, tissue fat droplets, or combinations of platelets and free fatty acids are released and migrate to the lungs or brain. Embolization can occur within the first 24 hours up to 72 hours after injury.

The first signs/symptoms are usually changes in the mental status, with apprehension, confusion and restlessness noted. Petechiae to the chest, anterior axillae, shoulders, conjunctiva and buccal membranes occur from capillary occlusion and are usually seen later. Respiratory distress with hypoxemia and hypoxia, pulmonary edema, and interstitial pneumonitis occur. The pulse rate increases, temperature elevates above 100 degrees and PaO_2 decreases.

MEDICAL CARE

Laboratory: serum lipase is elevated, sedimentation rate is increased; urine tests used to evaluate presence of free fat

Arterial blood gases: used to evaluate acid–base balance, presence of adequate oxygenation, and response to oxygen therapy

Electrocardiogram: used to evaluate changes in heart rate as well as cardiac changes, such as inversion of T waves and prominence of S wave in lead I showing myocardial and right ventricular failure

Corticosteroids: use is controversial, but may decrease inflammation and swelling

Heparin: use is controversial, but low dose heparin may be used to clear lipemic plasma and stimulate lipase activity

Dextran: low molecular weight dextran may be used to alter platelets and decrease intimal adhesions

X-rays: serial chest X-rays are used to evaluate pulmonary improvement or deterioration; X-rays of the bones involved in injury are used to evaluate healing process or alignment problems

NURSING DIAGNOSES

IMPAIRED GAS EXCHANGE

Related to: altered blood flow resulting from embolism, shunting

Defining Characteristics: abnormal acid–base balance, hypoxemia, hypoxia, tachypnea, tachycardia, air hunger, dyspnea, cyanosis, decreased oxygen saturation

Outcome Criteria

✔ Patient will be able to achieve and maintain adequate respiratory function with arterial blood gases within normal ranges and with no evidence of respiratory distress.

NOC: *Respiratory Status: Gas Exchange*

INTERVENTIONS	RATIONALES
Monitor vital signs, especially respiratory status; assess for dyspnea, use of accessory muscles, retractions, nasal flaring, or stridor.	Dyspnea and tachypnea may be early signs of respiratory insufficiency. Other signs usually result from advanced respiratory distress, and all require prompt intervention.
Observe for changes in mental status, irritability, apprehension, or confusion.	Changes in mental status often are the very first signs in respiratory insufficiency. As hypoxemia and acidosis worsen, the level of consciousness may deteriorate to the point of lethargy or stupor.

INTERVENTIONS	RATIONALES
Monitor pulse oximetry for oxygen saturation and notify physician for levels below 90%.	Oximetry may provide early warning of decreasing oxygenation and allow for prompt and timely intervention. In patients who have decreased peripheral circulation however, the accuracy of pulse oximetry will be compromised and cannot be relied on totally.
Administer oxygen via nasal cannula or mask as warranted.	Provides supplemental oxygen and increases available supply of oxygen to ensure optimal tissue oxygenation.
Obtain ABGs as warranted.	Decreased PaO_2 and increased $PaCO_2$ indicate impending respiratory failure and impaired gas exchange
Auscultate breath sounds for changes in equality and for presence of crackles (rales), rhonchi, wheezing, inspiratory stridor or crowing, or hyper-resonant sounds.	Adventitious breath sounds may indicate progression of respiratory insufficiency. Inspiratory crowing may indicate upper airway edema frequently seen with fat emboli.
Observe for presence of blood in sputum.	May indicate hemoptysis that occurs with pulmonary embolism.
Observe for petechiae to chest, axillae, buccal mucosa, and conjunctiva.	Petechiae to these areas are frequently seen with fat emboli, and may occur 2–5 days after injury.

INTERVENTIONS	RATIONALES
Encourage coughing, deep breathing exercises, and use of incentive spirometer.	Improves alveolar ventilation/oxygenation and helps to minimize atelectasis.
Prepare for placement on ventilator as warranted.	Deteriorating respiratory status may require mechanical ventilation to facilitate oxygenation.
Use great care in repositioning patient especially during the first days post-injury.	Gentle handling of injured bones and tissues may prevent the development of a fat embolism.
Monitor lab studies.	Patients with fat emboli frequently have anemia, elevated sedimentation rates, elevated lipase levels, fat in body fluids, hypocalcemia, and thrombocytopenia.
Administer corticosteroids as ordered.	Some physicians use steroids to prevent and treat fat emboli.

NIC: *Embolus Care: Pulmonary*

Discharge or Maintenance Evaluation

- Patient will have no respiratory dysfunction or distress.
- Patient will have arterial blood gases within his normal range.

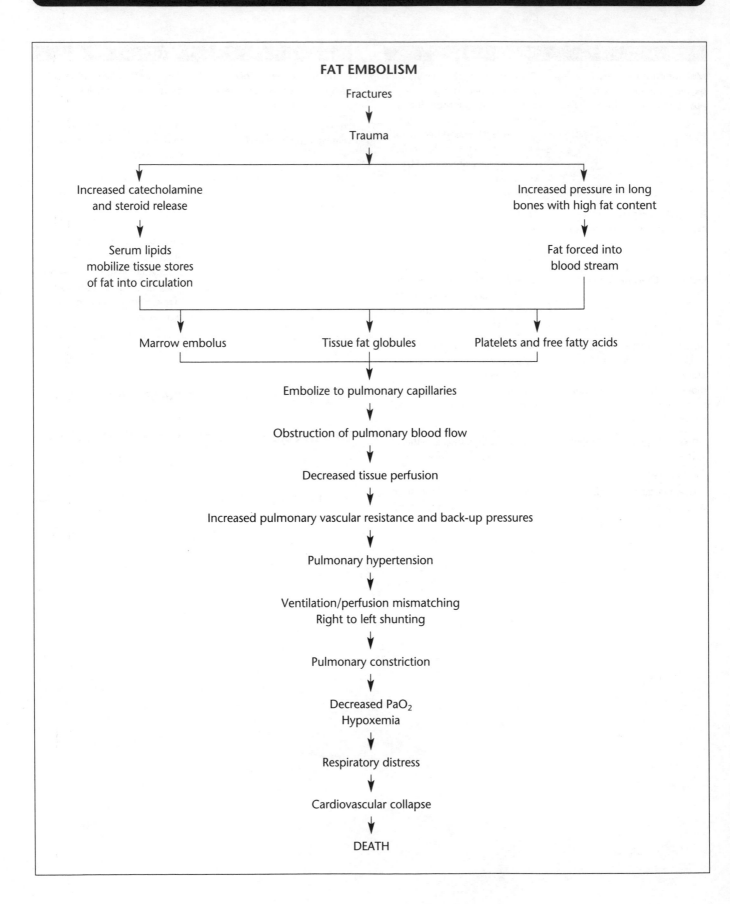

FAT EMBOLISM

Fractures

↓

Trauma

↓

Increased catecholamine
and steroid release

Increased pressure in long
bones with high fat content

↓

↓

Serum lipids
mobilize tissue stores
of fat into circulation

Fat forced into
blood stream

Marrow embolus   Tissue fat globules   Platelets and free fatty acids

↓

Embolize to pulmonary capillaries

↓

Obstruction of pulmonary blood flow

↓

Decreased tissue perfusion

↓

Increased pulmonary vascular resistance and back-up pressures

↓

Pulmonary hypertension

↓

Ventilation/perfusion mismatching
Right to left shunting

↓

Pulmonary constriction

↓

Decreased PaO$_2$
Hypoxemia

↓

Respiratory distress

↓

Cardiovascular collapse

↓

DEATH

UNIT 8

INTEGUMENTARY SYSTEM

CHAPTER 8.1

FROSTBITE/HYPOTHERMIA

Injuries from overexposure to cold, either air or water, occur in two types—localized injuries, such as frostbite, and systemic injuries, such as hypothermia. Untreated, both may be fatal.

Frostbite occurs after exposure to cold temperatures, usually below freezing. The severity of the injury is dependent on the amount of body heat lost, age, and exacerbating factors, such as wind chill, presence of wet clothing, and impairment of the circulatory status.

In frostbite, ice crystals form in the tissue fluids in and between the cells, causing injury to the red blood cells, which then develop sludging, and vascular damage. Blood is shunted to the heart and the brain. Skin is cold, hard, ashen white and numb, and with rewarming, becomes splotchy red or grayish in color, edematous, and very painful.

Frostbite can be either superficial, affecting skin and subcutaneous tissues, or deep, extending below subcutaneous tissues. With deep frostbite, the skin becomes white until thawed and then it becomes purplish-blue, with painful skin blisters, tissue necrosis, and development of gangrene when the tissue dies. At this point, amputation of the extremity may be required.

The most frequently seen sites that are involved with frostbite are the nose, ears, hands, and lower extremities. The goal of treatment is to restore body temperature to normal and prevent vascular damage to tissues. Supportive care is also important in restoring electrolyte imbalances and preventing hypovolemia.

Hypothermia occurs when the body's core temperature drops below 95° Fahrenheit and is noted by lethargy, mental dullness, decreasing level of consciousness, visual and auditory hallucinations, decreases in respirations and heart rate, and coma. The core temperature may be as low as 80° Fahrenheit and below 90°, the body loses its self-warming mechanisms.

Hypothermia may also preclude successful resuscitation. Cardiac arrest is difficult to overcome if the core temperature is less than 85° Fahrenheit because of the increased ventricular fibrillation threshold.

Treatment is aimed at rewarming the body to increase the core temperature to adequate ranges, and to preserve organ and tissue viability.

MEDICAL CARE

Laboratory: CBC may indicate infection with shift to left, hematocrit usually increases approximately 2–3% for every decrease in degree centigrade of body temperature; coagulation profiles used to identify coagulopathy may seem normal even when coagulopathies exist because of test performance at 37° C in the lab; at lower temperatures, fibrinogen may be decreased, and thrombocytopenia may occur; electrolyte levels used to identify imbalances, but hyperkalemia and hyponatremia may occur with damage to the ATPase pump; blood alcohol levels used to identify concurrent presence of alcohol; drug screens used to identify presence of drugs that are abused; myoglobin may be present when rhabdomyolysis occurs; BUN and creatinine increased because of renal deterioration and decreased perfusion

Electrocardiogram: used to identify cardiac rhythm, changes from tachycardia to bradycardia, atrial and ventricular dysrhythmias, conduction disorders, development of J waves (known as Osborne waves or hypothermic hump), or asystole as hypothermia progresses

IV fluids: used to restore circulating volume and prevent dehydration, and may be used to assist with rewarming

Dextran: low molecular weight dextran may be used to improve microcirculation to tissues

Reserpine: may be used to decrease sludging from injured cells and tissues

Antimicrobials: may be necessary to treat infection if patient has open wounds or systemic infection

Analgesics: morphine and other drugs may be used to relieve severe pain from cold injuries; aspirin may be used to decrease platelet aggregation and sludging

Surgery: fasciotomy may be required to reduce tissue pressure caused from edema; amputation may be necessary for gangrenous injuries, or debridement may be required for necrotic tissues

Dialysis: peritoneal or hemodialysis may be used, depending on severity of injury, in order to rewarm body

Rewarming techniques: warming blankets, warmed solutions for chest lavage or bladder irrigation, and warmed IV solutions may be utilized to increase temperature

COMMON NURSING DIAGNOSES

INEFFECTIVE AIRWAY CLEARANCE (see MECHANICAL VENTILATION)

Related to: obstruction of trachea, cognitive impairment from hypothermia

Defining Characteristics: dyspnea, apnea, cyanosis, decreased breath sounds, rhonchi, crackles, wheezing, ineffective or absent cough, restlessness, lethargy, orthopnea

DECREASED CARDIAC OUTPUT (see ARDS)

Related to: decreased venous return to the heart, decreased inotropic changes, changes in electrical rate, rhythm, and/or conduction caused by hypothermia

Defining Characteristics: heart rate changes, atropine-resistant bradydysrhythmias, decreased urinary output, decreased blood pressure, decreased preload, decreased afterload, atrial and ventricular dysrhythmias, increased lactate level, hypothermia, difficulty determining presence of pulse, hyperkalemia

ADDITIONAL NURSING DIAGNOSES

 ### HYPOTHERMIA

Related to: exposure to cold, suppressed shivering response, inadequate clothing

Defining Characteristics: temperature below 95° Fahrenheit, cold skin, mottling, cyanosis, pallor, poor judgment, apathy, decreased mental ability, level of consciousness changes, coma, lack of shivering, cardiopulmonary arrest, anuria, oliguria, decreased peripheral perfusion, piloerection, shivering, decreased capillary refill time, necrosis

Outcome Criteria

✔ Patient will achieve and maintain an acceptable temperature with no complications.

NOC: *Thermoregulation*

INTERVENTIONS	RATIONALES
Obtain baseline temperature, and monitor every 15 minutes until stable.	Temperatures below 90° F (32.2° C) result in suppression of normal body mechanisms to self-warming. Rewarming that is done too rapidly may cause peripheral vasodilation and may actually impede rewarming efforts. A hemodynamic catheter thermistor is the optimal monitoring apparatus because it measures actual core temperature. If a PA catheter is not utilized, rectal, esophageal, or tympanic routes may be used, but whichever method is used should be used consistently to facilitate accurate data.
Monitor ECG for heart rhythm, changes in conduction, dysrhythmias, and other changes. Treat per protocol.	Hypothermia that is mild in nature usually results in tachycardia, increased respiratory rate, increased blood pressure and cardiac output. Moderate hypothermia usually results in bradycardia, decreased blood pressure, and decreased cardiac output. Severe hypothermia usually results in apnea, ventricular dysrhythmias, the presence of J waves, progressing to ventricular fibrillation, and asystole. Hypothermia will conceal ECG changes that are normally associated with hyperkalemia.
Rewarm patient per hospital protocol. (Whole body or partial immersion into water that is 110°–118° F (43.4°–47.8° C),	Early rewarming decreases tissue damage from ice crystal formation, and helps to decrease cardiac instability and predisposition

(continues)

(continued)

INTERVENTIONS	RATIONALES
hypothermia blankets, gastric lavage with warmed solutions, peritoneal or hemodialysis, and IV infusions that are warmed are some methods currently used.)	to ventricular fibrillation. Heating blankets warm the patient decreasing the amount of heat loss from radiation and convection, but can cause tissue damage and burns at areas of pressure points if blanket is not properly covered. Radiant warmers generate heat close to the patient's skin, but may cause burns if sufficient circulation is not present to remove heat away from the skin. Convection air blankets prevent further loss of heat through convection, but the blanket must cover a large portion of the patient and the borders must be fastened securely. Rewarming the patient's airway by utilizing warmed, humidified gas via an artificial airway or through a mask affords only a small increase in core body temperature, and a rebound afterdrop may occur until the body temperature equilibrates with the environment. Rewarming utilizing peritoneal, pleural, or mediastinal lavage usually raises body temperature approximately 2° C per hour, but may not be a viable option if the patient also has an abdominal trauma. Mediastinal lavage has a high morbidity rate because of the need for a median sternotomy, and risk of infection. Heated IV fluids may be used, as well as blood products placed through a fluid warmer, but the fluid must be infused rapidly before the temperature drops, and if blood is warmed above 40° C, red blood cells will hemolyse. Cardiopulmonary bypass and extracorporeal venovenous rewarming techniques may be used to increase core temperature by approximately 4° C per hour, but may create bleeding complications from the necessary use of heparin, and requires expert technological equipment. Warming should be limited to a maximum of 2° C per hour except in the most extreme cases.

INTERVENTIONS	RATIONALES
Monitor patient for decreases in temperature after internal rewarming is discontinued.	An afterdrop of up to 2° C may occur after the blood circulates to the peripheral tissues, is cooled, and then returned to the heart.
Monitor patient for rewarming shock (decreased cardiac output, decreased blood pressure, cardiac dysrhythmias).	May indicate that the peripheral tissues were rewarmed prior to the core body, which may result in vascular collapse.
Observe for mental changes and return of shivering response.	Shivering is suppressed at temperatures below 90° F (32.2° C) and is the body's normal response to facilitate self-warming. Patients have decreased mental abilities and levels of consciousness dependent on severity of hypothermia/injury, with hypoxia and hypoxemia occurring because of decreased perfusion.
Monitor vital signs and cardiac rhythm. Treat aberrant cardiac rhythms per hospital protocol.	As the core body temperature decreases, peripheral vasoconstriction occurs, followed by increases in metabolic rate and muscle tone. As the temperature continues to fall, shivering, tachypnea, tachycardia, and hypertension will ensue. When the core temperature is lower than 95° F (35° C), metabolism, respiratory rate, and heart rate decrease. As the core temperature deteriorates, the rate of its decline accelerates, and heart rate, blood pressure, and respiratory rate decrease directly proportional to the temperature decline. When the core temperature goes below 86° F (30° C), repolarization aberrancies and atrial tachydysrhythmias begin followed shortly by ventricular fibrillation resulting from the inhibition of the Purkinje fiber velocity.
Administer IV thiamine as ordered.	If patient is alcoholic or malnourished, thiamine may help to decrease the chances of neurologic impairment from a thiamine deficiency, and should be given during rewarming efforts.
Monitor lab work for blood alcohol levels.	Alcohol impedes thermoregulatory function by suppressing the hypothalamus, decreasing perception of cold, and decreasing shivering.

INTERVENTIONS	RATIONALES
If patient has to walk for any substantial distance and has frozen feet, the feet should not be rewarmed prior to arriving to receive care.	If feet are partially warmed, and then pressure is exerted upon them during walking, it will result in tissue damage and necrosis.
Instruct patient/family on appropriate procedures for rewarming.	Provides knowledge and reduces anxiety.
Instruct patient/family regarding avoiding rubbing with or without snow.	This old method of slow rewarming is contraindicated because of increased tissue damage done by abrasion to already-impaired tissue.
Instruct patient/family, when appropriate, about alcohol or substance abuse strategies and community resources to use upon discharge.	Promotes knowledge of potential sources for treatment of alcoholism or drug problem and methods for getting help.

NIC: *Hypothermia Treatment*

Discharge or Maintenance Evaluation

- Patient will be normothermic, with stable vital signs.
- Patient will be awake, alert, and oriented, with no alterations in abilities.
- Patient will be able to maintain thermoregulation.
- Patient will exhibit no complications from hypothermia.

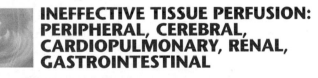

INEFFECTIVE TISSUE PERFUSION: PERIPHERAL, CEREBRAL, CARDIOPULMONARY, RENAL, GASTROINTESTINAL

Related to: exposure to cold temperatures, frozen body parts, hypothermia, tissue necrosis, sludging of red blood cells, tissue ischemia

Defining Characteristics: skin mottling, grayish skin color, purplish-blue color, cold skin, burning, tingling, numbness, pain, skin blisters, gangrene, diminished or absent pulses, decreased capillary refill, cardiac dysrhythmias, cardiac standstill, apnea, dyspnea, mental changes, unconsciousness, changes in consciousness level, coma, gangrene, oliguria, anuria, absent bowel sounds, ileus

Outcome Criteria

✔ Patient will achieve and maintain normal body temperature with no lasting complications of decreased perfusion.

NOC: *Tissue Perfusion*

INTERVENTIONS	RATIONALES
Assess patient's level of skin damage, if possible	The degree of severity of injury to the tissue may not be apparent for up to 72 hours after injury. Frequently, the patient may have varying degrees of frostbite in a single location. First degree frostbite is typically limited to the epidermis, and the skin is initially colored white or yellow. It may thaw quickly and become red and painful, with obvious wheals. The deeper tissues are not frozen, so mobility is normal. Second degree frostbite comprises the entire epidermis and may also involve the superficial dermis. It appears the same as first degree frostbite, but there will be some limitation of mobility. A bulla filled with clear fluid forms over the injured area during several hours after thawing. Usually these injuries create no permanent loss of tissue, but the patient may continue to always have cold sensitivity to those frostbitten areas. Third-degree frostbite occurs when the dermis is involved as well as the reticular layer. The tissue is stiff with restriction motion. After thawing, mobility may be restored briefly, but then the tissues begin to swell and hemorrhagic bullae occur because of the damage to the vascular plexus. Skin loss follows through a process of sloughing and mummification, and permanent tissue loss may occur. The most significant degree of frostbite, fourth degree, involves the full thickness of the skin as well as underlying tissue structures, including bones. Thawing may restore passive

(continues)

(continued)

INTERVENTIONS	RATIONALES
	mobility but the intrinsic muscle function is gone. Reperfusion is poor, and early necrosis evolves over several weeks to sloughing, mummification, and finally, auto-amputation. Corneal frostbite is rare, but can be noted and is an extremely disabling condition. Permanent opacification of the cornea occurs and will require corneal transplantation.
Monitor ECG for rhythm changes, dysrhythmias, and cardiac standstill, and treat according to hospital policy.	Hypothermia affects heart rate and rhythm and may cause heart irregularities from hypoxemia and conduction problems. Heart rhythm may be difficult to restore to sinus when body temperature is less than 85° F because of the increased ventricular fibrillation threshold. A 12-lead ECG may show an early J wave in the left ventricular leads.
Monitor vital signs every 15 minutes until stable, then every 1–2 hours.	During initial period after exposure, pulses and blood pressure may be too weak to be detectable. Rewarming too rapidly may result in heart irregularities.
Administer oxygen as ordered, with warmed humidification.	PaO_2 should be maintained above normal levels to treat hypoxia and hypoxemia that occurs with acidosis as a result of the injury and exposure.
Monitor pulse oximetry levels and notify physician if level drops below 90%. Monitor ABGs for changes.	Facilitates prompt identification of acid–base imbalances and changes in ventilation/oxygenation.
Monitor peripheral pulses for presence, character, quality, and changes.	Decreased or absent pulses may indicate impairment in circulation to extremities and may reflect tissue ischemia and necrosis.
Move and handle patient gently when required.	Excessive movement may trigger lethal dysrhythmias or may cause tissue damage.
Administer warmed IV solutions as ordered.	Restores circulating volume, helps to maintain hydration and output, assists with rewarming efforts, and assists with treatment of hypotension.
Administer low molecular weight dextran infusion (20 ml/kg/day), as ordered.	May be used to improve microcirculation.

INTERVENTIONS	RATIONALES
Administer reserpine IV as ordered.	May reduce sludging and improve microcirculation.
Monitor hourly intake and output, and notify physician for significant changes or abnormalities.	Anuria or oliguria may indicate decreased perfusion to renal vessels or dehydration.
Evaluate patient's level of consciousness and mental status, and notify physician for significant changes.	Patient may have weakness, incoordination, apathy, drowsiness, and confusion with hypothermia. When body temperature is below 90° F, stupor and coma are common.
Observe for muscle tremors, decreased reflexes, seizures, and Parkinson-like muscle tone.	Neurologic symptoms may occur due to hypothermic influences.
Remove constricting clothing and jewelry from patient.	Constriction especially in the presence of edema may impair circulation and perfusion.
Rewarm involved extremity in tepid water (37°–40° centigrade) until the tips of the injured part flush.	Prompt rewarming reverses ice crystal formation in tissues. Warmer water is not indicated due to the potential for burns. The appearance of skin flushing indicates that circulatory flow has been reestablished.
Avoid rubbing the injured extremity, and handle the area gently.	Helps to prevent further tissue damage.
Encourage patient to take warm liquids if possible.	Assists with rewarming.
Notify physician if pulse is absent after rewarming is accomplished.	When extremity has rewarmed, pulse should be able to be palpated. Absence of pulse may indicate decreased or absent circulation.
Prepare patient for fasciotomy or amputation as warranted.	Edema may impair circulation requiring a fasciotomy to relieve pressure. If gangrene is present, amputation of the involved area will be necessary.
Instruct patient regarding long-term effects: increased sensitivity to cold, tingling, burning, increased sweating, and so forth.	Provides knowledge and identifies symptoms that patient may be faced with during his lifetime.
Instruct patient to avoid smoking.	Smoking causes vasoconstriction and may inhibit healing process.

NIC: *Circulatory Precautions*

Discharge or Maintenance Evaluation

- Patient will achieve optimal circulation and peripheral perfusion with equal palpable pulses.
- Patient will be able to recall and adhere to instructions and avoid preventable complications.
- Patient will be able to recall instructions accurately.

ACUTE PAIN

Related to: tissue damage, surgical procedures, rewarming

Defining Characteristics: communication of pain, facial grimacing, moaning, guarding, abnormal focus on pain, anxiety

Outcome Criteria

✔ Patient will be free of pain, or pain will be controlled to patient's satisfaction.

NOC: *Pain Control*

INTERVENTIONS	RATIONALES
Evaluate pain level, and medicate with analgesics as ordered.	Rewarming process is extremely painful. Narcotics and NSAIDs should be given to control pain. NSAIDs, commonly ibuprofen, are used to decrease the release of eicosanoids that may further exacerbate tissue ischemia post-injury.
Elevate injured extremity on pillows as warranted.	Decreases edema which can result in pressure to tissues and pain.
Provide backrubs, repositioning, deep breathing exercises, visualization, guided imagery, and so forth.	Helps to refocus attention and enhances relaxation and ability to cope with pain.
Instruct patient to notify nurse of pain when discomfort is first noticed.	Because frostbite injuries are exceedingly painful, patient may be afraid of becoming addicted to narcotics, but if medication is given promptly before the pain has gotten out of control, smaller doses of analgesics are utilized.
Instruct patient to avoid smoking.	Nicotine causes vasoconstriction, which can worsen perfusion and pain.

NIC: *Medication Administration*

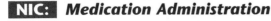

Discharge or Maintenance Evaluation

- Patient will be pain free or comfortable.
- Patient will be able to utilize comfort measures and techniques effectively to reduce or alleviate pain.

RISK FOR INFECTION

Related to: frozen tissue, open wounds, decreased tissue perfusion, edema, surgery

Defining Characteristics: elevated temperature, elevated white blood cell count, shift to left on differential, tachycardia, drainage, gangrene, edema

Outcome Criteria

✔ Patient will be free of open wounds and infection process, and/or wounds will heal in a timely manner.

NOC: *Tissue Integrity: Skin and Mucous Membranes*

INTERVENTIONS	RATIONALES
When extremity has been rewarmed, apply a bulky sterile dressing to the area. Place gauze between toes or fingers.	Dressings between digits reduce moisture and help prevent tissue damage. Dressings help protect the area to reduce further injury.
If blisters are present, avoid rupturing them.	Reduces the risk of infection.
Use sterile or strict aseptic technique for all dressing changes.	Frostbite makes the patient susceptible to infection.
Assist with whirlpool treatments for the injured extremity.	Treatments help to improve circulation, remove dead tissue, and help prevent infection.
Monitor vital signs and patient for presence of fever and chills.	Fever, tachycardia, and tachypnea may indicate presence of infection.
Administer alpha-adrenergic blockers as ordered.	May help to decrease postinjury vasospasms, especially if perfusion is limited. If the drug appears to improve blood flow, it should be continued at the minimally effective dose for several days and then tapered off.
Administer tetanus toxoid and tetanus immune globulin as ordered.	Frostbite is a tetanus-prone wound, and if immunization status is unknown, both medications should be given. If tetanus

(continues)

(continued)

INTERVENTIONS	RATIONALES
	immunization has been within the past five years, only the toxoid needs to be given.
Administer antimicrobials as ordered.	Antibiotics are routinely given prophylactically in the early management of frostbite because anaerobes and strepto-cocci are early causes of infection. Penicillin is usually the drug of choice, or clindamycin, if the patient is allergic to penicillins. If an infection develops during the healing of severe frostbite injuries, the infection can propagate systemically or cause gangrene.
Instruct patient/family regarding signs and symptoms to observe for, such as demarcated area changes, redness, change or presence of drainage, and so forth.	May indicate presence of infection or that tissue necrosis is extending.
Instruct patient/family regarding maintaining proper nutrition, with increased protein intake.	Adequate nutrition is required for maximum wound healing.
Instruct patient on all medications and procedures.	Promotes knowledge and helps to facilitate compliance with medical regimen.

NIC: *Infection Protection*

Discharge or Maintenance Evaluation

- Patient will be free of drainage from injury.
- Patient will be afebrile, with normal vital signs, and no symptoms of infection.
- Patient will have no systemic infection, or preventable complication.

IMPAIRED TISSUE INTEGRITY

Related to: frostbite, hypothermia, decreased perfusion, microemboli

Defining Characteristics: firm, white, cold areas on skin, peeling skin, fluid filled blisters, hemorrhagic bullae, necrosis, tissue sloughing, gangrene, autoamputation, mummification, edema, numbness, hyperesthesias, decreased mobility, lethargy, mental confusion, loss of consciousness, decreased respiratory rate, changes in cardiac rhythm, residual cold sensitivity

Outcome Criteria

✔ Patient will maintain optimal amount of tissue revascularization after rewarming.
✔ Patient will have minimal damaged tissues and tissue loss.

NOC: *Tissue Perfusion: Peripheral*

INTERVENTIONS	RATIONALES
Assess patient's level of tissue involvement.	Frostbite results when the tissue is cooled to a temperature at which ice crystals form, causing concentrations of some intravascular and extravascular fluids into a hypertonic solution. Once the tissue has been frozen solidly, injury is likely arrested, however, upon rewarming, a hyperfusion tissue injury occurs with the restoration of blood flow. Endothelial swelling in the thawed tissue causes a secondary loss of perfusion, ischemia, and infarction of tissues. All frozen tissue will appear the same— cold, hardened, bloodless— initially, and it is only after several hours to days later that the amount of true injury can be ascertained.
Avoid rewarming of tissue unless there is no risk of re-exposure to cold.	Refreezing of a frostbitten area worsens the injury to the point where irreparable damage occurs. Frostbitten tissue is highly susceptible to trauma, so care must be taken to handle patient as gently as possible.
Rewarm tissues per hospital protocol.	Active rewarming is done to decrease the amount of tissue that is destroyed.
Depending on the degree of frostbite, treatment may be aimed at avoiding additional injury, avoiding infection, and allowing the injury to evolve naturally. In severe injuries, patients are placed in the whirlpool for debridement of their wounds.	Dead tissue is removed by whirlpool debridement 1–2 times per day in a saline or diluted Betadine solution.

INTERVENTIONS	RATIONALES
Premedicate patient with analgesic prior to whirlpool treatment.	Debridement is extremely painful and premedication can help to decrease the patient's discomfort.
Perform ROM exercises gently while in the whirlpool.	Gentle exercises help to minimize tissue function loss.
After whirlpool treatment, patient should be dried gently, and a bulky dressing applied.	Some facilities use aloe vera ointments applied over the bullae to reduce the production of vasoconstrictive eicosanoids and to help with healing.
Culture wounds as ordered.	Provides for appropriate medication management utilizing the appropriate antimicrobial specific to the organism causing an infective process.
Instruct patient in all procedures, being honest about pain patient may experience.	Complete knowledge helps to facilitate compliance.
Prepare patient for surgical debridement if necessary.	Sometimes, even with the use of antibiotics, treatment of a local infection may require surgical procedures. Edema may require emergent fasciotomy, and gangrene that may lead to sepsis, may require amputation to be life-saving.
Instruct in ROM exercises, and postdischarge need for continuing therapy.	Contractures and tissue loss may require orthotics, prosthetics, and continued therapy to restore function to its maximal effort.

INTERVENTIONS	RATIONALES
Instruct patient/family regarding the need to avoid cold exposure.	Once the injury has healed, cold sensitivity will be present and must be managed by application of extra protection, or else the cold exposure may precipitate symptoms in a previously injured area.
Instruct patient that hyperhidrosis of the soles of the feet may occur, and care should be taken to keep feet warm and dry.	Increased sweating of the feet can result in infection and maceration of the skin.

NIC: *Wound Care*

Discharge or Maintenance Evaluation

- Patient will have minimal tissue loss with active, rapid rewarming.

- Patient will be able to recover from frostbite injury with the use of ancillary therapy services and orthotics or prosthetics.

- Patient will be able to accurately verbalize understanding of care being received and the need for painful procedures.

- Patient will be compliant with utilizing extra protection over previous frostbitten injury sites.

- Patient will have minimal amputation, and will exhibit no signs or symptoms of system infection.

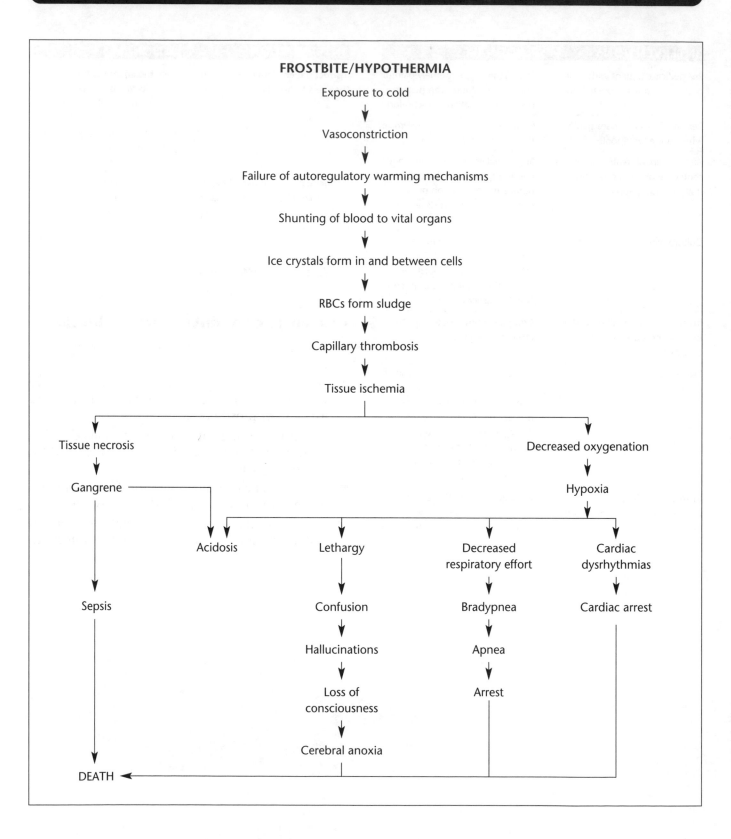

FROSTBITE/HYPOTHERMIA

CHAPTER 8.2

MALIGNANT HYPERTHERMIA

Malignant hyperthermia is a hypermetabolic condition involving skeletal muscle that is induced in susceptible patients by inhalation anesthetics and/or the use of succinylcholine. Although it occurs only about once in every 20,000 patients who may have an inherited autosomal genetic predisposition to this phenomenon, the consequences may be lethal.

In normal muscle nerve depolarization the release of acetylcholine from the nerve endings initiates the depolarization of the sarcolemma and proceeds through the transverse tubules that are next to the sarcoplasmic reticulum. It is here that the calcium ions are released by the dihydropyridine and ryanodine receptors. Calcium combines with troponin, releasing actin-myosin inhibitors, which then allow the actin and myosin filaments to move freely to initiate muscle contraction and utilize adenosine triphosphate (ATP). In patients who are susceptible to malignant hyperthermia, the dihydropyridine and ryanodine receptors are abnormal and lead to excessive calcium release, which in turn starts a cascade of other reactions, such as ATP breakdown and depletion, lactate production, increased carbon dioxide, myonecrosis, rhabdomyolysis, myoglobinemia, myoglobinuria, hyperkalemia, dysrhythmias, renal failure, and, ultimately, death, unless the cycle is stopped.

Malignant hyperthermia is a condition occurring from surgical procedures in which inhalation agents or muscle relaxants, such as succinylcholine, enflurane, fluroxene, ether, or halothane, are used. Malignant hyperthermia results from excessive stores of calcium in the intracellular spaces that causes a hypermetabolic state with increased muscle contractions.

The inherited trait for this condition can be identified by increased creatine phosphokinase levels and/or muscle biopsy for histochemistry and in vitro exposure to halothane. When this condition trait is identified in a patient who requires surgery, the preferred option is for local anesthesia.

The patient will notably have muscle rigidity, followed by tachycardia, dysrhythmias, rapidly increasing temperature, acidosis and shock. If left untreated, it has a mortality rate of 70%.

Treatment is aimed at recognition of the condition, with discontinuation of all anesthetic agents, and administration of dantrolene intravenously to slow down rate of metabolism. Supportive therapy to correct acidosis and fever should also be performed.

MEDICAL CARE

Electrocardiogram: used to identify conduction problems or dysrhythmias that may occur

Laboratory: electrolyte levels used to identify imbalances; usually has significant hyperkalemia; CPK increased because of muscle damage; myoglobinemia and myoglobinuria may be noted due to muscle breakdown; calcium usually increased

Arterial blood gases: used to identify hypoxia, hypoxemia, hyperventilation, and acid-base imbalances; usually has metabolic and respiratory acidosis, and frequently has base deficit >10 mmol; has increased end-tidal pCO_2 as initial sign

Oxygen: used to supplement oxygen supply because of increased metabolic state

Dantrium: drug used to reverse effects of excessive calcium in intracellular areas; usually given until symptoms abate

Sodium bicarbonate: may be used to treat severe acidosis

Hypothermic treatment: cooling blankets, iced lavages and enemas, infusions of cooled IV solutions may be required to reduce temperature

COMMON NURSING DIAGNOSES

DECREASED CARDIAC OUTPUT (see PHEOCHROMOCYTOMA)

Related to: hypermetabolic state, fluid shifting

Defining Characteristics: increased blood pressure and pulse, dyspnea, edema, confusion, restlessness, decreased urinary output, increased systemic vascular resistance, decreased cardiac output and cardiac index

IMBALANCED NUTRITION: LESS THAN BODY REQUIREMENTS (see PHEOCHROMOCYTOMA)

Related to: hypermetabolic state, anorexia

Defining Characteristics: inadequate food intake, weight loss, muscle weakness, fatigue

IMPAIRED GAS EXCHANGE (see PHEOCHROMOCYTOMA)

Related to: increased respiratory workload, impaired oxygen to the heart, hypoventilation, altered oxygen supply, altered blood flow, change in vascular resistance

Defining Characteristics: confusion, restlessness, hypercapnia, hypoxia, cyanosis, dyspnea, tachypnea, changes in ABG values, metabolic acidosis, respiratory acidosis, activity intolerance

ADDITIONAL NURSING DIAGNOSES

HYPERTHERMIA

Related to: reaction to anesthetic agents; hypermetabolic state

Defining Characteristics: elevated temperature, tachycardia, tachypnea, muscle rigidity, tetany, cyanosis, presence of heart failure, acidosis, dysrhythmias, shock

Outcome Criteria

✔ Patient will be free of fever, with stable vital signs, and will exhibit no evidence of muscle tetany.

 Thermoregulation

INTERVENTIONS	RATIONALES
Monitor vital signs frequently; if able, continuously monitor temperature for changes.	Provides for prompt identification of worsening condition and allows for observation for effectiveness of therapy.
Monitor ECG for changes and treat dysrhythmias per hospital protocol.	Dysrhythmias may occur as a result of the marked hyperkalemia or with electrolyte imbalances from fluid overload.
Administer dantrolene as ordered.	Normally given from 2–4 mg/kg IV rapidly through fast-running IV line; repeated every 15 minutes until a total of 10 mg/kg has been given, or symptoms subside. Dantrolene inhibits calcium release. Dantrolene (Dantrium) decreases the release of calcium from the sarcoplasmic reticulum and increases re-uptake. After initial dosing is given, dantrolene may be ordered at the rate of 1 mg/kg IV q 6 hours for up to 48 hours after insult.
Monitor ABGs for changes.	May indicate metabolic or respiratory acidosis, and patients frequently have noted base excess -10 mmol.
Administer cooled IV solutions as ordered, utilize iced solutions for gastric lavage or enema, and/or place patient on cooling blanket.	Methods may be required to decrease temperature to prevent further complication and body exhaustion.
Observe for shivering and administer Thorazine as ordered.	Shivering is a normal reaction to applications of cold, but is counterproductive because it increases metabolism to try to compensate for temperature changes. Thorazine is given to decrease shivering and reduce metabolic workload.
Assess patient for masseter muscle rigidity (MMR), or generalized muscle rigidity.	MMR is an initial symptom of malignant hyperthermia.
Ascertain what agent has been identified as the causative anesthetic, and provide patient with allergic labeling.	Known triggers for malignant hyperthermia include desflurane, enflurane, halothane, isoflurane, sevoflurane, and succinylcholine, and should be avoided for future use.

INTERVENTIONS	RATIONALES
Monitor patient for other medical problems that could show similar symptoms.	Several other medical conditions may mimic the symptoms of malignant hyperthermia and must be ruled out before a conclusive diagnosis is made. Those entities include: exertional heat stroke, cocaine toxicity, hypoxic encephalopathy, drug reactions, especially from meperidol, neuroleptic malignant syndrome, pheochromocytoma, serotonin syndrome, status epilepticus, and thyrotoxicosis.
Investigate for concurrent diagnoses of strabismus, club feet, hernias, scoliosis, and poor dentition.	Patients who are susceptible to malignant hyperthermia have been noted to be increased in prevalence when these disease states are also present.
Administer procainamide 15 mg/kg IV push over 10 minutes if ordered.	May be used in the treatment to prevent and treat hyperkalemic related dysrhythmias.
Do not give calcium channel blockers, such as verapamil, when administering dantrolene.	Concurrent administration of verapamil and dantrolene have been shown to cause severe hyperkalemia and myocardial depression.
Instruct patient/family in need of testing other members of the family for autorecessive trait.	May identify potential for anesthetic complications and avoid potentially life-threatening condition.
Instruct in utilization of hypothermic therapy methods.	Assists with understanding and facilitates compliance with discomfort.
Discuss with patient and/or family members about whether other reactions from anesthetic agents have occurred with	Because the incidence of malignant hyperthermia is based on a genetic autosomal gene, other family members have probably

INTERVENTIONS	RATIONALES
patient or other members of the blood-related family.	had some type of reaction, or may be in danger of having a reaction from specific anesthetics.
Instruct patient to always notify medical personnel of predisposition for malignant hyperthermia and/or wear a medic-alert bracelet.	Prevents future accidental use of anesthetic drugs that may induce this potentially-fatal condition.
Instruct patient/family that family members may want to be referred for testing prior to having surgical procedures.	Muscle biopsy testing may be done and is the only true way of knowing if the patient is susceptible to malignant hyperthermia. Cost of these tests may be prohibitive (approx $6,000) and are only done at certain centers that are familiar with the appropriate procedure.
Instruct patient/family that patient should be registered with the North American Malignant Hyperthermia Registry.	Registry can be contacted at (888) 274-7899, and keeps a large database for patients and providers.

NIC: *Anesthesia Administration*

Discharge or Maintenance Evaluation

- Patient will be normothermic with stable vital signs.
- Patient will have ECG with no rhythm aberrancies or conduction problems.
- Patient will exhibit no abnormal muscle contractions or tetany.
- Patient will be able to verbalize understanding of treatment and comply with regimen.
- Patient's family will comply and be tested for presence of trait that predisposes them to complications from anesthetic.

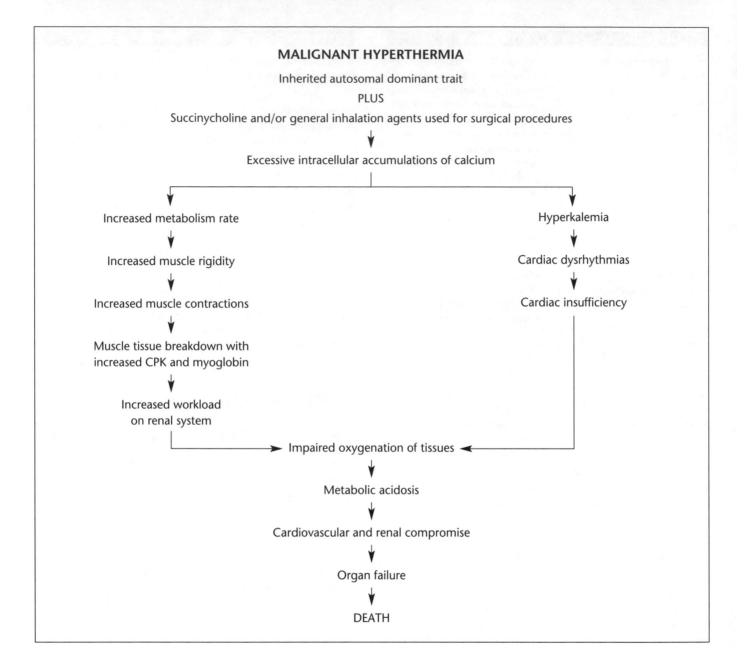

MALIGNANT HYPERTHERMIA

Inherited autosomal dominant trait

PLUS

Succinycholine and/or general inhalation agents used for surgical procedures

↓

Excessive intracellular accumulations of calcium

Increased metabolism rate   Hyperkalemia

↓   ↓

Increased muscle rigidity   Cardiac dysrhythmias

↓   ↓

Increased muscle contractions   Cardiac insufficiency

↓

Muscle tissue breakdown with
increased CPK and myoglobin

↓

Increased workload
on renal system

Impaired oxygenation of tissues

↓

Metabolic acidosis

↓

Cardiovascular and renal compromise

↓

Organ failure

↓

DEATH

CHAPTER 8.3

BURNS

Burns may be caused from thermal, chemical, electrical, or radioactive sources and may involve complex forms of trauma to multiple body systems. The depth of the injury is partially determined by the duration and intensity of exposure to the burning agent.

The initial treatment of a burn patient is to stop the burning process. This may be accomplished by cooling the skin, removal of contact with chemicals, removal from electrical current, or removal from radioactive environment. Often, inhalation injury also occurs because of inspiration of heated soot particles, chemicals and corrosives, or toxic fumes.

Burns are normally classified by depth of tissues involved. Superficial partial-thickness burns (formerly called first-degree) involved the epidermal skin layer and although the burn is uncomfortable, there is no blistering. Moderate partial-thickness burns (formerly called second-degree) involve the superficial dermal layer, have red to pink skin with blistering, with moist, weeping skin that is very painful. A second class of burns that were formerly called second degree, is the deep partial-thickness burns that involve deep dermal layers, and are pink to pale white, have blisters or bullae, and have no blanching with the application of pressure.

A severe burn, one in which the patient has 30% of the body involved, may take months to years to heal, and mortality is very high. Full-thickness, formerly third-degree, burns involve all the layers of the skin, and involve not only the epithelium, but fat, musculature, and bones, requiring extensive debridement and skin grafting.

There are several methods available for determination of the percentage of body burn involvement, but the "rule of nines" is frequently utilized. The body is sectioned off with each arm and head/neck area equaling 9%, front, back, and each leg equaling 18%, and the perineum equaling 1%. Extent of thickness, age, and other factors also play a significant role with treatment options. For acutely severe burns, transport to a burn center is recommended.

Shock may occur in adults who have burns covering greater than 15% of their body surface area, and with children when greater than 10% of their body surface area is involved. The burn injury causes dilation of the capillaries and small vessels which leads to increased capillary permeability and increased plasma loss. As edema increases, the destruction of the epidermis becomes a breeding ground for bacterial invasion and dead tissue sloughs off.

The initial response results in coagulation of cellular proteins, production of complement, histamine, and oxygen free-radicals, which lead to increased permeability. The oxygen free-radicals cause tissue injury by causing edema into the pulmonary interstitial spaces and intra-alveolar hemorrhage, and red blood cell lysis and intravascular hemolysis. A systemic response begins with the release of vasoactive substances, stress hormone production, and bacterial translocation. As fluid shifts tissue pressure is increased and may lead to compartment syndrome, or may lead to hemoconcentration, with increased hematocrit and blood viscosity. Cardiac output is decreased because of compensatory increases within the body trying to salvage major organs. If untreated, burns lead to hypovolemic shock, septic shock, metabolic acidosis, hyperkalemia, SIRS, and decreased perfusion to all body systems.

MEDICAL CARE

Laboratory: CBC will initially show elevated hematocrit due to hemoconcentration, and later decreased hematocrit may mean vascular damage to endothelium; white blood cell count may increase due to inflammatory response to the trauma and wound infection; WBC can be as high as 30,000/mm^3 initially, but resolves within 2 days; leukopenia may occur as a side effect from silver sulfadiazine or SIRS; thrombocytopenia may result within the first 72 hours because of hemodilution and potential microthrombi; protein and albumin are decreased because of protein loss from increased vascular permeability; coagulation studies usually will show increased prothrombin and partial thromboplastin time during the first 72 hours after injury as a result of leakage of clotting factors from the intravascular space; electrolytes may show initially hyperkalemia resulting from injury, later changing to hypokalemia when diuretic phase begins; sodium initially decreased with fluid loss and later changes to hypernatremia when renal system attempts to conserve water; alkaline phosphatase elevated, glucose elevated from stress reaction; albumin decreased; BUN and creatinine elevated because of renal dysfunction; carboxyhemoglobin may be done to identify carbon monoxide poisoning with inhalation injury

Radiography: chest X-rays used to identify complications that may occur as a result of inhalation injury or with fluid shifting from rapid replacement

Arterial blood gases: used to identify hypoxia or acid–base imbalances; acidosis may be noted because of decreased renal perfusion; hypercapnia and hypoxia may occur with carbon monoxide poisoning

Lung scans: may be used to identify magnitude of lung damage from inhalation injury

Electrocardiogram: used to identify myocardial ischemia or dysrhythmias that may occur with burns or electrolyte imbalances

Analgesics: required to reduce pain associated with tissue damage and nerve injury

Tetanus toxoid: required to provide immunity against infective organism

Antimicrobials: may be required to treat infection

Surgery: may be required for skin grafting, fasciotomy, debridement, or repair of other injuries

IV fluids: massive amounts of IV fluids may be required for fluid resuscitation immediately postburn, and will be required for maintenance of fluid balance as shifting occurs

COMMON NURSING DIAGNOSES

IMPAIRED GAS EXCHANGE (see MECHANICAL VENTILATION)

Related to: carbon monoxide poisoning, smoke inhalation, upper airway obstruction, burn

Defining Characteristics: increased work of breathing, dyspnea, abnormal arterial blood gases, hypoxemia, hypoxia, decreased oxygen saturation, inability to

effectively cough or clear secretions, viscous secretions, confusion, lethargy, restlessness, anxiety

ACUTE PAIN (see FROSTBITE)

Related to: burn injury, tissue destruction, wounds, debridement, surgery, invasive lines

Defining Characteristics: communication of pain, moaning, crying, facial grimacing, inability to concentrate, tension, anxiety

IMPAIRED SKIN INTEGRITY (see FROSTBITE)

Related to: burn injury, surgical procedures, invasive lines

Defining Characteristics: disruption of skin tissues, incisions, open wounds, drainage, edema

ANXIETY (see SNAKEBITE)

Related to: burn injury, threat of death, fear of disfigurement or scarring, hospitalization, mechanical ventilation

Defining Characteristics: expressions of apprehension, tension, restlessness, insomnia, expressions of concern, fear of unknown, tachypnea, tachycardia, inability to concentrate or focus

IMPAIRED PHYSICAL MOBILITY (see FROSTBITE)

Related to: burn injury, dressings, imposed physical inactivity

Defining Characteristics: inability to move at will, imposed inactivity, contractures, wounds, pain

RISK FOR INFECTION (see FROSTBITE)

Related to: burn injury, tissue destruction, open wounds, impaired skin integrity, ARDS

Defining Characteristics: elevated white blood cell count, differential shift to the left, fever, tachycardia, tachypnea, wound drainage, necrosis, presence of systemic infection

ADDITIONAL NURSING DIAGNOSES

DEFICIENT FLUID VOLUME

Related to: burn injury, loss of fluid through injured surfaces, hemorrhage, increased metabolic state, fluid shifts, third spacing, shock, increased cellular membrane permeability

Defining Characteristics: tachycardia, hypotension, changes in mental status, restlessness, decreased urine output, prolonged capillary refill, pallor, mottling, diaphoresis, poor turgor

Outcome Criteria

✔ Patient will achieve and maintain fluid balance with adequate urinary output.

NOC: *Fluid Balance*

INTERVENTIONS	RATIONALES
Monitor vital signs, and notify physician of significant changes or trends.	Hypotension may indicate that the circulating fluid volume is decreased. Changes in vital signs may indicate the amount of blood loss but may not change until loss is greater than 1000 cc. Hypovolemic shock may occur because of hemorrhage, third spacing, or coagulopathy.
Measure hemodynamics if pulmonary artery catheter has been placed. Notify physician for abnormal parameters.	CVP, or right atrial pressure, gives estimate of fluid volume status. Dehydration may be reflected by CVP of less than 5, while overhydration may be reflected at levels over 18 cm H_2O. Hemodynamic values may help to evaluate the body's response to the circulating volumes.
Observe for restlessness, anxiety, mental changes, changes in level of consciousness, or weakness.	Changes may reflect the severity of fluid loss.
Observe for bleeding from all orifices and puncture sites, and for presence/development of ecchymoses, hematomas, or petechiae.	May indicate impaired coagulation, impending or present DIC, or inadequate replacement of clotting factors.
Monitor intake and output hourly and notify physician for significant imbalances.	May indicate fluid volume deficit, and establishes a guide for fluid and blood product replacement. Fluid replacement is titrated to ensure urinary output of at least 30–40 cc/hr. Myoglobin may discolor the urine red to black, and if present, urinary output should be at least 75–100 cc/hr to reduce potential for renal tubular necrosis.

INTERVENTIONS	RATIONALES
Administer IV fluids as ordered. Two IV sites should be maintained.	Replaces fluid loss, allows for administration of vasoactive drugs, plasma extenders, and emergency medications, as well as the administration of blood products. Two sites are recommended to facilitate simultaneous fluid and blood resuscitation in critical settings. Crystalloids, such as Ringer's lactate, are used during the first 24 hours, then colloids are used because colloids help to mobilize extravascular fluids. Dextrose is usually not given during the first 24 hours after injury because dextrose does not remain in the vascular space where it is needed. Fluid resuscitation is initiated if the patient has more than 15–20% body surface area burned, and is given at a rate of 2–4 $cc/kg^3 \times$ the percentage of body surface area that has been burned. Half of this volume is given within the first 8 hours and the rest within the next 16 hours, and may be titrated per hospital protocol and patient response in maintaining urinary output.
Administer blood and/or blood products as ordered.	Whole blood may be required for acute bleeding episodes with shock due to the lack of clotting factors in packed red blood cells. Fresh frozen plasma and/or platelets may be required to replace clotting factors and to promote platelet function.
Prepare patient for placement of pulmonary artery catheter.	Provides knowledge to the patient, and catheter is invaluable for identifying changes in fluid status and hemodynamic responses to those changes.
Instruct patient, if he is able to take oral fluids, to increase intake.	Provides knowledge and gives patient some control over fluid intake to improve replacement of lost fluids from burns.
Instruct patient to notify nurse or physician of any dizziness, light headedness, or other symptoms.	May indicate worsening dehydration and allows for prompt intervention.

NIC: *Hypovolemia Management*

Discharge or Maintenance Evaluation

- Patient will have stable vital signs and urinary output.
- Patient will have balanced intake and output.
- Patient will have good turgor, moist membranes, and adequate capillary refill times.
- Patient will be free of hemorrhage or abnormal coagulation.
- Patient will have no transfusion reactions.

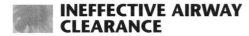

INEFFECTIVE AIRWAY CLEARANCE

Related to: airway obstruction, edema, burns to the neck and chest, trauma to upper airway, pulmonary edema, decreased lung compliance

Defining Characteristics: adventitious breath sounds, dyspnea, tachypnea, shallow respirations, apnea, cough with or without productivity, cyanosis, fever, anxiety, restlessness

Outcome Criteria

✔ Patient will have clear breath sounds with stable respiratory status.

NOC: *Respiratory Status: Airway Patency*

INTERVENTIONS	RATIONALES
Identify causative agent of burn.	May reflect type of exposure to toxic substances and potential for inhalation injury.
Monitor respiratory status for changes in rate, character, or depth; note tissue color changes with cyanosis, pallor, or cherry red color.	May indicate the presence or impending respiratory insufficiency and distress. Cherry red color may indicate carbon monoxide poisoning.
Auscultate lung fields for adventitious breath sounds.	Obstruction of airway and respiratory distress may happen quickly, but may be delayed up to 48 hours post-injury. Identification of abnormal crackles, wheezing, or stridor may indicate impending airway compromise and require immediate intervention.
Observe for presence of cough, reflexes, drooling, or dysphagia.	Inhalation injury may result in patient's inability to handle salivary or pulmonary secretions as a result of pulmonary edema.

INTERVENTIONS	RATIONALES
Observe sputum for color, characteristics, and the ability to expectorate mucus.	Smoke inhalation or breathing hot air may cause damage to the upper breathing passages and/or lungs. If sputum is dark black or charcoal gray, it should be suspected that the patient has lung involvement, and pneumonia is the cause of approximately half of all burn deaths.
Assess for reddened vocal cords or throat, stridor, singed nasal hairs, and wheezing.	Indicates that lung and upper respiratory injury has occurred. Stridor and wheezing may precede respiratory insufficiency and failure.
Elevate head of bed 30–45 degrees.	Promotes lung expansion and improves respiratory function.
Administer supplemental oxygen as warranted.	May be required to correct hypoxemia and acidosis; humidification of oxygen prevents drying out mucous membranes and keeps secretions less viscous.
Monitor ABGs and observe for trends or deterioration.	May facilitate timely identification of respiratory insufficiency and hypoxemia that requires intervention.
Monitor oximetry continuously.	Decreases in oxygen saturation may indicate impending hypoxemia or hypoxia.
Monitor ECG continuously and treat dysrhythmias per protocol.	Cardiac dysrhythmias may occur as a result of hypoxia or electrolyte imbalances, and some conduction problems may occur in response to rapid fluid resuscitation.
Instruct patient on coughing and deep breathing exercises.	Increases lung expansion and helps to mobilize secretions.
Prepare patient/family for potential placement on mechanical ventilation.	May be required for respiratory embarrassment and distress.

NIC: *Airway Management*

Discharge or Maintenance Evaluation

- Patient will be able to breathe spontaneously on his own with no adventitious breath sounds and adequate oxygen saturation.
- Patient will have arterial blood gases within normal limits.

- Patient will be able to comply with coughing and deep breathing exercises to help clear mucous secretions.
- Patient will not develop complications from injury.

IMBALANCED NUTRITION: LESS THAN BODY REQUIREMENTS

Related to: burn injury, increased metabolic rate, intubation

Defining Characteristics: intake less than output, weight loss, abnormal electrolytes, weakness, lethargy, catabolic state

Outcome Criteria

✔ Patient will have a positive nitrogen balance and stable body weight.

NOC: *Nutritional Status*

INTERVENTIONS	RATIONALES
Identify patient's caloric needs based upon body size and hypermetabolic state.	In burn injuries, fluids leak from the cells as well as energy, so patient requires at least twice their normal amount of calories. Up to 25% of the body weight is lost if the patient has a burn of 40% or more of the body.
Assess patient for presence of bowel sounds, and ability to eat.	Patient may be intubated, have throat burns and unable to eat, or gut may be paralyzed with ileus formation. Oral intake cannot be given in situations as these.
Insert nasogastric tube as ordered.	If patient has no intestinal motility, stomach contents will increase and must be removed to prevent vomiting and potential for aspiration.
Weigh patient every day, at same time, on same scale.	Allows for consistent data and accurate monitoring of patient's nutritional and fluid status.
Monitor all I&O q 1–2 hr. Notify physician of significant abnormalities.	Fluid resuscitation may result in fluid overload if the body is unable to handle the fluid shifting/third spacing. Deviations between intake and output can be used to validate weight discrepancies and assist in identifying imbalances.

INTERVENTIONS	RATIONALES
Administer enteral or parenteral nutritional support as ordered.	Enteral feedings are preferred, but a functional gut must be present, and in severe burns, initially intestinal motility is absent because of stress responses and administration of analgesics. Parenteral alimentation of a mixture of amino acids, lipids, glucose, vitamins, trace elements, and electrolytes may be required to meet the caloric needs in the hyperdynamic state of the burned patient. Their metabolic rate may be increased up to 200% over normal.
Monitor lab work, such as glucose levels, electrolytes, albumin, prealbumin, BUN and creatinine, and CBC.	May indicate the presence of developing hyperglycemia from too high concentrations of glucose solutions, electrolyte imbalances that can be altered by changing the solution of the hyperalimentation, renal dysfunction, the ability to utilize protein effectively, and the potential for impending infection and dehydration.
Provide site care for whichever type of line or tube has been inserted into patient.	Skin integrity is already impaired by burn injury, central lines should be assessed for drainage, redness, or malposition of the catheter that might signal infection. NG tubes can irritate the nasal mucosa and must be cleansed and retaped at least daily, ensuring that tube has not migrated from its original site to prevent infection from aspiration.
Instruct patient/family about increased caloric needs, and method to be used to facilitate ensuring nutritional support.	Provides knowledge about hyperdynamic state and need for increased calories and protein to allow body to heal.
Instruct patient/family regarding hand-washing and/or isolation precautions.	May be necessary to prevent infection, which in turn will require ever-increasing amounts of calories to meet metabolic demands.

NIC: *Nutrition Therapy*

Discharge or Maintenance Evaluation

- Patient will achieve a positive nitrogen balance and will have stable weight.
- Patient will exhibit no signs or symptoms of infection from IV lines or tubes.

- Patient will have normal lab values, indicative of electrolyte and protein balance.
- Patient will have equivalent intake and output.
- Patient/family will be able to accurately verbalize understanding of need for increased caloric regimen.

- Patient/family will exhibit no behavior that could preclude patient to infection.
- Patient will receive adequate nutrition to maintain and stabilize weight and condition to facilitate healing.

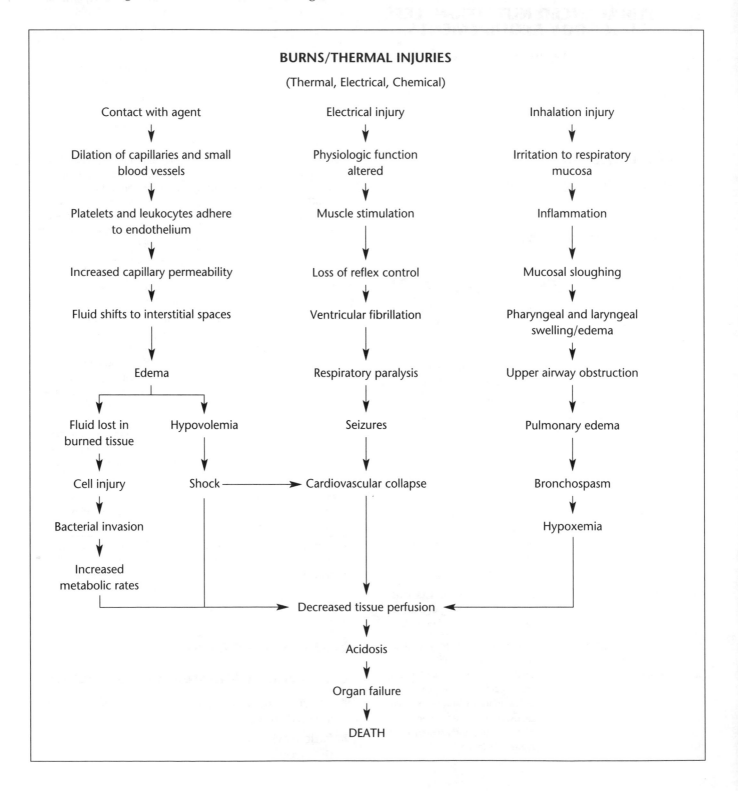

BURNS/THERMAL INJURIES

(Thermal, Electrical, Chemical)

Contact with agent	Electrical injury	Inhalation injury
↓	↓	↓
Dilation of capillaries and small blood vessels	Physiologic function altered	Irritation to respiratory mucosa
↓	↓	↓
Platelets and leukocytes adhere to endothelium	Muscle stimulation	Inflammation
↓	↓	↓
Increased capillary permeability	Loss of reflex control	Mucosal sloughing
↓	↓	↓
Fluid shifts to interstitial spaces	Ventricular fibrillation	Pharyngeal and laryngeal swelling/edema
↓	↓	↓
Edema	Respiratory paralysis	Upper airway obstruction
↓	↓	↓
Fluid lost in burned tissue — Hypovolemia	Seizures	Pulmonary edema
↓	↓	↓
Cell injury — Shock → Cardiovascular collapse		Bronchospasm
↓		↓
Bacterial invasion		Hypoxemia
↓		
Increased metabolic rates		

Decreased tissue perfusion

↓

Acidosis

↓

Organ failure

↓

DEATH

CHAPTER 8.4

LATEX ALLERGY

Hypersensitivity to latex is a growing concern, and becoming an increasingly more serious allergic hazard. Not only medical providers, such as physicians, nurses, and technicians, but also the general public are being frequently exposed to latex products. Patients who routinely catheterize themselves, suction themselves, or use latex products in any capacity are at risk for developing this hypersensitivity.

As the utilization of Universal Precautions has increased in the challenge of taking care of patients with HIV, hepatitis, and other diseases, so has the incidence of allergic response. When demand increased for gloves, the manufacturers were allowed to alter their production process to increase making enough to supply the growing demand, and one of the processes that was abandoned was the chemical rinsing of the gloves, which removed many of the protein allergens from the gloves. It has been hypothesized that with the increased residual proteins, allergies were more quickly identified.

Reactions to latex are not all the same. Irritant dermatitis is often noted, but this may not necessarily be an allergic response to latex because the powder in the gloves can also cause this reaction. Symptoms include urticaria and redness with dry, itchy, flaky skin.

Delayed hypersensitivity reactions, or type IV reactions, can occur anywhere from 30 minutes up to 3 days after exposure to latex. The cause may be the latex itself, chemicals used to treat the latex, or the powder in the gloves, and this type of reaction makes it difficult to diagnose the source because of the delayed reaction. Symptoms of this type of reaction include erythema, edema, urticaria, rhinitis, cough, and conjunctivitis.

The most severe reaction, or Type I, is an immediate reaction (<1 hour) to latex proteins, which is an IgE-mediated allergic response that occurs when IgE attaches to the mast cells in the respiratory and intestinal tracts. Results can be localized or systemic and deadly. Symptoms include urticaria, angioedema, dyspnea, pharyngeal edema, generalized edema, bronchospasm, dysrhythmias, flushing, conjunctivitis, diarrhea, and anaphylaxis. The symptoms may initially be mild, but increase in severity with each exposure, or anaphylaxis may be the first symptom noted.

Life-saving treatment is aimed at preserving the patient's airway and respiratory support. The source of the allergic response must be removed immediately, and subsequent treatment may include the use of antihistamines, corticosteroids, epinephrine, and IV fluids.

Once a patient has developed a severe reaction, they must be ever-vigilant about notifying family and coworkers, and avoiding all sources of latex. This can be quite difficult because latex is found not only in gloves, but in condoms, balloons, adhesive bandages, diapers, stethoscope tubing, and other products. They may also have a related allergy to bananas, kiwis, avocados, passion fruit, pineapple, and water chestnuts, which all are chemically similar to latex.

MEDICAL CARE

Laboratory: complement studies to identify IgE levels; CBC used to identify infection, anemia, and histamine reactions with differential; allergy testing used to identify concurrent allergens

Electrocardiogram: used to monitor cardiac rhythm and to identify potential dysrhythmias caused by hypoxia from anaphylaxis

Radiography: chest X-rays may be used to identify pleural effusions or infiltrates, and monitor for worsening pulmonary edema

IV fluids: used to restore circulating volume, prevent dehydration, and provide access for administration of emergency medications

Antihistamines: used to block histamine or bind to peripheral histamine receptors to help halt allergic reaction

Corticosteroids: used for serious allergy symptoms not relieved by other measures to reduce mucous flow, decrease inflammatory tissues, and decrease systemic response; used to decrease inflammation and for immunosuppression by inhibiting the migrating polymorphonuclear leukocytes, fibroblasts, increased capillary permeability, and lysosomal stabilization

Epinephrine: used in the treatment of anaphylaxis; beta-agonist action causes increased levels of cyclic AMP and produces bronchodilation, cardiac, and CNS stimulation

NURSING DIAGNOSES

LATEX ALLERGY RESPONSE

Related to: allergy to natural latex rubber products, contact with latex products, contact with foods that are chemically similar to latex

Defining Characteristics: dermatitis, eczema, chapped, dry skin, blisters, urticaria, edema of the lips, tongue, and/or throat, edema of eyelids or sclera, generalized edema, erythema, facial erythema, dyspnea, use of accessory muscles, tightness in chest, bronchospasm, wheezing, orthopnea, adventitious breath sounds, ineffective or absent cough, cyanosis, complaints of body warmth, restlessness, nasal congestion, rhinorrhea, hypotension, syncope, cardiac arrest, respiratory arrest, diarrhea, nausea, abdominal pain

Outcome Criteria

✔ Patient will have stable vital signs, respiratory status, and lab values will be within normal limits.

✔ Patient will recover and remain free of anaphylactic state.

✔ Patient will be able to avoid potential contact with latex-containing products.

NOC: *Symptom Severity*

INTERVENTIONS	RATIONALES
Monitor vital signs q 15 minutes until stable, then q 1 hour. Notify physician of significant changes.	Identification of respiratory changes or hypotension may indicate progression of localized reaction to systemic anaphylaxis, requiring emergent treatment.
Monitor respiratory status for changes in pattern, rate, use of	Detection of changes in status allows for timely response.

INTERVENTIONS	RATIONALES
accessory muscles, and work of breathing. Monitor oxygen saturation by oximetry and notify physician if <90%.	Wheezing and shortness of breath can deteriorate rapidly to respiratory distress and failure. Decreases in saturation may indicate that respiratory status is in danger of collapse and may require assisted ventilation.
Maintain patent airway per hospital protocol.	Airway maintenance is mandatory, and will be more difficult to maintain if edema progresses.
Administer IV fluids as ordered.	Provides IV access for emergency drugs, allows for hydration, and maintenance of circulating fluid volume in case of cardiovascular collapse.
When latex allergy is definite, remove all latex products from the room, and place signs in patient's room to this effect.	Prevents inadvertent use of allergy-causing equipment by caregivers.
Instruct patient/family regarding latex allergy, and give list of items and products that contain latex (rubber sink stoppers, sink mats, rubber-grip utensils, rubber electrical cords or hoses, bath mats and floor rugs with rubber backing, toothbrushes with rubber grip handles, undergarments or other clothing with elastic bands containing rubber, glue, paste, and art supplies, rubber bands, mouse and keyboard cords, rubber stamps, mouse and wrist pads containing rubber, keyboards and calculators with rubber keys, remote controls for TVs or VCRs that have rubber keys, camera, telescope, or binocular eye pieces, bathing caps, bathing suits with elastic, balloons, ATM machine buttons, grocery store checkout belts).	Provides opportunity for patient and family to remove potential harmful substances from home as well as to prevent future exposure to latex when away from home.
Instruct patient to seek medical assistance for any further allergic reactions.	Provides for timely intervention and potential life-saving treatment.
Instruct patient about wearing medical alert bracelet with allergy information specified.	Provides information to emergency providers should patient not be able to provide information.
Ensure that patient receives documentation of allergy for employer.	Assists with prevention of the patient having further contact with latex products and avoids reaction.

INTERVENTIONS	RATIONALES
Instruct patient never to travel alone.	The potential for coming into contact with some form of latex is very high, and if an anaphylactic reaction occurs, someone familiar with the condition needs to be available to provide emergency epinephrine and summon help.
Instruct patient/family in potential cross-over allergens with foods, such as bananas, avocados, kiwi, papaya, fig, pineapple, peach, plum, cherry, strawberry, melon, nectarine, grapes, tomato, celery, rye, wheat, hazelnut, and chestnuts.	These foods have proteins that act like latex proteins as they are metabolized in the body.

NIC: Latex Precautions

Discharge and Maintenance Evaluation

- Patient will have stable vital signs and unimpaired respiratory status.
- Patient will be free of edema and have no signs or symptoms of anaphylaxis.
- Patient will be able to verbalize understanding of latex allergy, signs/symptoms, and products to avoid.

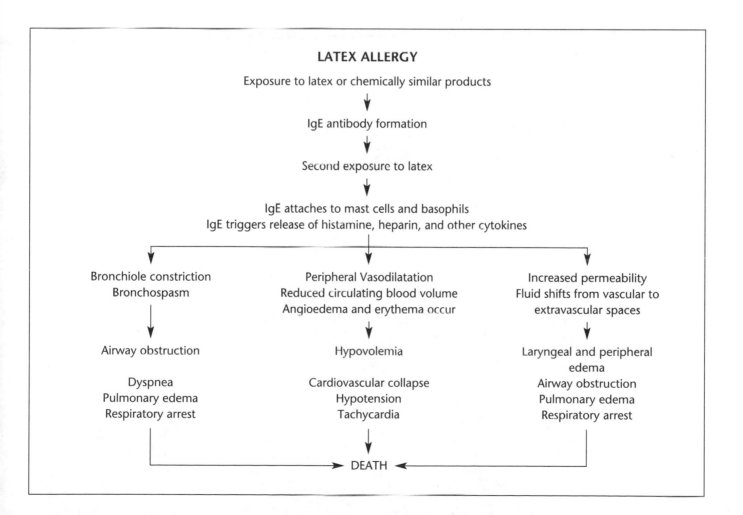

LATEX ALLERGY

Exposure to latex or chemically similar products
↓
IgE antibody formation
↓
Second exposure to latex
↓
IgE attaches to mast cells and basophils
IgE triggers release of histamine, heparin, and other cytokines

Bronchiole constriction Bronchospasm	Peripheral Vasodilatation Reduced circulating blood volume Angioedema and erythema occur	Increased permeability Fluid shifts from vascular to extravascular spaces
↓	↓	↓
Airway obstruction	Hypovolemia	Laryngeal and peripheral edema
Dyspnea Pulmonary edema Respiratory arrest	Cardiovascular collapse Hypotension Tachycardia	Airway obstruction Pulmonary edema Respiratory arrest

DEATH

UNIT 9

OTHER

CHAPTER 9.1

MULTIPLE ORGAN DYSFUNCTION SYNDROME

Multiple organ dysfunction syndrome, or MODS, is also referred to as multiple system organ failure (MSOF) and multisystem failure (MSF), and basically is defined as a state in which organ dysfunction in an acutely ill and compromised patient occurs to such an extent that normal homeostasis is unable to be preserved without medical intercession. When advancements in technology enabled hospitals to be able to support critical patients, the incidence of MODS began. Inadequate resuscitation accounts for approximately half of all MODS cases, and MODS accounts for approximately 70–80% of all ICU fatalities.

Sepsis denotes the presence of microorganisms or their byproducts in the bloodstream that create a fulminating infection with resultant systemic involvement and shock. The hemodynamic changes that occur during septic shock may result in inadequate perfusion and the development of multiple organ dysfunction syndrome. Another syndrome that may lead to MODS is systemic inflammatory response syndrome (SIRS). Both sepsis and SIRS utilize the same inflammatory cascade with differing sources of infectious versus noninfectious causes, and can both potentially lead to MODS.

As the bacterial infection progresses, the immune system attempts to destroy the causative microorganism, and the endotoxins within the cell membrane are released into the vascular system. The endotoxins then trigger systemic inflammation, activation of the complement cascade, and histamine release. This results in vasodilation, increased capillary permeability, and leakage of the protein-rich plasma into the interstitial tissues.

As the plasma seeps into the alveoli, and platelets and white blood cells embolize in the microcirculation, resulting in release of more vasoactive materials, the lung's compliance decreases and ARDS develops. The liver is unable to detoxify the circulating endotoxins because of microembolization in the liver itself as well as sludge in the hepatic system. As fluid volume decreases, the heart rate increases and cardiac output is raised. As the abdominal organs are constricted from emboli in the microcirculation, myocardial toxic factor (MTF) is released and blocks the calcium ion action and contractility decreases. As more and more endotoxins are circulating, more and more body systems are affected with decreased perfusion, hypoxia, and anaerobic mechanisms that the body tries to use to maintain metabolic function.

The goal of treatment is to support cardiopulmonary function and to identify and eradicate the organisms responsible for the infection in the first place. With two organ systems involved, mortality is 50–60% despite treatment, with the percentage increasing to 90–100% mortality with four or more systems involved. In 1995, J.C. Marshall, D. J. Cook, and N.V. Christou developed a reliable descriptive algorithm chart that predicted mortality for patients with MODS. It utilized six different organ systems with physiologic measurements of respiratory, renal, hepatic, cardiovascular, hematologic, and neurologic indicators, and was associated with predictable mortality rates ranging from 25% to 75%.

The most frequent precipitating factor is usually a temporary episode of a shock state that results in body cell ischemia. The typical pattern of MODS includes a hypotensive episode that is apparently successfully resuscitated, with elevation of heart rate and progressive respiratory failure. The patient is then intubated and appears to be doing better, but is in a hypermetabolic and hyperdynamic state that produces progressive changes in lab work. Eventually liver failure occurs, leading to bleeding and coagulopathies, until finally microbial growth progresses, causing renal failure and involvement of all systems, with death ensuing approximately one month after the initial event.

MEDICAL CARE

Laboratory: CBC used to identify hemorrhage, platelet dysfunction, infection, shifts to the left on differential; electrolytes with sodium decreased; renal profiles used to evaluate renal dysfunction and therapeutic response to treatment; hepatic profiles to evaluate hepatic dysfunction; coagulation profiles to identify clotting dysfunction and DIC; fibrinogen elevated with DIC; cultures done to identify causative organism and determine appropriate antimicrobial therapy; glucose elevated because of metabolic state; lactate level increased with metabolic acidosis, shock, or hepatic dysfunction

Electrocardiogram: used to identify conduction disturbances or cardiac dysrhythmias; may have ST and T wave changes mimicking MI

Arterial blood gases: used to identify hypoxia, hypoxemia, acid–base imbalances and evaluate effectiveness of therapy; initially may have respiratory alkalosis and hypoxemia, and in later stages, metabolic and respiratory acidosis with compensatory mechanism failure

Radiography: chest X-rays used to identify pulmonary or cardiac changes in vasculature, edema, complications; abdominal X-rays used to identify potential sources of infection, for example, free air in abdomen

Antimicrobials: may be used to treat infectious causes of sepsis

Narcan: has been used to counteract some of the endotoxins that are circulating in system

Corticosteroids: have been used to decrease inflammatory response to toxins

COMMON NURSING DIAGNOSES

RISK FOR INFECTION (see RENAL FAILURE)

Related to: progression of sepsis to septic shock, broken skin, tissue trauma, incompetent secondary defenses, compromised immune system, invasive lines, malnutrition, debilitation

Defining Characteristics: increased white blood cell count, shift to the left, fever, chills, cough with or without sputum production, wound drainage, hypotension, tachycardia, impaired skin integrity, wounds, positive blood, urine or sputum cultures, cloudy concentrated urine

HYPERTHERMIA (see PHEOCHROMOCYTOMA)

Related to: circulating endotoxins, dehydration, hypermetabolic state

Defining Characteristics: increased temperature, fever, flushed, warm skin, tachypnea, tachycardia

IMPAIRED GAS EXCHANGE (see MECHANICAL VENTILATION)

Related to: endotoxins in circulation, hyperventilation, hypoventilation, respiratory alkalosis, increased capillary permeability, alterations in blood flow caused by microembolism, capillary damage, changes in alveolar-capillary membrane

Defining Characteristics: dyspnea, tachypnea, hypoxia, hypoxemia, hypercapnia, confusion, restlessness, cyanosis, inability to move secretions, tachycardia, dysrhythmias, abnormal ABGs, decreased oxygen saturation

DEFICIENT FLUID VOLUME (see GI BLEEDING)

Related to: vasodilation, third spacing, fluid shifting, increased capillary permeability

Defining Characteristics: weight loss, output greater than intake, hypotension, tachycardia, decreased central venous pressure, decreased hemodynamic pressures, increased temperature, dilute urine with low specific gravity, oliguria with high specific gravity, weakness, stupor, lethargy

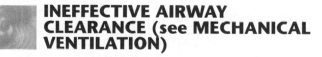

INEFFECTIVE AIRWAY CLEARANCE (see MECHANICAL VENTILATION)

Related to: decreased level of consciousness, secretions, obstruction, pulmonary congestion

Defining Characteristics: dyspnea, apnea, cyanosis, decreased breath sounds, rhonchi, crackles, wheezing, ineffective or absent cough, restlessness, lethargy, orthopnea, abnormal arterial blood gases, tachycardia, hypertension

IMBALANCED NUTRITION: LESS THAN BODY REQUIREMENTS (see BURNS)

Related to: increased metabolic rate, decreased intake of nutrients, changes in normal eating pattern

Defining Characteristics: hyperthermia, increased metabolic rate, sepsis, weight loss, loss of muscle mass, altered taste, lack of interest in eating, diarrhea, hair loss, capillary fragility, pale mucous membranes, sore, inflamed oral cavity, muscle weakness

ANXIETY (see MECHANICAL VENTILATION)

Related to: threat of death, sensory impairment, sepsis, change in environment, change in support status, change in health status, life-threatening crises

Defining Characteristics: fear, restlessness, muscle tension, apprehension, helplessness, communication of uncertainty, sense of impending doom, worry

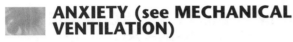

ADDITIONAL NURSING DIAGNOSES

INEFFECTIVE TISSUE PERFUSION: CEREBRAL, CARDIOPULMONARY, GASTROINTESTINAL, RENAL, AND PERIPHERAL

Related to: vasoconstriction, microembolism, vascular occlusion, hypovolemia, increased oxygen consumption, inadequate oxygen delivery, alteration in utilization of oxygen by tissues, bleeding

Defining Characteristics: decreased peripheral pulses, prolonged capillary refill time, pallor, cyanosis, erythema, paresthesias, pain, tissue edema, lethargy, confusion, oliguria, anuria, abnormal ABGs, decreased hemoglobin and hematocrit

Outcome Criteria

✔ Patient will have adequate perfusion to all body systems.

NOC: *Tissue Perfusion*

INTERVENTIONS	RATIONALES
Monitor vital signs q 1 hour, noting trends.	Hypotension occurs when microorganisms enter the bloodstream and activate chemical substances that result in vasodilation, decreased systemic vascular resistance, and hypovolemia. Tachypnea may be the first symptom of sepsis as the body responds to endotoxins and developing hypoxia. Bradycardia and hypotension may indicate increasing arteriovenous exchange, which can result in decreased tissue perfusion.
Monitor hemodynamic pressures if available, at least every 1–2 hours and prn.	When shock progresses to cold stage, cardiac output decreases in response to decreased contractility and alterations in afterload and preload. Decreased CVP and PA pressures may indicate hypovolemic state and hypoperfusion. Increases in PA pressures and CVP may indicate too rapid fluid or blood resuscitation and fluid overload as a result, or cardiac decompensation. Fluid shifting may cause third spacing and fluid overload, and monitoring hemodynamics can facilitate early identification of changes in trends.
Monitor ECG for changes and treat according to hospital protocol.	Tachycardia occurs in response to hypovolemia and circulating endotoxins. Dysrhythmias may occur from hypoxia, acid–base imbalances, electrolyte imbalances, or shock. Emergent treatment may be required to sustain life if lethal dysrhythmias occur.
Monitor mental status and level of consciousness for changes.	May indicate impending or present hypoxia or acidosis leading to decreased cerebral perfusion.
Auscultate lung fields for adventitious breath sounds.	May indicate fluid overload in response to fluid resuscitation or presence of congestive failure.
Observe for changes in peripheral skin color and temperature.	Vasodilation may occur in the early phase of shock with warm, pink, dry skin, but as shock progresses, vasoconstriction occurs and reduces peripheral blood flow resulting in mottling, or pale to dusky skin that is cold and clammy.
Monitor intake and output every hour. Notify physician if urine <30 cc/hr.	As renal perfusion is compromised by vasoconstriction or microemboli, oliguria or anuria may develop.

INTERVENTIONS	RATIONALES
Palpate abdomen and auscultate for bowel sounds.	Absence of bowel sounds may indicate decreased perfusion to the mesentery from vasoconstriction that may result in paralytic ileus.
Administer IV fluids as ordered.	Large volumes may be required to maintain circulating volume from hypovolemic state, but must be monitored to identify and treat fluid overloading.
Administer oxygen as ordered.	Provides supplemental oxygen necessary for cellular perfusion and to relieve hypoxia.
Administer vasoactive drugs as ordered.	May be required to maintain pressure and hemodynamics at adequate levels to maintain perfusion to body systems.
Turn patient every 2 hours and prn.	Changing position may help avoid lung congestion, skin breakdown, and improve vital capacity.
Monitor lab work and notify physician of significant abnormalities.	Abnormal creatine kinase, and lactate dehydrogenase may indicate tissue damage and decreased oxygen exchange in lungs. Decreased hemoglobin and hematocrit may result in ischemia to tissues, and should be monitored to help establish fluid and blood replacement requirements, and WBC should be monitored with differentials to identify infection and efficacy of treatment being given. Coagulation profiles may be altered by endotoxins, administration of anticoagulants, and so forth, and should be monitored to help guide correct dosing of medications. BUN, creatinine, creatinine clearance and urine osmolality may change as renal function is impaired.
Observe for oozing at puncture sites, petechiae, ecchymoses, or bleeding from any area.	May indicate presence or impending DIC or coagulation problem.
Monitor for drug toxicity signs and symptoms.	Decreased perfusion may increase half-life and decrease metabolism of therapeutic drugs and cause toxic reactions.
Instruct patient/family in medical diagnosis and treatment as warranted.	Patient may be too ill to comprehend information. Information promotes knowledge and assists

INTERVENTIONS	RATIONALES
	family to take active role in patient's health status and maintenance.
Instruct patient to notify nurse if increased rest periods are needed between activities.	Resting helps to conserve energy and lessens tissue hypoperfusion.
Involve therapists in patient care as ordered/warranted.	May be required to increase ability to function independently if patient survives.
Instruct patient/family regarding dietary changes and needs.	Patient may require higher nutrient content that can be obtained orally, and may require enteral or parenteral nutrition because of impairment of gastrointestinal perfusion.
Instruct patient in relaxation techniques, guided imagery, and so forth.	Helps to improve vasodilation and prevents vasoconstriction that may result from anxiety.
Instruct patient in signs/symptoms to report to nurse/physician such as bleeding, pain, numbness, and so forth.	May be signs of impending or present hypoperfusion of an organ system which requires immediate treatment to promote effective and beneficial treatment.
Instruct patient/family regarding avoidance of over-the-counter medications unless authorized by physician.	Some drugs can be nephrotoxic, or can accentuate or negate effects of other drugs being taken for medical regime.

NIC: *Shock Management*

Discharge or Maintenance Evaluation

- Patient will have stable vital signs and hemodynamic parameters.
- Patient will have warm skin, with palpable peripheral pulses that are equal bilaterally.
- Patient will be neurologically stable, and have adequate perfusion to all body systems.

INEFFECTIVE THERMOREGULATION

Related to: trauma, sepsis, hemorrhage, systemic reaction to infection

Defining Characteristics: warm or cool skin, temperature elevation, temperature below normal, flushed skin, pallor, cyanosis, decreased capillary refill time, tachycardia, tachypnea, shivering, seizures, increased or decreased metabolic rates

Outcome Criteria

✔ Patient will have stable vital signs, with normothermic temperature.

✔ Patient will have warm and dry skin, with no further complications.

NOC: *Thermoregulation*

INTERVENTIONS	RATIONALES
Monitor vital signs q 1–2 hours, and prn. Notify physician of significant abnormalities. Use consistent method of temperature evaluation, with optimal use of pulmonary artery thermistor.	Evaluation of temperature establishes need for further intervention, allows for accurate data comparisons, and identifies efficacy of treatment protocol. Hyperthermia may produce hypoxia by increasing oxygen demand and consumption that occurs because of increased tissue metabolism. This increase may result in dyspnea, tachypnea, and tachycardia with dysrhythmias.
Assess neurologic status q 4 hours and prn, and notify physician of any significant changes.	Alterations in level of consciousness or orientation may be a result of tissue hypoxia. Hyperthermia increases cerebral edema and intracranial pressure, and hypothermia decreases metabolic rate.
Administer antipyretics as ordered, but avoid aspirin-containing products when possible.	Medication helps to decrease fever, and aspirin and aspirin-containing medications may result in hemorrhage.
Administer tepid sponge baths, or utilize cooling blankets to lower hyperthermia.	Helps to reduce excessive fever.
Administer IV fluids as ordered. If patient is allowed, provide oral fluids.	Maintains fluid hydration and balance. Utilization of oral fluids encourages patient to participate in care.
If patient is hypothermic, utilize warming blankets and adjust environmental temperature.	Temperature of the environment affects body temperature regulation.
Instruct patient/family regarding signs/symptoms of changes in body temperature, and methods to avoid hyperthermia or hypothermia.	Provides knowledge, plan of action, and includes patient in helping to take an active role in his own care.

NIC: *Temperature Regulation*

Discharge or Maintenance Evaluation

■ Patient will be normothermic, with stable vital signs.

■ Patient will exhibit no neurological symptoms of complications that might be associated with temperature fluctuations.

■ Patient and family will be able to accurately verbalize understanding of instructions and information given.

IMPAIRED URINARY ELIMINATION

Related to: renal hypoperfusion, disseminated intravascular coagulation, cellular injury, inability to metabolize toxins from kidneys, nephrotoxic antimicrobial treatment

Defining Characteristics: dysuria, urgency, urinary retention, incontinence, urinary frequency, nocturia

Outcome Criteria

✔ Patient will maintain fluid balance and intake will equal output.

✔ Patient will exhibit no complications with urinary system.

NOC: *Urinary Elimination*

INTERVENTIONS	RATIONALES
Monitor patient's ability to urinate and note voiding pattern, I&O, and complaints of nocturia, dysuria, or frequency.	Intake and output data is indispensable for identifying fluid imbalances and for providing appropriate treatment. If patient is unable to urinate, an indwelling catheter should be placed to ensure accuracy of output information.
Assist with bladder training as needed.	Adaptation to routine and normal physiologic function may result with treatment plan.
If patient requires catheterization on an intermittent basis, catheterize patient as ordered, recording amounts voided spontaneously and residual amounts via catheter.	Catheterization based on a schedule can help to promote normal voiding, prevent infection, and preserve ureterovesical functioning.
If indwelling catheter is required, provide good perineal care at least every shift. Change dressing	Reduces risk of infection, provides feeling of cleanliness, and ensures observation for complications.

INTERVENTIONS	RATIONALES
and clean catheter site for supra-pubic catheters per protocol.	Suprapubic catheters provide increased mobility for patient and decrease risk for bladder infections.
Encourage oral intake up to 3 L/day if condition tolerates.	Adequate oral hydration dilutes chemical materials within body, and helps to maintain hydration status.
Instruct patient in all procedures.	Provides knowledge, decreases fear, and facilitates compliance with treatment regimen.
Instruct patient/family regarding techniques for catheterization if these are to be utilized post discharge.	Knowledge of procedures and ability to perform return demon-stration accurately reduces anxiety and allows for independence.
Instruct patient/family on signs/symptoms of urinary infections, and to notify physician of complications.	Provides troubleshooting plan of care, and facilitates knowledge to provide for timely intervention for prompt recognition of problems.

NIC: *Urinary Elimination Management*

Discharge or Maintenance Evaluation

- Patient will be able to have equivalent intake and output.
- Patient will be free of infection, and urinalysis will be within normal limits.
- Patient/family will be able to accurately perform procedures, accurately verbalize signs and symp-toms to be aware of, and methods of trou-bleshooting problems.

INTERRUPTED FAMILY PROCESSES

Related to: family members unable to meet patient's physical needs, patient unable to meet family's emo-tional needs, trauma, situational crisis, change in health status of family member, changes in family's financial situation, changes in family's social status, threat of death, threat of loss of family member

Defining Characteristics: unavailability of response to family members, inability to meet family's needs or expectations, changes in power alliances, increased somatic complaints, increased stress behaviors, expres-sion of conflict with family or others, changes in sup-port status, unavailability of emotional support, inability to express feelings, inability to accept feelings of family members, inability of family members to relate to each other, rigidity of role function, inability to constructively cope with traumatic experience

Outcome Criteria

- ✔ Family members will be able to agree on a primary decision maker and spokesman for the family.
- ✔ Family members will develop tools for construc-tively responding to patient and to other family members.
- ✔ Family members will assume duties carried out by the patient and will provide emotional support to other family members.

NOC: *Family Coping*

INTERVENTIONS	RATIONALES
Assist family to identify person who will be assuming the role as head of household.	Helps to establish family hierarchy and ensures ability to function on a day-to-day basis.
Emphasize role and position of patient within the family.	Helps family members to under-stand changes within family dynamics.
Provide head of family with updated information on patient's condition and information required for decision making.	Avoids misinterpretation and places responsibility for commu-nication within the family unit.
Provide adequate time with head of family and support regarding changes in role and additional responsibilities.	Encourages family member to ask questions, discuss feelings, and ask for help in decision making process.
Provide opportunities for all family members to participate in family conferences, if possible.	Helps family identify goals and work toward common goals to facilitate effective family dynamics.
Instruct family members in com-munity resources, social services, support groups, and so forth.	Provides access to additional coping resources.
Instruct family members regard-ing patient's disease process, updates, and information on procedures.	Provides information and knowl-edge to allay fears and to assist in making decisions.

NIC: *Family Mobilization*

Discharge or Maintenance Evaluation

- Family members will be able to identify an individual to take on head of household responsibilities.

- Family members will rally together and assume responsibilities formerly carried out by patient.

- Family members will be able to share feelings and communicate with each other effectively.

- Family members will be able to access community resources.

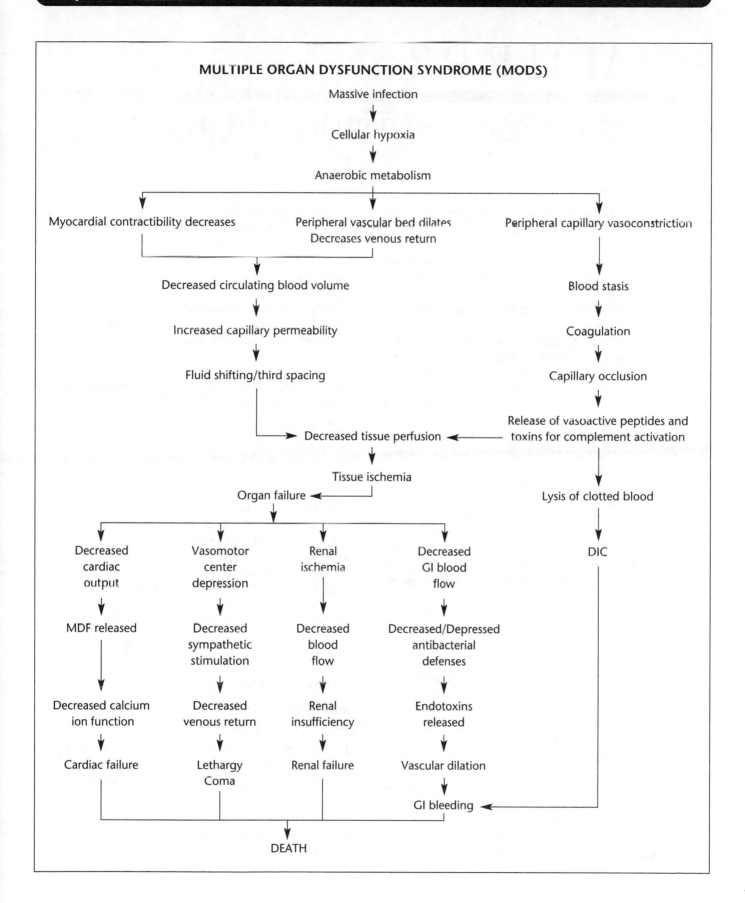

CHAPTER 9.2

ACUTE POISONING/DRUG OVERDOSE

Attempts to end one's life by use of excessive amounts of medication may be executed for many reasons. Active self-destructive behavior usually results from the patient's perception of an overwhelming catastrophic event in his life, in conjunction with the lack of appropriate coping strategies, and is visualized as a means of escape from the sensed threat to self.

Suicidal patients are frequently ambivalent about wanting to die, and may have visions of last-minute rescue. The suicidal person may feel despair, guilt, shame, hopelessness, boredom, depression, weariness, or dependency, and when the point is reached when the person perceives that life no longer has meaning and despair is overwhelming, the patient acts on those emotions. Suicide may be considered the last logical step when the person perceives that others do not want him or her around or that the problem can never be reconciled.

Usually, an attempt at causing death is the culmination of a process in which the person had ideations about suicide, verbal or nonverbal threats of that intention, and gestures which included attempts of causing self-injury without actual intention to cause death.

Suicide is the eighth leading cause of death in this country today, and the second leading cause of death in young people. Drug ingestion is the most frequent method utilized with suicide attempts, partially because of the availability of medications, and partially to avoid more violent means of death, such as with weapons or by hanging.

There are instances in which the person is not attempting suicide, but experiences an accidental toxic ingestion level. If the chemical concentration of a substance does not exceed a dangerous measurement, the effects of the ingestion are usually reversible. Organ dysfunction, such as renal insufficiency or failure, or liver hypoperfusion, may cause a normal dosage of medication, such as analgesics or cardiovascular drugs, to reach a toxic level.

Cleaning solutions are the most frequently implicated substances in accidental exposure that are reported to poison control centers, followed by analgesics, cosmetics, plants, cold medications, animal bites, pesticides, topical medications, foreign bodies, and then food. The most common sources of lethal ingestion include analgesics, antidepressants, sedatives, recreational drugs, alcohol, fumes and gases, asthmatic medications, and automobile products.

MEDICAL CARE

Laboratory: drug screens may be used to identify agent used in an accidental or purposeful poisoning; alcohol level to assess concurrent use or toxicity; electrolytes may be abnormal because of trauma or interaction with medication; hematocrit may be decreased with hypovolemia; drug levels, such as phenobarbital or acetaminophen, may be elevated because of toxicity; renal profile may show renal insufficiency; liver profile may show hepatic dysfunction, especially with acetaminophen overdose; coagulation profiles may be abnormal; urinalysis may show low specific gravity, increased protein, hematuria, oxalate crystals, or metabolic by-products from drug overdose; pregnancy test performed on all females of childbearing age, including girls 12–17 years of age, to determine if morbidity is also involved for fetus

Radiography: chest X-rays may show aspiration pneumonia or pulmonary edema complications

Electrocardiogram: used to identify conduction problems or dysrhythmias that may occur from drug overdosage, electrolyte disturbances, or with congestive failure

Dialysis: hemodialysis or hemoperfusion may be performed to remove some drugs when levels are severely elevated

Diuretics: may be required to force osmotic diuresis with agents such as mannitol, to manage certain forms of overdose

Acetylcysteine: Mucomyst is treatment of choice with acetaminophen overdose

Charcoal: used to bind poisons, toxins, or other irritants, increases absorption in the GI tract, and helps to inactivate toxins until excreted

COMMON NURSING DIAGNOSES

INEFFECTIVE BREATHING PATTERN (see MECHANICAL VENTILATION)

Related to: neurologic impairment, respiratory depression from drug, obstruction, pulmonary edema, pneumonia

Defining Characteristics: apnea, dyspnea, lethargy, stupor, coma, abnormal arterial blood gases, decreased oxygen saturation, shallow respirations, tachypnea, stridor, adventitious breath sounds

INEFFECTIVE AIRWAY CLEARANCE (see PNEUMONIA)

Related to: obstruction of trachea, cognitive impairment from drug ingestion

Defining Characteristics: dyspnea, apnea, cyanosis, decreased breath sounds, rhonchi, crackles, wheezing, ineffective or absent cough, restlessness, lethargy, orthopnea, abnormal arterial blood gases

INEFFECTIVE INDIVIDUAL COPING (see MECHANICAL VENTILATION)

Related to: crisis, drug overdose, loss of control, depression

Defining Characteristics: verbal manipulation, inability to meet basic needs, inability to effectively deal with crisis, ineffective defense mechanisms, irritability, hostility

ADDITIONAL NURSING DIAGNOSES

RISK FOR INJURY

Related to: toxic effects of ingested drugs

Defining Characteristics: respiratory arrest, pulmonary edema, shock, cardiac dysrhythmias, conduction changes, encephalopathy, amblyopia, edema, bronchoconstriction, blindness, blurring of vision, hypotension, hypothermia, seizures, hypertension, rhabdomyolysis, oliguria, anuria, heart failure, mental status changes, impaired airway, breathing, and/or circulation, hyperthermia, nausea, vomiting, diarrhea, report by self or others of ingestion of toxic substance

Outcome Criteria

✔ Patient will achieve and maintain function of all organ and body systems and be able to eliminate ingested drug.

NOC: *Risk Detection*

INTERVENTIONS	RATIONALES
Obtain past health history, with names of medications taken, allergies, past illnesses, last meal eaten, and events occurring prior to ingestion of the toxic substance. Assess patient for patent airway, breathing, circulation, level of consciousness, other injuries or signs via visual examination, and consult with poison control center.	Provides information that may be invaluable to discerning what substance has been taken or used, possible reasons (i.e., terminal illness), and information that will be necessary should surgical procedures be required. Adequacy of perfusion and airway is primary goal, and maintenance of perfusion of all body systems may be related to observations of nurse during initial critical time.
Monitor vital signs every 1-2 hours and prn.	Facilitates early identification of changes and prompt interventions. Drug overdose may cause CNS depression with hypothermia, cardiac dysfunction from toxic drug levels, and pressure changes with volume imbalances.
Monitor core body temperature, ideally with hemodynamic catheter thermistor.	Provides accurate core body temperature information and can be used to identify thermoregulatory problems and correct them promptly.
Monitor ECG for changes in rhythm, dysrhythmias, or conduction problems, and treat according to hospital protocol.	Overdoses of tricyclic antidepressants may cause prolongation of PR, QT, and QRS complex; ST segment and T wave abnormalities, intraventricular conduction defects, bundle branch blocks, and dysrhythmias that may lead to cardiac arrest.

(continues)

(continued)

INTERVENTIONS	RATIONALES
Maintain airway and provide supplemental oxygen as warranted.	Patients with overdoses may be unable to protect their own airway and have bronchoconstriction or obstruction leading to respiratory arrest and death. Supplemental oxygen may be required to offset acid–base imbalances that result from overdosage.
Auscultate lung fields for breath sounds and presence of adventitious sounds.	Pulmonary edema may result from overdoses of barbiturates, sedatives, hypnotics, and tranquilizers. Changes in breath sounds may identify impending edema or heart failure.
Auscultate heart for tones and presence of abnormal sounds.	Gallops, murmurs, and rubs may indicate the presence or impending presence of complications such as pulmonary edema or heart failure.
Administer IV fluids as ordered.	Crystalloid solutions are normally used to treat hypovolemia which may occur because of compromised circulatory status.
Administer naloxone as ordered.	Reverses effects of narcotic agents and may be required to manage CNS depression or respiratory depression.
Administer 100 cc of 50% dextrose IV as ordered.	May be given to rule out hypoglycemia as cause for comatose state. Hypoglycemia can occur from exposure to insulin, oral hypoglycemics, ethanol, or salicylates.
Administer thiamine 100 mg IV as ordered.	Routinely given to avert precipitation of Wernicke–Korsakoff syndrome, an encephalopathy that occurs in chronic alcoholism caused by damage to the medial aspects of the temporal lobes, especially the hippocampal gyri and hippocampi.
Administer antidote, once substance is identified.	Some of the more commonly known antidotes include: Mucomyst for acetominophen, Flumazenil for benzodiazepines, sodium bicarbonate for cyclic antidepressants, amyl nitrate for cyanide, Pyridoxine for INH, and naloxone for opioids.
If no antidote is known or available for particular substance ingested, maintain organ function, and attempt to limit	Lavage removes any nonabsorbed substance, and general management of cleansing of system should occur to limit effects on

INTERVENTIONS	RATIONALES
the absorption of any remaining substance.	specific organs and tissues to prevent long-term damage.
Monitor intake and output every 2 hours; compare 24-hour totals, and observe for changes in urine character and color.	Assists with estimation of fluid balance within body. Myoglobin may be present if rhabdomyolysis occurs as a result of overdose.
Insert nasogastric tube, aspirate fluid for analysis, lavage stomach, and administer activated charcoal as ordered.	Lavage is done to remove any drugs that may be left in stomach to prevent further absorption of the drug. Aspirate may be sent to lab for analysis of drugs ingested to provide identification for appropriate treatment. Charcoal is given to absorb drugs from gastric contents to prevent systemic absorption.
Administer osmotic diuretics as ordered.	May be required to manage overdoses of ethanol, methanol, ethylene glycol, and isoniazid, but must be done using caution to avoid fluid overload and electrolyte imbalances.
Administer sodium bicarbonate as ordered.	May be required for management of salicylate poisoning to alkalinize urine.
Administer ascorbic acid or ammonium chloride as ordered.	May be required for management of amphetamine or PCP overdoses to acidify urine.
Administer Mucomyst as ordered.	May be required for management of acetaminophen overdose to decrease absorption and limit hepatic dysfunction.
Administer physostigmine as ordered.	May be required for management of tricyclic antidepressant overdoses to reverse the anticholinergic effects, but should be given cautiously to prevent cholinergic toxicity.
Administer polyethylene glycol with electrolytes for complete bowel irrigation.	Helps to clear the gastrointestinal tract without causing emesis or fluid or electrolyte imbalance. Medication is indicated only for slowly dissolving and sustained-release drugs, and is contraindicated if the patient has a gastrointestinal obstruction, perforation, or bleeding.
Assist with hemodialysis, hemoperfusion, or hemofiltration, as warranted.	Hemodialysis may be required to correct metabolic acid-base disturbances, with hyperkalemia, and fluid overload. Hemoperfusion is superior to dialysis for clearing substances that are

INTERVENTIONS	RATIONALES
	bound to plasma proteins. Hemofiltration use is investigational; it can eliminate larger molecules and can be utilized after the other modalities to prevent toxic level rebound.
Monitor patient for cardiovascular compromise if he is suspected of body stuffing or body packing.	If patient has hurriedly tried to hide illicit drugs and either swallow them, or stuff containers in body cavities, the potential for a massive and sudden reaction is high if the containers break.
Prepare patient for surgery if patient has become symptomatic while in police custody.	May indicate that the patient has attempted "body packing", which includes swallowing containers, condoms, balloons, or bags filled with illegal substances, and when one of these packages contacts the alkaline environment of the small intestine, the contents burst, causing a massive overdose. Laparotomy or other surgical intervention to remove the container and remainder of drug may be a lifesaving procedure.
Prepare patient/family for dialysis procedures.	Hemodialysis or hemoperfusion may be required for removal of drugs from system in severe intoxication when levels are potentially lethal or the toxin may be metabolized to a more lethal substance.
Ensure suicide precautions are exercised—removal of all potentially dangerous items from room and reach, close observation at all times, keeping exiting windows and doors impenetrable, providing all medications in liquid form, accompanying the patient to other ancillary areas, and avoidance of secret pacts with patient.	Maintenance of precautions facilitate a safe environment and allows for identification of potential problems. A patient who has made one attempt at suicide may attempt to complete the job and may be quite resourceful with items to perform the deed. Medications should be given in liquid form to ensure that the patient has swallowed the medication rather than saving it to use as suicide attempt later.
Provide padded side rails, with rails elevated at all times.	Provides safe environment and reduces risk of injury, especially if patient has a seizure.
Provide information to patient/family regarding community resources, therapists, detox centers, counselors, and so forth.	May be required for postdischarge care to seek further help for care in handling problems.

NIC: *Substance Use Treatment: Overdose*

Discharge or Maintenance Evaluation

- Patient will have stable vital signs and neurological status.
- Patient will have stable function of all body systems.
- Patient will have absorption of drugs minimized and maximal elimination of absorbed drugs.
- Patient will remain free of other injury.

RISK FOR VIOLENCE SELF-DIRECTED

Related to: drug overdose, psychological status, dysfunctional family, excessive stress or anxiety, history of suicide attempts, threatened loss of important person or possession, low self-esteem, chronic illness, terminal disease

Defining Characteristics: feelings of loneliness, hopelessness, helplessness, perceived or real loss of significant person, job, health status, or control, unpredictable behavior, threats, low self-esteem, dependence on drugs or alcohol, withdrawal from substances, communication of suicidal ideations, depression, hostility, loss of interest in appearance, acting out behaviors, low energy level, insomnia, self-destructive behavior, self-mutilation, social isolation, feelings of rejection by others

Outcome Criteria

✔ Patient will achieve and maintain psychologic stability and seek assistance with mental health providers.

NOC: *Distorted Thought Control*

INTERVENTIONS	RATIONALES
Respond to all suicidal threats seriously.	Prompt intervention decreases possibility of suicide attempt.
Ask patient directly if he or she has thought about suicide, and if patient responds affirmatively, ask what he or she plans to do.	Potential for suicide increases if the patient has a viable plan. Bringing up the subject of suicide does not place the idea into the patient's head, but allows for the patient to express feelings he or she may have not been able to verbalize to anyone else.
Ensure environment is calming, darkened, with enough light for observation of patient.	Facilitates decreased fear and anxiety which may result with violent behavior.
Approach patient in a nonjudgmental, nonthreatening manner.	May have a calming effect on patient.

(continues)

(continued)

INTERVENTIONS	RATIONALES
Listen to patient and what he has to say about his current situation without reacting emotionally.	Allows patient to verbalize problems. Emotional responses from caregivers may exacerbate hostile reactions from patient.
Confirm understanding of patient's problem, but do not reinforce denial.	Fosters communication and facilitates realistic feelings and methods for coping.
Assist patient to verbalize emotions, anger, and other stressors, and to develop a plan for dealing with them.	Provides safe outlets for patient to express feelings and helps to work out realistic solutions for solving problems.
Remove objects from room, such as razors, belts, glass objects, and pills.	Items may be used by patient to injure self, and removal of these items ensures patient's safety.
Monitor patient closely, placing patient next to nurse's station, arranging for one-on-one care when possible.	Assists to protect patient from harming self.
Supervise all medication administration, making sure patient does swallow medication. Be alert for any reactions to these drugs.	Prevents hoarding of doses of medication by patient to try suicidal attempt again.
Instruct patient/family on community resources, hot lines, crisis centers, ministerial counselors, etc.	Provides knowledge and assistance of resources available once patient is discharged.
Consult mental health provider/professional as warranted.	Allows for effective therapeutic psychological treatment to discern appropriate methods of coping with crisis.

INTERVENTIONS	RATIONALES
Encourage family members to discuss their feelings and methods of coping.	Validates their feelings and responses and may assist them in finding more appropriate methods to cope with crisis.
Discuss actions to take if patient expresses suicidal ideations or attempts.	Patient may be more likely to try suicidal attempt again if situations or coping strategies are not changed. Understanding that if the patient has a definite plan for suicide, the more likely it is that he will be successful at ending his life, and that immediate intervention will be required.

NIC: *Suicide Prevention*

Discharge or Maintenance Evaluation

- Patient will achieve psychological equilibrium and have no further suicidal attempts/gestures.
- Patient will be able to cope with crises in an appropriate manner, and will be able to effectively search out community resources for assistance.
- Patient and family will be able to verbalize feelings and effectively achieve therapeutic communication.
- Patient and family will be able to access available resources.

ACUTE POISONING/DRUG OVERDOSE

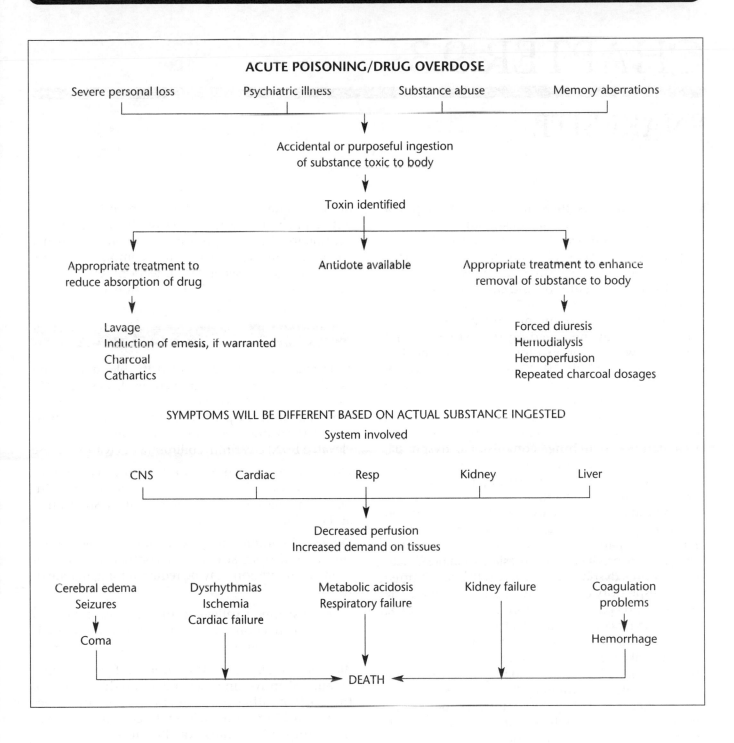

Severe personal loss   Psychiatric illness   Substance abuse   Memory aberrations

Accidental or purposeful ingestion
of substance toxic to body

Toxin identified

Appropriate treatment to
reduce absorption of drug

Antidote available

Appropriate treatment to enhance
removal of substance to body

Lavage
Induction of emesis, if warranted
Charcoal
Cathartics

Forced diuresis
Hemodialysis
Hemoperfusion
Repeated charcoal dosages

SYMPTOMS WILL BE DIFFERENT BASED ON ACTUAL SUBSTANCE INGESTED

System involved

CNS   Cardiac   Resp   Kidney   Liver

Decreased perfusion
Increased demand on tissues

Cerebral edema
Seizures

Coma

Dysrhythmias
Ischemia
Cardiac failure

Metabolic acidosis
Respiratory failure

Kidney failure

Coagulation
problems

Hemorrhage

DEATH

CHAPTER 9.3

SNAKEBITE

In the United States, there are actually two types of poisonous snakes—coral snakes and pit vipers, which include rattlesnakes, water moccasins, and copperheads. Coral snakes are usually nocturnal creatures and less active than pit vipers, but tend to bite with a chewing motion and cause significant tissue damage.

Snakebites may occur on any portion of the body, but usually are noted on the extremities. Pit viper bites with envenomation result in immediate pain and edema within 10–20 minutes. Other symptoms include fever, ecchymoses, blisters, and local necrosis, as well as nausea, vomiting, diarrhea, metallic or rubbery taste, tachycardia, hypotension, and shock. Neurotoxins may cause numbness, tingling, fasciculations, twitching, convulsions, dysphasia, occasional paralysis, respiratory distress, coma, and death. Pit viper bites may also impair coagulation and cause internal bleeding.

Coral snake bites usually have a delayed reaction up to several hours, and may result in very little or no tissue pain, edema, or necrosis. The neurotoxic venom produces paresthesias, weakness, nausea, vomiting, dysphagia, excessive salivation, blurred vision, respiratory distress and failure, loss of muscle coordination, paralysis, abnormal reflexes, shock, cardiovascular collapse, and death. Coral snake bites may also result in coagulopathy problems.

The snake venom is a mixture of several proteins, enzymes, and polypeptides, and may produce several toxic reactions in patients who have been bitten. Correct diagnosis is imperative to treat the specific envenomation accurately and in a timely manner. Snakebites are critical emergencies and require precise identification of the snake as well as presence of envenomation. Designation of severity of the bite is commonly rated as minor, moderate, or severe, and depends on the presence of symptoms, depth of envenomation, and laboratory findings.

Treatment of snakebite involves administration of antivenin after a test dose for horse serum sensitivity is performed. If this sensitivity is present, diphenhydramine may be given prior to the antivenin. Swelling may necessitate surgical intervention to relieve the pressure and to prevent further vascular damage, and ensuing complications are usually related to secondary infection, renal failure, disseminated intravascular coagulation, or gangrene.

MEDICAL CARE

Laboratory: CBC used to identify blood loss and hemoconcentration; fibrinogen level, platelets, PT, PTT, and APTT to evaluate clotting; blood type and cross-matching to provide blood products as warranted; renal and liver studies to identify dysfunction; elevated BUN, creatinine, bilirubin, or creatine kinase

Electrocardiogram: used to establish a baseline for identification of problems that may occur with hemodynamic changes and to identify dysrhythmias and conduction problems

Surgery: fasciotomy may be required to relieve pressure caused from swelling or compartmental syndrome; amputation may be required for gangrene or necrosis

Analgesics: used to alleviate and/or control the pain related to envenomation and swelling; morphine is usually not given because of its vasodilator action

Antivenin: required as the antidote for snakebite; amount of antivenin is dependent on the severity of the reaction rather than patient weight, and ranges from 3 to 15 or more vials; children usually require more antivenin because of the ratio of venom to body size

Sedation: may be required to alleviate anxiety and to facilitate compliance with treatments

Tetanus toxoid: given to prevent complication that may be induced with infection from snakebite

Corticosteroids: usually are not recommended in the initial phase after snakebite because of the enhancement of the venom action and blocking of anti-venin; may be warranted to treat shock or allergic reactions

Diphenhydramine: used when the patient has a reaction to the horse serum used for antivenin, or for other anaphylactic reactions

COMMON NURSING DIAGNOSES

ACUTE PAIN (see FROSTBITE)

Related to: snakebite, swelling, edema, surgical procedures, decreased tissue perfusion, anxiety, envenomation

Defining Characteristics: communication of pain, moaning, crying, facial grimacing, inability to concentrate

FEAR/ANXIETY (see MECHANICAL VENTILATION)

Related to: snakebite, threat of death, fear of disfigurement or scarring, hospitalization, mechanical ventilation, envenomation

Defining Characteristics: expressions of apprehension, tension, restlessness, insomnia, expressions of concern, fear of unknown, tachypnea, tachycardia, inability to concentrate or focus

ADDITIONAL NURSING DIAGNOSES

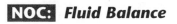 RISK FOR DEFICIENT FLUID VOLUME

Related to: hemorrhage, third spacing, altered coagulation, increased cellular membrane permeability, shock

Defining Characteristics: tachycardia, hypotension, changes in mental status, restlessness, decreased urine output, prolonged capillary refill, pallor, mottling, diaphoresis, poor turgor

Outcome Criteria

✔ Patient will achieve and maintain fluid balance with adequate urinary output.

NOC: *Fluid Balance*

INTERVENTIONS	RATIONALES
Monitor vital signs q 1 hour, and notify physician of significant changes or trends.	Hypotension may indicate that the circulating fluid volume is decreased. Changes in vital signs may indicate the amount of blood loss but may not change until loss is greater than 1000 cc. Hypovolemic shock may occur resulting from hemorrhage, third spacing, and the release of vasoactive substances and coagulopathy from the snakebite.
Measure hemodynamics if pulmonary artery catheter has been placed. Notify physician for abnormal parameters.	CVP, or right atrial pressure, gives estimate of fluid volume status. Dehydration may be reflected by CVP of less than 5, while overhydration may be reflected at levels over 18 cm H_2O. Hemodynamic values may help to evaluate the body's response to the circulating volume and bleeding status.
Observe for restlessness, anxiety, mental changes, changes in level of consciousness, or weakness.	Changes may reflect the severity of fluid loss.
Observe for bleeding from all orifices and puncture sites, and for presence/development of ecchymoses, hematomas, or petechiae.	May indicate impaired coagulation, impending or present DIC, or inadequate replacement of clotting factors.
Monitor intake and output hourly and notify physician for significant imbalances or urinary output less than 30 cc/hr for two hours.	May indicate fluid volume deficit, and establishes a guide for fluid and blood product replacement.
Administer IV fluids as ordered. Two IV sites should be maintained.	Replaces fluid loss, allows for administration of vasoactive drugs, plasma extenders, and emergency medications, as well as the administration of antivenin. Two sites are recommended to facilitate simultaneous fluid and blood resuscitation in critical settings. Crystalloids do not work as well as colloids because of the increased capillary permeability.
Administer blood and/or blood products as ordered.	Whole blood may be required for acute bleeding episodes with shock due to the lack of clotting factors in packed red blood cells. Fresh frozen plasma and/or platelets may be required to replace clotting factors and to promote platelet function.

(continues)

(continued)

INTERVENTIONS	RATIONALES
Instruct on use of antivenin, effects, side effects. Test dose for horse serum.	Provides knowledge and decreases anxiety. Skin test is required to identify hypersensitivities to the antivenin and frequently is repeated to ensure that the results are not false. If a reaction is noted, the antivenin is still given but is preceded by diphenhydramine.
Prepare patient for placement of pulmonary artery catheter.	Provides knowledge to the patient, and catheter is invaluable for identifying changes in fluid status and hemodynamic responses to those changes.

NIC: *Hemorrhage Control*

Discharge or Maintenance Evaluation

- Patient will have stable vital signs and urinary output.
- Patient will have balanced intake and output.
- Patient will have good turgor, moist membranes, and adequate capillary refill times.
- Patient will be free of hemorrhage or abnormal coagulation.
- Patient will have no transfusion reactions.

INEFFECTIVE TISSUE PERFUSION: PERIPHERAL, CARDIOPULMONARY, RENAL, CEREBRAL, GASTROINTESTINAL

Related to: envenomation, edema, compartmental syndrome, coagulopathy, hemorrhage, hypovolemia, neurotoxins

Defining Characteristics: hypotension, tachycardia, edema, decreased or absent pulses, inflammation, reddened or cyanotic skin, necrosis, gangrene, mental changes, restlessness, anxiety, abnormal hemodynamic parameters, abnormal arterial blood gases, dysphagia

Outcome Criteria

✔ Patient will have adequate tissue perfusion to all organ systems.

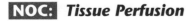

NOC: *Tissue Perfusion*

INTERVENTIONS	RATIONALES
Observe puncture wound for bleeding, color, temperature, and note changes from baseline.	Skin normally changes after a snakebite from inflamed to a dark, cyanotic color. Changes in the wound and local tissues may reflect the action of the venom and potential complications.
Measure the circumference of the extremity involved initially and then every 2–4 hours.	Monitors for swelling and inflammation, and helps to identify the need for fasciotomy.
Palpate, or use doppler, to discern peripheral pulses distal to the snakebite, and notify physician for absence or decrease.	Edema may result in compartmental syndrome and obstruct circulation to the extremity causing ischemia, necrosis, and gangrene.
Assist with fasciotomy or insertion of catheter into the tissues of the edematous extremity.	Reduces tissue pressure and prevents tissue dehiscence and other complications.
Administer oxygen as warranted.	Provides supplemental oxygen which may be decreased because of hemorrhage or oxygen-carrying capability.
Evaluate extremity and site of snakebite for pain, ecchymoses, blisters, or blebs.	Venom effects may jeopardize tissue perfusion. Swelling and discoloration usually begin to dissipate after 48 hours, and continued problems may indicate the presence of other complications.
Apply ice packs over dressings as warranted. *Do not* apply ice directly over snakebite and surrounding tissues.	May reduce swelling. Ice packs may increase damage to skin tissues and cause necrosis.
Monitor for complaints of paresthesias, weakness, muscle incoordination, or fasciculations.	May indicate advancement of neurotoxic venom.
Observe for increases in salivation, dysphasia, dysphagia, or lethargy.	May indicate advancement of venom and further complications that will require life-saving treatment.
Observe for changes in respirations, increased work of breathing, nasal flaring, retractions, dyspnea.	May indicate impending respiratory distress and may lead to cardiovascular failure and death.
Prepare patient for fasciotomy.	Provides knowledge and reduces anxiety. Incision may be required to prevent skin dehiscence from edema.
Instruct patient in signs to notify physician or nurse: swelling, paresthesias, color changes, temperature changes, and so forth.	Provides for prompt identification of problem and prompt intervention to prevent further complications.

INTERVENTIONS	RATIONALES
Prepare patient for amputation.	Provides knowledge and facilitates understanding of need for procedure, risks, and benefits, and allows the patient to make an informed choice. Amputation may be required for gangrene/necrosis.

NIC: Circulatory Precautions

Discharge or Maintenance Evaluation

- Patient will achieve and maintain adequate perfusion to all body systems.
- Patient will have palpable, equal peripheral pulses, with no paresthesias or evidence of ischemia.
- Patient will have adequate urine output and balanced intake/output.
- Patient will have adequate cerebral perfusion with no mental status changes.
- Patient will be able to accurately recall all information.
- Patient will be able to make an informed consent for procedures and will comply with treatment modalities.
- Patient will not exhibit any preventable complications.

IMPAIRED SKIN INTEGRITY

Related to: snakebite, envenomation, surgical procedures, invasive lines, necrosis, gangrene

Defining Characteristics: disruption of skin tissues, incisions, open wounds, drainage, edema

Outcome Criteria

✔ Patient will have wound healing occurring in a timely manner.

NOC: Wound Healing: Primary Intention

INTERVENTIONS	RATIONALES
Assess wound and surrounding tissues for appearance, drainage, swelling, healing, deterioration, and so forth.	Provides baseline for comparison and for identification of deterioration.

INTERVENTIONS	RATIONALES
Cleanse wound with soap and water, or other agents per hospital protocol, as warranted.	Removes debris and drainage from skin surfaces and helps to prevent infection.
Apply gauze dressing as warranted and change every day utilizing sterile technique.	Dressing may help to control bleeding, absorbs drainage, and provides barrier for wound. Using proper technique for wound care prevents potential complications.
Elevate extremity as warranted.	Reduces swelling and pain, and helps to keep skin tissues free of pressure that might cause ischemia or necrosis.
Monitor extremity and wound for changes.	Swelling and discoloration should begin to subside by 48 hours. If swelling increases, or tissue perfusion is impaired, surgical intervention may be required.
Prepare patient for fasciotomy or amputation, as warranted.	Provides knowledge to patient to facilitate an informed choice, and reduces anxiety.

NIC: Wound Care

Discharge or Maintenance Evaluation

- Patient will have healed wounds with no circulatory impairment.
- Patient will be able to circumvent preventable complications.

IMPAIRED GAS EXCHANGE

Related to: envenomation, ARDS, neurotoxins, cardiotoxins, hematotoxins, lactic acidosis, edema, snakebite, anaphylactic reactions, bronchospasm

Defining Characteristics: dyspnea, tachypnea, air hunger, abnormal arterial blood gases, altered acid–base balances, cyanosis, inadequate oxygen saturation levels

Outcome Criteria

✔ Patient will maintain own airway and have optimal ventilation and perfusion.

NOC: Respiratory Status: Gas Exchange

INTERVENTIONS	RATIONALES
Monitor respiratory status for changes: dyspnea, tachypnea, decreased oxygen saturation levels, cyanosis, decreases in mentation, restlessness, and so forth.	May indicate hypoxemia and hypoxia.
Administer oxygen as ordered.	Provides supplemental oxygen to increase availability, and to saturate red blood cells with oxygen.
Observe for laryngeal spasm, bronchospasm, or excessive salivation.	May indicate worsening respiratory status which may require mechanical ventilation.
Obtain ABGs as warranted for signs of respiratory distress.	Will identify acid–base imbalances as well as hypoxemia, hypercarbia, and other ventilatory problems.
Prepare for intubation and mechanical ventilation, as warranted.	Hypoxemia that is not able to be corrected will require mechanical ventilation to facilitate adequate oxygenation.

INTERVENTIONS	RATIONALES
Instruct patient in notifying nurse if changes in respiratory status occur.	The patient will be able to identify increasing work of breathing, which can lead to timely intervention to minimize hypoperfusion to other body systems.
Instruct patient/family regarding need for mechanical ventilation, if warranted.	Venomous toxins may impair respiratory centers and patient may require mechanical ventilation for perfusion. Knowledge decreases fear and anxiety, and improves compliance.

NIC: *Acid–Base Management*

Discharge or Maintenance Evaluation

- Patient will be free of respiratory distress and able to maintain own airway and oxygenation on room air.
- Patient will have no respiratory complications.

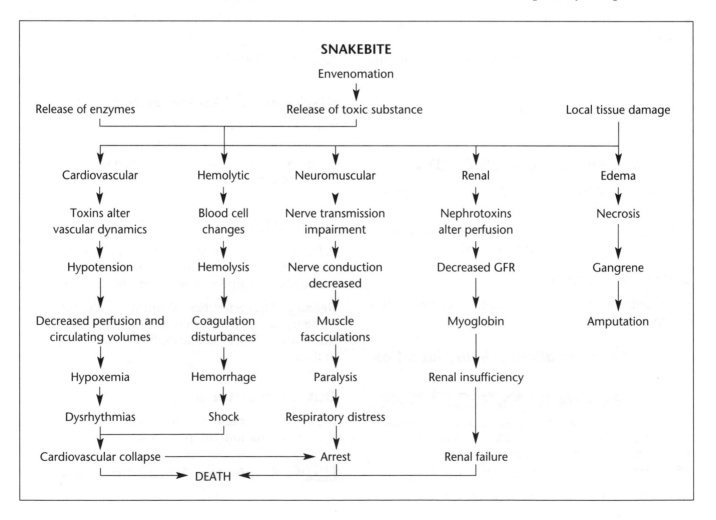

CHAPTER 9.4

TRANSPLANTS

Transplantation of living tissues, cells, or organs from one individual to another is one method of treatment for several end-stage organ diseases. Often, transplantation is the last resort for a variety of disorders after conventional medical or surgical therapies have failed to provide adequate function ing. Recent advances in technique and treatment have improved the rate of success, and transplantation has improved the quality of life for many patients who otherwise would either die or be resigned to lives of dialysis or suffering.

Transplants are categorized by the relationship between the donor and the recipient. An autograft relates to the transplantation of tissue from one location to another in the same person. An isograft is a graft between identical twins, and an allograft, or homograft, is a graft between members of the same species. A xenograft, or heterograft, is a graft between members of different species.

Bone marrow transplants are performed in order to restore immunologic and hematologic function to patients who have aplastic anemia, leukemia, or severe combined immunodeficiency disorder. Multiple aspirations of bone marrow are obtained and then infused intravenously with red blood cells.

Heart transplants are performed to attempt to restore function in end-stage cardiac failure that has been unresponsive to other medical therapeutics, and usually involve patients who have cardiomyopathy, rheumatic heart disease, congenital heart disease, or coronary artery disease. After the patient is placed on cardiopulmonary bypass and the diseased heart is removed, the donor allograft heart is implanted. Frequently, a combined heart–lung transplant is performed because of the increased success rate as a result of fewer vascular anastomoses being required.

Renal transplants are performed to restore kidney function in end-stage renal disease. Allografts are usually obtained from living relatives or cadavers. The kidney is usually implanted in a retroperitoneal position against the psoas muscle in the iliac fossa.

When cadaver kidneys are used approximately half of the recipients may require dialysis because of the presence of acute tubular necrosis.

Liver transplants are performed to restore function in patients with chronic active hepatitis, hepatitis B antigen-negative postnecrotic cirrhosis, primary hepatocellular tumor, or congenital anomalies of the bile duct or inborn errors of metabolism in children. The liver is implanted into the right upper abdominal quadrant and the vasculature is anastomosed. Biliary drainage anastomosis problems often result in bacteremia.

Pancreas transplants are performed on patients with insulin-dependent diabetes mellitus to provide insulin-producing tissue. The pancreas, either total with a small amount of duodenum, or partial segment of the distal pancreas, is transplanted. This type of transplant is performed as a life-enhancing procedure and is most successful prior to the development of severe secondary diabetic complications.

Bone marrow transplants (BMT) and peripheral blood stem cell transplants (PBSCT) are measures used to help reactivate the immunologic and hematologic systems following chemotherapy or radiation therapy performed to permanently destroy all malignant cells within the bone marrow. Bone marrow or stem cells that have been obtained are given intravenously, in the hope that the cells will be transported to the marrow and reestablish a normal hematopoiesis. BMT can be allogenic or autologous. Siblings have a one in four chance of being an HLA match, so frequently, a patient that is planning to undergo radiation or chemotherapy, may have bone marrow harvested prior to the procedure, and then transfused afterwards. Using the patient's own bone marrow decreases the chance of rejection and graft-versus-host disease, but the potential for recurring malignancy is higher.

With PBSCT, which is frequently performed in conjunction with BMT, the patient's own bone marrow is stimulated and then the peripheral stem cells are harvested during repeated phereses. As with the autologous BMT, once the chemotherapy or radiation treatments are over, the cells are reinfused. Potential complications of both BMT and PBSCT include immunocompromise for at least a year, profound thrombocytopenia, renal insufficiency, veno-occlusive disease, and acute or chronic graft-versus-host disease.

The goal in transplantation is to maintain optimal functioning of the organ and to prevent rejection. This goal is facilitated by antigen matching, tissue typing for histocompatibility, tests for prior sensitization, transfusions of whole blood, and immunosuppressive therapy.

Despite a small increase in the available donor organs, the number of candidates for transplant far exceeds the organs available, and many patients die prior to undergoing transplantation. Complications of infection, rejection, and immunosuppressive drugs are a very real part of the process.

Transplantation of almost any tissue is feasible but rejection is the most frequent complication when the body tries to destroy the graft tissue. Rejection occurs when the immune system recognizes the graft as being foreign to the body and begins a responsive action to the antigens of the graft. Thus begins a cell-mediated immune response in the lymph tissues. Antibody-mediated immune responses, inflammatory responses, and complement activation also play a significant role in the rejection process.

Rejection may occur immediately after transplantation or up to years later, and most transplant patients experience at least one rejection episode during their lives. Signs/symptoms of rejection vary depending on the type of graft. Corneal transplant rejection is evidenced by corneal clouding, corneal edema, or conjunctival hyperemia. Cardiac transplant rejection is evidenced by decreased QRS, right axis shift, atrial dysrhythmias, conduction defects, S_3 gallop, jugular vein distention, decreased exercise tolerance, low grade fever, malaise, weight gain, dyspnea, right-ventricular failure, and peripheral edema. Liver transplant rejection may be manifested with changes in urine or stool color, jaundice, hepatomegaly, ascites, pain in the center of the back, right flank, or right upper quadrant of the abdomen, low grade fever, malaise, or anorexia. Renal transplant rejection may involve low-grade fever, decreased urine output, pain, swelling and/or tenderness in the kidney, increased blood pressure, malaise, weight gain, or peripheral edema. Pancreas transplant rejection may show symptoms of increased glucose levels, polyuria, polydipsia, polyphagia, weight loss, low-grade fever, and tender or enlarged pancreas. Bone marrow transplantation rejection is usually evident by severe diarrhea, jaundice and skin changes.

Rejection can be classified as being acute, hyperacute, or chronic depending on the mechanisms of rejection and the duration of time prior to the appearance of symptoms. Acute reactions may occur anywhere from 7 days to several weeks after transplant. A cell-mediated acute reaction occurs when the graft develops interstitial edema, ischemia, and necrosis, but high dose steroid therapy may reverse the reaction. Antibody-mediated acute reactions occur when fibrin, platelets, and polymorphonuclear cells adhere to the graft cells, resulting from recipient antibody–donor antigen responses. This aggregation produces ischemia and eventually necrosis. Hyperacute reactions develop immediately after the transplant up to a few days later. Immediate hyperacute reactions happen when the recipient has preformed antibodies against the donor antigens and is usually caused by previous blood transfusions, previous transplants, or from pregnancy. An accelerated hyperacute reaction happens when the recipient's lymphocytes and neutrophils infiltrate the graft and may be prevented with the use of antisera to T lymphocytes. Chronic reactions occur over many months and eventually lead to loss of graft function. This occurs when the vascular endothelium becomes inflamed, and the arterial lumen decreases. Fibrin and platelets aggregate and over time, result in decreased blood flow to the organ, and ischemia and dysfunction prevail.

The principal mechanism of rejection is GVHD (graft versus host disease). This occurs when an immunocompetent donor graft is transplanted into an immune-impaired recipient. If the donor and the recipient are not histocompatible, foreign cells will initiate an attack against the host cells, which are then unable to reject them. This usually occurs with bone marrow or liver transplants.

MEDICAL CARE

Laboratory: renal profiles used to assess kidney function; hepatic profiles used to assess liver function; CBC used to evaluate anemia, infection, and blood loss; glucose levels used to monitor pancreatic function; ABO blood grouping; Lewis antigens used to evaluate compatibility for kidney transplants; micro-toxicity assays for evaluation of bone marrow; tissue typing for histocompatibility; lymphocyte antibody screen to evaluate preformed antibodies; lymphocyte cross-matching used after a suitable donor is found; serology, HIV, hepatitis screens to evaluate suitability for transplantation

Surgery: required for transplantation of tissues/organs

Biopsy: tissue biopsies used as the most accurate diagnostic tool to determine the extent of lymphocyte infiltration and potential tissue damage; serial biopsies can be used to monitor course of treatment

Immunosuppressive drugs: used to decrease or elimi-nate the body's ability to reject new transplanted tissues; can increase the risk for opportunistic organisms; usually a combination of drugs are used rather than just one

Blood transfusions: used to improve graft survival of certain organisms

Radiation therapy: used in some instances for pre-transplantation immunosuppression

Thoracic duct drainage: used in some instances for pretransplantation immunosuppression

COMMON NURSING DIAGNOSES

 ### INEFFECTIVE TISSUE PERFUSION: CARDIOPULMONARY, CEREBRAL, RENAL, GASTROINTESTINAL, PERIPHERAL (see RENAL FAILURE)

Related to: transplant rejection, allergic reactions, infection, pulmonary edema, DIC

Defining Characteristics: oliguria, anuria, polyuria, fever, chills, increased white blood cell count, differential shift to the left, bleeding, ecchymoses, hema-turia, guaiac positive stools, DIC, blood dyscrasias, decreased platelet count, headache, mental status changes, adventitious breath sounds, gallops, abnor-mal heart tones, dysrhythmias, rashes, ulcerations, nausea, vomiting

ACUTE PAIN (see CARDIAC SURGERY)

Related to: transplant operation, invasive lines and catheters, immobility

Defining Characteristics: communication of pain, facial grimacing, increased blood pressure, increased heart rate, diaphoresis, moaning, splinting

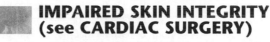 ### IMPAIRED SKIN INTEGRITY (see CARDIAC SURGERY)

Related to: transplant operation, invasive lines and catheters, biopsies, wounds

Defining Characteristics: surgical incisions, disruption of skin surfaces, abrasions, redness, warmth, drainage

DEFICIENT KNOWLEDGE (see RENAL FAILURE)

Related to: transplant operation, changes in health status, anxiety

Defining Characteristics: lack of knowledge, presence of preventable complications, verbalized questions

ADDITIONAL NURSING DIAGNOSES

RISK FOR INFECTION

Related to: immunosuppression, effects of transplan-tation, invasive procedures, invasive lines/catheters, trauma, surgery, disease

Defining Characteristics: increased immature white blood cells, differential with a shift to the left, fever, chills, cough, hypotension, tachycardia, presence of wounds, positive blood, urine, or sputum cultures, cloudy urine, purulent drainage

Outcome Criteria

✔ Patient will have no signs/symptoms of infection after transplant surgery.

 NOC: *Immune Status*

INTERVENTIONS	RATIONALES
Patient should be in private room, with appropriate isolation techniques in use. Visitors with illness must be restricted from visiting.	Decreases potential of infection when patient is already immunocompromised.
Observe for signs/symptoms of infection to all body systems.	Provides for prompt identification of complication and facilitates timely intervention.

(continues)

(continued)

INTERVENTIONS	RATIONALES
Provide diet with appropriate nutrients and fluids. Restrict fresh fruits and vegetables.	Proper nutrition facilitates antibody formation and prevents dehydration. Fresh fruits/vegetables may harbor parasitic spores or bacteria that may result in an infection.
Monitor CBC, especially WBC count for abrupt changes in neutrophils.	Sudden decreases in mature WBCs may result from chemotherapy and further compromise the immune response.
Use sterile/aseptic technique with dressing changes, IV site changes, or other invasive care.	Immunosuppressive drugs or effects of the patient's disease process may slow wound healing. Drainage is a potential medium for bacterial growth.
Observe mouth and oral cavity for presence of lesions or thrush. Use nystatin as warranted.	Steroid and antibiotic administration may result in an overgrowth of fungal colonization resulting in candidiasis.
Administer prophylactic antimicrobials as ordered.	Prophylactic use of fluconazole may reduce the occurrence of Candida albicans in BMT patients, and use of acyclovir can lower the incidence of reactivation of the herpes simplex virus and cytomegalovirus in BMT patients who are seropositive.
Instruct patient/family in signs/symptoms to report that indicate infection.	Prompt recognition of potential signs of infection allows for timely intervention.
Instruct patient/family regarding all medications, effects, side effects, and method/timing of dosing.	Provides knowledge and enhances compliance.

NIC: *Infection Protection*

Discharge or Maintenance Evaluation

- Patient will exhibit no signs of infection post-transplant.
- Patient will have stable vital signs and hemodynamics.
- Patient will not develop any complication.

RISK FOR INJURY

Related to: rejection of transplanted organ, tissue, or bone marrow, allergic reaction to transplant

Defining Characteristics: fever, chills, diaphoresis, peripheral edema, weight gain, decreased urine output, hypertension, urticaria, enlargement of the graft, oliguria, anuria, hypotension, right-sided heart failure, right flank pain, light-colored stools, anorexia, sore throat, cough, malaise, dysuria, diarrhea, erythema, swollen areas, flushing, warm skin, white blood cell count <1500/μl, ANC <500/μl, organ failure, dysrhythmias, dyspnea, abnormal arterial blood gases

Outcome Criteria

✔ Patient will not experience rejection of new transplant.

NOC: *Risk Detection*

INTERVENTIONS	RATIONALES
Monitor patient for fever, chills, hypotension, flushing, inflammation, thrush, cough, urinary changes.	May indicate impending rejection of transplant, or adverse reaction to immunosuppressants. Acute rejection is common and usually occurs during the first weeks or months following the transplant.
Monitor for increased bilirubin levels, hepatomegaly, encephalopathy, or heart failure.	May indicate complication as a result of bone marrow transplant and is usually seen in 25% of patients.
Observe for rash or skin ulcerations.	May indicate presence of graft-versus-host disease (GVHD) and may occur up to 2 weeks post-transplant.
Administer immunosuppressive therapy as ordered.	Drugs interfere with some step in the body's response against the graft to decrease the immune response. Imuran suppresses DNA and RNA synthesis; cyclosporine blocks the release of interleukin-1 and gamma-interferons and blocks activated T lymphocytes; prednisone and other corticosteroids inhibit T-cell proliferation, decrease production of interleukin-2 and gamma-interferons, and decrease IgG synthesis; muromonab blocks T cells that foster renal rejection; cyclophosphamide, used when azathioprine is contraindicated, decreases the production of antibodies, and begins destruction of lymphocytes in circulation; monoclonal antibody

INTERVENTIONS	RATIONALES
	(OKT3) suppresses or inactivates an antigen-recognition site on T cells; FK-506, the latest drug approved for liver transplants and is approved for renal transplants, with some exceptions, has actions comparable to cyclosporine.
Administer blood products as warranted.	Anemia and blood dyscrasias may be present after bone marrow transplants and require supplementation of blood products until transplantation is successful and may occur up to 2 weeks after infusion. Granulocyte infusion may be deemed necessary if antimicrobials therapy is not effective to treat infections.
Monitor lab studies for significant changes.	Provides data that may be indicative of impending or present rejection.
Prepare patient for biopsies as warranted.	Cardiac transplants require periodic endomyocardial biopsies to identify cellular rejection.
Instruct patient/family on signs/symptoms of rejection of particular transplanted organ/tissue.	Promotes knowledge, facilitates compliance, and allows for prompt notification to decrease severity of complications or rejection episode.
Prepare patient for surgery as warranted.	If excessive immunosuppression is required or if rejection is inevitable, kidney transplants may require removal and patient will need placement back on dialysis.
Instruct patient on all medications taken, side effects, adverse effects, contraindications, and potential drug interactions.	Decreases risk of self-medication, and provides for prompt notification of adverse reactions that may require further intervention.

NIC: *Emergency Care*

Discharge or Maintenance Evaluation

- Patient will have minimal rejection of transplanted organ/tissue.
- Patient will be able to comply with drug regimen to prevent rejection.
- Patient will be able to verbalize understanding of signs/symptoms to report to physician, and will be able to seek prompt medical care.

- Patient will be cognizant of all medications being taken, purposes, and potential side effects, and will have no adverse reactions.
- Patient will avoid further surgery.

SOCIAL ISOLATION

Related to: changes in health status, changes in physical status, imposed physical isolation, inadequate support system

Defining Characteristics: feelings of loneliness, feelings of rejection, absence of family members/friends, sad, dull affect, inappropriate behaviors

Outcome Criteria

✔ Patient will be able to participate in activities as tolerated and be able to have effective interaction with people within confines of medical disease process.

NOC: *Social Involvement*

INTERVENTIONS	RATIONALES
Determine patient's comprehension of medical situation and rationales.	Identifies potential misconceptions and allows for realistic input to facilitate understanding.
Utilize appropriate isolation techniques based on patient's condition, and when possible, limit use of protective equipment.	Facilitates providing safe environment for patient yet providing social interaction to decrease feelings of social isolation. Appropriate use of gowns, masks, and gloves may be required because of patient's suppressed immune system.
Encourage visitation of family as much as possible. Provide a telephone so that patient may contact family and friends.	Transplantation costs are high and done in major hospital settings, so family members may not be able to travel great distances for the length of time the patient may be hospitalized. Methods of communication are important to promote feelings of inclusion in family matters.
Identify significant family members or friends who are important to patient and involve them in care.	Support systems decrease sense of isolation and loneliness and help to reestablish communication.
Assist patient to develop strategies for coping with isolation.	Promotes feelings of self-control while developing goals for achievement.

(continues)

(continued)

INTERVENTIONS	RATIONALES
Instruct patient/family regarding health care needs and treatment plan.	Encourages optimal health and well-being, and allows for improved social activity
Contact social services, counselors, organizations, ministers, or other resources.	May be helpful to continue care once patient is discharged, and may be able to facilitate supportive encounters.

NIC: *Socialization Enhancement*

Discharge or Maintenance Evaluation

- Patient will be able to verbalize understanding of necessity for isolation procedures and will comply.

- Patient will have fewer feelings of loneliness and isolation.

- Patient will be able to meet sensory demands by family and friends.

- Patient will be able to effectively access community resources for referrals.

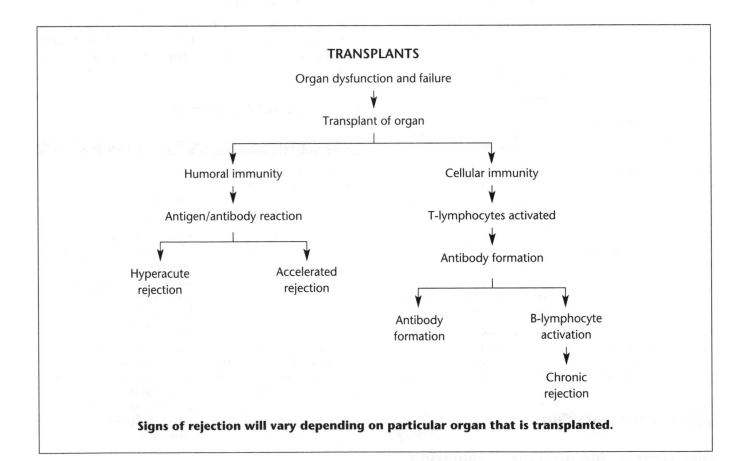

TRANSPLANTS

Organ dysfunction and failure

↓

Transplant of organ

Humoral immunity   Cellular immunity

↓   ↓

Antigen/antibody reaction   T-lymphocytes activated

↓

Antibody formation

Hyperacute rejection   Accelerated rejection

Antibody formation   B-lymphocyte activation

↓

Chronic rejection

Signs of rejection will vary depending on particular organ that is transplanted.

CHAPTER 9.5

SYSTEMIC INFLAMMATORY RESPONSE SYNDROME

Septic shock, or septic syndrome, has previously been classified as presence of infection, tachypnea, and tachycardia that is accompanied by hyperthermia or hypothermia, and major organ dysfunction. With the identification that noninfectious causes also have a major part in sepsis, the terminology was changed to systemic inflammatory response syndrome (SIRS) to underscore that infection is not the restricted cause of the changes noted in the patient, and also that the inflammatory reaction of the patient is crucial in determining the severity of the disease. End-stage organ failure and mortality increase with each phase of the progressing inflammatory process. SIRS can result from not only infectious, but noninfectious trauma, such as burns, pancreatitis, ischemia, reperfusion, or multitrauma. SIRS is an uncontrollable inflammatory response to an assortment of clinical insults, and is defined by the presence of at least two of the following: temperature above 38° C or below 36° C, heart rate over 90 beats/minute, respiratory rate greater than 20 breaths/minute, $PaCO_2$ less than 32 mm Hg, and white blood cell count above 12,000/mm^3 or below 4,000/mm^3, or above 10% bands. Sepsis is still a correct term when SIRS is a result of an active infection. Septic shock occurs when sepsis is advanced, with hypotension, and organ dysfunction, and is unresponsive to fluid resuscitation.

SIRS has four phases of development. In Stage I, a local response occurs with the release of pro-inflammatory mediators (cytokines, eicosanoids, platelet-activating factors, etc.) that create elaborate reactions. They destroy injured tissues, promote new tissue growth, and help combat pathogenic organisms, neoplastic cells, and foreign antigens. The body initiates an anti-inflammatory response of its own with interleukin-4, 10, and 11, tumor necrosis factor receptors, interleukin-1 receptor antagonists, transforming growth factor, and other substances to ensure the effects of the proinflammatory mediators do not become detrimental.

In Stage II, there is an initial systemic response. In patients who have a severe infection, foreign antigens or pathogens enter the bloodstream directly and create more proinflammatory mediators, that help to engage neutrophils, platelets, lymphocytes, and coagulation factors to the local site. Eventually, a compensatory systemic anti-inflammatory response should cause the proinflammatory reaction to decrease. Few clinical signs are noted at this time and organ dysfunction is very rare.

By Stage III, there is massive systemic inflammation. Some patients have lost the inflammatory response regulation and a massive reaction occurs. Usually, this is proinflammatory and creates hypotension, abnormal temperatures, and tachycardia. As endothelial dysfunction progresses, microvascular permeability increases and platelet sludging blocks the microvasculature. Blood flow is impeded and causes ischemia and may cause reperfusion injury. Dysfunction of the regulatory vasoactive mechanisms creates severe vasodilatation, causing severe shock, and compromising blood flow to vital organs.

In Stage IV, patients have excessive immunosuppression with persistent overwhelming inflammation and usually die from shock. In those patients who do manage to survive, the anti-inflammatory mechanisms may be able to control the inflammation.

MEDICAL CARE

Laboratory: CPK, AST, and amylase used to evaluate specific organ/tissue destruction; BUN, creatinine, bilirubin, and ammonia used to evaluate renal and hepatic function; CBC used to identify occult bleeding or hemorrhage, and to discern presence of infection, especially with shift to the left on differential; coagulation studies used to identify coagulopathy, also present with DIC; cultures of blood, urine, and sputum used to identify pathogenic cause and appropriate antimicrobial therapy; urinary electrolytes, osmolality, and creatinine clearance help to identify renal or metabolic dysfunction; glucose levels usually elevated from stress response; serum enzymes used to identify cardiac impairment

Radiography: chest X-rays used to identify presence of pulmonary infiltrates, pulmonary edema, and changes in vasculature

Electrocardiogram: used to identify baseline cardiac rhythm, to identify conduction aberrancies, dysrhythmias, and cardiovascular compromise caused by hypoxia, hypoperfusion, or electrolyte imbalances

Arterial blood gases: used to evaluate hypoxia and hypoxemia; usually respiratory alkalosis attempting to compensate for metabolic acidosis, with pH below 7.35 and decreased bicarbonate level; in late SIRS, respiratory acidosis with $PaCO_2$ <45 mm Hg; shows progressive intrapulmonary shunting, with increasing FIO_2 required to maintain oxygen saturation

IV fluids: used to attempt fluid resuscitation and increase cardiac output and to maintain hydration

Vasoactive drugs: used when fluid resuscitation fails; used to improve contractility and increase systemic vascular resistance to maintain organ perfusion; inotropic agents help to increase cardiac index, decrease pulmonary capillary wedge pressures, and decrease afterload; in severe cases, alpha-adrenergic drugs may be required to maintain a minimal blood pressure to temporarily stabilize the patient

Antimicrobial therapy: used in the management of sepsis to eradicate the pathogenic cause of infection; frequently two antimicrobials will be used in conjunction for broad coverage, polymicrobial infections, and potential for antibacterial synergy

Glucocorticosteroids: current trend is that these drugs are of no benefit for treatment of septic shock

Naloxone: has been shown to alter endotoxic shock, increase stroke volume and heart rate, and improved hemodynamics in animal studies

J5 antiserum: used experimentally and found to reduce mortality from gram-negative sepsis by 50%, but it has adverse effects on the serum donor, variability of antiserum activity, and the need to use human blood created risk for transmission of viral disease

Monoclonal antibodies: anti-endotoxin E5 has been shown in clinical trials to reduce mortality in bacteremic and nonbacteremic patients; Ha-1A, which is derived from *Escherichia coli*, reduced mortality almost by half in patients with bacteremia and shock

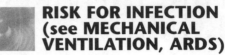

COMMON NURSING DIAGNOSES

RISK FOR INFECTION (see MECHANICAL VENTILATION, ARDS)

Related to: inadequate primary defenses, inadequate secondary defenses, immunosuppression, trauma, multisystem trauma, invasive procedures, malnutrition

Defining Characteristics: fever, tachycardia, elevated white blood cells with shift to the left on differential, broken skin, immunosuppression, hypothermia, hyperthermia, tachycardia, tachypnea, hypotension, decreased hemodynamic pressures

IMPAIRED GAS EXCHANGE (see MECHANICAL VENTILATION)

Related to: SIRS, sepsis, altered oxygen-carrying capability, altered oxygen supply

Defining Characteristics: dyspnea, nasal flaring, tachycardia, pale, dusky skin, confusion, diaphoresis, hypoxia, hypoxemia, irritability, restlessness, abnormal arterial blood gases

IMBALANCED NUTRITION: LESS THAN BODY REQUIREMENTS (see MECHANICAL VENTILATION)

Related to: increased metabolic rate, decreased intake of nutrients, changes in normal eating pattern

Defining Characteristics: hyperthermia, increased metabolic rate, sepsis, weight loss, loss of muscle mass, altered taste, lack of interest in eating, diarrhea, hair loss, capillary fragility, pale mucous membranes, sore, inflamed oral cavity, muscle weakness

ADDITIONAL NURSING DIAGNOSES

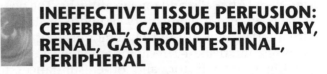

INEFFECTIVE TISSUE PERFUSION: CEREBRAL, CARDIOPULMONARY, RENAL, GASTROINTESTINAL, PERIPHERAL

Related to: hypovolemia, SIRS, sepsis, septic shock, bacteremia, endotoxins, DIC, immunosuppression, trauma, burns, multisystem injury, pancreatitis

Defining Characteristics: increased cardiac output and increased cardiac index initially, increased arterial lactate levels, cellular acidosis, decreased bowel sounds, ileus, decreased systemic vascular resistance, hypotension, hypothermia, hyperthermia, tachycardia, tachypnea, PCWP normal to low, oxygen delivery and consumption variable but usually decreased as shock progresses, rapid, weak, and thready peripheral pulses, warm skin initially, then cool skin, atelectasis, crackles, wheezing, changes in pulse pressure, respiratory alkalosis, metabolic acidosis, respiratory acidosis, increasing intrapulmonary shunting, increased WBC, shift to the left on differential, positive cultures, increased BUN and creatinine, increased enzymes

Outcome Criteria

✔ Patient will have normal oxygen delivery and consumption.

✔ Patient will have systolic blood pressure at least 90 mm Hg, with normal hemodynamic parameters.

✔ Patient will have perfusion to all body systems.

NOC: *Tissue Perfusion*

INTERVENTIONS	RATIONALES
Monitor vital signs q 1 hour and prn.	Tachypnea, tachycardia, and hypotension will occur with hypoperfusion and decreased cardiac output.
Monitor hemodynamic parameters q 1 hour.	Indicates fluid status as well as changes in perfusion status to allow for timely intervention.
Administer oxygen as ordered. Prepare for intubation and mechanical ventilation as required.	Supplemental oxygen will be required as hypoxia and hypoxemia increase. As shock progresses, the ability to maintain oxygen saturation will decrease, and the only method of maintaining adequate respiratory perfusion may be with mechanical ventilation.
Administer IV fluids as ordered.	Fluid resuscitation may be required when blood pressure drops in order to maintain at least the minimum adequate blood flow. At least 2 IV lines should be in place with large gauge needles to handle rapid infusion.
Administer blood products as ordered.	May be required to increase circulating blood volume,

INTERVENTIONS	RATIONALES
	increase oxygen-carrying capability, and to treat complications, such as DIC.
Administer vasoactive medications as needed once fluid resuscitation is tried.	Dopamine is used frequently in low doses for its ability to improve renal and splanchnic blood flow, but may be used in higher doses to support blood pressure. Dobutamine may be used for myocardial depression but should be used with caution in hypotensive patients because it also reduces SVR. Norepinephrine is used for septic shock patients who do not respond to fluid resuscitation in order to maintain renal function, to increase renal and splanchnic blood flow, and can be used with other drugs in combination to improve blood pressure. Epinephrine increases myocardial oxygen consumption and demand, but may be needed to manage low oxygen delivery and consumption with younger patients.
Monitor ECG for cardiac rhythm, conduction defects, and dysrhythmias, and treat per protocol.	As SIRS and sepsis progress, fluid shifting can create electrolyte imbalances and cardiac hypoperfusion that may result in cardiac rhythm irregularities. Treatment of these may be life-saving.
Auscultate lung fields and heart tones q 2–4 hours and prn. Notify physician of significant changes.	Fluid resuscitation may result in pulmonary edema, with wheezing and crackles audible. New gallops or murmurs may indicate impending cardiac failure, cardiac hypoperfusion, or impending tamponade.
Assess patient's level of consciousness and orientation.	As SIRS progresses, the patient may have decreased sensorium reflecting decreasing cerebral perfusion.
Auscultate abdomen for presence and character of bowel sounds. Observe for abdominal distention.	Decreasing or absent bowel sounds may indicate presence of ileus, obstruction, or hypoperfused state.
Palpate peripheral pulses, and observe extremities for color, capillary refill, and sensation.	Hypoperfusion causes the body to shunt blood from the periphery to vital organs, leading to decreased or absent peripheral pulses, cold extremities that are mottled or cyanotic.

(continues)

(continued)

INTERVENTIONS	RATIONALES
Control hyperthermia with cooling blankets, antipyretics, or tepid baths.	Hyperthermia adds to oxygen consumption and demand, worsening perfusion to all organs.
Avoid Trendelenburg's position for decreased blood pressure.	Position impairs gas exchange, increases pulmonary blood flow, and may decrease cerebral perfusion.
Administer medications to sedate/paralyze patient as warranted/ordered.	Medication may be required to reduce the work of breathing with mechanical ventilation in order to maintain adequate ventilation and perfusion.
Instruct patient and/or family regarding disease process.	Patient may be too ill or comatose from hypoperfusion to be instructed. Family needs information and updates as condition changes.
Instruct family regarding all procedures, equipment, and medications.	Facilitates knowledge and helps to decrease fear.

NIC: *Circulatory Care*

Discharge or Maintenance Evaluation

- Patient will have vital signs and hemodynamic parameters within normal range.
- Patient will have peripheral pulses present with no signs of hypoperfusion.
- Patient will be able to breathe on his own, with clear lung fields to auscultation, and oxygen saturation maintained.
- Patient will have adequate urinary output.
- Patient will be awake, alert, and oriented in all spheres.
- Patient's family will be able to understand instructions and information presented to them.

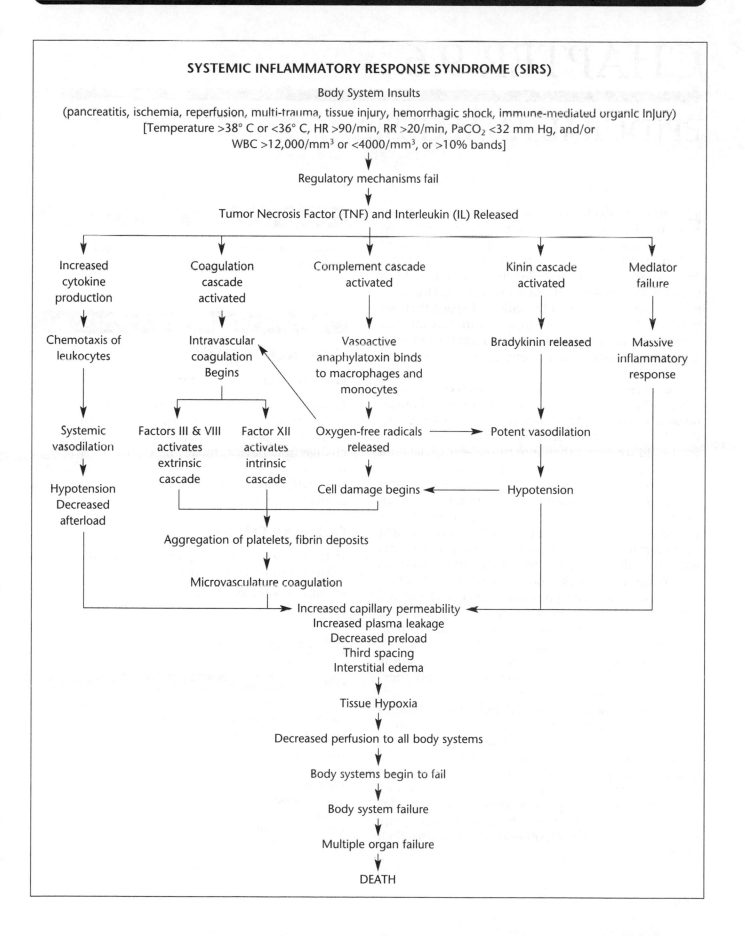

SYSTEMIC INFLAMMATORY RESPONSE SYNDROME (SIRS)

Body System Insults

(pancreatitis, ischemia, reperfusion, multi-trauma, tissue injury, hemorrhagic shock, immune-mediated organic injury)
[Temperature >38° C or <36° C, HR >90/min, RR >20/min, $PaCO_2$ <32 mm Hg, and/or
WBC >12,000/mm^3 or <4000/mm^3, or >10% bands]

Regulatory mechanisms fail

Tumor Necrosis Factor (TNF) and Interleukin (IL) Released

| Increased cytokine production | Coagulation cascade activated | Complement cascade activated | Kinin cascade activated | Mediator failure |

Chemotaxis of leukocytes → Intravascular coagulation Begins → Vasoactive anaphylatoxin binds to macrophages and monocytes → Bradykinin released → Massive inflammatory response

Systemic vasodilation

Factors III & VIII activates extrinsic cascade   Factor XII activates intrinsic cascade   Oxygen-free radicals released → Potent vasodilation

Hypotension Decreased afterload

Cell damage begins ← Hypotension

Aggregation of platelets, fibrin deposits

Microvasculature coagulation

Increased capillary permeability
Increased plasma leakage
Decreased preload
Third spacing
Interstitial edema

Tissue Hypoxia

Decreased perfusion to all body systems

Body systems begin to fail

Body system failure

Multiple organ failure

DEATH

CHAPTER 9.6

EPIDURAL ANALGESIA

Epidural analgesia was once only used in major medical centers for pain control, but currently, most hospitals utilize this type of pain management technique for both acute and chronic types of pain. Because of its efficacy in consistent pain relief, it has become a common form of pain control. Drugs are injected or infused into the epidural space that lies between the dura and the ligamentum flavum, just outside the subarachnoid space, via a catheter that is placed there under aseptic conditions, usually by an anesthesiologist.

Analgesia delivered in this manner facilitates pain relief without sensory, motor, or sympathetic changes, because of the ability to bypass the blood–brain barrier. The medication disperses slowly into the subarachnoid space and then into the cerebrospinal fluid and onward to the spinal nervous system.

A continuous infusion of an anesthetic and/or analgesic solution through the epidural catheter can usually reduce the amount of analgesia required by the patient after surgery or procedures, and can assist in shorter lengths of stay postoperatively. In patients with chronic pain, a continuous infusion controls pain without the peaks and troughs related to intermittent injections, and has minimal central and system circulation of the medication. Infusions of bupivacaine and/or fentanyl usually relieve pain completely, and a new anesthetic, Ropivacaine, has less cardiovascular toxicity. Morphine is commonly used for epidural infusions because it is fairly inexpensive and causes few adverse reactions.

There are some disadvantages to this type of management, however; because of the catheter's proximity to the spinal nerves and canal, there is danger of migration of the catheter. It requires skilled and accurate placement technique and verification of placement prior to each intermittent injection. Some of the most frequent adverse reactions are leg weakness, numbness, and itching, and these symptoms can be treated with other drugs to control their effect.

MEDICAL CARE

Surgical placement: placement of the catheter is done aseptically usually by an anesthesiologist into the lower back at a specific site from T10 to L4

NURSING DIAGNOSES

ACUTE PAIN

Related to: surgical procedures, tissue damage, trauma

Defining Characteristics: communication of pain, facial grimacing, diaphoresis, hypertension, tachycardia, tachypnea, dilated pupils, change in appetite, change in behavior, moaning, crying, muscle rigidity, guarding, inability to focus on anything but oneself, withdrawal from social contact, insomnia, impaired thought process, confusion

Outcome Criteria

✔ Patient will have no pain, or pain will be controlled to patient's satisfaction.

✔ Patient will have no complications from epidural analgesia.

NOC: *Pain Level*

INTERVENTIONS	RATIONALES
Assess patient and have him describe pain characteristics, rating pain on 0–10 scale.	Each patient's pain level and response to it will be different.
Ensure that epidural catheter is in correct place prior to intermittent injection by aspirating gently. If blood is noted or more than 1 ml of clear fluid can be aspirated, withhold injection and notify physician.	Indicates that catheter has migrated potentially into the spinal column.

INTERVENTIONS	RATIONALES
Maintain strict aseptic technique when injecting medication through the epidural catheter.	Minimizes risk of pathogenic entry and infection.
Assess patient frequently to ensure that pain has been relieved.	Facilitates prompt identification of complications or need for concurrent use of low dose anesthetic agents to potentiate effects of analgesia.
Instruct patient regarding placement of epidural catheter, medications being used, and signs and symptoms to report to nurse/physician.	Facilitates patient knowledge, compliance, and prompt identification of any complications.
Encourage coughing and deep breathing exercises.	Epidural analgesia will facilitate better chest expansion and decrease risk of atelectasis.
Instruct patient/family in distracting activities, guided imagery, and so forth.	Assists patient to keep from focusing on pain and allows for other avenues of pain relief to be utilized.

NIC: *Analgesic Administration: Intraspinal*

Discharge or Maintenance Evaluation

■ Patient will be free of pain.

■ Patient will be able to identify signs and symptoms of which to notify nurse and/or physician to avert potential complications.

RISK FOR INFECTION

Related to: invasive epidural catheter, intermittent injections of analgesic agent, entrance site to spinal area

Defining Characteristics: redness at site, drainage around insertion site, odor, fever, tachycardia, elevated white blood cells with shift to the left on differential, broken skin, immunosuppression

Outcome Criteria

✔ Patient will have stable vital signs and remain free of signs and symptoms of infection.

NOC: *Risk Control*

INTERVENTIONS	RATIONALES
Identify concurrent physiological conditions that may contribute to risk of infection.	Nursing assessment ensures appropriate plan of care.
Ensure proper handwashing and wearing gloves when caring for patient.	Handwashing is the primary action to decrease risk of infection as the body is the foremost source of microbial contamination.
Use aseptic technique while caring for epidural lines and catheter.	Minimizes risk of cross contamination and infection.
Monitor vital signs every 1–2 hours.	Tachycardia and tachypnea may indicate presence of infection.
Change epidural analgesic solution every 24 hours, including tubing.	Microbial colonization may result if solution is not changed frequently.
Observe dressing to back every 2–4 hours, noting position change of catheter, drainage, redness around site. Notify physician for significant changes.	Epidural catheter should be marked as to placement, and documented every shift. Dressings should be occlusive and dry to maintain catheter placement and integrity.
Change dressing to epidural site every 24 hours and prn, using aseptic technique, and being extremely careful not to dislodge or move catheter.	Changing dressing is the number one cause of catheter placement change, so extreme caution must be used to prevent migration. Observation of wound site, and wound care provide nurse with opportunity to ensure correct placement and help facilitate securing of catheter. Redness or drainage from site should be immediate indication of infection and will require removal after notification of physician.
Culture site per protocol.	Helps to identify specific pathogens to allow for proper antimicrobial therapy to eradicate infection.
Instruct patient in procedures prior to performing them.	Provides knowledge of what to expect and lessens anxiety.
Instruct patient of signs/symptoms of which to notify nurse/physician.	Facilitates prompt recognition of complications to allow for timely intervention.

NIC: *Infection Precautions*

Discharge or Maintenance Evaluation

■ Patient will have stable vital signs.

■ Patient will exhibit no signs of infection from epidural catheter.

- Patient will experience no adverse reactions to epidural catheter and medication.

RISK FOR INJURY

Related to: presence of epidural catheter, potential for catheter migration

Defining Characteristics: itching, nausea, respiratory depression, numbness of legs, weakness to legs, urinary retention, hypotension, pain

Outcome Criteria

✔ Patient will exhibit no signs of catheter migration and be free of pain.

NOC: *Symptom Control*

INTERVENTIONS	RATIONALES
Assess epidural catheter dressing for occlusiveness and catheter for change in documented position.	Dressings that are wet, loosened, or missing may indicate that catheter is no longer in appropriate position to provide pain relief. Catheter should be marked so changes in location of marked catheter indicate movement of catheter within subarachnoid space, and potential migration to spinal canal.
Assess patient for complaints of weakness or numbness to legs.	Indicates that catheter is no longer in correct position.
Monitor vital signs, especially blood pressure and heart rate.	Vital signs may increase from sympathetic agents being utilized in solution, and if catheter has

INTERVENTIONS	RATIONALES
	migrated, disbursement of these drugs may cause vasodilation.
Monitor patient for complaints of onset of itching all over.	May indicate side effects of drugs being utilized in infusion.
Administer naloxone as ordered/indicated.	Reverses narcotic-related side effects.
Administer diphenhydramine as ordered/indicated.	Assists with histamine blockade to reduce pruritis.
Monitor I&O q 2 hours and notify physician if <30 cc/hr.	May indicate oliguria or urinary retention resulting from migration of epidural catheter.
Instruct patient to notify nurse for complaints of nausea, itching, leg weakness or numbness, or difficulty breathing.	May indicate migration of catheter, which will require intervention.
Instruct patient to notify nurse if pain is not relieved.	May indication malposition of catheter, or need for different analgesic solution, or possibly extra bolus of analgesic/ anesthetic agent.

NIC: *Risk Identification*

Discharge or Maintenance Evaluation

- Patient will exhibit no signs of epidural catheter migration.
- Patient will have stable vital signs and be pain-free.
- Patient will be able to accurately verbalize understanding of symptoms to report to nurse/physician.

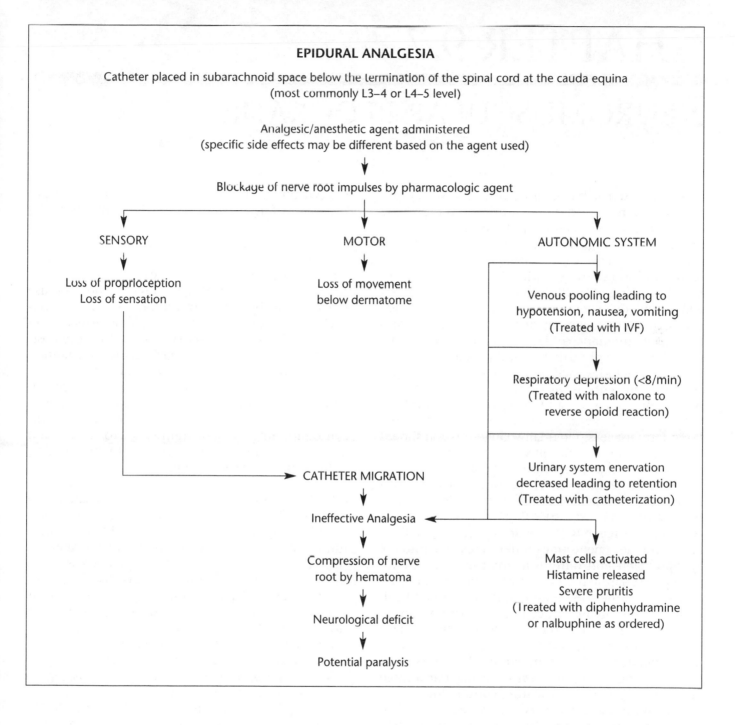

EPIDURAL ANALGESIA

Catheter placed in subarachnoid space below the termination of the spinal cord at the cauda equina
(most commonly L3–4 or L4–5 level)

Analgesic/anesthetic agent administered
(specific side effects may be different based on the agent used)

Blockage of nerve root impulses by pharmacologic agent

SENSORY

Loss of proprioception
Loss of sensation

MOTOR

Loss of movement
below dermatome

AUTONOMIC SYSTEM

Venous pooling leading to
hypotension, nausea, vomiting
(Treated with IVF)

Respiratory depression (<8/min)
(Treated with naloxone to
reverse opioid reaction)

Urinary system enervation
decreased leading to retention
(Treated with catheterization)

CATHETER MIGRATION

Ineffective Analgesia

Compression of nerve
root by hematoma

Mast cells activated
Histamine released
Severe pruritis
(Treated with diphenhydramine
or nalbuphine as ordered)

Neurological deficit

Potential paralysis

CHAPTER 9.7

NEUROMUSCULAR BLOCKADE

Neuromuscular blocking agents, or NMBs, originally were used in the operating room to provide complete muscle relaxation and preclude any movement during surgical procedures. Today they are used in the intensive care setting to produce muscle relaxation and manage critical illnesses or injuries. Short-term uses of NMBs include assisting with emergent problems, such as the need for endotracheal intubation, management of life-threatening agitation, or maintenance of lack of motion for patients who are undergoing therapeutic procedures. Long-term use includes facilitation of mechanical ventilation, prevention of activity-induced rises in intracranial pressure, and assistance in controlling movement in patients that could be life-threatening. Long-term usage is potentially dangerous and should be used cautiously and only by personnel who are appropriately trained in the drugs' usage and actions.

Normal neuromuscular transmission starts with an action potential or impulse that travels through a motor nerve toward a specific target muscle. When the impulse reaches the neuromuscular junction, acetylcholine, a neurotransmitter, is released into the synaptic cleft and diffuses across this area to bind with postsynaptic receptors on the motor end plate. The ion channels open and allow sodium and calcium to enter the muscle cell, and potassium ions to exit the cells and enter the blood plasma. This exchange of ions results in muscle depolarizations and generates muscle contraction. The NMBs work by inhibiting the impulses from being transmitted and preventing the muscle from contracting.

Neuromuscular blockers can be categorized as depolarizing or nondepolarizing, based on their mechanism of action. Succinylcholine is the only depolarizing NMB in the United States at this time, and it imitates the acetylcholine effect that occurs at the postsynaptic receptors, and opens the ion channels that allow sodium and calcium to flow into the cells. This movement causes the muscle cell membrane to depolarize and contract. As the drug withdraws from the postsynaptic receptors, the muscle fibers remain depolarized. Any further muscle action is disabled until the drug recedes from the neuromuscular junction and is metabolized. NMB with a depolarizing drug results in a short phase of muscular fasciculations that is then followed by paralysis of the muscle.

Nondepolarizing drugs prevent the impulse transmission by blocking the postsynaptic acetylcholine receptors. This maintains a muscle relaxation and flaccid paralysis. There is no effect on the postsynaptic receptor after binding to it, the ion channels remain closed, and the presynaptic receptors are blocked, which may reduce the production of acetylcholine. These drugs are further divided into groups based upon their chemical structure, such as benzylisoquinolines (tubocurarine, metocurine, and atracurium) and aminosteroids (pancuronium, vecuronium, and rocuronium).

Neuromuscular blocking agents are contraindicated in patients who have not received sedation and analgesia first, in patients who cannot have a protected airway, in patients with unstable bone fractures, or in patients with known history of malignant hyperthermia. Usage of NMBs in patients with an intracranial injury is controversial because the potential for chemical paralyzation prior to sedation is high and can result in increases in cerebral blood flow and further injury. Neurologic examinations cannot be performed and a progressive injury may worsen without notice, and seizure activity may be difficult, if not impossible, to detect, leading to increased cerebral metabolism and injury.

Complications resulting from the use of NMBs include post-traumatic stress disorder, prolonged weakness and paralysis, myopathy, polyneuropathy, bronchoconstriction, barotraumas, hypoxemia, pneumonia, hemodynamic compromises, and renal dysfunction.

The level of neuromuscular blockade should be monitored, and can be accomplished by clinical assessment and peripheral nerve stimulation using several methods. This test is usually performed by placing electrodes over the ulnar nerve in the wrist and applying an electrical stimulus consisting usually of a series of four electrical impulses called the "train-of-four," (TOF) stimulus. A desired response from this stimulation is the flexion or adduction of the thumb from the contraction of the adductor pollicis muscle. The degree of blockade is approximated by the number of twitches, from no twitches approximating 100% of the neuroreceptors being blocked, to four twitches representing zero to 75% blockage. Another pattern of stimulation that has been recently developed to identify neuromuscular blockade is the double burst stimulation (DBS 3/3). This consists of three pulses spaced 20 milliseconds apart followed $\frac{3}{4}$ of a second later by a second group of three pulses similarly spaced. If the muscle is not paralyzed, the response to DBS 3/3 will be two short muscle contractions of equal strength, but in the partially paralyzed muscle, the second response will be weaker than the first.

MEDICAL CARE

Mechanical ventilation: required with the administration of any NMB agent because of paralysis of respiratory musculature; patent airway and sufficient oxygenation must be provided to ensure appropriate ventilation and to prevent hypoxia and hypoxemia

Analgesics: opioids, usually morphine or fentanyl, are used in conjunction with sedatives to ensure maximal protection from noxious stimuli, and should be titrated to reduce pain while the patient is paralyzed to produce a state of unconsciousness

Sedatives: used in conjunction with analgesics, to provide aggressive sedation to ensure unconsciousness and patient relaxation; benzodiazepines, such as midazolam, diazepam, lorazepam, and propofol, are frequently used and titrated to maintain unconsciousness

Neuromuscular blocking agents: drugs used to block presynaptic impulses, impair release and binding of acetylcholine, and interfere with impulse transmission; succinylcholine is a depolarizing agent that mimics acetylcholine's effect and causes paralysis; benzylisoquinolines, such as tubocurarine, metocurine, and atracurium, are similar to curare, and aminosteroids, such as pancuronium, vecuronium, and rocuronium, are nondepolarizing drugs that pre-

vent the transmission of the nerve impulses, block presynaptic receptors, and decrease acetylcholine production

Neuromuscular blockade reversal agents: drugs, such as edrophonium, pyridostigmine, and neostigmine used to inhibit cholinesterase, increasing acetylcholine, and displacing the NMBs from the receptor sites allowing motor function to return; anticholinergic agents, such as atropine or glycopyrrolate, used in conjunction with cholinesterase inhibitors resulting from potential bradycardia, salivation, bronchospasm, and cardiac arrest

Electrocardiogram: used to identify heart rhythm, dysrhythmias, conduction defects, changes due to electrolyte imbalances

Arterial blood gases: used to identify acid–base imbalances, oxygenation status, ventilation/perfusion mismatching due to bronchoconstriction

Radiography: chest X-rays used to identify worsening or improvement of pulmonary infiltrates, increases in cardiac size, accurate placement and maintenance of correct position of endotracheal tube, identify barotraumas that may result from increased inspiratory pressures, or the presence of a nosocomial pneumonia; abdominal X-rays used to identify abscess formation, perforation, free air, or other abdominal complications

Laboratory: used to identify electrolyte function and imbalance, renal and liver function resulting from metabolization of NMBs; CBC used to identify presence of infection, anemia, or histamine release; specific drug levels used to identify therapeutic levels versus toxicity

Electroencephalographic-based technology: used in some institutions to monitor sedation levels and patient response to anesthetic agents; new bispectral index monitor also uses analysis of the patient's electromyographic activity from the facial muscles that change with the effect of sedative and NMBs

Peripheral nerve stimulation testing: method used to identify level of neuromuscular blockade; usually done by the Train-of-Four (TOF) stimulus, with notations of how many twitches of a particular nerve pathway from zero to four correlates with the percentage of receptors that are occupied by a NMB agent; helps to prevent overdosage with NMBs and to identify level of blockade

COMMON NURSING DIAGNOSES

IMPAIRED SPONTANEOUS VENTILATION (see MECHANICAL VENTILATION)

Related to: inability to breathe spontaneously caused by neuromuscular blocking agent administration

Defining Characteristics: paralysis of respiratory musculature, apnea, apprehension, tachycardia, elevated blood pressure, decreased PaO_2, decreased SaO_2, increased $PaCO_2$

ADDITIONAL NURSING DIAGNOSES

IMPAIRED PHYSICAL MOBILITY

Related to: administration of neuromuscular blocking agents, sedatives, and analgesics

Defining Characteristics: inability to move at will, paralysis, partial paralysis, muscle twitching, fasciculations, decreased range of motion, incoordination, prolonged weakness or paralysis, atrophy, pressure areas, decreased muscle tone, difficulty weaning from mechanical ventilation

Outcome Criteria

✔ Patient will be adequately paralyzed using neuromuscular blocking drugs and will exhibit no evidence of avoidable side effects.

✔ Patient will maintain muscle and joint range of motion, with no evidence of complications, such as contractures or skin breakdown.

NOC: *Mobility Level*

INTERVENTIONS	RATIONALES
Obtain baseline vital signs and physical assessment prior to the administration of NMBs.	These baseline values help to establish parameters to monitor, oxygenation and ventilation status, and hemodynamic status. The NMBs affect the function of the entire body system and may cause multiple effects—both desirable and undesirable, and the nurse should be aware of significant changes in the patient who is paralyzed and cannot communicate adverse reactions.
Administer ordered sedatives and analgesics.	NMB drugs *must not* be administered until these drugs are given and have elicited an unconscious state. To do otherwise puts the patient at risk for severe anxiety and pain, and potential post-traumatic stress syndrome. The NMBs do nothing to affect consciousness, so the patient is awake and aware, yet completely unable to move or breathe on his own.
Administer ordered neuromuscular blocking agent per protocol after unconsciousness has been obtained in patient.	Bolus dosing of NMBs should be given after monitoring of patient's clinical status has been established, and may be repeated in 1–2 minutes to allow for minimal histamine releases. Infusion dosing of NMBs should be titrated to ordered parameters, with the ideal amount being the smallest amount used to achieve the desired result for the shortest time to obtain the desired clinical goals. Bolus dosing of NMBs usually begin at 0.1–0.2 mg/kg IV for drugs such as pancuronium, vecuronium, pipecuronium, rocuronium, dosacurium, mivacurium, and cisatracurium. The drugs that are used for infusion titration include pancuronium, vecuronium, pipecuronium, rocuronium, atracurium, mivacurium, and cisatracurium, and vary according to the specific drug.
Assess patient closely, observing for signs of consciousness. Monitor vital signs q 1 hour and prn.	Opioids produce vasodilation, reduce preload, decrease cardiac output, and decrease blood pressure. Some NMBs trigger the release of histamine, which can cause bronchoconstriction, vasoconstriction, or vasodilation. Pancuronium can create a hyperdynamic state affecting myocardial oxygen supply and demand, and has significant vagolytic effects. If the patient is not adequately placed in an unconscious state prior to or during NMB administration, the patient will have pain and anxiety leading to increased stress responses from

INTERVENTIONS	RATIONALES
	increased catecholamine levels, with associated hemodynamic changes.
Monitor ECG for rhythm changes or dysrhythmias, and treat per hospital protocol.	Use of haloperidol may prolong the QT and cause Torsades des pointes dysrhythmias. Electrolyte imbalances, overdosage of drugs, or interactions with drugs may produce cardiac changes.
Speak softly and treat patient as if he is awake, explaining all care and procedures.	The patient may have break-through awareness despite levels of sedation and analgesia. Being paralyzed and unable to respond, yet being able to feel, think, and hear can be extremely frightening for the patient, and a calming manner helps to reduce potential anxiety.
Ensure patient has at least 2 intravenous lines prior to the administration of NMBs.	Multiple access lines should be available for management of any adverse reactions, such as decreased blood pressure, and to administer fluids and medications. Frequently a "sedation cocktail," composed of differing medications such as analgesics, benzodiazapines, and so forth, will be utilized, depending on the institution's protocol, which can be titrated for changing levels of consciousness, and may be all that is needed to achieve the desired goals. Multiple lines are also required because of potential interactions of medications, that may result in precipitation of the fluid, or inactivation of the drug.
Monitor pulse oximetry levels and ABGs prn.	With the administration of NMBs and a reduction in respiratory drive, patients who are on the ventilator can develop changes in oxygenation and ventilation because of the reduction in respiratory rate and minute ventilation. This can compromise oxygenation and increasing carbon dioxide levels within the body. Attention to the oxygen saturation can help avoid harmful reductions with the patient's oxygenation status.

INTERVENTIONS	RATIONALES
Assess the patient for development of reddened areas to the skin, ulcerations, or abrasions to all parts of the patient's body at least every 4 hours and prn.	Prompt recognition of redness or irritation of the skin, especially over bony prominences, facilitates prompt intervention to prevent further skin deterioration and allows for immediate skin care to be performed.
Reposition the patient at least every 2 hours and prn. Use special types of beds as ordered, such as specialty airflow beds.	The patient is unable to move at all, and requires repositioning to avoid risk of skin breakdown and pressure sores.
Provide range of motion to all extremities at least every 4 hours and prn.	This helps to prevent joint contractures and muscle atrophy.
Monitor the patient's level of sedation. Depending on the hospital protocol and physician's orders, these levels can be assessed by use of hemodynamics, allowing the patient to recover from NMB blockade on a daily basis, or with the use of electro-encephalographic technology.	Hemodynamics, such as increased pulse rate and blood pressure, may be noted if the patient is having pain or anxiety. The patient may also experience diaphoresis and lacrimation because of the sympathetic nervous system response, but these signs are not always reliable because they can vary from patient to patient and can be affected by use of concurrent medication therapy or their other disease states. Allowing the patient to "wake up" once per day to allow for the determination of the patient's sensorium, and need for continued NMB blockade can be helpful if the patient can communicate, and will help to titrate sedation for a particular patient's needs. This may be contraindicated based on the patient's clinical diagnosis and need for immobility. An EEG may help to correlate brain activity with the effects of drugs, such as midazolam and propofol, but is impractical because of the difficulty in the application of electrodes, the bulkiness of machinery, and the problems in determining the interpretation of the EEG results. A bispectral index monitor is a specially designed machine that allows for measurement of patient's response to sedation and blockade by using electrodes on the patient's forehead and temple

(continues)

(continued)

INTERVENTIONS	RATIONALES
	and incorporates electromyographic activity in the facial muscles. This equipment is easier to use than standard EEG monitors and allows for improved assessment of an arousal response and assessment of sedation.
Assess patient for level of neuromuscular blockade by clinical assessment accompanied by peripheral nerve stimulation. Document level of blockade per hospital protocol frequency. Testing is usually done at the ulnar nerve in the wrist by placing electrodes over this nerve and applying an electrical stimulus, normally a sequence of four impulses, called the "train-of-four" stimulus (TOF). The desired reaction from the TOF stimulus is either flexion or adduction of the thumb from contraction of the adductor pollicis muscle.	The number of responses from the TOF stimulus is related to a percentage of receptor sites that are affected by the NMB drugs. If the patient has four twitches, it means that the NMB occupies less than 75% of the receptors, three twitches means approximately 75% blockade, two twitches means 75% to 80% blockade, one twitch means 90% blockade, and no twitching designates 100% neuromuscular blockade. Traditional TOF testing has definite limitations insofar that the muscle twitches can be missed by visual or tactile assessments, which could result in incorrectly estimating the patient's level of neuromuscular blockade. Muscle groups also vary in their response to the specific NMB agent being utilized. For example, a peripheral nerve stimulation that occurs at the ulnar nerve may not reflect the responses of the chest wall or diaphragm because the sensitivity of the muscle groups differ with each agent. The TOF response can potentially be zero, but the patient could still have muscle movement. Edema of the patient, impaired nerve function, and poor electrical contact with the electrodes are also a significant factor. Although the ulnar nerve is the most traditionally used area for TOF monitoring, other sites can also be used for electrode placement. These include the ulnar nerve between the elbow and wrist (expected response would be thumb adduction), facial nerve (expected response would be ipsilateral eye and facial movement), posterior

INTERVENTIONS	RATIONALES
	tibial nerve (expected response would be plantar flexion of the great toe), and the peroneal nerve (expected response would be dorsiflexion of the foot).
If the patient suffers from hemiplegia, ensure that monitoring is performed at the correct location on the unaffected side.	Hemiplegics have a marked resistance to neuromuscular blockade in their affected limbs and incorrect monitoring can lead to NMB overdose.
Administer reversing agents for neuromuscular blockade as ordered.	Cholinesterase inhibitors, such as edrophonium, pyridostigmine, and neostigmine, impede acetylcholinesterase, the enzyme responsible for the degradation of acetylcholine, that ultimately increases the amount of acetylcholine and moves the NMBs from the receptor sites and allows the neuromuscular function to be restored.
Administer anticholinergic agents, such as atropine or glycopyrrolate, as ordered.	These drugs are usually administered concurrently with the anticholinesterase drugs because they can result in bradycardias, hypersalivation, bronchospasm from muscarinic receptor stimulation, or cardiac arrest. The half-life of the NMBs is usually greater than that of the anticholinesterase drug, so the patient may develop a rebound blockade, weakness, or paralysis.
Assess patient following reversal of NMB blockade for prolonged neuromuscular blockade and/or weakness.	Overdosing with an NMB or accumulation of the drug or metabolites can result in prolongation of the paralysis and weakness. If the patient has renal dysfunction, agents, such as vecuronium, and its metabolites accumulate and can lead to a delayed recovery. Concurrent use of other medications, such as aminoglycoside antibiotics, beta-blockers, calcium channel blockers, nitroglycerin, diuretics, and immunosuppressants can result in prolonged weakness from potentiation of neuromuscular blockade. Use of corticosteroids with NMBs may result in diffuse flaccid weakness that will interfere with mechanical ventilatory weaning. Nerve changes and

INTERVENTIONS	RATIONALES
	changes in the neuromuscular junction and tissues of the patient may result in prolonged weakness, resulting in atrophy and muscle deconditioning. Other clinical states, such as acidosis, muscular dystrophies, and collagen diseases can interfere with neuromuscular transmission and potentiate neuromuscular blockade.
Instruct patient/family regarding need for use of neuromuscular blockade, describe what to expect, that the patient will not be left alone, and stress that the patient will be given medication to keep him or her unconscious during the process.	Provides information, reduces anxiety, and assures patient he or she will not be conscious yet not able to breathe, communicate, or move.
Instruct family in the need and appropriate performance of range of motion exercises.	Involves patient's family in patient's care and reduces anxiety and frustration by allowing them to help.
Instruct patient/family regarding the need for frequent repositioning, as well as use of any special airflow bed/mattress.	Reduces hazards of immobility, such as pressure formation.

NIC: *Anesthesia Administration*

Discharge or Maintenance Evaluation

- Patient will achieve adequate sedation and unconsciousness prior to and during administration of neuromuscular blockade.
- Patient will exhibit no signs of complications of mobility.
- Patient will recover from neuromuscular blockade when accomplished without any prolonged weakness or paralysis.
- Patient will have no complications from therapy.
- Family will be able to participate in patient's care and improve their self-esteem.
- Patient's clinical goals will be achieved with the use of neuromuscular blockade drugs.

RISK FOR INJURY

Related to: neuromuscular blockade administration, immobility, drug interactions

Defining Characteristics: apnea, bradycardia, hypotension, bronchospasm, cardiac arrest, persistent weakness or paralysis, muscle atrophy, myopathy, neuropathy, increased intracranial pressure, damage to tissues or blood vessels, malignant hyperthermia, increased myocardial oxygen consumption and demand, dysrhythmias

Outcome Criteria

✔ Patient will exhibit no adverse reactions with neuromuscular blockade administration, and will have no complications as a result of immobility and paralysis.

NOC: *Risk Control*

INTERVENTIONS	RATIONALES
Identify other medications that patient may be receiving, or has received, that may interact with NMBs.	Medications, such as clindamycin and lithium, can affect the neuromuscular transmission of presynaptic blockade. Calcium channel blockers and aminoglycosides can impair the movement of calcium ions and decrease the release of acetylcholine. Ketamine, propranolol, and amphetamines may interfere with postsynaptic receptor binding of acetylcholine and allow impulse generation at the motor end plate. Metocurine, pancuronium, and vecuronium have an increased resistance to nondepolarization if the patient is on phenytoin or carbamazepine, and may require up to a 50% increase in dosage requirements. Dantrolene and clindamycin may interfere in muscle contraction by interfering with the impulse propagation to a specific muscle. Single-dose clindamycin and irrigation of the peritoneal cavity with neomycin fluid can result in extended neuromuscular blockade. Corticosteroid therapy in conjunction with NMBs may create an acute myopathy with diffuse, flaccid weakness that frequently interferes with mechanical ventilatory weaning.
Monitor vital signs for changes q 1 hour and prn. Monitor ECG	Pancuronium has significant vagolytic effects and can result in

(continues)

(continued)

INTERVENTIONS	RATIONALES
for changes and treat per hospital protocol.	a hyperdynamic state in which the myocardium is compromised because of the increased oxygen consumption and demand. Changes in heart rhythm may occur as imbalances between supply of oxygen is decreased for the heart's increased workload. If patient is not adequately sedated or given analgesics prior to the administration of NMBs, their awareness of noxious stimuli and anxiety-producing states will cause changes in blood pressure and heart rate. Opioids result in vasodilation, decreasing cardiac output and blood pressure. Benzodiazepines lower the levels of circulating catecholamines and may induce hypotension, especially in volume-depleted patients.
Monitor respiratory status q 2 hours and prn. Monitor oxygen saturation and ABGs prn.	When the diaphragm is paralyzed, abdominal contents can result in pressure exerted against the chest cavity altering lung excursion. Use of NMBs preclude mobilization of secretions that may result in nosocomial infections, such as pneumonia. As the paralyzed patient has no control of inspired tidal volume, the mismatching between perfusion of the dependent and nondependent areas of the lung, as well as histamine's pulmonary vasoactive reactions, may result in hypoxemia. Some NMBs activate a histamine response that can result in bronchoconstriction, especially if the patient is asthmatic. This bronchoconstriction may result in increased inspiratory pressures that enhance the potential for the occurrence of barotrauma.
Ensure that adequate use of sedation and analgesia is done prior to any administration of NMBs.	Helps to decrease the patient's awareness and fear of his or her surroundings and inability to move at will. Frequently, NMBs may not be necessary if adequate sedation is given.
Avoid administration of NMBs in patients who present with unstable bone fractures.	The muscle relaxation that is obtained with these drugs has the potential to release bone

INTERVENTIONS	RATIONALES
	fragments that may injure adjoining tissues or vasculature.
Assess patient for signs and symptoms of malignant hyperthermia: increased temperature, metabolic acidosis, dysrhythmias, and muscle breakdown.	Succinylcholine is one of the known drugs that can produce this life-threatening disorder in patients who have a genetic predisposition for the disorder.
Monitor ICP in patients who have head injuries.	Succinylcholine may cause a temporary increase in ICP, so its use is only justified in emergency situations. If necessary, treatment with hyperventilation, barbiturates, and nondepolarizing agents in small doses may decrease the potential for increasing pressures and decreased CPP.
Monitor all body systems and perform as thorough an assessment as possible at least q 2–4 hours and prn.	Neuromuscular blockade masks the clinical ability to assess for progressive injury or seizure activity, as well as abdominal pathology leading to complications.
Monitor lab work, especially electrolytes, renal profiles, kidney function tests, and serum creatine kinase, blood glucose, and CBC.	Most sedatives and analgesics and several NMBs are metabolized in the liver and excreted through the kidneys, so if renal or hepatic function is impaired, the actions of the drugs being given could result in complications, such as overdosage and prolonged paralysis. Changes in electrolytes can increase or decrease the NMB's effect. Succinylcholine is contraindicated in patients with increased serum potassium levels because the drug can increase potassium levels by 0.5–1.0 mEq/L. In patients who have burn or crush type injuries, an increase in the release of potassium may result in a hyperkalemic cardiac arrest. Myopathy or the use of corticosteroids may increase serum CK and glucose levels. CBC may be useful to identify potential infections and blood dyscrasias.
If propofol is utilized, ensure that aseptic technique is used when preparing the medication, and that the vial is disposed of within 12 hours.	This drug is lipid-based and has an increased risk for infection. The amount of preservative that is added to the drug is not of sufficient content to make the drug bacteriostatic.

INTERVENTIONS	RATIONALES
Ensure that the drugs required to reverse the neuromuscular blockade are readily available.	Cholinesterase inhibitors and anticholinergics reverse the action of the drug upon acetylcholinesterase and acetylcholine.
Ensure that the patient receives artificial tears and/or eye lubricants q 2–4 hours and prn.	The paralyzed patient is unable to blink, and these artificial agents must be used to prevent complications, such as corneal drying, ulceration, or abrasions.
Never leave patient unattended.	Patients who are paralyzed are totally dependent on others for their physical, emotional, and safety needs.
Instruct patient/family in use of neuromuscular blocking agents, need for use, and what to expect. Inform family to speak to patient when they visit.	Reduces fear and increases knowledge. Knowing that the patient may be able to hear what is being said may assist family in coping with patient's disease process and recovery.
Ascertain from family members any history of adverse reaction from anesthetic agents.	May provide information regarding the potential for malignant hyperthermia.
If possible, allow family members to see patient when patient is not paralyzed.	Allows for family to observe patient in a more realistic state of consciousness and assuages fears that patient is comatose.

NIC: *Infection Protection*

Discharge or Maintenance Evaluation

- Patient will exhibit no signs of malignant hyperthermia.
- Patient will exhibit no signs or symptoms of infection because of decreased lung excursion and immobility of secretions.
- Patient will experience no adverse reactions to neuromuscular blockade agents.
- Patient will have stable renal and hepatic function, with normal electrolytes.
- Patient will have stable vital signs and hemodynamic parameters.

RISK FOR POST-TRAUMA SYNDROME

Related to: neuromuscular blockade use if patient was not adequately sedated prior to administration

Defining Characteristics: feelings of fear, helplessness, re-experiencing the event or perception, avoidance of stimuli associated with the event, increased anxiety, increased startle response, distress with social, occupational, or other areas of previous normal function, changes in sleep pattern, changes in self-image, lack of coping ability, substance abuse, isolation

Outcome Criteria

✔ Patient will not experience any post-traumatic stress syndrome because of adequate analgesia and sedation prior to neuromuscular blockade.

NOC: *Risk Detection*

INTERVENTIONS	RATIONALES
Obtain information/assessment of prior mental status and monitor for changes in function once patient no longer is receiving NMBs.	Provides baseline information in order to identify potential problems that may require intervention.
Actively listen to patient regarding perceptions of time spent paralyzed and on the ventilator.	Helps to establish a trusting relationship in order to explore patient's feelings and identify methods to help patient cope with trauma.
Avoid stimuli that may aggravate patient's symptoms, such as loud noises, bright lights, and painful procedures, when possible.	May assist patient to avoid flashbacks to the traumatic event.
Always warn patient prior to touching and avoid approaching patient unaware.	These actions may be misinterpreted and trigger flashbacks to the trauma.
Discuss potential methods of coping with the trauma, including stress-reduction techniques, biofeedback, guided imagery, and so forth.	Helps patient to strengthen own ability to cope and establish a sense of control when facing fear and anxiety.
Instruct patient/family that a post-traumatic response may occur anytime from immediately following the trauma, up to years afterwards.	Alerts patient and family of potential for risk of response to remembrance of drug-induced paralysis.
Instruct family and friends about signs and symptoms of post-traumatic responses and interventions they can use.	Helps family to understand patient's problem and enables them to become involved, rather than withdraw from patient.
Instruct patient/family in obtaining community resources and referrals for support.	Provides information to ensure that patient will be able to receive care and reduce feelings of isolation.

NIC: *Risk Identification*

Discharge or Maintenance Criteria

- Patient will not develop chronic post-traumatic stress syndrome, substance abuse, or other mental health dysfunction.

- Patient will be able to verbalize understanding of risk of post-traumatic stress syndrome and use coping strategies to decrease anxiety.

- Patient and family will be able to obtain community referrals and assistance to decrease isolation and improve ability to cope with situation.

NEUROMUSCULAR BLOCKADE

NORMAL NEUROMUSCULAR TRANSMISSION

Action potential impulse occurs and travels toward a specific muscle

↓

Acetylcholine released at the neuromuscular junction if calcium ions are present

↓

Acetylcholine binds with post-junctional or synaptic receptors on motor end plate

↓

Ion channels open
Sodium and calcium enter the muscle
Potassium leaves the muscle and enters the plasma

↓

Motor end plate depolarizes

↓

Muscle contraction occurs

NEUROMUSCULAR BLOCKADE BY NONDEPOLARIZING AGENTS

Action potential impulse occurs and travels toward a specific muscle

↓

Administration of NMB

↓

Presynaptic receptors blocked
Amount of acetylcholine production decreased

↓

Acetylcholine released at the neuromuscular junction

↓

NMBs block postsynaptic acetylcholine receptors and prevent acetylcholine from binding

↓

Ion channels remain closed

↓

Muscle remains relaxed

Neuromuscular Blockade can be influenced by concurrent use of other drugs in these ways:

Interference with nerve impulse transmission by presynaptic blockade
[Clindamycin, Lithium]

Impairment of acetylcholine release because of dysfunction with calcium ions
[Calcium channel blockers, Aminoglycosides]

Impairment of acetylcholine binding to postsynaptic receptors that prevent impulse generation
[Ketamine, Propranolol, Amphetamines]

Interference with impulse transmission within the target muscle producing full neuromuscular blockade
[Dantrolene, Clindamycin, Neomycin]

BIBLIOGRAPHY

BOOKS

Alfaro-LaFevre, R. (2004). *Critical thinking in nursing: A practical approach* (3rd ed.). Philadelphia: W.B. Saunders Co.

Apple, S., & Lindsay, J. (1999). *Principles and practices of interventional cardiology*. Philadelphia: Lippincott Williams & Wilkins.

Barnum, B.S. (1999). Teaching nursing in the era of managed care. New York: Springer Publishing.

Baron, R.B. (Ed.). (2001). *Current medical diagnosis and treatment 2001* (40th ed.). New York: McGraw–Hill Publishers.

Beers, M., & Berkow, R. (Eds.). (1999). *The Merck manual* (17th ed.). Rahway, NJ: Merck, Sharp, & Dohme, Inc.

Black, J., Hawks, J., & Keene, A. (2001). *Medical–Surgical nursing: Clinical management for positive outcomes* (6th ed.). Omaha, NE: W.B. Saunders Co.

Blanchard, R., & Loeb, S. (2001). *Nurses drug looseleaf*. Blue Bell, PA: Blanchard & Loeb Publishers, Inc.

Bucher, L., & Melander, S. (1999). *Critical care nursing*. Newark, NJ: W.B. Saunders Co.

Carlson, K., Eisenstat, S., & Ziporyn, T. (1997). *The Harvard guide to women's health* (2nd ed.). Cambridge, MA: Harvard University Press.

Carpenito, L.J. (2004). *Handbook of nursing diagnosis* (10th ed.). Philadelphia: Lippincott Williams & Wilkins.

Carpenito, L.J. (2004). *Nursing diagnosis: Application to clinical practice* (10th ed.). Philadelphia: Lippincott Williams & Wilkins.

Carpenito, L. (1999). *Nursing care plans and documentation: Nursing diagnosis and collaborative problems* (3rd ed.). Chester, PA: Lippincott Williams & Wilkins.

Chocan, N., Comerford, K., & Jones, L. (Eds.). (2002). *Nursing 2002 drug handbook* (22nd ed.). Springhouse, PA: Springhouse Corporation.

Daniels, R. (2002). *Delmar's manual of laboratory and diagnostic tests*. Clifton Park, NY: Delmar Learning.

DeLaune, S.C., & Ladner, P.K. (2002). *Fundamentals of nursing: Standards and practice* (2nd ed.). Clifton Park, NY: Thomson Delmar Learning.

Dochterman, J.M., & Bulechek, G.M. (2004). *Nursing interventions classificaton (NIC)* (4th ed.). St. Louis: Mosby, Inc.

Doengens, M., & Moorhouse, M.F. (2000). *Nursing care plans. Guidelines for individualizing patient care* (5th ed.). Philadelphia: F.A. Davis Co.

Gardner, P. (2003). *Nursing process in action*. Clifton Park, NY: Thomson Delmar Learning.

Gomella, L., & Haist, S. (Eds.). (1997). *Clinician's pocket reference* (8th ed.). Philadelphia: McGraw–Hill Publishing.

Grif Alspach, J. (Ed.). (1998). *Core curriculum for critical care nursing* (5th ed.). Philadelphia: W.B. Saunders Co.

Gulanick, M. (1998). *Nursing care plans: Nursing diagnosis and intervention* (4th ed.). St. Louis, MO: Mosby Year Book.

Guyton, A., & Hall, J. (2000). *Textbook of medical physiology* (10th ed.). Philadelphia: W.B. Saunders Co.

Harkreader, H. (2004). *Fundamentals of nursing: Caring and clinical judgment* (2nd ed.). Philadelphia: W.B. Saunders Co.

Harvey, M. (2000). *Study guide to core curriculum for critical care nursing* (3rd ed.). Philadelphia: W.B. Saunders Co.

Kelly-Heidenthal, P. (2003). *Nursing leadership and management*. Clifton Park, NY: Thomson Delmar Learning.

Kozier, B., Erb, G., Blais, K., & Wilkinson, J. (2004). *Fundamentals of nursing: Concepts, process and practice*. Upper Saddle River, NJ: Pearson Education.

Lewis, S.M., Collier, I.C., & Heitkemper, M.M. (1999). *Medical-Surgical nursing: assessment and management of clinical problems* (5th ed.). St. Louis, MO: Mosby Year Book.

Maas, M., Johnson, M., & Moorhead, S. (Eds.). (1999). *Nursing outcomes classification (NOC)*. St. Louis, MO: Mosby Year Book.

McCloskey, J.C., & Bulechek, G.M. (2000). *Nursing interventions classification (NIC)*. St. Louis, MO: Mosby Year Book.

Medical-Surgical Nursing (10th ed.). Philadelphia: Lippincott Williams & Wilkins.

Minssen, B. (1995). *Critical care core curriculum* (6th ed.). Lubbock, TX: Panhandle Education for Nurses.

Minssen, B. (1995). *Multiple organ failure syndrome* (2nd ed.). Lubbock, TX: Panhandle Education for Nurses.

Moorhead, S., Johnson, M., & Maas, M. (2004). *Nursing outcomes classification (NOC)* (3rd ed.). St. Louis: Mosby, Inc.

Nettina, S. (Ed.). (2002). *Lippincott's pocket manual of nursing practice* (2nd ed.). Philadelphia: Lippincott Williams & Wilkins.

Nettina, S. (2001). *The Lippincott manual of nursing practice* (7th ed.). Philadelphia: Lippincott Williams & Wilkins.

Nettina, S. (Ed.). (2001). *Lippincott manual of nursing practice* (7th ed.). Philadelphia: Lippincott Williams & Wilkins.

North American Nursing Diagnosis Association (2003). *Nursing diagnoses: Definitions and classifications 2003–2004*. Philadelphia: North American Nursing Diagnosis Association.

Organon, Inc. (1998). *Train of four: Peripheral nerve stimulation*. West Orange, NJ: Author.

Rippe, J.M., & Irwin, R.S. (Eds.). (2000). *Manual of intensive care medicine*. (3rd ed.). Boston: Lippincott Williams & Wilkins.

Smeltzer, S., & Bare, B. (2004). *Brunner and Suddarth's textbook of medical-surgical nursing* (10th ed.). Philadelphia: Lippincott Williams & Wilkins.

Smeltzer, S., & Bare, B. (Eds.). (2000). *Brunner and Suddarth's textbook of medical–surgical nursing* (9th ed.). Philadelphia: Lippincott Williams & Wilkins.

Sparks, S., & Taylor, C. (2001). *Nursing diagnosis reference manual* (5th ed.). Springhouse, PA: Springhouse Corporation.

Spratto, G.R., & Woods. A.L. (2002). *2003 Edition PDR Nurse's drug handbook*. Clifton Park, NY: Thomson Delmar Learning.

Swearingen, P., & Keen, J. (2001). *Manual of critical care nursing: Nursing interventions and collaborative management* (4th ed.). St. Louis, MO: Mosby Year Book.

Ulrich, S., & Canale, W. (2001). *Nursing care planning guides: For adults in acute, extended and home care settings* (5th ed.). Philadelphia: W.B. Saunders Co.

Urden, L., Diann, S., Lough, M., and Urden, M. (2002). *Thelan's critical care nursing: Diagnosis and management*. St. Louis: Mosby, Inc.

Woods, S., Mozer, S., Underhill, S., Sivarajan, E. (2000). *Cardiac nursing*. Philadephia: Lippincott Williams & Wilkins.

White, L. (2003). *Documentation and the Nursing Process*. Clifton Park, NY: Thomson Delmar Learning.

PERIODICALS

Alcoser, P., & Burchett, S. (1999). Bone marrow transplantation. *American Journal of Nursing, 99* (6), 26–31.

American College of Cardiology and American Heart Association, Inc. (2001). ACC/AHA Guidelines for the evaluation and management of chronic heart failure in the adult: Executive summary. *JACC, 38* (7), 2101–2113.

Arbour, R. (2000). Mastering neuromuscular blockade. *Dimensions of Critical Care Nursing, 19* (5), 4–25.

Ball, C., Adams, J., Boyce, S., et al. (2001). Clinical guidelines for the use of the prone position in acute respiratory distress syndrome. *Intensive Critical Care Nursing, 17* (2), 94–104.

Barr, J., Zomorodi, K., Bertaccini, E.J., et al. (2001). A double-blind randomized comparison of IV lorazepam versus midazolam for sedation of ICU patients via a pharmacological trial. *Anesthesiology, 95* (2), 286–292.

Barker, E. (1999). Brain attack! A call to action. *RN, 62* (5), 54–62.

Behbehani, N.A., Al-Mane, F., D'Yachkova, Y., et al. (1999). Myopathy following mechanical ventilation for acute severe asthma: The role of muscle relaxants and corticosteroids, *Chest, 115* (6), 1627–1631.

Bockhold, K. (2000). Who's afraid of Hepatitis C? *American Journal of Nursing, 100* (5), 26–31.

Booij, LHDJ. (1997). Neuromuscular transmission and its pharmacological blockade, Part 1: Neuromuscular transmission and general aspects of its blockade. *Pharmacy World and Science, 19* (1), 1–12.

Booij, LHDJ. (1997). Neuromuscular transmission and its pharmacological blockade, Part 2: Pharmacology of neuromuscular blocking agents. *Pharmacy World and Science, 19* (1), 13–34.

Booij, LHDJ. (1997). Neuromuscular transmission and its pharmacological blockade, Part 3: Continuous infusion of relaxants and reversal and monitoring of relaxation. *Pharmacy World and Science, 19* (1), 35–44.

Carroll, P. (2000). A new way to monitor paralyzing drugs. *RN, 63* (5), 62–66.

Chua Patel, C., Kinsey, G., Koperski-Moen, K., & Bungum, L. (2000). Vacuum-assisted wound closure. *American Journal of Nursing, 100* (12), 45–48.

Cole, L. (2002). Unraveling the mystery of acute pancreatitis. *Dimensions in Critical Care Nursing, 21* (3), 86–89.

Coplin, W.M., O'Keefe, G.E, Grady, M.S., et al. (1997). Thombotic, infectious, & procedural complications of the jugular bulb catheter in the intensive care unit. *Neurosurgery, 41* (1), 101–109.

Covington, H. (1998). Use of propofol for sedation in the ICU. *Critical Care Nursing, 98* (18), 34–39.

DeDeyne, C., Struys, M., Decruyenaere, J., et al. (1998). Use of continuous bispectral EEG monitoring to assess depth of sedation in ICU patients. *Intensive Care Medicine, 24* (12), 1294–1298.

Dilanchian, P. (2001, October 15). Hypertension—Staying informed about drug therapy, *Nurseweek*.

Eagle, K., & Guyton, R., Davidoff, R., et al. (1999). ACC/AHA guidelines for CABG surgery. *Journal of the American College of Cardiology, 34* (4), 1262–1347.

Gattinoni, L., Tognoni, G., Pesenti, A., et al. (2001). Effect of prone positioning on the survival of patients with acute respiratory failure. *New England Journal of Medicine, 345* (8), 568–573.

Goldstein. L.E., & Henderson, D.C. (2000). Atypical antipsychotic agents and diabetes mellitus. *Primary Psychiatry, 7* (5), 65–68.

Gray, M. (2000). Urinary retention: Management in the acute care setting. *American Journal of Nursing, 100* (8), 36–42.

Habel, M. (2001, March 19). Brain attack—New stroke treatments, education can limit disabilities. *Nurseweek.*

Halm, M., & Penque, S. (1999). Heart disease in women. *American Journal of Nursing, 99* (4), 26–31.

Hill, L. (1998). ICU sedation: A review of its pharmacology and assessment. *Journal of Intensive Care Medicine, 13,* 174–183.

Holcomb, S.S. (2002). Thyroid diseases: a primer for the critical care nurse. *Dimensions in Critical Care Nursing, 21* (4), 127–133.

Holcomb, S.S. (2002). Diabetes insipidus. *Dimensions in Critical Care Nursing, 21* (3), 94–97.

Hopkins, P.M. (2000). Malignant hyperthermia: Advances I clinical management and diagnosis. *British Journal of Anaesthia, 85,* 118–128.

Horne, C., & Derrico, D. (1999). Mastering ABGs. *American Journal of Nursing, 99* (8), 26–33.

Howard, L., Gopinath, S.P., Uzura, M., et al. (1999). Evaluation of a new fiberoptic catheter for monitoring jugular venous oxygen saturation. *Neurosurgery, 44* (6), 1280–1285.

Kearney, K. (2000). Digitalis toxicity. *American Journal of Nursing, 100* (6), 51–52.

King, M., & Tomasic, D. (1999). Treating TB today. *RN, 62* (6), 26–30.

Kitabchi, A.E., Umpierrez, G.E., Murphy, M.B., et al. (2001). Management of hyperglycemic crises in patients with diabetes mellitus. *Diabetes Care, 24,* 131–153.

Kozuh, J. (2000). NSAIDs & antihypertensives: An unhappy union. *American Journal of Nursing, 100* (6), 40–42.

Lewis, K.L., & Rothenberg, D.M. (1999). Neuromuscular blockade in the intensive care unit. *American Journal of Health-System Pharmacy, 56,* 72–75.

Low, W.C. (2002). Bone marrow stem cells help rats after CVA. *Experimental Neurology, 174,* 11–20.

Mancini, M., & Kaye, W. (1999). AEDs: Changing the way you respond to cardiac arrest. *American Journal of Nursing, 99* (5), 26–30.

McCormick, J., & Blackwood, B. (2001). Nursing the ARDS patient in the prone position: The experience of qualified ICU nurses. *Intensive Critical Care Nursing, 17* (6), 331–340.

Meistleman, C., & Plaud, B. (1997). Neuromuscular blockade: Is it still useful in the ICU? *European Journal of Anesthesiology, 14* (15), 53–56.

Mitchell, R. (1999). Sickle cell anemia. *American Journal of Nursing, 99* (5), 38–39.

Nestel, P.J., Shinge, H., Pomeroy, S., et al. (2001). High-fat meals impair arterial elasticity and increase heart attack risk. *Journal of the American College of Cardiology, 37* (7), 1929–1935.

O'Hanlon-Nichols, T. (1999). Neurologic assessment: The basics of a comprehensive examination. *American Journal of Nursing, 99* (6), 44–50.

Ohlinger, M.J., & Rhoney, D.H. (1998). Neuromuscular blocking agents in the neurosurgical intensive care unit. *Surgical Neurology, 49,* 217–221.

Orhon Jeck, A. (2001, April 2). Of human bondage—Alternatives to restraints help reduce risks to patients. *Healthweek.*

Osterman, M.E., Keenan, S.P., Seiferling, R.A., et al. (2000). Sedation in the intensive care unit: A systematic review. *Journal of the American Medical Association, 283* (11), 1451–1459.

Pasero, C. (2000). Continuous local anesthetics. *American Journal of Nursing, 100* (8), 22–23.

Poznanski Hutchison, C. (1999). Healing touch: An energetic approach. *American Journal of Nursing, 99* (4), 43–48.

Ramsburg, K. (2000). Rheumatoid arthritis. *American Journal of Nursing, 100* (11), 40–43.

Roark, D. (2000). Overhauling the organ donation system. *American Journal of Nursing, 100* (6), 44–48.

Rosenberg, H., Antognini, J., Muldoon, S., et al. (2002). Testing for malignant hyperthermia. *Anesthesiology, 96* (1), 232–237.

Rowlee, S.C. (1999). Monitoring neuromuscular blockade in the intensive care unit: The peripheral nerve stimulator. *Heart & Lung, 28* (5), 352–363.

Rudis, M.I., Sikora, C.A., Angus, E., et al. (1997). A prospective randomized controlled evaluation of peripheral nerve stimulation versus standard clinical dosing of neuromuscular blocking agents in critically ill patients. *Critical Care Medicine, 25* (4), 575–583.

Schoofs, N. (1999). Sjogren's syndrome? *RN, 62* (4), 45–47.

Shovein, J., Damazo, R., & Hyams, I. (2000). Hepatitis A: How benign is it? *American Journal of Nursing, 100* (5), 43–47.

Sinisalo, J., Mattila, K., Valtonen, V., et al. (2002). Effect of 3 months of antimicrobial treatment with clarithromycin in acute non-q-wave coronary syndrome. Lowered risk of death or serious cardiovascular events. *Circulation: Journal of the American Heart Association, 105* (13), 1555–1560.

Soltesz, S., Silomon, M., Biedler, A., et al. (2001). Gamma-hydroxybutyric acid-ethanolamide (LK 544). The suitability of LK 544 for sedation of patients in intensive care in comparison with midazolam. *Anaesthesist, 50* (5), 323–328.

Valsa, M., & Lawrence, M. (2001, Sept. 3). Post-acute care—Where does the money come from? *Nurseweek.*

Wilson, D., & Tracy, M.F. (2000). CABG and the elderly. *American Journal of Nursing, 100* (5), 24AA–24UU.

Wong, F. (1999). A new approach to ABG interpretation. *American Journal of Nursing, 99* (8) 34–36.

APPENDIX A

NANDA NURSING DIAGNOSES

Activity Intolerance
Acute Confusion
Acute Pain
Adult Failure To Thrive
Anticipatory Grieving
Anxiety
Autonomic Dysreflexia

Bathing/Hygiene Self-Care Deficit
Bowel Incontinence

Caregiver Role Strain
Chronic Confusion
Chronic Low Self-Esteem
Chronic Pain
Chronic Sorrow
Compromised Family Coping
Constipation

Death Anxiety
Decisional Conflict (specify)
Decreased Cardiac Output
Decreased Intracranial Adaptive Capacity
Defensive Coping
Deficient Diversional Activity
Deficient Fluid Volume
Deficient Knowledge (specify)
Delayed Growth And Development
Delayed Surgical Recovery
Diarrhea
Disabled Family Coping
Disorganized Infant Behavior
Disturbed Body Image
Disturbed Energy Field
Disturbed Personal Identity
Disturbed Sensory Perception (specify: visual, auditory,
    kinesthetic, gustatory, tactile, olfactory)
Disturbed Sleep Pattern
Disturbed Thought Processes
Dressing/Grooming Self-Care Deficit
Dysfunctional Family Processes: Alcoholism
Dysfunctional Grieving
Dysfunctional Ventilatory Weaning Response

Effective Breast-Feeding
Effective Therapeutic Regimen Management
Excess Fluid Volume

Fatigue
Fear
Feeding Self-Care Deficit
Functional Urinary Incontinence

Health-Seeking Behaviors (specify)
Hopelessness
Hyperthermia
Hypothermia

Imbalanced Nutrition: Less Than Body Requirements
Imbalanced Nutrition: More Than Body Requirements
Impaired Adjustment
Impaired Bed Mobility
Impaired Dentition
Impaired Environmental Interpretation Syndrome
Impaired Gas Exchange
Impaired Home Maintenance
Impaired Memory
Impaired Oral Mucous Membrane
Impaired Parenting
Impaired Physical Mobility
Impaired Skin Integrity
Impaired Social Interaction
Impaired Spontaneous Ventilation
Impaired Swallowing
Impaired Tissue Integrity
Impaired Transfer Ability
Impaired Urinary Elimination
Impaired Verbal Communication
Impaired Walking
Impaired Wheelchair Mobility
Ineffective Airway Clearance
Ineffective Breast-Feeding
Ineffective Breathing Pattern
Ineffective Community Coping
Ineffective Community Therapeutic Regimen
    Management
Ineffective Coping

Ineffective Denial
Ineffective Family Therapeutic Regimen Management
Ineffective Health Maintenance
Ineffective Infant Feeding Pattern
Ineffective Protection
Ineffective Role Performance
Ineffective Sexuality Patterns
Ineffective Therapeutic Regimen Management
Ineffective Thermoregulation
Ineffective Tissue Perfusion (specify type: renal, cerebral, cardiopulmonary, gastrointestinal, peripheral)
Interrupted Breast-Feeding
Interrupted Family Processes

Latex Allergy Response

Nausea
Noncompliance (specify)

Parental Role Conflict
Perceived Constipation
Post-Trauma Syndrome
Powerlessness

Rape-Trauma Syndrome
Rape-Trauma Syndrome: Compound Reaction
Rape-Trauma Syndrome: Silent Reaction
Readiness for Enhanced Communicaton
Readiness for Enhanced Community Coping
Readiness for Enhanced Coping
Readiness for Enhanced Family Coping
Readiness for Enhanced Family Processes
Readiness for Enhanced Fluid Balance
Readiness for Enhanced Knowledge (specify)
Readiness for Enhanced Nutrition
Readiness for Enhanced Organized Infant Behavior
Readiness for Enhanced Parenting
Readiness for Enhanced Self-Concept
Readiness for Enhanced Sleep
Readiness for Enhanced Spiritual Well-Being
Readiness for Enhanced Therapeutic Regimen Management
Readiness for Enhanced Urinary Elimination
Reflex Urinary Incontinence
Relocation Stress Syndrome
Risk for Activity Intolerance
Risk for Aspiration
Risk for Autonomic Dysreflexia
Risk for Caregiver Role Strain
Risk for Constipation

Risk for Deficient Fluid Volume
Risk for Delayed Development
Risk for Disorganized Infant Behavior
Risk for Disproportionate Growth
Risk for Disuse Syndrome
Risk for Falls
Risk for Imbalanced Body Temperature
Risk for Imbalanced Fluid Volume
Risk for Imbalanced Nutrition: More Than Body Requirements
Risk for Impaired Parent/Infant/Child Attachment
Risk for Impaired Parenting
Risk for Impaired Skin Integrity
Risk for Infection
Risk for Injury
Risk for Latex Allergy Response
Risk for Loneliness
Risk for Other-Directed Violence
Risk for Perioperative-Positioning Injury
Risk for Peripheral Neurovascular Dysfunction
Risk for Poisoning
Risk for Post-Trauma Syndrome
Risk for Powerlessness
Risk for Relocation Stress Syndrome
Risk for Self-Directed Violence
Risk for Self-Mutilation
Risk for Situational Low Self-Esteem
Risk for Spiritual Distress
Risk for Sudden Infant Death Syndrome
Risk for Suffocation
Risk for Suicide
Risk for Trauma
Risk for Urge Urinary Incontinence

Self-Mutilation
Sexual Dysfunction
Situational Low Self-Esteem
Sleep Deprivation
Social Isolation
Spiritual Distress
Stress Urinary Incontinence

Toileting Self-Care Deficit
Total Urinary Incontinence

Unilateral Neglect
Urinary Retention
Urge Urinary Incontenance

Wandering

APPENDIX B

NURSING OUTCOMES CLASSIFICATIONS (NOC)

Abuse Cessation
Abuse Protection
Abuse Recovery Status
Abuse Recovery: Emotional
Abuse Recovery: Financial
Abuse Recovery: Physical
Abuse Recovery: Sexual
Abusive Behavior Self Restraint
Acceptance: Health Status
Activity Tolerance
Adaptation to Physical Disability
Adherence Behavior
Aggression Self-Control
Allergic Response: Localized
Allergic Response: Systemic
Ambulation
Ambulation: Wheelchair
Anxiety Level
Anxiety Self-Control
Appetite
Aspiration Prevention
Asthma Self-Management

Balance
Blood Coagulation
Blood-Glucose Level
Blood Loss Severity
Blood Transfusion Reaction
Body Image
Body Mechanics Performance
Body Positioning: Self-Initiated
Bone Healing
Bowel Continence
Bowel Elimination
Breastfeeding Establishment: Infant
Breastfeeding Establishment: Maternal
Breastfeeding: Maintenance
Breastfeeding: Weaning

Cardiac Disease Self-Management
Cardiac Pump Effectiveness
Caregiver Adaptation to Patient Institutionalization

Caregiver Emotional Health
Caregiver Home Care Readiness
Caregiver Lifestyle Disruption
Caregiver-Patient Relationship
Caregiver Performance: Direct Care
Caregiver Performance: Indirect Care
Caregiver Physical Health
Caregiver Stressors
Caregiver Well-Being
Caregiving Endurance Potential
Child Adaptation to Hospitalization
Child Development: 1 Month
Child Development: 2 Months
Child Development: 4 Months
Child Development: 6 Months
Child Development: 12 Months
Child Development: 2 Years
Child Development: 3 Years
Child Development: 4 Years
Child Development: Middle Childhood
Child Development: Adolescence
Circulation Status
Client Satisfaction: Access to Care Resources
Client Satisfaction: Caring
Client Satisfaction: Communication
Client Satisfaction: Continuity of Care
Client Satisfaction: Cultural Needs Fulfillment
Client Satisfaction: Functional Assistance
Client Satisfaction: Physical Care
Client Satisfaction: Physical Environment
Client Satisfaction: Protection of Rights
Client Satisfaction: Psychological Care
Client Satisfaction: Safety
Client Satisfaction: Symptom Control
Client Satisfaction: Teaching
Client Satisfaction: Technical Aspects of Care
Cognition
Cognitive Orientation
Comfort Level
Comfortable Death
Communication
Communication: Expressive

Communication: Receptive
Community Competence
Community Disaster Readiness
Community Health Status
Community Health Status: Immunity
Community Risk Control: Chronic Disease
Community Risk Control: Communicable Disease
Community Risk Control: Lead Exposure
Community Risk Control: Violence
Community Violence Level
Compliance Behavior
Concentration
Coordinated Movement
Coping

Decision Making
Depression Level
Depression Self-Control
Diabetes Self-Management
Dignified Life Closure
Discharge Readiness: Independent Living
Discharge Readiness: Supported Living
Distorted Thought Self-Control

Electrolyte and Acid/Base Balance
Endurance
Energy Conservation

Fall Prevention Behavior
Falls Occurrence
Family Coping
Family Functioning
Family Health Status
Family Integrity
Family Normalization
Family Participation in Professional Care
Family Physical Environment
Family Resiliency
Family Social Climate
Family Support During Treatment
Fear Level
Fear Level: Child
Fear Self-Control
Fetal Status: Antepartum
Fetal Status: Intrapartum
Fluid Balance
Fluid Overload Severity

Grief Resolution
Growth

Health Beliefs
Health Beliefs: Perceived Ability to Perform
Health Beliefs: Perceived Control
Health Beliefs: Perceived Resources
Health Beliefs: Perceived Threat

Health Orientation
Health-Promoting Behavior
Health-Seeking Behavior
Hearing Compensation Behavior
Hemodialysis Access
Hope
Hydration
Hyperactivity Level

Identity
Immobility Consequences: Physiological
Immobility Consequences: Psycho-Cognitive
Immune Hypersensitivity Response
Immune Status
Immunization Behavior
Impulse Self-Control
Infection Severity
Infection Severity: Newborn
Information Processing

Joint Movement: Ankle
Joint Movement: Elbow
Joint Movement: Fingers
Joint Movement: Hip
Joint Movement: Knee
Joint Movement: Neck
Joint Movement: Passive
Joint Movement: Shoulder
Joint Movement: Spine
Joint Movement: Wrist

Kidney Function
Knowledge: Body Mechanics
Knowledge: Breastfeeding
Knowledge: Cardiac Disease Management
Knowledge: Child Physical Safety
Knowledge: Conception Prevention
Knowledge: Diabetes Management
Knowledge: Diet
Knowledge: Disease Process
Knowledge: Energy Conservation
Knowledge: Fall Prevention
Knowledge: Fertility Promotion
Knowledge: Health Behavior
Knowledge: Health Promotion
Knowledge: Health Resources
Knowledge: Illness Care
Knowledge: Infant Care
Knowledge: Infection Control
Knowledge: Labor and Delivery
Knowledge: Medication
Knowledge: Ostomy Care
Knowledge: Parenting
Knowledge: Personal Safety
Knowledge: Postpartum Maternal Health
Knowledge: Preconception Maternal Health

Knowledge: Pregnancy
Knowledge: Prescribed Activity
Knowledge: Sexual Functioning
Knowledge: Substance Abuse Control
Knowledge: Treatment Procedure(s)
Knowledge: Treatment Regimen

Leisure Participation
Loneliness Severity

Maternal Status: Antepartum
Maternal Status: Intrapartum
Maternal Status: Postpartum
Mechanical Ventilation Response: Adult
Mechanical Ventilation Weaning Response: Adult
Medication Response
Memory
Mobility
Mood Equilibrium
Motivation

Nausea & Vomiting Control
Nausea & Vomiting: Disruptive Effects
Nausea & Vomiting Severity
Neglect Cessation
Neglect Recovery
Neurological Status
Neurological Status: Autonomic
Neurological Status: Central Motor Control
Neurological Status: Consciousness
Neurological Status: Cranial Sensory/Motor Function
Neurological Status: Spinal Sensory/Motor Function
Newborn Adaptation
Nutritional Status
Nutritional Status: Biochemical Measures
Nutritional Status: Energy
Nutritional Status: Food and Fluid Intake
Nutritional Status: Nutrient Intake

Oral Health
Ostomy Self-Care

Pain: Adverse Psychological Response
Pain Control
Pain: Disruptive Effects
Pain Level
Parent-Infant Attachment
Parenting: Adolescent Physical Safety
Parenting: Early/Middle Childhood Physical Safety
Parenting: Infant/Toddler Physical Safety
Parenting Performance
Parenting: Psychosocial Safety
Participation in Health Care Decisions
Personal Autonomy
Personal Health Status
Personal Safety Behavior

Personal Well-Being
Physical Aging
Physical Fitness
Physical Injury Severity
Physical Maturation: Female
Physical Maturation: Male
Play Participation
Post Procedure Recovery Status
Prenatal Health Behavior
Preterm Infant Organization
Psychomotor Energy
Psychosocial Adjustment: Life Change

Quality of Life

Respiratory Status: Airway Patency
Respiratory Status: Gas Exchange
Respiratory Status: Ventilation
Rest
Risk Control
Risk Control: Alcohol Use
Risk Control: Cancer
Risk Control: Cardiovascular Health
Risk Control: Drug Use
Risk Control: Hearing Impairment
Risk Control: Sexually Transmitted Diseases (STDs)
Risk Control: Tobacco Use
Risk Control: Unintended Pregnancy
Risk Control: Visual Impairment
Risk Detection
Role Performance

Safe Home Environment
Seizure Control
Self-Care Status
Self-Care: Activities of Daily Living (ADL)
Self-Care: Bathing
Self-Care: Dressing
Self-Care: Eating
Self-Care: Hygiene
Self-Care: Instrumental Activities of Daily Living (IADL)
Self-Care: Nonparenteral Medication
Self-Care: Oral Hygiene
Self-Care: Parenteral Medication
Self-Care: Toileting
Self-Direction of Care
Self-Esteem
Self-Mutilation Restraint
Sensory Function Status
Sensory Function: Cutaneous
Sensory Function: Hearing
Sensory Function: Proprioception
Sensory Function: Taste and Smell
Sensory Function: Vision
Sexual Functioning
Sexual Identity

Skeletal Function
Sleep
Social Interaction Skills
Social Involvement
Social Support
Spiritual Health
Stress Level
Student Health Status
Substance Addiction Consequences
Suffering Severity
Suicide Self-Restraint
Swallowing Status
Swallowing Status: Esophageal Phase
Swallowing Status: Oral Phrase
Swallowing Status: Pharyngeal Phase
Symptom Control
Symptom Severity
Symptom Severity: Perimenopause
Symptom Severity: Premenstrual Syndrome (PMS)
Systemic Toxin Clearance: Dialysis

Thermoregulation
Thermoregulation: Neonate

Tissue Integrity: Skin and Mucous Membranes
Tissue Perfusion: Abdominal Organs
Tissue Perfusion: Cardiac
Tissue Perfusion: Cerebral
Tissue Perfusion: Peripheral
Tissue Perfusion: Pulmonary
Transfer Performance
Treatment Behavior: Illness or Injury

Urinary Continence
Urinary Elimination

Vision Compensation Behavior
Vital Signs

Weight: Body Mass
Weight Control
Will to Live
Wound Healing: Primary Intention
Wound Healing: Primary Intention

APPENDIX C

NURSING INTERVENTIONS CLASSIFICATIONS (NIC)

Abuse Protection Support
Abuse Protection Support: Child
Abuse Protection Support: Domestic Partner
Abuse Protection Support: Elder
Abuse Protection Support: Religious
Acid-Base Management
Acid-Base Management: Metabolic Acidosis
Acid-Base Management: Metabolic Alkalosis
Acid-Base Management: Respiratory Acidosis
Acid-Base Management: Respiratory Alkalosis
Acid-Base Monitoring
Active Listening
Activity Therapy
Acupressure
Admission Care
Airway Insertion And Stabilization
Airway Management
Airway Suctioning
Allergy Management
Amnioinfusion
Amputation Care
Analgesic Administration
Analgesic Administration: Intraspinal
Anaphylaxis Management
Anesthesia Administration
Anger Control Assistance
Animal-Assisted Therapy
Anticipatory Guidance
Anxiety Reduction
Area Restriction
Aromatherapy
Art Therapy
Artificial Airway Management
Aspiration Precautions
Assertiveness Training
Asthma Management
Attachment Promotion
Autogenic Training
Autotransfusion

Bathing
Bed Rest Care
Bedside Laboratory Testing
Behavior Management

Behavior Management: Overactivity/Inattention
Behavior Management: Self-Harm
Behavior Management: Sexual
Behavior Modification
Behavior Modification: Social Skills
Bibliotherapy
Biofeedback
Bioterrorism Preparedness
Birthing
Bladder Irrigation
Bleeding Precautions
Bleeding Reduction
Bleeding Reduction: Antepartum Uterus
Bleeding Reduction: Gastrointestinal
Bleeding Reduction: Nasal
Bleeding Reduction: Postpartum Uterus
Bleeding Reduction: Wound
Blood Products Administration
Body Image Enhancement
Body Mechanics Promotion
Bottle Feeding
Bowel Incontinence Care
Bowel Incontinence Care: Encopresis
Bowel Irrigation
Bowel Management
Bowel Training
Breast Examination
Breastfeeding Assistance

Calming Technique
Capillary Blood Sample
Cardiac Care
Cardiac Care: Acute
Cardiac Care: Rehabilitative
Cardiac Precautions
Caregiver Support
Care Management
Cast Care: Maintenance
Cast Care, Wet
Cerebral Edema Management
Cerebral Perfusion Promotion
Cesarean Section Care
Chemical Restraint
Chemotherapy Management

Chest Physiotherapy
Childbirth Preparation
Circulatory Care: Arterial Insufficiency
Circulatory Care: Mechanical Assist Device
Circulatory Care: Venous Insufficiency
Circulatory Precautions
Circumcision Care
Code Management
Cognitive Restructuring
Cognitive Stimulation
Communicable Disease Management
Communication Enhancement: Hearing Deficit
Communication Enhancement: Speech Deficit
Communication Enhancement: Visual Deficit
Community Disaster Preparedness
Community Health Development
Complex Relationship Building
Conflict Mediation
Constipation/Impaction Management
Consultation
Contact Lens Care
Controlled Substance Checking
Coping Enhancement
Cost Containment
Cough Enhancement
Counseling
Crisis Intervention
Critical Path Development
Culture Brokerage
Cutaneous Stimulation

Decision-Making Support
Delegation
Delirium Management
Delusion Management
Dementia Management
Dementia Management: Bathing
Deposition/Testimony
Developmental Care
Developmental Enhancement: Adolescent
Developmental Enhancement: Child
Dialysis Access Maintenance
Diarrhea Management
Diet Staging
Discharge Planning
Distraction
Documentation
Dressing
Dying Care
Dysreflexia Management
Dysrhythmia Management

Ear Care
Eating Disorders Management
Electroconvulsive Therapy (ECT) Management
Electrolyte Management
Electrolyte Management: Hypercalcemia

Electrolyte Management: Hyperkalemia
Electrolyte Management: Hypermagnesemia
Electrolyte Management: Hypernatremia
Electrolyte Management: Hyperphosphatemia
Electrolyte Management: Hypocalcemia
Electrolyte Management: Hypokalemia
Electrolyte Management: Hypomagnesemia
Electrolyte Management: Hyponatremia
Electrolyte Management: Hypophosphatemia
Electrolyte Monitoring
Electronic Fetal Monitoring: Antepartum
Electronic Fetal Monitoring: Intrapartum
Elopement Precautions
Embolus Care: Peripheral
Embolus Care: Pulmonary
Embolus Precautions
Emergency Care
Emergency Cart Checking
Emotional Support
Endotracheal Extubation
Energy Management
Enteral Tube Feeding
Environmental Management
Environmental Management: Attachment Process
Environmental Management: Comfort
Environmental Management: Community
Environmental Management: Home Preparation
Environmental Management: Safety
Environmental Management: Violence Prevention
Environmental Management: Worker Safety
Environmental Risk Protection
Examination Assistance
Exercise Promotion
Exercise Promotion: Strength Training
Exercise Promotion: Stretching
Exercise Therapy: Ambulation
Exercise Therapy: Balance
Exercise Therapy: Joint Mobility
Exercise Therapy: Muscle Control
Eye Care

Fall Prevention
Family Integrity Promotion
Family Integrity Promotion: Childbearing Family
Family Involvement Promotion
Family Mobilization
Family Planning: Contraception
Family Planning: Infertility
Family Planning: Unplanned Pregnancy
Family Presence Facilitation
Family Process Maintenance
Family Support
Family Therapy
Feeding
Fertility Preservation
Fever Treatment
Financial Resource Assistance

Fire-Setting Precautions
First Aid
Fiscal Resource Management
Flatulence Reduction
Fluid/Electrolyte Management
Fluid Management
Fluid Monitoring
Fluid Resuscitation
Foot Care
Forgiveness Facilitation

Gastrointestinal Intubation
Genetic Counseling
Grief Work Facilitation
Grief Work Facilitation: Perinatal Death
Guilt Work Facilitation

Hair Care
Hallucination Management
Health Care Information Exchange
Health Education
Health Policy Monitoring
Health Screening
Health System Guidance
Heat/Cold Application
Heat Exposure Treatment
Hemodialysis Therapy
Hemodynamic Regulation
Hemofiltration Therapy
Hemorrhage Control
High-Risk Pregnancy Care
Home Maintenance Assistance
Hope Instillation
Hormone Replacement Therapy
Humor
Hyperglycemia Management
Hypervolemia Management
Hypnosis
Hypoglycemia Management
Hypothermia Treatment
Hypovolemia Management

Immunization/Vaccination Administration
Impulse Control Training
Incident Reporting
Incision Site Care
Infant Care
Infection Control
Infection Control: Intraoperative
Infection Protection
Insurance Authorization
Intracranial Pressure (ICP) Monitoring
Intrapartal Care
Intrapartal Care: High-Risk Delivery
Intravenous (IV) Insertion
Intravenous (IV) Therapy
Invasive Hemodynamic Monitoring

Kangaroo Care

Labor Induction
Labor Suppression
Laboratory Data Interpretation
Lactation Counseling
Lactation Suppression
Laser Precautions
Latex Precautions
Learning Facilitation
Learning Readiness Enhancement
Leech Therapy
Limit Setting
Lower Extremity Monitoring

Malignant Hyperthermia Precautions
Mechanical Ventilation
Mechanical Ventilatory Weaning
Medication Administration
Medication Administration: Ear
Medication Administration: Enteral
Medication Administration: Eye
Medication Administration: Inhalation
Medication Administration: Interpleural
Medication Administration: Intradermal
Medication Administration: Intramuscular (IM)
Medication Administration: Intraosseous
Medication Administration: Intraspinal
Medication Administration: Intravenous (IV)
Medication Administration: Nasal
Medication Administration: Oral
Medication Administration: Rectal
Medication Administration: Skin
Medication Administration: Subcutaneous
Medication Administration: Vaginal
Medication Administration: Ventricular Reservoir
Medication Management
Medication Prescribing
Meditation Facilitation
Memory Training
Milieu Therapy
Mood Management
Multidisciplinary Care Conference
Music Therapy
Mutual Goal Setting

Nail Care
Nausea Management
Neurologic Monitoring
Newborn Care
Newborn Monitoring
Nonnutritive Sucking
Normalization Promotion
Nutrition Management
Nutrition Therapy
Nutritional Counseling
Nutritional Monitoring

Oral Health Maintenance
Oral Health Promotion
Oral Health Restoration
Order Transcription
Organ Procurement
Ostomy Care
Oxygen Therapy

Pain Management
Parent Education: Adolescent
Parent Education: Childrearing Family
Parent Education: Infant
Parenting Promotion
Pass Facilitation
Patient Contracting
Patient Controlled Analgesia (PCA) Assistance
Patient Rights Protection
Peer Review
Pelvic Muscle Exercise
Perineal Care
Peripheral Sensation Management
Peripherally Inserted Central (PIC) Catheter Care
Peritoneal Dialysis Therapy
Pessary Management
Phlebotomy: Arterial Blood Sample
Phlebotomy: Blood Unit Acquisition
Phlebotomy: Cannulated Vessel
Phlebotomy: Venous Blood Sample
Phototherapy: Mood/Sleep Regulation
Phototherapy: Neonate
Physical Restraint
Physician Support
Pneumatic Tourniquet Precautions
Positioning
Positioning: Intraoperative
Positioning: Neurologic
Positioning: Wheelchair
Postanesthesia Care
Postmortem Care
Postpartal Care
Preceptor: Employee
Preceptor: Student
Preconception Counseling
Pregnancy Termination Care
Premenstrual Syndrome (PMS) Management
Prenatal Care
Preoperative Coordination
Preparatory Sensory Information
Presence
Pressure Management
Pressure Ulcer Care
Pressure Ulcer Prevention
Product Evaluation
Program Development
Progressive Muscle Relaxation
Prompted Voiding

Prosthesis Care
Pruritus Management

Quality Monitoring

Radiation Therapy Management
Rape-Trauma Treatment
Reality Orientation
Recreation Therapy
Rectal Prolapse Management
Referral
Religious Addiction Prevention
Religious Ritual Enhancement
Relocation Stress Reduction
Reminiscence Therapy
Reproductive Technology Management
Research Data Collection
Resiliency Promotion
Respiratory Monitoring
Respite Care
Resuscitation
Resuscitation: Fetus
Resuscitation: Neonate
Risk Identification
Risk Identification: Childbearing Family
Risk Identification: Genetic
Role Enhancement

Seclusion
Security Enhancement
Sedation Management
Seizure Management
Seizure Precautions
Self-Awareness Enhancement
Self-Care Assistance
Self-Care Assistance: Bathing/Hygiene
Self-Care Assistance: Dressing/Grooming
Self-Care Assistance: Feeding
Self-Care Assistance: IADL
Self-Care Assistance: Toileting
Self-Care Assistance: Transfer
Self-Esteem Enhancement
Self-Hypnosis Facilitation
Self-Modification Assistance
Self-Responsibility Facilitation
Sexual Counseling
Shift Report
Shock Management
Shock Management: Cardiac
Shock Management: Vasogenic
Shock Management: Volume
Shock Prevention
Sibling Support
Simple Guided Imagery
Simple Massage
Simple Relaxation Therapy

Skin Care: Donor Site
Skin Care: Graft Site
Skin Care: Topical Treatments
Skin Surveillance
Sleep Enhancement
Smoking Cessation Assistance
Socialization Enhancement
Specimen Management
Spiritual Growth Facilitation
Spiritual Support
Splinting
Sports-Injury Prevention: Youth
Staff Development
Staff Supervision
Subarachnoid Hemorrhage Precautions
Substance Use Prevention
Substance Use Treatment
Substance Use Treatment: Alcohol Withdrawal
Substance Use Treatment: Drug Withdrawal
Substance Use Treatment: Overdose
Suicide Prevention
Supply Management
Support Group
Support System Enhancement
Surgical Assistance
Surgical Precautions
Surgical Preparation
Surveillance
Surveillance: Community
Surveillance: Late Pregnancy
Surveillance: Remote Electronic
Surveillance: Safety
Sustenance Support
Suturing
Swallowing Therapy

Teaching: Disease Process
Teaching: Foot Care
Teaching: Group
Teaching: Individual
Teaching: Infant Nutrition
Teaching: Infant Safety
Teaching: Infant Stimulation
Teaching: Preoperative
Teaching: Prescribed Activity/Exercise
Teaching: Prescribed Diet
Teaching: Prescribed Medication
Teaching: Procedure/Treatment
Teaching: Psychomotor Skill
Teaching: Safe Sex
Teaching: Sexuality
Teaching: Toddler Nutrition
Teaching: Toddler Safety

Teaching: Toilet Training
Technology Management
Telephone Consultation
Telephone Follow-Up
Temperature Regulation
Temperature Regulation: Intraoperative
Temporary Pacemaker Management
Therapeutic Play
Therapeutic Touch
Therapy Group
Total Parenteral Nutrition (TPN) Administration
Touch
Traction/Immobilization Care
Transcutaneous Electrical Nerve Stimulation (TENS)
Transport
Trauma Therapy: Child
Triage: Disaster
Triage: Emergency Center
Triage: Telephone
Truth Telling
Tube Care
Tube Care: Chest
Tube Care: Gastrointestinal
Tube Care: Umbilical Line
Tube Care: Urinary
Tube Care: Ventriculostomy/Lumbar Drain

Ultrasonography: Limited Obstetric
Unilateral Neglect Management
Urinary Bladder Training
Urinary Catheterization
Urinary Catheterization: Intermittent
Urinary Elimination Management
Urinary Habit Training
Urinary Incontinence Care
Urinary Incontinence Care: Enuresis
Urinary Retention Care

Values Clarification
Vehicle Safety Promotion
Venous Access Device (VAD) Maintenance
Ventilation Assistance
Visitation Facilitation
Vital Signs Monitoring
Vomiting Management

Weight Gain Assistance
Weight Management
Weight Reduction Assistance
Wound Care
Wound Care: Closed Drainage
Wound Irrigation

APPENDIX D

ABBREVIATIONS

α	alpha
β	beta
°	degree
° C	degrees Celsius, degrees centigrade
° F	degrees Fahrenheit
%	percent, percentage
<	less than
>	greater than
AAA	abdominal aortic aneurysm
abd	abdomen, abdominal
ABGs	arterial blood gases
ACE	angiotension-converting enzyme
ADH	antidiuretic hormone
ALT	alanine aminotransferase
ANA	antinuclear antibody
APTT	activated partial thromboplastin time
ARDS	adult respiratory distress syndrome, acute respiratory distress syndrome
ARF	acute renal failure
ASA	acetylsalicylic acid, aspirin
ASCVD	arteriosclerotic (or atherosclerotic) cardiovascular disease
ASHD	arteriosclerotic (or atherosclerotic) heart disease
AST	aspartate aminotransferase
ATN	acute tubular necrosis
AV	atrioventricular
BP	blood pressure
BS	blood sugar, blood glucose
BUN	blood urea nitrogen
C	Celsius, centigrade
C&S	culture and sensitivity
CABG	coronary artery bypass graft
CAD	coronary artery disease
cAMP	cyclic adenosine monophosphate
CAVH	continuous arteriovenous hemofiltration

CAVHD	continuous arteriovenous hemodialysis, or hemodiafiltration
cc	cubic centimeter
CHF	congestive heart failure
CI	cardiac index
CK, CPK	creatine kinase, creatine phophokinase
cm	centimeter
CNS	central nervous system
CO	cardiac output
CO_2	carbon dioxide
COPD	chronic obstructive pulmonary disease
CPAP	continuous positive airway pressure
CRRT	continuous renal replacement therapies
CSF	cerebrospinal fluid
cTnI	cardiac specific troponin I
cTnT	cardiac specific troponin T
CV	cardiovascular
CVA	cerebrovascular accident, stroke
CVP	central venous pressure
CVVHD	continuous venovenous hemodialysis, or hemodiafiltration
DI	diabetes insipidus
DIC	disseminated intravascular coagulation
DKA	diabetic ketoacidosis
DLV	differential lung ventilation
DTRs	deep tendon reflexes
ECG	electrocardiogram
EDH	epidural hematoma
EF	ejection fraction
ETT	endotracheal tube
F	Fahrenheit
FIO_2	fraction of inspired oxygen
FRC	functional residual capacity
Fx	fracture
GCS	Glasgow Coma Scale
GFR	glomerular filtration rate

GI	gastrointestinal		mmol	millimole
GVHD	graft-versus-host disease		MODS	multiple organ dysfunction syndrome
h, hr	hour		MSOF	multisystem organ failure
Hct	hematocrit		NANDA	North American Nursing Diagnosis Association
HELLP	hemolysis, elevated liver enzymes, low platelets		NIC	nursing interventions classifications
HF	heart failure		NIF	negative inspiratory force
HHS	hyperosmolar hyperglycemic state		NMB	neuromuscular blockade
HI	head injuries		NOC	nursing outcomes classification
HITT	heparin-induced thrombopenia and thrombosis		NPO	nothing by mouth
HIV	human immunodeficiency virus (AIDS)		NS	normal saline
Hmg	hemoglobin		NTG	nitroglycerin
HOB	head of bed		O_2	oxygen
HR	heart rate		OD	overdose
HTN	hypertension		OPCAB	off-pump coronary artery bypass
I&O	intake and output		OTC	over-the-counter
IAB	intra-aortic balloon		PA	pulmonary artery
IABP	intra-aortic balloon pump		PAT	paroxysmal atrial tachycardia
ICP	intracranial pressure		pCO_2, $PaCO_2$	partial pressure of arterial carbon dioxide tension
IE	infective endocarditis		PCWP	pulmonary capillary wedge pressure
ITP	idiopathic thrombocytopenic purpura		PE	pulmonary embolism
IV	intravenous		PEEP	positive end-expiratory pressure
IVF	intravenous fluids		pH	hydrogen ion concentration
IVP	intravenous push		PIH	pregnancy induced hypertension
kg	kilogram		pO_2, PaO_2	partial pressure of arterial oxygen tension
LDH	lactic dehydrogenase		Postop	postoperative
LFTs	liver function tests		PPD	purified protein derivative (TB testing)
LMWH	low molecular weight heparin		PRN, prn	as needed
LOC	level of consciousness		PS	pressure support
LR	lactated Ringer's		PSV	pressure support ventilation
LVSW	left ventricular stroke work		PT	prothrombin time
LVSWI	left ventricular stroke work index		PTCA	percutaneous transluminal coronary angioplasty
m^2	square meter		PtiO$_2$	oxygen saturation of peripheral cerebellar tissues
MAO	monoamine oxidase			
MAOI	monoamine oxidase inhibitor		PTT	partial thromboplastin time
MAP	mean arterial pressure, mean arterial blood pressure		PVC	premature ventricular contraction
mEq	milliequivalent		PVR	peripheral vascular resistance
MH	malignant hyperthermia		q	every
MI	myocardial infarction		RF	renal failure
MIDCAB	miniminally invasive direct coronary artery bypass		RL	Ringer's lactate
			ROM	range of motion
ml	milliliter		RVSW	right ventricular stroke work
mm Hg	millimeters of mercury		RVSWI	right ventricular stroke work index

SB	Sengstaken–Blakemore tube	SVT	supraventricular tachycardia
SCUF	slow continuous ultrafiltration	TEE	transesophageal echocardiography
SGOT	see AST	TOF	train of four
SGPT	see ALT	TPN	total parenteral nutrition
SIADH	syndrome of inappropriate antidiuretic hormone	TPR	total peripheral resistance
		u/L	units per liter
SIMV	synchronized intermittent mandatory ventilation	U/O	urinary output
		UA	urinalysis
SIRS	systemic inflammatory response syndrome	UTI	urinary tract infection
$SjvO_2$	oxygen saturation of the jugular venous bulb	VAD	ventricular assist device
		VMA	vanillylmandelic acid
SL	sublingual	VS	vital signs
SMV	synchronized mandatory ventilation	V_T	tidal volume
SVR	systemic vascular resistance		

INDEX

Note: **Bold** type indicates main entries which are nursing diagnoses.

NOTES

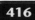

License Agreement for Delmar Learning, a division of Thomson Learning, Inc.

Educational Software/Data

You the customer, and Delmar Learning, a division of Thomson Learning, Inc. incur certain benefits, rights, and obligations to each other when you open this package and use the software/data it contains. BE SURE YOU READ THE LICENSE AGREEMENT CAREFULLY, SINCE BY USING THE SOFTWARE/DATA YOU INDICATE YOU HAVE READ, UNDERSTOOD, AND ACCEPTED THE TERMS OF THIS AGREEMENT.

Your rights:

1. You enjoy a non-exclusive license to use the software/data on a single microcomputer in consideration for payment of the required license fee, (which may be included in the purchase price of an accompanying print component), or receipt of this software/data, and your acceptance of the terms and conditions of this agreement.

2. You acknowledge that you do not own the aforesaid software/data. You also acknowledge that the software/data is furnished "as is," and contains copyrighted and/or proprietary and confidential information of Delmar Learning, a division of Thomson Learning, Inc. or its licensors.

There are limitations on your rights:

1. You may not copy or print the software/data for any reason whatsoever, except to install it on a hard drive on a single microcomputer and to make one archival copy, unless copying or printing is expressly permitted in writing or statements recorded on the diskette(s).

2. You may not revise, translate, convert, disassemble or otherwise reverse engineer the software/data except that you may add to or rearrange any data recorded on the media as part of the normal use of thesoftware/data.

3. You may not sell, license, lease, rent, loan or otherwise distribute or network the software/data except that you may give the software/data to a student or an instructor for use at school or, temporarily at home.

Should you fail to abide by the Copyright Law of the United States as it applies to this software/data your license to use it will become invalid. You agree to erase or otherwise destroy the software/data immediately after receiving note of termination of this agreement for violation of its provisions from Delmar Learning.

Delmar Learning, a division of Thomson Learning, Inc. gives you a LIMITED WARRANTY covering the enclosed software/data. The LIMITED WARRANTY follows this License.

This license is the entire agreement between you and Delmar Learning, a division of Thomson Learning, Inc. interpreted and enforced under New York law.

LIMITED WARRANTY

Delmar Learning, a division of Thomson Learning, Inc. warrants to the original licensee/purchaser of this copy of microcomputer software/data and the media on which it is recorded that the media will be free from defects in material and workmanship for ninety (90) days from the date of original purchase. All implied warranties are limited in duration to this ninety (90) day period. THEREAFTER, ANY IMPLIED WARRANTIES, INCLUDING IMPLIED WARRANTIES OF MERCHANTABILITY AND FITNESS FOR A PARTICULAR PURPOSE, ARE EXCLUDED. THIS WARRANTY IS IN LIEU OF ALL OTHER WARRANTIES, WHETHER ORAL OR WRITTEN, EXPRESS OR IMPLIED.

If you believe the media is defective please return it during the ninety (90) day period to the address shown below. Defective media will be replaced without charge provided that it has not been subjected to misuse or damage.

This warranty does not extend to the software or information recorded on the media. The software and information are provided "AS IS." Any statements made about the utility of the software or information are not to be considered as express or implied warranties.

Limitation of liability: Our liability to you for any losses shall be limited to direct damages, and shall not exceed the amount you paid for the software. In no event will we be liable to you for any indirect, special, incidental, or consequential damages (including loss of profits) even if we have been advised of the possibility of such damages.

Some states do not allow the exclusion or limitation of incidental or consequential damages, or limitations on the duration of implied warranties, so the above limitation or exclusion may not apply to you. This warranty gives you specific legal rights, and you may also have other rights which vary from state to state. Address all correspondence to: Delmar Learning, a division of Thomson Learning, Inc., 5 Maxwell Drive, P.O. Box 8007, Clifton Park, NY 12065-8007. Attention: Technology Department.

SYSTEM REQUIREMENTS

The CD-ROM version will be developed to run on client systems with the following minimum configuration:

- Operating System: Microsoft Windows 98 SE, Windows 2000, Windows XP
- Processor: Pentium PC 120 MHz or higher
- RAM: 64 MB of RAM or better
- Free Drive Space: 25 MB free disk space
- CD-ROM Drive—necessary for installation only
- Internet Connection Speed: 56K or better in order to view web links provided in program but is not required.
- Screen Resolution: 800 × 600 pixels or better
- Color Depth: 16-bit color (thousands of colors) or 24-bit color (millions of colors)
- Sound card: N/A

SET UP INSTRUCTIONS

To install the program, simply run the "X:\setup.exe", where X is the drive letter of you CD-ROM drive. Follow the on screen prompts to complete the installation. You may also:

1. Double click My Computer
2. Double click the Control Panel icon
3. Double click Add/Remove Programs
4. Click the Install button and follow the on screen prompts from there.